The
Journal of Infectious Diseases

Published by the John McCormick Institute for Infectious Diseases

Volume 43

1928

Chicago, 1928

Composed and Printed by
American Medical Association Press
Chicago, Illinois, U. S. A

THE PATHOLOGY OF THE MEMBRANES OF BRAIN AND SPINAL CORD

1. THE HISTOLOGY OF NORMAL DURA MATER AND PIA-ARACHNOID

THOR ROTHSTEIN, L. W. AVERY AND R. RICHTER

From the Department of Neurology of Rush Medical College, Chicago

For more than two years we have collected observations of the pathologic conditions of dura mater and pia-arachnoid. During our studies we gradually formed an opinion about the microscopic anatomy of these membranes which materially differs from the current descriptions of their normal microscopic structure. It therefore seems necessary to give an account of our conception of their normal histology before we enter upon a description of our findings of their pathological conditions. Our remarks, in the main, will be limited to the cellular constituents of the meninges.

Technique.—The material used was, for the most part, fixed initially in solution of formaldehyde. However, material fixed immediately in chrome, Zenker's fluid, alcohol and combinations of chrome and osmic acid were also used. Formalin-fixed material was also treated with chrome and combinations of chrome and osmic acid.

In order to study the protoplasmic structures it was necessary to find staining methods which would stain the protoplasm, leaving the collagen and reticulum fibers unstained or faintly stained. Modification of iron-hematoxylin, thionin and silver stains were found suitable, though many other stains were tried. The iron-hematoxylin method can be managed so that different degrees of contrast between collagen, reticulum and protoplasm are obtained, making it possible to distinguish the various types of fibers and protoplasmic structures. This is especially true when chromitized material is used.

Sections from formalin material were treated for 24 hours in a week, aqueous solution of pyridin, washed in running water for 12 to 24 hours and placed in 3% aqueous solution of tannic acid. They were again washed in running water for a day or two after which they were ready to stain. It was found that the whole pieces could be treated as above if pure pyridin was used instead of the weak, aqueous solution and if the time for each step was lengthened to two or three days. With some tissue it was found to be advantageous to add an equal amount of picric acid to the solution of tannic acid.

The sections can be stained in iron-hematoxylin by the usual methods or in thionin. When the latter is used the sections, after being treated as above, are placed in a very weak ammonia water until they regain their transparency They are then washed in water and stained from 15 to 40 minutes or longer. Decolorization is accomplished with creosote and controlled under the microscope.

Sections from chrome material made either after embedding or by the freezing method are first dechromitized and then stained with iron-hematoxylin or thionin.

Received for publication, Jan. 10, 1928.

The degree of dechromitization was found to be important and had to be determined for each material.

The silver methods used were the Bielschowsky method for sections and a modification of Cajal's silver impregnation. In the latter process formalin-fixed material was washed in running water for 24 hours, treated for a like period of time in pure pyridin and again washed very well. Frozen sections were placed in 10% silver nitrate for one to three days, passed quickly through water and developed in a solution containing 2% hydroquinon and 7% formalin. They were then decolorized by one-half solution of potassium ferricyanid in 70% alcohol, washed and fixed in hyposulphite. A troublesome precipitate may occur but this can be avoided by first embedding the sections in a 10% solution of gum mastic in 95% alcohol as described by Dieterle[1] in staining for spirochetes. The sections are then treated as above and after developing the gum mastic is removed by acetone.

In all the methods it was found that when the membranes were well stained the mitochondria and the intracellular fibrillae were faintly stained. On the other hand when mitochondria were brought out sharply the intracellular fibrillae as well as the membranes were seen only faintly or not at all. However, preparations were obtained in which all structures could be distinctly identified in the same cell.

Preparations made by teasing fresh material as well as that treated with the various fixing fluids were also studied.

DURA MATER

The cells of the dura mater are more or less similar to a membrane and could very properly be called membranous. On cross sections vertical to the surface one sees long, narrow, oblong or baton-like nuclei, and in both directions of the nucleus a narrow line of granular protoplasm which latter may not be observed without appropriate staining. In sections parallel to the surface the cells present a very different appearance. Their nuclei are oval and the membranous protoplasm has considerable extension. The cell forms are so varied that we would not even attempt to describe them but a faint expression of such variations is given by drawings 1 to 5. The extension of the cell is, in the main, parallel to the surface but not exclusively so. The cells show either wing-formed projections or are curved in such a way that their membranous protoplasm lies in two or more planes.

Another striking fact about the cells is that they anastomose with each other. Sometimes the connections between two cells are very broad. At other times they are long, slender bridges but then the connections are usually numerous. Often the picture is such that one would rather speak about a net or mesh-form protoplasmic membrane instead of communicating cells. This impression depends upon the finding of areas of membranes which anastomose with cells, but the

1. Arch. Neurol. & Psychiat., 1927, 18, p. 73.

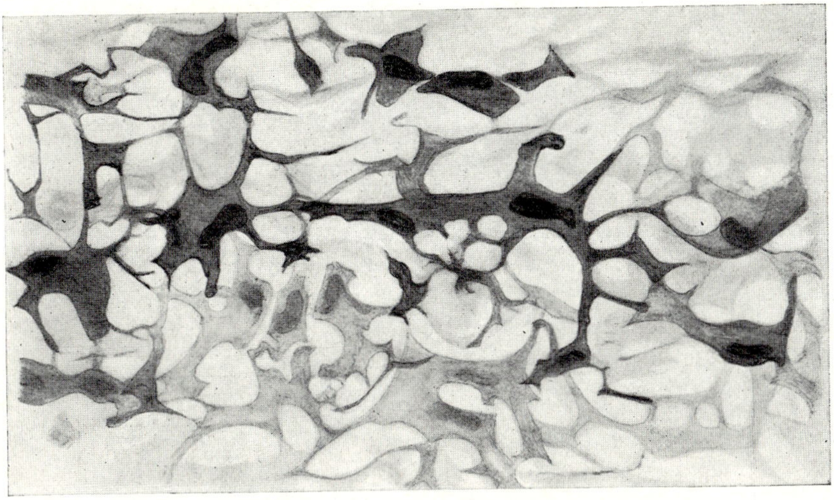

Fig. 1.—Dura of dog: tangential section; the syncytial cells stained dark; collagenic fibers not stained; formalin, frozen section, silver stain, magnification × 900.

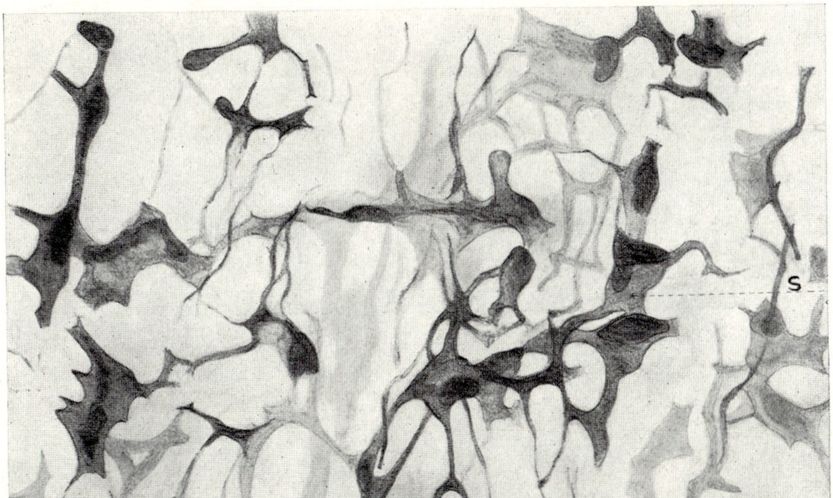

Fig. 2.—Dura of dog: tangential section, syncytial cells, method as in figure 1.

area does not show any nucleus (a of drawing 5 may give a faint idea of this condition). Also the cells may be connected with such broad anastomoses that several cells form one whole (s of drawing 2 shows somewhat of this condition).

There are no borderlines between the cells. The membranous protoplasm of one cell continues without interruption into the protoplasm of another cell, forming a syncytial network spinning through the whole thickness and extent of the dura.

The arrangement of the nuclei is such that they generally, but not always, are found where the meshes are of their greatest width. Seldom is a nucleus found lying alone. Generally they lie in groups of two,

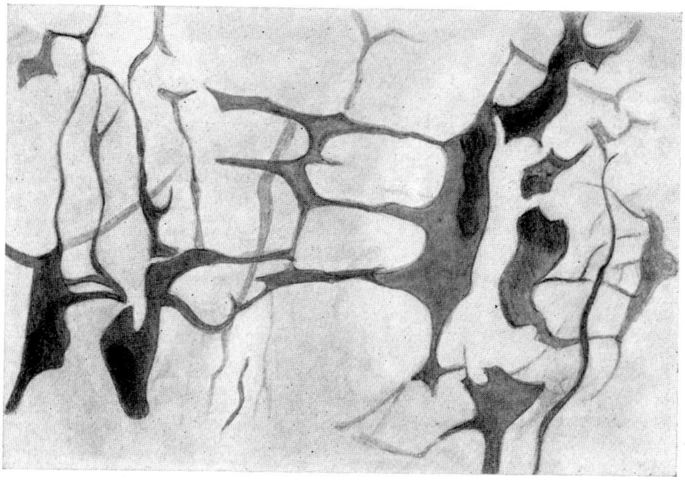

Fig. 3.—Dura of dog: tangential section, syncytial cells, method as in figure 1.

four or even more, and close together. Often they are found so close together that they cover each other, and only distinct staining makes it possible to recognize that more than one nucleus is present (fig. 6). Seen from the edge they present a rod-like appearance, but seen from the surface most of them have the oval shape of the usual connective tissue nucleus. Their size, however, varies considerably. In some groups one may find, besides nuclei of the usual size, others which are much smaller and may be round in shape, or one may find nuclei which are twice or even thrice as large as the most commonly seen nucleus. On cross sections of dura one may see rod-like nuclei two, three or even four times as large as the other nuclei, but the explanation of this is, as a rule, that several nuclei lie in a row close together.

In iron-hematoxylin stained sections the nuclei present a very different degree of attraction to the stain. Some nuclei are intensely dark stained, others so faintly that they could easily be overlooked. In one and the same group of nuclei one may find nuclei of different degree of staining, but the smaller, round nuclei seem to hold the stain stronger. However, even the oval nuclei do not stain uniformly.

The membranous protoplasm of the dura cells when observed under low magnification and from the edge, presents itself as a thin line, and when seen from the surface appears as a membrane with no thickness. However, under higher magnification (1800) it is found to have considerable volume. With mitochondria stains these cytologic constituents can readily be demonstrated. They are found in considerable number

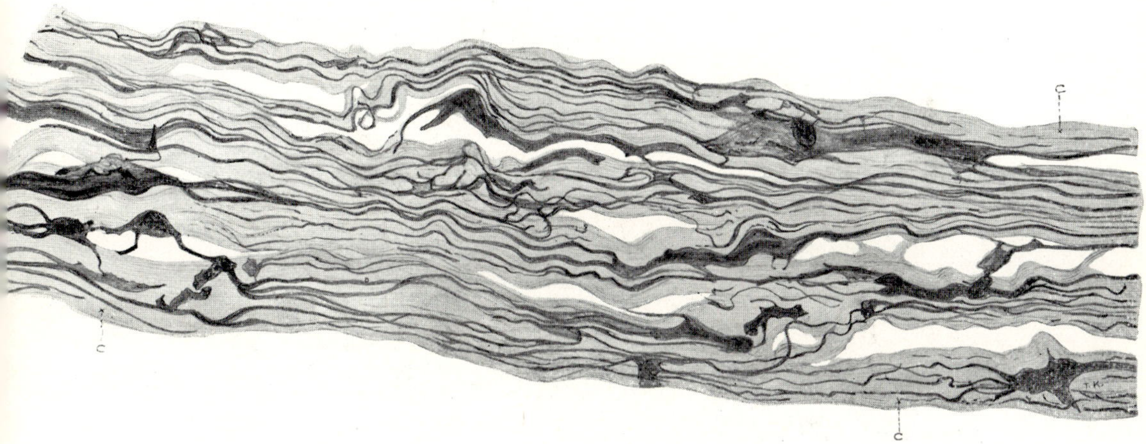

Fig. 4.—Human dura: tangential section (hernia cerebri), syncytial cells with long anostomosing projections forming a network on collagenic fibers; c—collagenic fiber bundle; Bielchowsky's stain, magnification × 980.

in the cells. They are found more densely in the neighborhood of the nuclei, while the protoplasm further away shows a more or less rich sprinkling of these elements. Wherever the protoplasmic network exists, whether or not nuclei are present, mitochondria are found in the protoplasm. It seems, therefore, necessary to consider the whole membranous network as a living, active membrane (probably of very important functions) and not as a structure serving only as support for cells. In other words, if one speaks of cells, the membrane and the whole of the membrane has to be considered as the protoplasm of the cells.

Another formation found in the protoplasm is fibrillae. They can be followed through a whole cell and into the protoplasm of another cell.

They are of the kind Mallory has described as fibroglia.[1a] They differ in no way from the fibroglia found in pia arachnoid and will be mentioned later.

It has already been said that the membranous protoplasm (cellular membranes) is, in the main, extended in a plane parallel to the surface of the dura. As cross sections show the dura to have many layers of cells with bundles of collagenic fibers separating the cell layers, one could consider the dura to be formed by layers of cell membrane and layers of collagenic fibers. Dura, as a fact, corresponds to this structural for-

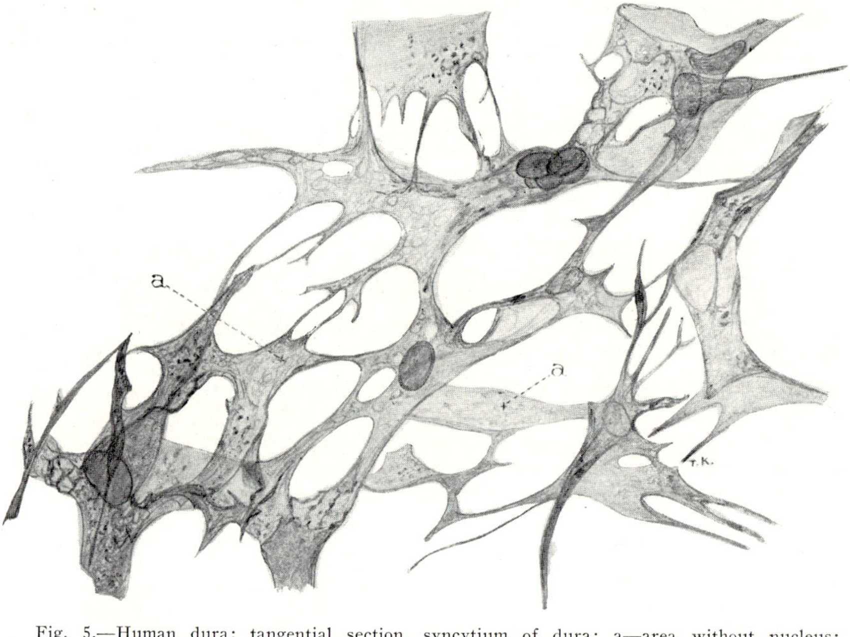

Fig. 5.—Human dura: tangential section, syncytium of dura; a—area without nucleus; formalin, Champy fluid, iron-hematoxylin, magnification × 1800.

mation to a certain extent. One can usually split a piece of dura (at least partly, whatever part it is taken from) parallel to it's surface into two or three lamellae. In doing so one can observe that much tissue is torn. The different layers of cellular membrane and collagenic fibers anastomose with each other. A cross section of dura in which the cellular membranes are stained clearly demonstrates anastomosis by cells and anastomosis by collagenic fibers between the different layers.

1a. Mallory, F. B.: A hitherto undescribed fibrillar substance produced by connective tissue cells, J. M. Research, 1903, 10, p. 334.

In between the collagenic fibers lie the cellular membranes. In material well fixed without shrinkage one sees the membranous protoplasm in close proximity, we would say adherent, to the collagenic bundles. Where the protoplasmic membrane is broad it lies as a sheet upon the bundle or surrounds it more or less, forming at least a part of a cylinder (fig. 5). Where the cells lie far apart one sees the protoplasmic connections between the cells lying close to the collagenic bundle, and following every kink or wrinkle of the bundle. The forms which the cells and their anastomosing protoplasmic strands take are so manifold that any description is hopeless.

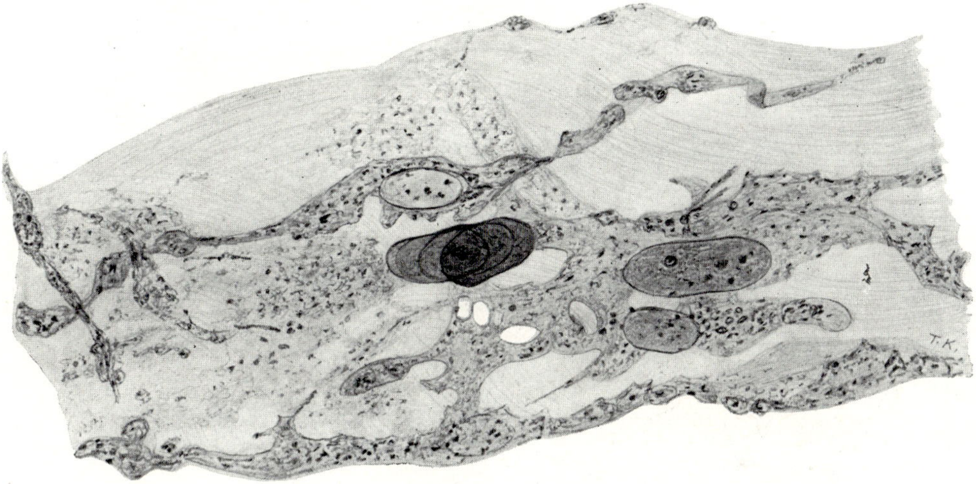

Fig. 6.—Human dura: tangential section, mitochondria are shown in the protoplasm; formalin, Champy's fluid, iron-hematoxylin, magnification × 1800.

We do not feel it probable that we have succeeded in staining the protoplasmic membranes throughout their full extension. We feel rather that our technique has not been able to demonstrate the thinnest part of the membranes, and also not the finest protoplasmic projections. Here and there in the preparations we find pictures which may mean that a fine membrane exists, but the delicacy of the structure makes it impossible to decide.

In silver preparations showing long and slender protoplasmic anastomosis between cells (fig. 4) we frequently have seen slender, faintly stained strands which seemed to bury themselves in the collagenic fiber bundle. Sometimes we have got the impression that there existed a substance in between the fibrillae constituting the collagenic bundle which was a direct continuation of the protoplasmic membrane.

A few times we have observed fibroglia fibers leaving the protoplasmic membrane and joining the collagenic fiber bundle. The relation of the fibrillae to the cells will be mentioned again in the discussion of the pia-arachnoid.

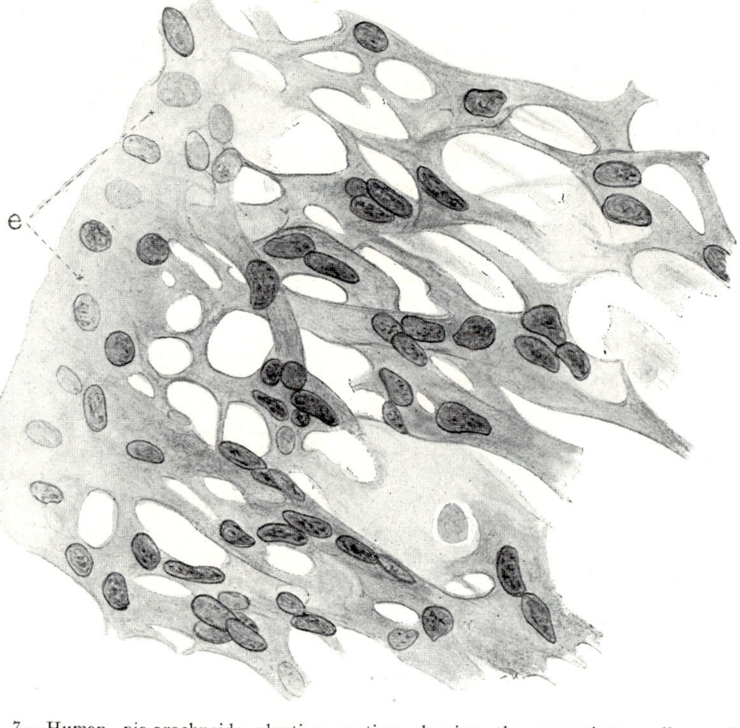

Fig. 7.—Human pia-arachnoid: slanting section showing the syncytium, collagen fibers unstained; c—surface endothelium; formalin, Müller's fluid, iron-hematoxylin, magnification × 600.

A layer of endothelial cells is described on the outer surface of the dura, and another layer of endothelial cells on the inner surface of the dura. The endothelial layer on the outside of the dura, in such places where it remains after loosening the dura from the skull, is a single layer of cells. On the inner side of the dura, on the other hand, it presents itself in some places as being a single layer of cells, in other places it consists of several layers. The so-called endothelium has the same characters as the endothelial cells of pia-arachnoid and bears the same relation to the dura cells (fibroblasts) as the endothelium of pia-arachnoid bears to the cells (fibroblasts) of these membranes. We will, therefore, speak of the endothelial cells later.

Besides the syncytium formed by the fibroblasts, one finds cells in the dura which do not form protoplasmic connections with the syncytium. They are free cells and to them belong the plasma cells, the wandering cells and some pigment cells. They will be discussed in the report of the observations of pathologic tissue.

PIA-ARACHNOID

One may study the cellular structure of the pia-arachnoid by teasing after fixation in various fluids. This method has formerly been used to a great extent but has, however, many objections. For our purpose we have gained the best information from sections made more or less parallel to the surface. The sections were treated to prevent the staining of the collagenic fibers. On such sections the protoplasm of the endothelial cells is seen to be like a membrane which has its greatest extension in a plane parallel to the surface. The cells have, however, wing-formed projections from their lower surface which lie in a plane forming more or less of an angle to the surface plane. The wing-formed projections connect with the protoplasm of a cell lying directly under it, and this cell again with one lying still deeper, etc. (fig. 8). At the same time the cells are connected with neighboring cells on the sides by bridges of protoplasm. In this way the cells form a net or meshwork of protoplasm which is continuous throughout the whole section. The protoplasm of all the cells, those on the surface (endothelial cells) as well as the cells in the depth of the tissue, is membrane-like, and gives the impression that the endothelial membrane of the surface continues as a network through the whole thickness of the tissue

The membranous protoplasmic network lying immediately below the surface presents narrow meshes. Toward the deeper parts of the arachnoid the meshes grow gradually wider. In no place in the protoplasmic network have we been able to detect any borderline between the cells. The protoplasm of one cell is a direct continuation of that of another cell and the surface endothelium forms a part of the protoplasmic network. In this network nuclei are irregularly distributed but mostly found arranged in groups. A true syncytium is formed by the cells and it seems therefore even more inappropriate to speak about cells here than in the dura. A protoplasmic membrane with groups (or centers) of nuclei seems better to describe the picture. In the description of the protoplasmic structure it does not seem to us of great importance whether one or the other term is used.

The syncytial protoplasmic membrane follows the trabeculae of the spider-webbed subarachnoidal tissue down to and spins through the more dense pia and pia intima. In this way is formed a net-like proto-

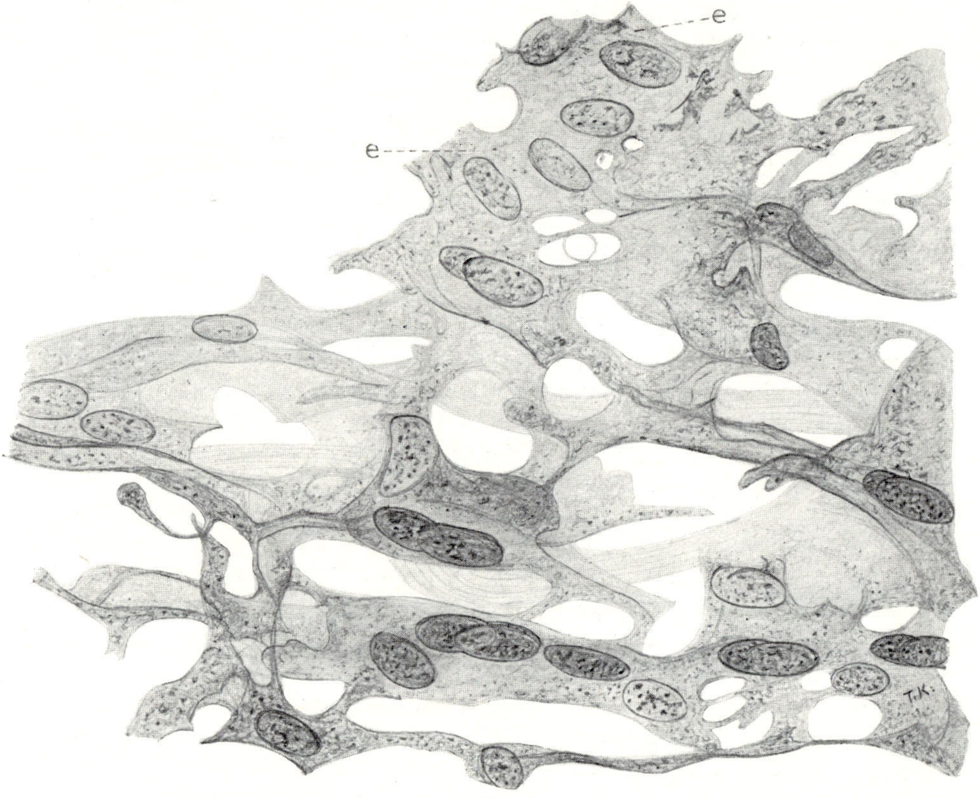

Fig. 8.—Human pia-arachnoid: the syncytium and the endothelial cells in direct connection with the underlying cells, the nuclei are in groups; collagen fibers not stained; e—surface endothelium; formalin, iron-hematoxylin, magnification × 1800.

plasmic membrane (syncytium) extending from the surface of the arachnoid to the surface and even into the substance of the brain with the pial projections which surround the vessels entering the brain substance. In the spider-webbed part of the arachnoid the syncytium (mesenchyme network) follows the trabeculae more or less surrounding them but here it may also spread out to become more or less fenestrated membranes of wide extension. Partially enclosed chambers of varying size are formed by the membranes bridging spaces between fibrillae.

The nuclei are arranged in groups. Especially in places where the protoplasm has spread out forming membranes is this group arrangement of nuclei striking (figs. 11, 12 and 15). Drawing 15 shows a group containing nine nuclei arranged around the centrosome. Such a number of nuclei in one group, although uncommon, cannot be considered exceptional. The nuclei frequently lie so close together that they cover each other and make it impossible to count their number with any accuracy. Where the syncytium takes the form of a network of more narrow protoplasmic strands and large meshes the group arrangement of the nuclei is not so marked but can easily be recognized (figs. 9 and 10). The size and shape of the nuclei varies considerably. Although the greatest number of them have the usual form and size of the connective tissue nuclei one meets with many nuclei of considerable smaller size and then usually round or nearly so. On the other hand one not so seldom sees nuclei of much larger size and one may even meet with nuclei which, with good reason, could be called giant nuclei (figs. 9, 10, 11, 12 and 13) give an idea of the variety of form and size of nuclei. None of the observed giant nuclei have been reproduced. In preparations stained with iron-hematoxylin the nuclei stain with different intensity. Some are very dark, others are faintly stained and nuclei in the same group may show varying intensity of staining.

The protoplasm of the syncytium contains numerous mitochondria (fig. 11). They are most numerous in the neighborhood of the nuclei while in the rest of the protoplasm they are found in varying amounts. However thinly the membrane is spread out mitochondria can be found. We have never found the syncytium to present the appearance of a membrane without structure. In the protoplasm rounded bodies are also regularly found which are much larger than the mitochondria and have other staining properties than the mitochondria. The bodies are distributed in rather an orderly fashion though the protoplasm, being more numerous around the nuclei and more scarcely found the further away from the nuclei. They are brought out at times in preparations stained with silver or anilin stains. With iron-hematoxylin they stain poorly but are partially stained and visible as ring-shaped formations in the preparations reproduced in figure 11.

As mentioned under technique one can manage the iron-hematoxylin staining in such a way that the collagenic fibers are not stained, but in the protoplasm one frequently finds both the mitochondria and struc-

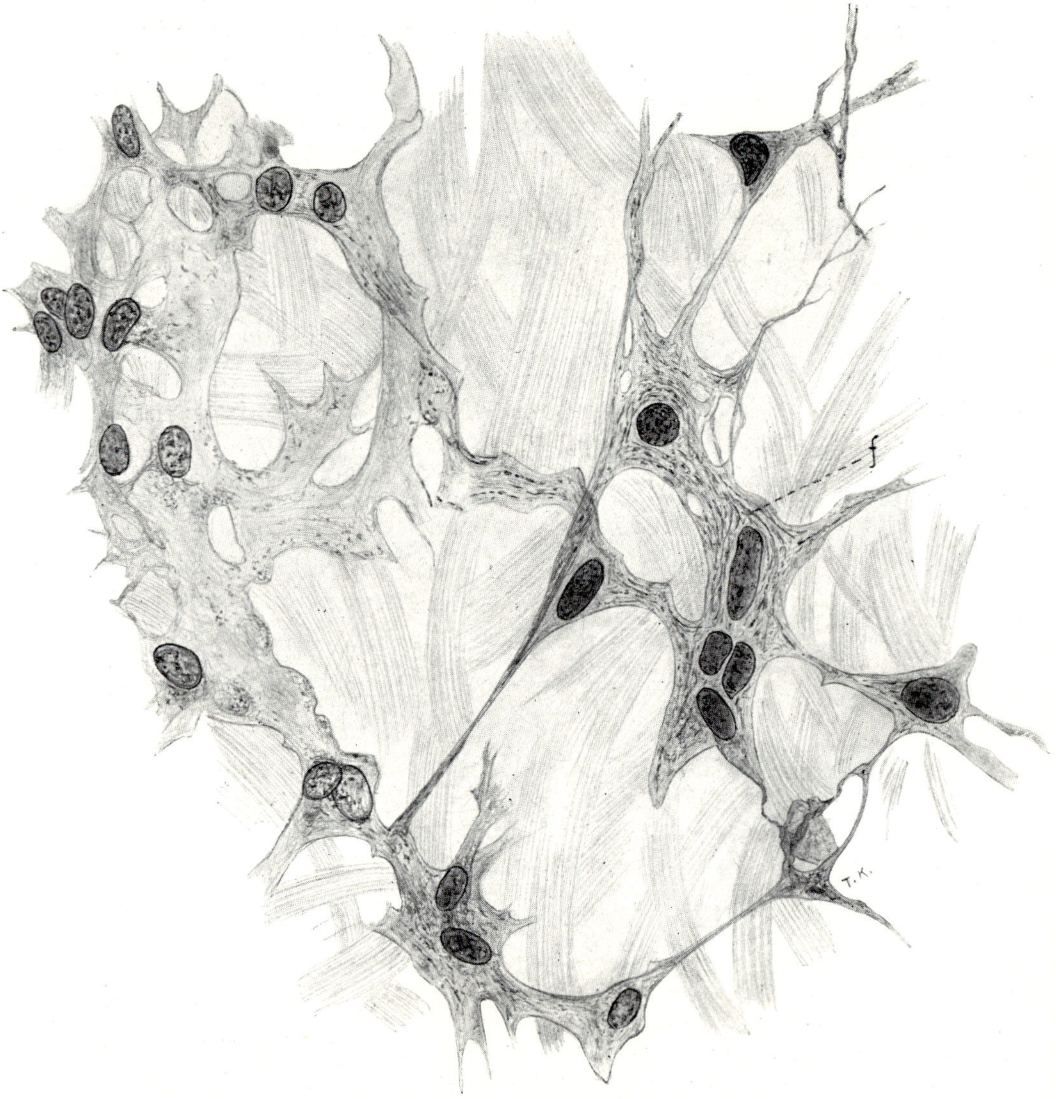

Fig. 9.—Human pia-arachnoid: syncytium with large meshes from deeper layer of the pia-arachnoid, the collagenic fibers faintly indicated, many collagenic bundles seen not to be in contact with syncytium (incomplete staining); f—fibrillae in the cells; formalin, iron-hematoxylin, magnification × 1200.

tures which, with good reason, can be called fibrillary. They give the impression of fibrillae having been formed by the mitochondria arranging themselves in a row. Meves [2] studying the connective tissue cells of chicken embryos came to the conclusion that the collagen fibrillae

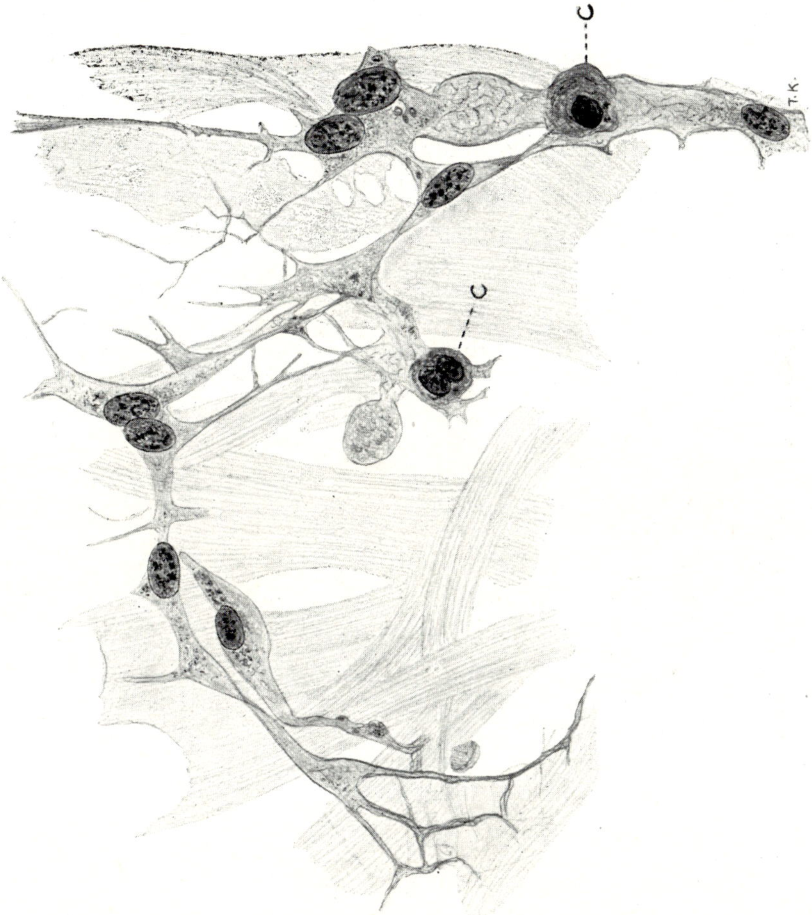

Fig. 10.—Human pia: syncytium from pia in a sulcus; c—cells becoming free from the syncytium; formalin, iron-hematoxylin, magnification × 1200.

were formed by the mitochondria. We have seen many pictures from which we think it possible that intracellular fibrillae are formed in this way. On account of their localization and their beaded appearance we

2. Archiv. Mikr. Anat., 1910, vol. 71, p. 149.

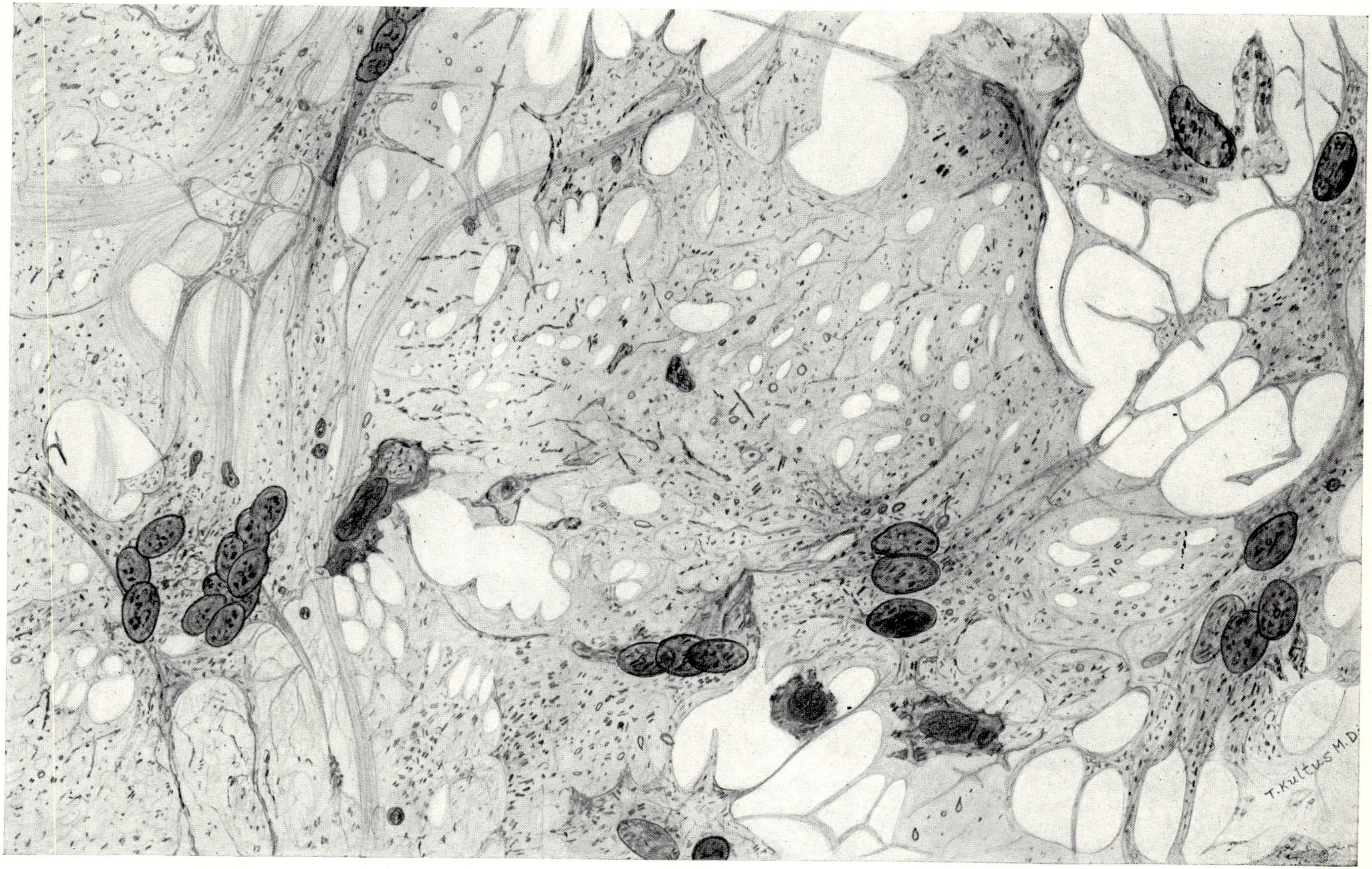

Fig. 11.—Human pia (child): pial syncytium which has formed fenestrated membranes, mitochondria through the whole membrane, in places mitochondria seem to have arranged themselves to fibrillary structure; some collagenic fibers in one part of the drawing; formalin, iron-hematoxylin, magnification × 1800.

will call them the protoplasmic or cytoplasmic fibrillae. We designate them thus simply to have a short expression when speaking of them. In the parts of the syncytium which are spread out to membranes of large extension the cytoplasmic fibrillae show an arrangement corresponding to the one presented in figures 11 and 14. (The last figure is, however, taken from the pia of a chronic syphilitic meningitis. Most of the other protoplasmic constituents have degenerated, leaving fibrillary

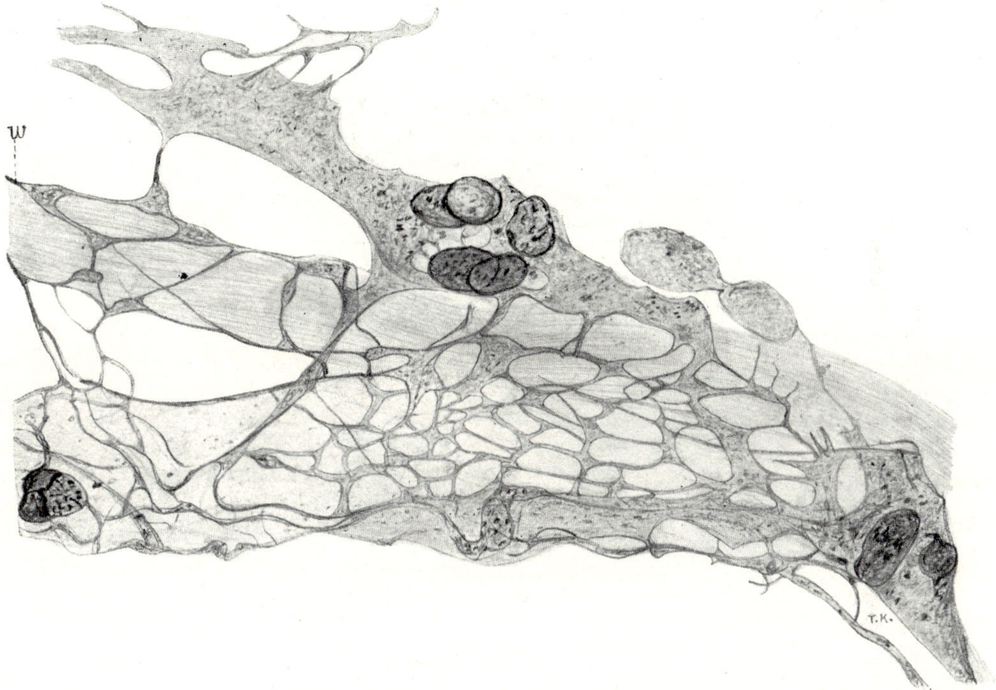

Fig. 12.—Human pia-arachnoid: syncytial membranes forming a spider web; w—spider web spinning around collagenic bundle; in the protoplasmic meshwork the cytoplasmic fibers are not stained; formalin, iron-hematoxylin, magnification × 1800.

structures more plainly visible. In some silver-gold stained preparations from normal meninges we have seen corresponding pictures.) Where the syncytium forms a more open network and only a narrow extension of protoplasm surrounds the nuclei the cytoplasmic fibrillae show, as a rule, a more orderly course as may be seen in figure 9. They run parallel and can be followed from one nucleary center to another. They continue even into the narrowest and longest protoplasmic branches and enter with them into other cells (nucleary centers).

The thionin method is by far the best for studying the cytoplasmic fibrillae. The masses of collagenic fibers are decolorized or stained a pale green, while the cytoplasmic fibrillae are stained very sharply, bluish or violet. The nuclei are stained deep blue, the remainder of the protoplasm faintly or not at all. The cytoplasmic fibrillae may run parallel through the whole protoplasm but most commonly their course does not seem to be parallel in the neighborhood of the nuclei. There they run in different directions and give the appearance of a network although it is unlikely that any real network exists. In the

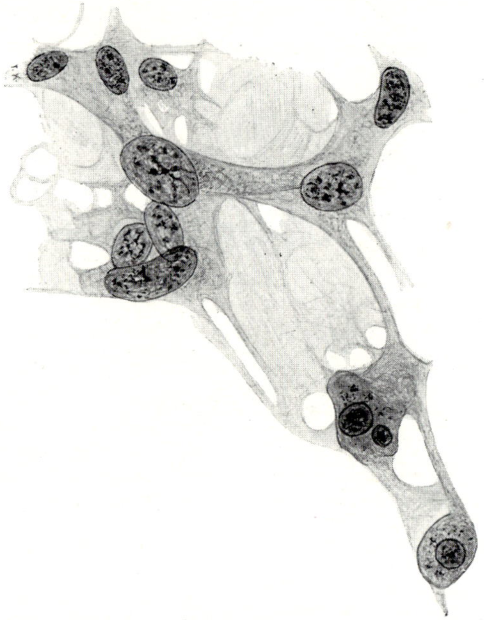

Fig. 13.—Human pia: pial syncytium, grouped nuclei; formalin, thionin, magnification × 1200.

edge of the protoplasm and in the protoplasmic projections the course of the cytoplasmic fibrillae is distinctly parallel. The individual fibrils are not smooth; they seem to be built up of small, intensely stained nodules which appear to be connected by a substance that is faintly stained. The nodules are not equally large. Here and there nodules are found two or three times as large as others. This may depend upon a juxtaposition of the nodules. With thionin staining these fibrillae seem finer than in iron hematoxylin. In the edge of the protoplasm, however, one sees coarser fibrillae but these, to all appearances, are formed by the juxtaposition of two or more finer fibrillae. One frequently sees two or more fine fibrillae leave the edge or surface of the protoplasm and join, forming a coarser fibrilla which then crosses the space between two nucleary centers or cells. They then separate again and enter the protoplasm of another nucleary center. Where these join or separate one can discern a slight membrane which holds them together. Many times one sees a coarse fibrilla spread out and reveal itself to consist of several small fibrillae between which a membrane exists. This indicates that the protoplasm is actually present in the coarse part

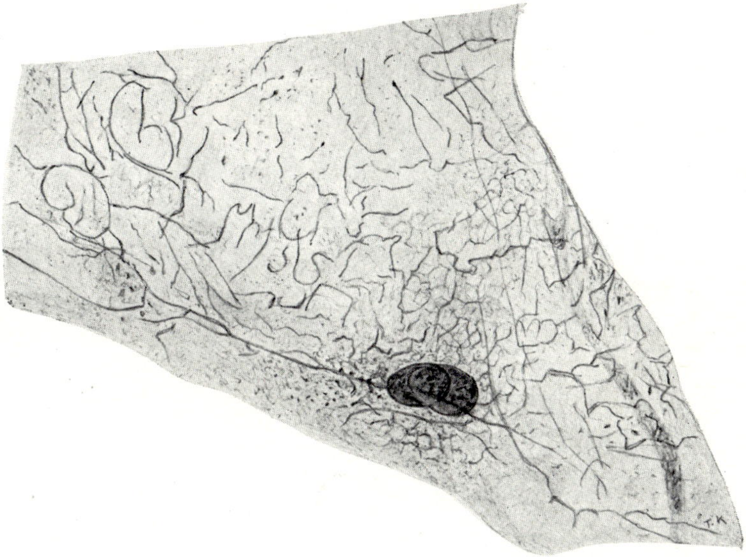

Fig. 14.—Human pia (chronic syphilitic meningitis): syncytial membrane from pia, degenerative cell, making the fibrillary structure in the protoplasm more visible; formalin, iron-hematoxylin, magnification × 1800.

even though such fibrillae appear to be without it. In the joined part, however, no protoplasmic membrane can be seen. The cytoplasmic fibrillae which in considerable numbers arise from different cells or nucleary centers, form a rich network. This network constitutes the reticulum (fig. 16). The whole reticulum is formed by the cytoplasmic fibrillae which lie in protoplasmic membranes. Nearly all the strands in the reticulum are formed by several cytoplasmic fibrillae. The net-formed effect is not due to the splitting of individual fibers but to one or several individual fibers changing their course and leaving one strand to join another. Where the individual fibrilla spread out from each other one can plainly see a membrane (protoplasm). Therefore we do not hesitate to say that this protoplasmic membrane exists in greater or lesser amounts where reticulum exists.

Several times we have observed how a fine collagenic fiber comes to a cell and apparently combines directly with the cytoplasmic fibrillae. When a bundle of collagenic fibers splits up so that finer bundles are formed one sees that the individual fibers stain in the same tone as the reticulum fibers. Furthermore they have the same nodular appearance. However, the distances between the nodules are greater and more

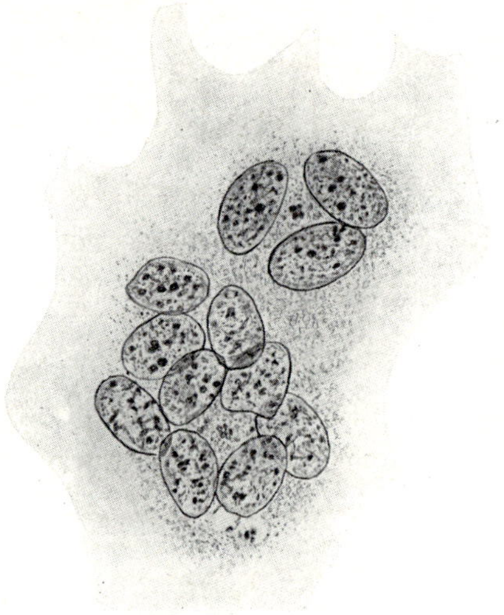

Fig. 15.—Human pia: groups of nuclei in syncytial membrane; formalin thionin, magnification × 1200.

irregular than in the cytoplasmic fibrillae, and this gives the collagenic fibers and the fibers of the reticulum a different appearance. Whether these nodes on the collagen fibers are really of mitochondrial nature we are unable to decide, but in preparations with mitochondria well stained one finds mitochondria along the reticulum fibrillae and also at times along the collagenic fibers, some seeming to lie in the collagenic fiber bundles.

Besides the fine protoplasmic fibrillae one finds coarser fibrillae which correspond to those described by Mallory as fibroglia. One may see them divide and reveal themselves as many or fewer fine nodulated fibrillae of the same appearance as the cytoplasmic or reticulum fibrillae.

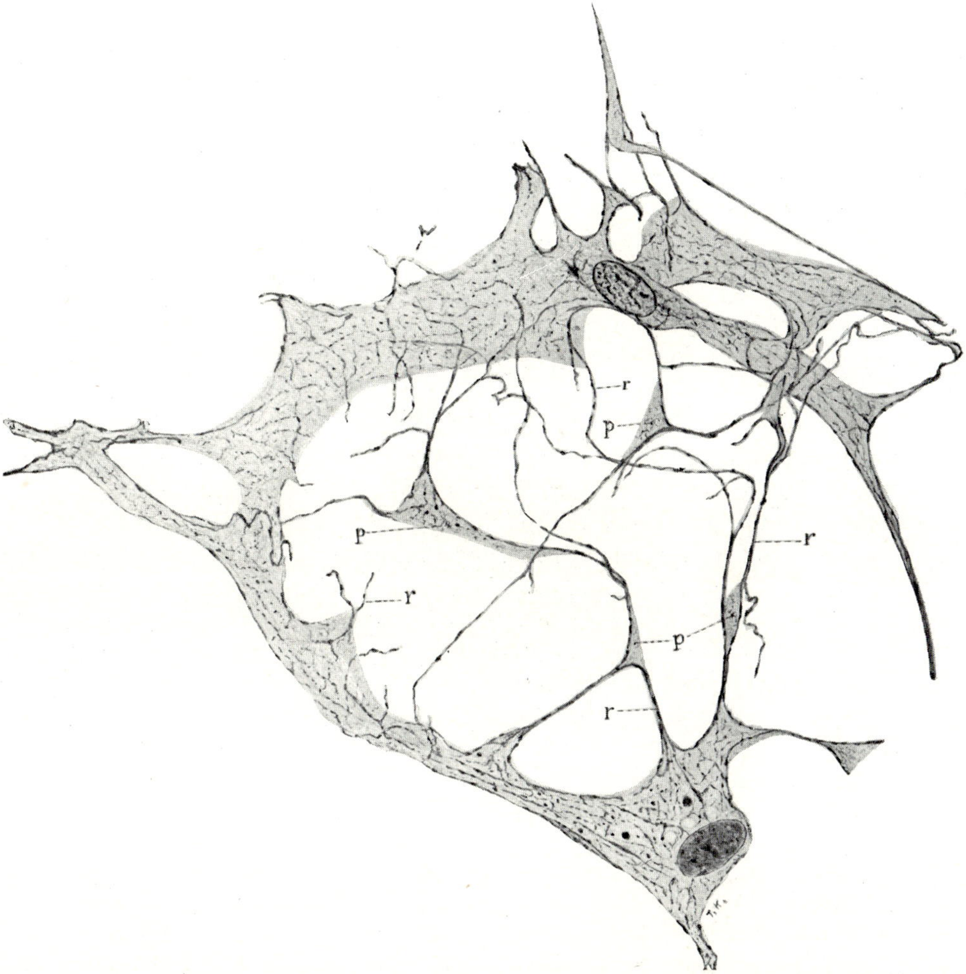

Fig. 16.—Human pia-arachnoid: syncytium showing the fibrillary structure, the cytoplasmic fibrillae plainly seen entering into protoplasm, and going out into the projections of the protoplasm forming the reticulum—r; p—protoplasmic membrane is seen where reticular fibers separate; formalin, Müller's solution, thionin, magnification × 1800.

During our studies we have come to the conclusion that fibroglia, reticulum fibers, and collagenic fibers are all the same kind of fibrillae, originating from the cytoplasmic fibrillae. Rössle and Yoshida,[3] Miller,[4] Foot,[5] and above all Mallory,[6] have given excellent reasons for considering the collagenic fibers and reticulum as one and the same kind of fibrillae differing only in their anatomical arrangement.

In between the syncytial protoplasmic membranes run the collagenic fibers. They are found in the narrow meshes immediately under the so-called endothelium. They adhere closely to or stand in close contact with the syncytial membranes. Where the collagenic fibers form a reticulum of great meshes one sees the syncytial membranes follow them and sometimes surround them. Where the syncytium is an unbroken membrane it seems to lie as a sheet upon the collagenic bundles. Where the syncytium is more in the form of a spider web (fig. 12) one sees the protoplasmic strands spinning on or around the collagenic fibers (fig. 12-w).

Iron-hematoxylin preparations give the impression that there exist many collagenic bundles which are not in touch with any syncytium. One has, however, no right to draw that conclusion from these preparations for the reason that the staining is uncertain in such places where collagenic fibers lie close together. It has been impossible for instance to stain the syncytium in the dura in more than parts of the section; so that the syncytium is seen in one part of the section and not in another. Silver-gold method applied to sections from the same material gives at times a much more complete staining of the syncytium. From the study of such sections it seems probable that every collagenic fiber bundle stands in close contact with the syncytium either by being in contact with a membrane or with a fine network of protoplasm spinning over its surface (figs. 6 and 12).

It remains for us to speak about the endothelium. It has already been stated that the endothelial cells stand in direct continuity with the syncytial membranes through wing-formed processes (figs. 7 and 8). In tangential sections strongly stained with iron-hematoxylin the endothelial cells appear to be a continuous membrane containing nuclei. In this protoplasm can be seen numerous mitochondria. Besides the mitochondria one finds in preparations appropriately stained cytoplasmic fibrillae as described in the syncytial membrane, and these fibrillae

3. Beitr. z. path. anat. u. z. allg. path., 1909, 14, p. 110.
4. Am. Rev. Tuberc., 1923, 7, p. 141.
5. Am. J. Path., 1925, vol. 1, p. 341; J. Lab. & Clin. Med., 1924, 9, p. 777.
6. Ibid., 1927, 17, p. 515.

can be seen passing into the deeper lying syncytial membranes. Even coarser fibers of the thickness and appearance of fibroglia are seen (fig. 17). The coarser fibers spin through long stretches of the membrane, crossing above and below nuclei and apparently lying in the protoplasm of the cells. Here and there lines may be seen that simulate cell borderlines but closer inspection always reveals them as fibrillae. The nuclei are not distributed evenly, rather

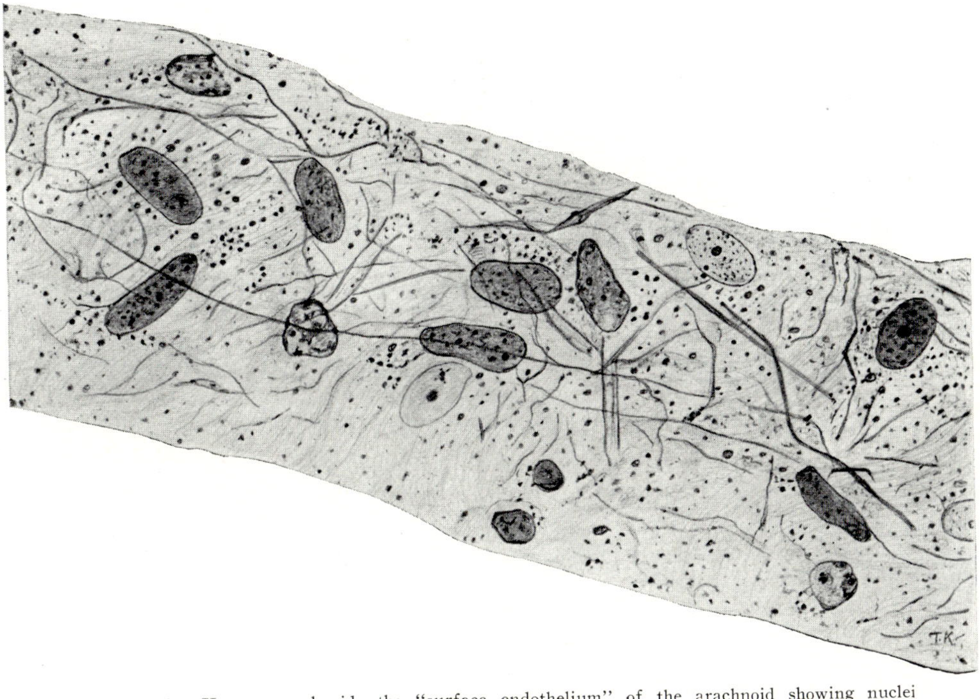

Fig. 17.—Human arachnoid: the "surface endothelium" of the arachnoid showing nuclei in groups and fibrillae in the endothelium, formalin, chrome, iron-hematoxylin, magnification × 1800.

they are arranged in groups in the same way as the nuclei lie in the deeper syncytium.

One may study the endothelium of membranes which are split off from the pia-arachnoid, but this is not a satisfactory method on account of the thickness of the membrane and the shrinkage that occurs due to the elasticity and to the hardening. It seems to us that the cell borderlines that have been described depend on the staining of fibrillae and on wrinkles that occur from shrinkage and contraction of the membranes. However, in the split-off membranes one can study the different types of nuclei of the surface layer. One is struck by the great number of nuclei which evidently belong to wandering cells which travel just beneath or seemingly in the membraneous protoplasm itself. Many of them lie in exactly the same focus as the nuclei of the superficial layer. One will find these wandering cells especially numerous if one kills an animal by injecting into the spinal canal hardening fluid containing osmic acid such as Champy's fluid.

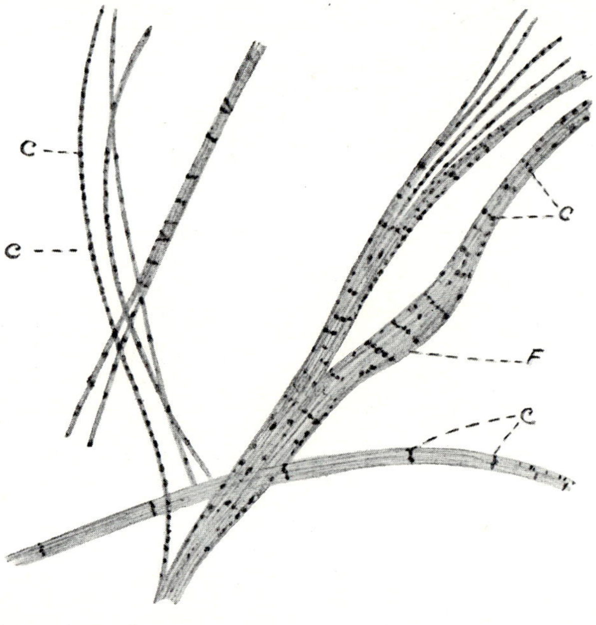

Fig. 18.—Human pia: c—chromaphilic granules probably of mitochondrial nature; f—collagen fiber bundle; formalin, Müller's solution, thionin, magnification × 1800.

The endothelial cells form a part of the syncytium, that is, they are the most superficial layer. Like the cells which form the syncytium they are fibroblastic in nature. Maximow [7] has described how in cultures endothelial cells may change into fibroblasts. It may be that the cells of the surface layer (endothelium) are, to a certain degree, modified but they certainly show the same characteristics as the fibroblasts of the syncytial membranes. All the different so-called endothelial membranes

7. Archiv. f. Mikr. Anat., 1922, 96, p. 494.

which have been described in arachnoidal pia and intimal pia are all formed by fibroblasts which have taken the form of membranes. The endothelium of the dura shows the same relation and the same characteristics as the endothelial cells of pia-arachnoid.

Of the cellular elements of the pia-arachnoid we have only described the fixed cells, that is, cells which are a part of the syncytium and all of fibroblastic nature. One finds even in normal meninges, cells which have no connection whatever with the syncytium and are free cells. As they are intimately connected with the different pathological processes we shall describe them in the report about such conditions.

Controversy has long been active with respect to the origin, structure and function of connective tissue and its various derivatives. It is not our intention to enter into an historical discussion of these matters, but only to note that in several quarters there has been a trend away from the older and still prevalent conceptions of the nature of the connective tissue.

Key and Retzius [8] in 1875 described cells in the dura which possessed extended and frequently anastomosing processes. These correspond in many ways to some of our observations.

From studies on early embryonic connective tissue with reference to the development of the vitreous v. Szily [9] concludes that embryonic connective tissue is laid down in a noncellular fibrillary supporting network which is present at the earliest stages between all primitive epithelial layers. This structure, he considers, is made up of protoplasmic processes derived from the epithelial cells themselves and forming intercellular bridges between their layers. Mesenchymal cells wander into this network, and become very closely associated with the fiber system to make up the embryonic connective tissue.

Ranke [10] on the basis of his observations on pathologic alteration in arteries and some embryological studies is lead to the conclusion that the prototype of all connective tissue is a protoplasmic network. Nuclei migrate into this protoplasmic structure forming a syncytium, within which two fundamental histiogenic processes occur: the liberation of free cells (blood cells, histiogenic wandering cells), and the formation of fibrillary differentiation products within the bridges of the plasma network.

8. Studien in der Anatomie des Nervensystems und des Bindegewbes, 1875, p. 157.

9. Ueber das Enstehen eines fibrillären Stützgewebes und desen Verhaltnis zus Glaskörperfrage. Merkel-Bonnet's Anat. Hefte., 1908, 35, p. 651.

10. Ztschr. f. d. Neurol. u. Psychiat., 1914, 27, p. 221.

Following the views of Ranke in many respects, Hueck [11] also attacks the prevailing view that connective tissue is merely an inert supporting substance and that it is formed by amalgamation of the products of discrete cells. This observer, too, considers that all connective tissue has for its original model a net-like or sponge-like protoplasm and that in it fibrillae and other differentiated formations are elaborated. He emphasizes that mesenchymal tissue is vital and active especially, in adult connective tissue, that portion of plasmatic "Grundsubstanz" which persists.

Concerning the formation of the fibrillae in the protoplasmic net. Ranke and Hueck both take the view that a morphologic differentiation of an indifferent type of fiber first occurs, probably chiefly in the surface portions of the network as a result of stresses and other physical factors. Later there is a chemical differentiation of the indifferent fibers into elastic or collagenic fibrillae. Meves,[2] however, presents evidence to show that the mitochondria, numerous in all embryonic cells, form the collagenic fibers in the developing tendons of chick embryos.

CONCLUSIONS

The cells of the dura mater and of the pia-arachnoid form a syncytial membrane spinning through the whole thickness of the respective meninges, which demonstrates that the original mesenchymal syncytium remains permanent through life, so far as dura and pia are concerned. The so-called "membranes" of the meninges instead of being only supporting structures are protoplasm having the constituents for highly important functions.

The so-called surface endothelium forms an integral part of the syncytium and has fibroblastic characteristics.

Reticulum consists of protoplasm with cytoplasmic fibrillae. In the protoplasm which contains or accompanies the reticular fibers mitochondria can be demonstrated. Fibroglia is formed from the cytoplasmic fibrillae, and collagenic fibers also arise from cytoplasmic fibrillae.

11. Beitr. path. Anat. u. allg. Path., 1920, 66, p. 330.

BACTERICIDAL PROPERTIES OF THE ACYL AND ALKYL DERIVATIVES OF RESORCINOL

Bettylee Hampil

From the Department of Bacteriology, School of Hygiene and Public Health, Johns Hopkins University, Baltimore

Resorcinol, a diphenol $C_6H_4(OH)_2$, has long been known to possess bactericidal properties. It has also been definitely established that the substitution of alkyl groups in the nucleus of phenol has the effect of increasing its disinfectant strength.[1] The same has been demonstrated in reference to resorcinol which is less toxic to laboratory animals than phenol.

In 1913 Johnson and Hodge[2] reported the synthesis of ethyl resorcinol and n-propyl resorcinol. The biological examination of these substances by Rettger and Leonard[3] showed that n-propyl resorcinol possessed distinctly more bactericidal activity than either resorcinol or ethyl resorcinol and that it might be administered to laboratory animals without toxic effect. Johnson and Lane in 1921[4] reported the synthesis of n-butyl resorcinol. This derivative was found to be more active as a bactericide than the propyl compound. In cooperation with Leonard in his investigations in urinary antisepsis, Dohme, Cox, and Miller[5] have prepared in pure crystalline form the alkyl resorcinols together with their intermediate ketones from n-propyl resorcinol to n-tridecyl resorcinol. They have also synthesized the iso-butyl, iso-amyl and iso-hexyl derivatives as well as their corresponding ketones.

In 1924 Leonard[6] reported the experimental properties of the alkyl resorcinols as urinary antiseptics. The results of this investigation are in accord with the orignial hypothesis that in these componds there is a marked rise in bactericidal efficiency accompanying the increased sum of the atomic weights in the alkyl chain. Leonard found, further, that no increase in toxicity accompanied these large increases in bactericidal power. According to this work, n-hexyl resorcinol was placed at the peak of the series, n-heptyl resorcinol showed a distinct drop in bactericidal efficiency, and the n-octyl derivative was found to be entirely devoid of germicidal properties. Leonard and Frobisher[7] in 1926 observed that n-hexyl resorcinol is a powerful surface tension reducent. This observation was brought about in attempting to explain why this drug, although equally as bactericidal in alkaline and in acid urine in vitro, apparently lost its activity as an antiseptic in vivo when sodium bicarbonate was administered at the same time. It was definitely determined that the administration of sodium bicarbonate was contraindicated

Received for publication, Jan. 10, 1928.

1. Tilley, F. W., and Schaeffer, J. M.: J. Bact., 1926, 12, p. 303.
2. J. Am. Chem. Soc., 1913, 35, p. 1014.
3. Leonard, Veader: Science, 1925, 62, p. 408.
4. J. Am. Chem. Soc., 1921, 18, p. 348.
5. Ibid., 1926, 48, p. 1688.
6. J. Urol., 1924, 12, p. 585.
7. Trans. Am. A. G.-U. Surgeons, 1925, 18, p. 333.

simply because of its diuretic action with the consequent rise in the surface tension of the urine through the dilution accompanying diuresis. As a result of these and other experimental observations, the general conclusion was drawn that surface tension plays an important rôle in disinfection by chemical substances and that germicides which have the property of lowering the surface tension of their solvents are more powerful, other things being equal, than those which do not lower this tension.[8] In a recent investigation Frobisher[9] found this property to be common to both the acyl and alkyl series of resorcinol compounds. It was also found to be considerably increased in each successive derivative of each series. A measurement of the germicidal activity of the compounds by the U. S. Hygienic Laboratory method for testing disinfectants confirmed the original hypothesis only to a certain degree, since there was a sudden drop in the bactericidal effectiveness of the derivative beyond the n-heptyl and n-hexyl resorcinols. This was so in spite of the fact that the surface tension was progressively lowered, and was explained on the grounds of decreased water solubility; these relatively insoluble compounds enter into solution in water in too low a concentration to destroy organisms but even smaller amounts than this are nevertheless sufficient to depress surface tension.

Since the work of Leonard[6] on n-hexyl and n-heptyl resorcinol has been the only comprehensive study of members of this very important group of germicides, this investigation was undertaken to study the bactericidal activity of further members of the series. The problem resolved itself into systematic inquiry along four definite lines, namely: the effect of elevation of temperature on their bactericidal activity; their bactericidal power in the presence of organic material; the effect of alkalization on their bactericidal properties; and finally, the determination of a gram-positive specificity of the higher members of the alkyl series.

EFFECT OF ELEVATION OF TEMPERATURE ON RELATIVE ACTIVITY OF THE COMPOUNDS AS MEASURED BY PHENOL COEFFICIENTS

The compounds used in the investigation were prepared in the Research Laboratories of Sharp and Dohme of Baltimore in pure crystalline form, and were kindly furnished by them. The method followed was that indicated by the U. S. Hygienic Laboratory for the testing of disinfectants, 1921[10] differing only in certain details. Two brands of peptone were used, Difco and Witte, and the results are considered separately. The compounds were tested at 20 C., 37 C., and 45 C.

The term phenol coefficient is used throughout this work to express the relative bactericidal strength of the compound and of phenol in 15

8. J. Urol., 1926, 15, p. 1.
9. J. Bact., 1927, 13, p. 163.
10. Public Health Reports, 1921, 36, p. 1559.

minutes. The choice of this 15 minute period was made necessary because of the variability and fluctuations in the results characteristic of the compounds when the shorter time intervals are employed. In general, the figures thus obtained are lower than when the five and ten minute intervals are included in the average. The coefficients reported are based on the minimum figures observed.

Results.—It will be readily seen on examination of table 1 that with the increase in the length and weight of the alkyl chain, there is a pronounced rise in germicidal efficiency of each successive compound in each series. In the original work reported by Leonard, n-hexyl resorcinol was placed at the peak of the efficiency curve of the alkyl derivatives, and

TABLE 1.—COMPARISON OF ALKYL AND ACYL DERIVATIVES OF RESORCINOL AT 20 C. AND 37 C.

DIFCO BROTH

Compound	Phenol Coefficient at 20 C.	Phenol Coefficient at 37 C.	Percentage* Increase in Efficiency	Compound	Phenol Coefficient at 20 C.	Phenol Coefficient at 37 C.	Percentage* Increase in Efficiency
Propyl	5	5	81	Propylyl	Not tested†	Not tested	
N-butyl	25.4	17.5	25	N-butyryl	16.3	10	11
Iso-butyl	14.5	12.5	56	Iso-butyryl	2.2	2.7	116
N-amyl	54	40	33	N-amylyl	45.4	25	0
Iso-Amyl	50	35	27.2	Iso-Amylyl	2.7	2.5	66.6
N-hexyl	80	120	172	N-hexylyl	45.8	60	130
Iso-hexyl	75	110	106				
Heptyl	127	280	300	Iso-hexylyl, heptylyl, octylyl, nonylyl, decylyl, undecylyl, dodecylyl, and tridecylyl were not tested †			
Octyl	63.6	300	755				
Nonyl	—36 **	20	Not estimated				
Decyl, undecyl, dodecyl, tridecyl, and meristyl were not tested†							
Phenol	1:110 dilution kills	1:200 dilution kills	81.8				

* These figures were calculated from bactericidal dilutions in 15 minutes at 20 C. and at 37 C.
** —36 indicates 1:4000 emulsion is inactive.
† "Not tested" means substances can not be tested because of insolubility.

n-octyl was found to be devoid of bactericidal effects at 20 C. Since the products used at that time contained considerable amounts of impurities, it is to be expected that the two results might differ somewhat. The phenol coefficients for the acyl derivatives at 20 C. check very closely with those reported by Frobisher.[9] In this instance, the solutions were made from the same samples of substances. Great variations in phenol coefficiency are shown from day to day, especially in the higher compounds, even where the stock dilutions have been identical. This is in accord with the reports of other workers who have experimented with these compounds.

As shown by the percentage increase in efficiency column of table 1, elevation of temperature enhances the activity of each compound throughout the two series. This percentage increase is less than that shown by phenol until the six carbon atom alkyl chain is reached in each series. A pronounced rise in effectiveness is then noted. This is especially true of the alkyl derivatives. N-octyl resorcinol, which occupies a position below the n-hexyl derivatives at 20 C. is found to be twice as efficient as the latter at body temperature, while nonyl resorcinol, which is apparently inert at 20 C., becomes 20 times as efficient as phenol under these conditions. Among the acyl derivatives n-hexlyl resorcinol is found to retain its position at the high point of the curve but with a pronounced increase in activity. The isomeric compounds are likewise increased in bactericidal potency by the elevation of temperature. Each isomer occupies a position just below its corresponding normal homologue.

TABLE 2.—COMPARISON OF PHENOL COEFFICIFNTS OF ALKYL RESORCINOLS WITH DIFCO AND WITTE PEPTONE BROTHS

Compound	Phenol Coefficients at 20 C. Difco	Phenol Coefficients at 20 C. Witte	Phenol Coefficients at 37 C. Difco	Phenol Coefficients at 37 C. Witte	Phenol Coefficients 45 C. Witte
Propyl	5	5	5	5	5
N-butyl	25.4	22	17.5	17.5	15
Iso-butyl	14.5	12.7	12.5	12.5	....
N-amyl	54	54	40	40	40
Iso-amyl	50	40.9	35	30	....
N-hexyl	80	72	120	90	81.2
Iso-hexyl	75	40.9	110	50	....
Heptyl	127	49	280	100	133.3
Octyl	63.6	—36	300	110	200
Nonyl	—36	—36	20	—36	233.3
Decyl	—36	—36	—36	—36	30
Undecyl	—36	—36	—36	—36	....
Dodecyl	—36	—36	—36	—36	....
Tridecyl	—36	—36	—36	—36	....
Meristyl	—36	—36	—36	—36	....
Phenol	1:200 dilution kills		1:110 dilution kills		1:400 dilution kills

A comparison of the phenol coefficients of the alkyl resorcinols with Difco and Witte peptone broths is indicated in table 2. The results obtained for the lower members of the alkyl series with Witte broth are practically identical with those obtained with Difco broth. However, with the hexyl derivative striking differences are manifested. The phenol coefficients are less for n-hexyl, n-heptyl and n-octyl resorcinol. Nonyl resorcinol, which had exhibited bactericidal activity in Difco broth with the elevation of temperature is again found apparently inert. A further elevation of temperature to 45 C. produces a higher germicidal efficiency in the series above n-hexyl in comparison with phenol than did n-hexyl and the lower derivatives. Most striking is the behavior of both nonyl and decyl resorcinol. At 20 C. and at 37 C. these two substances were inactive as disinfectants, but with elevation of the temperature to 45 C., nonyl resorcinol becomes the most powerful member of the series. The action of the n-butyl derivative is also rather unusual. In comparison with phenol, this substance becomes less active, giving a lower phenol coefficient at 37 C. and at 45 C. than at 20 C.

Discussion.—Before attempting to interpret the results of experiments designed to bring out the chief characteristics and properties of the alkyl and acyl resorcinols, it is well to keep in mind a general idea of the nature and structure of these compounds. As has already been explained, they are built upon a diphenolic nucleus—the variant being the sum of the atomic weights of the alkyl chain introduced into the ring. The lower homologues are relatively simple, but as each series is ascended, the opportunity for complexity becomes more and more pronounced. It is reasonable to suppose that in the case of n-butyl resorcinol, for instance, the alkyl configuration remains under all circumstances a straight chain resulting in a relatively simple compound showing less variable and uncertain properties. However, when n-hexyl resorcinol is reached, the molecule becomes much more complex; with each succeeding derivative the chances that we are dealing with a compound in which the carbon atoms of the alkyl chain are linked in the exact spacial relationship presented in the structural formula become successively diminished. It is possible that the configuration of the alkyl radical may not be fixed but may be constantly shifting and changing. Such a condition might account for many of the perplexing difficulties encountered in the study of the compounds.

A discussion of the results derived from the study of the alkyl resorcinols at body temperature may be divided into two phases. The first concerns the effect of the elevation of temperature upon the efficiency of the compounds, and the second, the use of culture media showing differences in nitrogenous content as represented by Difco and Witte peptones.

It may be assumed that the manner of distribution of the chemical substances between the bacteria and the solvent and its subsequent activity upon the protoplasm of the test organisms is the same in homologous compounds. For that reason, if the bactericidal efficiency of each member of the two series of derivatives of resorcinol had shown a definite or fixed percentage of increase upon the elevation of temperature, the effect might be due altogether to what is termed a lessening of the inherent resistance of the organisms. The results as shown by table 1 do not bear this out. The members below hexyl resorcinol in the alkyl series show a percentage increase in efficiency less than that of phenol, while hexyl resorcinol and the next three above it show an extraordinary rise in germicidal value. The explanation of this phenomenon probably lies not in a change in resistance of the bacterial cells but in the effect of the elevated temperature on the chemicals themselves and on those factors affecting their bactericidal powers.

As the sum of the atomic weights in the alkyl chain becomes larger in successive derivatives, there are changes in two properties which have been previously observed to accompany this increase. The first is a lessening of the degree of solubility. Some of the higher alkyl resorcinols are dissolved in water at 20 C. with difficulty while at 37 C. and 45 C. they are much more soluble. The second change in activity common to the two series is the enhancement of their ability to lower surface tension. Leonard and Frobisher [8] first observed this and concluded that the high degree of bactericidal efficiency of the compounds probably depends to a great extent upon the ready permeability of the bacteria due to this characteristic. These workers noted a fall in germicidal value at 20 C. after the derivative showing six carbon atoms in the alkyl chain had been passed.

It is known that heat tends to decrease the intensity of adsorption of substances dissolved in solutions which are of low surface tension. This was experimentally demonstrated by Bayliss.[11] It would be expected therefore, that an elevation of temperature to 37 C. or 45 C. would by dissociation of the adsorption complex tend to decrease the effectiveness of the higher alkyl derivatives to a greater degree than that of the simpler homologues since the higher derivatives are greater surface tension reducents than the lower ones. However, since the results are contrary to this expectation, the extraordinary increase in the efficiency of the heavier resorcinols at high temperatures appears to depend to a large degree upon their increased solubility. At body temperature and at 45 C. there is actually more of the compound in solution, hence it exists in a higher concentration on the surface of the bacterial cell, and therefore, permeates the cell more readily and exerts its toxic action on the bacterial proteins. This is conditional upon the assumption that the toxic action of resorcinols is due to toxic action upon the bacterial proteins proof of which is now under investigation.

The action of octyl, nonyl and decyl resorcinols against Bacillus typhosus grown in Witte broth is probably the best evidence found to substantiate the idea that bactericidal activity in the resorcinols depends

11. Biochem. J., 1906, 1, p. 173.

on their water solubility (table 2). The three compounds are apparently inert as germicides when tested at 20 C. At 37 C octyl resorcinol becomes 110 times as powerful as phenol. The other two are still inert. At 45 C. however, nonyl resorcinol shows a bactericidal effectiveness in excess of the other derivatives of resorcinol and 233.3 times that of phenol. The activity of decyl resorcinol is less pronounced though it also is bactericidal under these conditions.

The divergent results in the phenol coefficients at 20 C. and at 37 C. when Witte peptone broth is used both for growing the test organisms and for the subcultures rather than Difco peptone broth, are pronounced with the higher alkyl resorcinols (table 2). The fact is illustrated that organisms may show a difference in resistance to certain disinfectants, depending on the composition of the nitrogenous material in which they are grown. N-octyl and nonyl resorcinol are striking examples. When tested at 37 C. against Bacillus typhosus cultured in Difco peptone broth, the disinfecting power of octyl resorcinol is estimated to be 300 times that of phenol. When the test organism is grown in Witte broth, the compound is only 110 times more powerful than phenol. Nonyl resorcinol gives a phenol coefficient of 20 when Difco broth is used while it is apparently inactive as a disinfectant against bacteria cultivated in Witte broth.

It is evident therefore that there is some protective mechanism against the action of the compounds in one case which is not present in the other. Whether this mechanism is within the organism itself or in the surrounding fluid remains an open question. Wright [12] in 1917 observed that phenol coefficients estimated when Witte broth is used were uniform, while results obtained with Difco broth were variable. This was attributed to the high H-ion concentration of the Digestive Ferments Co. peptone produced at that time, which necessitated an adjustment of the P_H value to between 6.0 and 7.0 and resulted in a medium of less nutritive value. However, in the work reported in this paper, the H-ion concentration of both peptones in unadjusted mediums is practically the same, ranging between P_H 6.6 and 6.8 after sterilization. The differences obtained are therefore not due to variations in H-ion concentrations of the two mediums.

It was thought that a difference in buffer indices might account for the higher protective qualities induced in Witte peptone, but a titration of several batches of mediums of each type showed relatively little variation in this respect.

12. J. Bact., 1917, 2, p. 315.

BACTERICIDAL ACTIVITY OF ACYL AND ALKYL RESORCINOLS AT 37 C. IN PRESENCE OF STANDARDIZED ORGANIC MATERIAL

The method used was that prescribed by the United States Hygienic Laboratory for estimating the phenol coefficients of disinfectants in the presence of organic material.[13] The temperature of medication was 37 C. Difco and Witte peptones were used in the culture mediums instead of the peptomum siccum of Armour.

The presence of standardized organic material (2% peptone, 1% gelatin) causes a decisive drop in the efficiency of each of the compounds with the exception of n-butyl resorcinol. N-hexyl resorcinol is found to be the most active germicide of the series with both Difco broth and Witte broth. N-hexyl and n-octyl resorcinol, which had occupied the

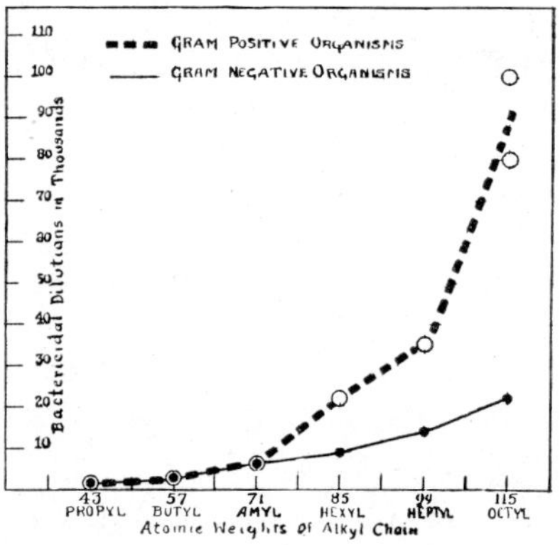

peaks of the acyl and alkyl curves respectively in water at 37 C. show no germicidal value with Difco broth when interpreted by the results of this type of experiment. When Witte broth was used, n-octyl and n-heptyl resorcinol exhibited a complete loss in effectiveness. Just as in the previous work when the two peptones were used, the organisms grown in Witte broth proved more resistant to disinfection.

The reduction of the efficiency of disinfectants in the presence of organic matter has been recognized since the earliest studies in germicides were made by Krönig and Paul,[14] Chick and Martin [15] and others. Where the disinfection is known to occur as a relatively simple chemical reaction, as in the case of corrosive sublimate and formaldehyde, the

13. Anderson, J. F., and McClintic, T. B.: Hyg. Lab. Bull. 82, 1912.
14. Ztschr. f. Hyg., 1897, 25, p. 1.
15. J. Hyg., 1908, 8, p. 654.

reason for this diminution in efficiency is obvious since the disinfectant forms a chemical combination with the organic material as well as the bacteria. There exists, in this instance, a definite quantitative relationship between the amount of the disinfectant in solution and that of the organic material present. In the case of phenol and phenolic substances, however, there are physiochemical factors involved which are less readily understood.

TABLE 3.—LOSS OF EFFICIENCY OF ALKYL AND ACYL RESORCINOLS IN 3% ORGANIC MATERIAL AT 37 C. AS SHOWN BY PHENOL COEFFICIENTS

Compound	Dilution in H_2O: Phenol Coefficient	3% Organic Material: Phenol Coefficient	Percentage Loss in Efficiency	Dilution in H_2O: Phenol Coefficient	3% Organic Material: Phenol Coefficient	Percentage Loss in Efficiency
ALKYL SERIES						
Propyl	5	4.5	10	5	4	20
N-butyl	17.5	16.9	2.8	17.5	14	20
Iso-butyl	....	....	....	12.5	10	25
N-amyl	40	30	33.3	40	30	33.3
Iso-amyl	35	26.9	22.8	30	25	16.6
N-hexyl	120	31	74	90	40	55.5
Iso-hexyl	110	24.8	77	50	25	50
N-heptyl	280	28.9	89	100	—36	100
N-octyl	300	—36	100	110	—36	100
N-nonyl	20	—36	100	—36	—36	
N-decyl	—36	Not tested		—36	—36	
N-undecyl	—36	Not tested		Not tested		
N-dodecyl	—36	Not tested		Not tested		
N-tridecyl	—36	Not tested		Not tested		
Meristyl	—36	Not tested		Not tested		
ACYL SERIES						
Propylyl	Not tested	Not tested		Not tested		
N-butyryl	10	5.2	48	Not tested		
Iso-butyryl	2.7	1.4	48	Not tested		
N-amylyl	25	12.9	48	Not tested		
Iso-amylyl	2.5	1.2	52	Not tested		
N-hexylyl	60	—36	100	Not tested		
Iso-hexylyl	Not tested			Not tested		
N-heptylyl	Not tested			Not tested		
N-octylyl	Not tested			Not tested		
N-decylyl	Not tested			Not tested		
N-undecylyl	Not tested			Not tested		
N-dodecylyl	Not tested			Not tested		
N-tridecylyl	Not tested			Not tested		
Phenol	1:200 dilution kills	1:200 dilution kills	0	1:200 dilution kills	1:200 dilution kills	0

A 3% gelatin-peptone mixture consists of a suspension of sticky material the larger particles of which may settle to the bottom of the seeding tube on standing. In this particular type of experiment, phenol is not diminished in bactericidal activity at 37 C. The alkyl and acyl resorcinols, however, become progressively less active with each ascending compound of the two series. Beyond n-hexyl and n-hexylyl, the derivatives show complete loss of bactericidal power. When a more complex material was used, such as 10% normal horse serum, the same general results were manifested, despite the fact that the material affords a more homogeneous and uniform suspension. As has been pointed out previously, one of the most outstanding characteristics of this series of compounds is their ability to lower surface tension. Because of this property, it is possible that there may be a rapid adsorption of the chemical substances to the particles of organic material present, thus leaving a diminished quantity free in solution to accomplish the disinfection.

EFFECT OF ALKALI ON THE BACTERICIDAL POWER OF THE ALKYL RESORCINOLS

In carrying out the details of the phenol coefficient technic it was observed that the addition of the broth culture to dilutions of n-heptyl resorcinol and the succeeding higher alkyl derivatives produced a distinct opalescence. The longer and heavier the alkyl chain, the more noticeable was this characteristic. These compounds are all readily soluble in alkali. It was thought, therefore, that the addition of alkali would dissolve the turbidity, since it was assumed that the substances had been partially thrown out of the solution. This was found to be the case. At the same time dilutions of n-octyl resorcinol, which were ordinarily inert, could be rendered toxic to bacteria by the addition of .2 cc. N 40/KOH, an amount of alkali itself inactive as a germicide. With the higher alkyl resorcinols, however, the amount of KOH necessary to dispel the opalescence formed was found to be slightly toxic for Bacillus typhosus. Various other alkalies were then tried and .2 cc. of 1% sodium carbonate was found suitable. This amount of sodium carbonate in dilutions of phenol did not enhance its germicidal properties.

The result of the addition of alkali on the germicidal activity of the compounds was tested by observing its effect in aqueous solutions and in the presence of the standard organic mixture. In aqueous solution, the technic used was the same as that employed in determining the phenol coefficients at 37 C. except for the addition of .2 cc. of 1% sodium carbonate to each seeding tube. Phenol to which the same amount of alkali had been added was used as a control. In determining the effect of the alkali in the presence of organic material, certain changes in making up the test dilutions were necessary. One cc. of the organic mixture was made neutral to phenolphthalein. An excess of .4 cc. of the alkali was then added. This same amount of alkali in phenol dilutions in organic material showed no effect on the resistance of the bacteria.

In making up the test dilutions the following scheme was used:

Dilution of Chemical	1% Na_2CO_3	Organic Material	Final Solution
3.2 cc.	0.8 cc.	1 cc.	5 cc.

As can be seen, it became necessary to make the original solution of the compound $\frac{3.2}{5}$ stronger than the desired final dilution. Since the higher alkyl derivatives of resorcinol are extremely insoluble, homogeneous emulsions of decyl and undecyl resorcinol cannot be made up in concentrations of less than 1 : 7000. Although they showed bactericidal activity in water with the addition of alkali, their efficiency in the presence of organic material cannot be measured by means of this technic. Under these circumstances, it is hardly justifiable to record their bactericidal power in comparison with phenol as less than 1 for the reason that they are probably potentially active.

Results and Discussion.—The precise effect of alkali on the bactericidal power of the various alkyl derivatives of resorcinol is not easily

TABLE 4.—EFFECT OF ADDITION OF ALKALI ON PHENOL COEFFICIENTS OF ALKYL RESORCINOLS AT 37 C.

Compound	Dilution in H_2O : Phenol Coefficient	Dilution in H_2O + Alkali : Phenol Coefficient	Dilution in 3% Organic Material : Phenol Coefficient	Dilution in 3% Organic Material + Alkali Phenol Coefficient
Propyl	5	4.5	4	4.5
N-butyl	17.5	14	14	17.5
Iso-butyl	12.5	7.5	10	12.5
N-amyl	40	20 to 25	30	40
Iso-amyl	30	20	25	30
N-hexyl	90	60	40	60 to 70
Iso-hexyl	50	50	25	35
N-heptyl	100	175	—36	90
N-octyl	110	350	—36	140
N-nonyl	—36	450	Not tested	25
N-decyl	—36	200	Not tested	—36
N-undecyl	—36	30	Not tested	—36
N-dodecyl	Not tested	—36	Not tested	—36
N-tridecyl	Not tested	Not tested	Not tested	—36
Meristyl	Not tested	Not tested	Not tested	—36

explained. In aqueous solutions, homologues below n-heptyl resorcinol suffer distinct diminution in bactericidal activity, while the peak of the germicidal efficiency of the series is extended to nonyl resorcinol, whose phenol coefficient was estimated at 450. Decyl and undecyl resorcinol, which had been entirely inert in previous experiments, become active. In 1913 Cooper [16] had observed that the germicidal power of phenol was decreased when there was a small amount of sodium hydroxide present. This was explained on the theory that the alkali formed salts with phenol, which became partly hydrolysed in solution. With the addition of sodium carbonate, however, phenol shows no change in microbicidal activity. With the lower resorcinols, which are phenolic substances possessing two hydroxyl groups instead of one as in phenol, it is probable

16. Biochem. J., 1913, 7, p. 175.

that a di-sodium salt is formed which is less active as a germicide than the original compound.

With the compounds above n-hexyl resorcinol, the effect of the addition of the alkali is entirely different. The compounds are markedly increased in their bactericidal activity. Here again, the question of water solubility and the reduction of surface tension may enter. The opalescence observed upon the addition of the broth culture to solutions of these higher derivatives may be due to an adsorption or association between the molecules of peptone and those of the chemical substances, and the addition of the alkali may be supposed to have a two-fold effect.

TABLE 5.—BACTERICIDAL AND NONBACTERICIDAL DILUTIONS OF SIX ALKYL RESORCINOLS FOR SIX TEST ORGANISMS AT 37 C.

Phenol used as a standard of comparison

Compound	Dilutions	Bacillus aerogenes		Bacillus coli		Bacillus typhosus		Bacillus dysenteriae (Shiga)		Staphylococcus albus		Bacillus xerosis
	Exposure Hours	1	24	1	24	1	24	1	24	1	24	1
Propyl	Bactericidal....	1000	1100	1000	1700	1000	2000	1400	2400	1000	2000	1200
	Nonbactericidal	1300	2000	1200	2200	1600	2600	2000	3600	1300	2400	....
Butyl	Bactericidal....	3000	4000	2500	5000	2500	5000	3500	5000	2500	5000	2500
	Nonbactericidal	4000	5000	3000	10000	3000	9000	6000	8500	3500	9000	....
Amyl	Bactericidal....	6000	7000	6000	15000	6000	12000	8000	12000	5000	12000	6000
	Nonbactericidal	8000	14000	8000	20000	8000	17000	11000	18000	7000	18000	....
Hexyl	Bactericidal....	8000	15000	9000	14000	9000	17000	12000	15000	20000	38000	20000
	Nonbactericidal	13000	22000	14000	28000	20000	27000	21000	26000	34000	60000	....
Heptyl	Bactericidal....	10000	18000	14000	20000	15000	32000	18000	21000	30000	52000	35000
	Nonbactericidal	15000	25000	22000	46000	28000	52000	26000	28000	50000	85000	....
Octyl	Bactericidal....	20000	36000	22000	36000	22000	40000	35000	48000	100000	200000	80000
	Nonbactericidal	25000	50000	32000	56000	30000	60000	45000	58000	130000	290000	....
Phenol	Bactericidal....	225	475	175	350	175	400	300	600	175	600	150
	Nonbactericidal	250	525	200	400	200	450	325	625	250	800	....

It may increase the water solubility to such an extent that more of the compound is actually in solution and therefore in a condition to permeate the bacterial cells. At the same time it may also decrease the extent of the adsorption or association between the peptone and the resorcinol derivative.

In the presence of organic material with alkali a general enhancement of each member of the series occurs. The percentage increase in effectiveness becomes greater after n-hexyl resorcinol is reached. N-heptyl and n-octyl resorcinol, which had been previously recorded as ineffective, become far more active. N-octyl resorcinol occupies the peak of power under these conditions with a bactericidal activity 140 times that of phenol. Nonyl resorcinol is also effective. Unfortunately the other members of the series could not be tested owing to their insolubility.

BACTERICIDAL ACTION OF THE ALKYL RESORCINOLS AGAINST CERTAIN ORGANISMS IN VITRO

In the original work reported by Leonard[17] on the secretion of bactericidal urine following the oral administration of n-hexyl resorcinol it was demonstrated that in vitro Staphylococcus albus is killed by this compound at a decidedly higher dilution than Bacillus coli both in water and in human urine. This drug was also found to exhibit in general a greater clinical efficiency in clearing up cases of pyelitis and cystitis caused by Staphylococcus albus, Staphylococcus aureus and Streptococcus anhemolyticus than those of Bacillus coli origin. Since in most instances of urinary infection where Bacillus coli is the causative agent, the organism is found to be present in large numbers, the factor of mass action was considered responsible to a great extent for lengthening the time necessary to complete disinfection.

The bactericidal activity of the resorcinol derivatives, other than the n-hexyl and n-heptyl compounds, has not been tested up to the present time except against Bacillus typhosus. Experiments were, therefore, undertaken to determine the bactericidal strength of certain of the alkyl resorcinols against six different organisms to ascertain whether any one compound might manifest a selective action against a certain type of organisms.

Method.—The organisms used were Bacillus typhosus (Hopkins strain), Bacillus coli from urinary infection, Bacillus lactis-aerogenes, Bacillus dysenteriae (Shiga), Staphylococcus albus from urinary infection and Bacillus xerosis from normal eye. The bacteria were grown in plain broth consisting of 1% Difco peptone, 0.5% NaCl and 0.3% Liebig beef extract, tubed 10 cc. to each tube with a P_H value between 6.6 and 6.8 after sterilization. Daily transfers of one standard loopful were made for five days prior to use to insure an active and uniform rate of growth. For the tests each day a 24 hour filtered culture was diluted in such a manner that 0.1 cc. contained between 10 and 12 million organisms. Controls were run to insure the addition of the correct number of bacteria. Plain agar was used for plates to determine the viability of all strains of bacteria except Bacillus xerosis. For this organism infusion agar was used. Stock solutions of the chemical compounds were made in sterile distilled water, and the dilutions of each compound made from these. Dilutions of the compounds were tested in 5 cc. portions to which was added 0.1 cc. of the bacterial culture. After an

17. J. Am. M. A., 1924, 83, p. 2005.

exposure at 37 C. for one hour and 24 hours respectively 0.1 cc. was transferred to a petri plate, and the agar previously cooled to 42 C. was poured over it.

Results and Discussion.—There are two dilutions of each compound recorded in table 5. One is termed the bactericidal dilution; the other the nonbactericidal dilution. The former indicated the dilution of the compound including and below which the bacteria are always killed. The nonbactericidal dilution is that dilution above which the organisms are never destroyed. As can be noted, this difference between the two dilutions ranges from 300 to 30,000. This has been designated as the zone of variability.

The data accumulated in this phase of the study bring out several significant facts concerning the alkyl derivatives of resorcinol. The first is a recognized specificity of n-hexyl, n-heptyl and n-octyl resorcinol for the disinfection of Gram positive organisms in vitro at 37 C. Coincidently, evidence is presented which lends further support to our hypthesis that there is a difference between the configuration of the alkyl chains of the lower and higher members of this series of phenolic substances. A second consideration has to do with the extended information concerning the zone in which fluctuations in bactercidal activity are manifested.

The selective microbicidal action of the higher alkyl resorcinols at 37 C. against gram-positive organisms is graphically represented in chart 1. In the chart two compositive curves were drawn. One represents the data obtained with three gram-negative bacteria, Bacillus lactis-aerogenes, Bacillus coli, and Bacillus typhosus; the other, with two species retaining Gram's stain, Staphylococcus albus and Bacillus xerosis. As is indicated, the lower derivatives, n-propyl, n-butyl and n-amyl resorcinol, possess practically the same disinfecting power against these five organisms. On the other hand, the higher derivatives, n-hexyl, n-heptyl and n-octyl resorcinol, show a bactericidal effectiveness from three to five times greater against Staphylococcus albus and Bacillus xerosis than the three gram-negative bacilli.

Bacillus dysenteriae (Shiga) although a gram-negative organism, is shown to be more highly sensitive to the action of the compounds than the other Gram negative bacilli. This sensitivity, however, is by no means so marked with the higher derivatives when compared with the results obtained against Staphylococcus albus and Bacillus xerosis.

The question of the variability in microbicidal potency of the high dilutions of the alkyl resorcinols has for some time been very perplexing.

As has been stated, this was first observed in determining phenol coefficients at 20 C. The same difficulty was encountered when the phenol coefficient tests were done at 37 C. Elevating the temperature, therefore, does not seem to mitigate the condition. In this study, the zone of variability is even more clearly demonstrated. The lower homologues show a comparatively small degree of variability, though, in comparison with phenol, the characteristic is decidedly pronounced. N-hexyl resorcinol and the two following derivatives, however, exhibit a wide zone in which the disinfection property of the dilutions cannot be accurately established. In other words, dilutions within this zone may or may not destroy the bacteria with which they come in contact. This variability is just as extensive if not more so, after 24 hours of exposure as after one hour. It is also pronounced regardless of the type of bacteria used, and it appears to be wider against the less resistant organisms. No explanation for this can be offered at the present time, but the conclusion may be drawn that this characteristic is neither corrected nor controlled by elevation of temperature, increased length of exposure, or a combination of the two.

SUMMARY

The bactericidal properties of the alkyl resorcinols and their intermediate ketones have been studied in detail. The higher alkyl derivatives of resorcinol in comparison with phenol are less effective as bactericides against Bacillus typhosus grown in Witte peptone broth than against the same organism grown in Difco peptone broth. In the presence of organic material at 37 C. the alkyl resorcinols progressively lose a portion of their bactericidal activity. Beginning with n-butyl resorcinol, the percentage of inhibitory effect increases until at n-heptyl and n-octyl resorcinol there is a total loss of disinfecting power. An elevation of temperature from 20 C. to 37 C. increases the bactericidal properties of each member of the alkyl series from the n-propyl to the n-octyl derivative. A further elevation from 37 C. to 45 C. renders nonyl and decyl resorcinol also potent as bactericides in aqueous solution.

Because of the increased solubility of the alkyl resorcinols in alkali, the addition of 1% Na_2Co_3 to these compounds causes a pronounced rise in microbicidal action beyond the hexyl derivative both in the presence and in the absence of organic material. The disinfecting properties of the alkyl resorcinols in vitro depend to a great extent upon their water solubility.

Each member of the acyl series of derivatives of resorcinol is increased in bactericidal power by an elevation of temperature from 20 C. to 37 C. from the n-butyryl to the n-hexylyl compound. These derivatives are practically ineffective as bactericides at 37 C. in a standard organic mixture.

N-hexyl, n-heptyl and n-octyl resorcinol appear to possess a specificity in disinfection action against the vegetative forms of gram-positive organisms in vitro at 37 C.

In high dilutions of the compound, the alkyl resorcinols show a wide zone in which their toxicity to bacteria is fluctuating and uncertain. This zone is progressively increased as the alkyl chain is extended.

NOTE.—Since the completion of this investigation, Schaeffer and Tilley[18] have reported phenol coefficients for the normal alkyl resorcinols and their intermediate ketones. The general results showing the marked increase in the germicidal efficiency of the heavier resorcinols at higher temperatures and their selective action for Micrococcus aureus (Staphylococcus aureus) are in accord with results indicated in this paper.

18. J. Bact., 1927, 14, p. 259.

THE NATURE OF DIPHTHERIA TOXIN

Arthur Locke and E. R. Main

From the Henry Baird Favill Laboratory of St. Luke's Hospital, Chicago

This is a report of our investigations into the physiochemical nature of diphtheria toxin.

I

The first section is a study of the conditions which favor the production of toxin in cultures of the diphtheria bacillus and was undertaken with the object of inquiring into the mechanism by which the toxin is produced. The plan of presentation is: a brief summary of the work which has been done relevant to the conditions which favor the production of toxin in cultures of toxicogenic organisms; a record of the writers' efforts to arrive at a more precise knowledge of these conditions; and finally a discussion of the various hypotheses which have been advanced relative to the nature and origin of the toxin principle.

The majority of the published investigations into the optimum conditions for toxin production have been concerned with the practical problem of preparing high titer diphtheria toxin in a simple, reproducible, and economical fashion. They have covered, from the bacteriological angle: variations in the toxicogenicity of different strains of the diphtheria bacillus [1] variations in the toxicogenicity of the generally used Park 8 strain in different laboratories, during different seasons, and upon different mediums,[2] and variations in morphologic character paralleling variations in toxicogenicity.[3] Little of this work has been undertaken in a sufficiently critical way to yield conclusions as to the mechanism of toxin production.

From the chemical angle, investigations have been reported covering: the character of the meat used for the preparation of the infusion, its content of fats and substances capable of producing surface-tension lowering soaps,[4] its age, the effect of storage, etc. (Davis [1]); the elution procedure used in making the infusion, the temperature, P_H, and mineral content of the water used, and the duration of the elution [5, 6] the physical character of the infusion extract, its viscosity [7] and salt content [5]; and the influence of sugar fermentation during the

Received for publication, Jan. 14, 1928.

1. (a) Park and Williams: J. Exper. Med., 1896, 1, p. 164; (b) Hartley and Hartley: J. Path. and Bact., 1922, 25, pp. 458, 462, 479; (c) Davis: J. Bact., 1920, 5, p. 477.
2. Schmidt, M. S.: Ann. de l'Inst. Pasteur, 1925, 39, p. 875; MacConkey: J. Hyg., 1912, 12, p. 507.
3. Heinemann: J. Bact., 1917, 2, p. 361; Crowell: J. Bact., 1926, 11, p. 65; Cowan: Brit. J. Exper. Path., 1927, 8, p. 6.
4. Larson: Proc. Soc. Exper. Biol. & Med., 1921, 19, p. 62.
5. Walbum: Abderhalden Handb. d. biol. Arbeitsmethoden, 1925, 13 (2), p. 595.
6. Dean: Bacteriology of Diphtheria, 1908.
7. Godoy: Compt. rend Soc. de Biol., 1926, 95, p. 998.

elution procedure,[1b, 8, 9] It seems probable that the chief function of the meat infusion is to supply the inorganic requirements for bacterial growth.[10]

The influence of the type of peptone used has been examined in mediums of the auto-digest or Martin type,[11] the trypsin digest or Douglas type,[1b, 12] and in mediums prepared from peptones representing protein-split products in varying stages of hydrolysis.[1b, 1c, 13] The necessity for the presence of the so-called proteoses has been established. The value of the presence of the various inorganic and organic accessory substances whose addition has been recommended[5, 7, 14] is not established.

The influence of the initial P_H of the broth medium on toxin production has been studied exhaustively,[1b, 13] but very little more has been discovered than was reported by Park and Williams in 1896.[1] The optimum initial P_H would seem to depend in part on the composition of the medium.[15] It is generally near P_H 7.8. No toxin appears to be produced after the alkalinity exceeds P_H 8.1 to 8.3. The variations in P_H accompanying autoclaving, particularly when large amounts of bicarbonate are present in the broth, accompanying growth, and accompanying aeration, have also been studied.[16]

The manner of sterilization of the medium before inoculation has proved to be important. When dried, already partly-denatured proteoses have been used for the medium, the effect of a careful, minimum autoclaving at P_H 7.8 has been negligible, but when fresh, nascent proteoses of the Douglas medium type have been used, although considerably more toxin has been produced, it has been necessary to autoclave at P_H 4.0 or to sterilize the medium by Seitz filtration.[1b, 1c, 17]

It has been recommended that 0.1 per cent of sterile dextrose be added to the broth[8] that the temperature of incubation be 35 C.,[5] that inoculation be made with a single loopful of an 18-hour culture already habituated to the broth medium, and that ordinary Erlenmeyer flasks, loosely plugged with cotton,[17] be used as containers. The cultures should be protected from strong illumination or undue agitation.[18]

Our own studies of the conditions favoring toxin production are summarized in table 1 and in figures 1 to 6. The curves in figure 1 represent the toxin production of a Park 8 strain of the diphtheria bacillus: (I) on peptone-meat infusion medium; (II) on proteose peptone medium; (III) on the proteose peptone medium after enrichment with dextrose, and (IV) on the dextrose enriched medium after a second addition of dextrose during the period of maximum growth. The mediums were prepared as follows.

8. Smith, Th.: J. Exper. Med., 1899, 4, p. 373.
9. Spronck and van Furenhout: Ann. de l'Inst. Pasteur, 1895, 9, p. 758.
10. Wheeler: Am. J. Path., 1927, 3, p. 540.
11. Martin: Ann. de l'Inst. Pasteur, 1898, 12, p. 26.
12. Douglas: Lancet, 1914, 2, p. 891.
13. Bunker: J. Bact., 1919, 4, p. 379.
14. Robinson and Meader: J. Infect. Dis., 1920, 27, p. 106; Calcaterra: Centralbl. f. Bakt., O., 1911, 60, p. 15; Davis and Ferry: J. Bact., 1919, 4, p. 217.
15. Abt. and Loiseau: Ann. de l'Inst. Pasteur, 1922, 36, p. 535.
16. Plastridge and Rettger: Proc. Soc. Exper. Biol. & Med., 1927, 24, p. 752; Dernby and David: J. Path. & Bact., 1921, 24, p. 150.
17. Watson and Langstaff: J. Path. & Bact., 1927, 30, p. 383.
18. Roux and Yersin: Ann. de l'Inst. Pasteur, 1888, 2, p. 629; 1889, 3, p. 273.

An 8 per cent suspension of "Bacto-veal" was warmed for one hour at 38 C., with continuous stirring. Eighteen hours later, the suspension was warmed at 80 C. for 5 minutes, again with stirring, and filtered warm through a Buchner suction filter. The clear filtrate was then enriched with 2 per cent of the peptone

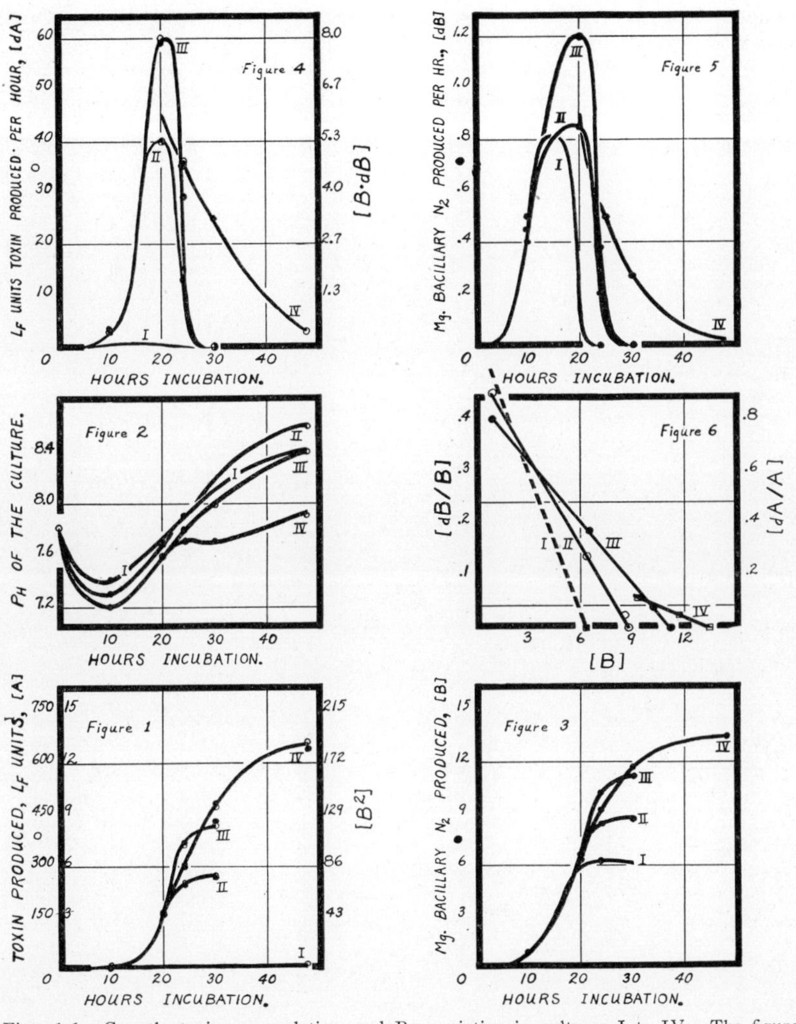

Figs. 1-6.—Growth, toxin accumulation, and PH variation in cultures I to IV. The figures are explained in the text.

and 0.5 per cent of salt, cooled to 5 C. adjusted to PH 7.8 to 8.0 with N/1 NaOH, boiled for 5 minutes, and filtered repeatedly through a good paper until brilliantly clear. After readjustment of the PH, if this became necessary, the filtrate was dispensed in 50 cc. quantities in 250 cc. Pyrex, Erlenmeyer flasks and autoclaved for 30 min. at 10 lbs. steam pressure. A slight precipitate separated which was almost entirely redissolved upon standing for 18 hrs. at 35 C. in a dark, vibration-free incubator. After this interval, 0.1 per cent dextrose was added to the flasks in series III and IV, and all of the flasks were inoculated

Table 1.—Accumulation of Toxin, Bacillary Nitrogen and Filtrable, Acid-Precipitable Nitrogen in Cultures I-Iv

Medium	Hours Incubation	PH ±0.1	Toxin Produced, Lf Units: Observed Value In Toto (50 cc.)	Toxin Produced, Lf Units: Selected Value In Toto (A)	Toxin Produced, Lf Units: Selected Value Per Hour (dA)	Bacillary N_2 Produced, Mg.: Observed Value In Toto (50 cc.)	Bacillary N_2 Produced, Mg.: Selected Value In Toto (B)	Bacillary N_2 Produced, Mg.: Selected Value Per Hour (dB)	Precipitable N_2 Mg. In Toto
I, (peptone without sugar)	10	7.4				1.0	1.0	....	0.12
	10	7.4				1.3			0.12
	24	7.9				6.3	6.3	0	0.43
	24	7.8				6.4			0.42
	48	8.4	10	10	0	6.1	5.8	0	0.37
	48	8.4				5.5			0.45
II, (proteose without sugar)	10	7.3	10	10	2.8	0.8	1.0	0.45	0–0.02
	10	7.3				1.0			....
	20	7.7	165	165	40	5.7	6.3	0.85	....
	20	7.7	165			6.7			0.23
	24	7.9	250	250	13	8.5	8.5	0.20	0.35
	24	7.9	200			7.7			....
	30	8.2	275	275	0	8.4	8.7	....	0.46
	30	8.2	275			8.7			0.49
	48	8.5	275	275	0	...	...	0	0.8
	48	8.6	275			...			0.7
III, (proteose with sugar addition at 0 hours)	10	7.2	8	8	2.8	0.9	1.0	0.40	....
	10	7.2				1.2			0–0.02
	20	7.6	165	165	60	6.3	6.5	1.20	0.20
	20	7.6	165			7.1			0.17
	24	7.8	360	360	29	10.6	10.2	0.38	0.40
	24	7.8	360			10.0			0.40
	30	8.0	385	415	$\neq 0$	11.2	11.2	....	0.40
	30	7.9	415			12.1			0.38
	48	8.3	415	415	0	....	....	0	0.55
	48	8.4	415			....			0.60
IV, (proteose with sugar additions at 0 and 20 hours)	24	7.7	305	305	36	10.6	9.2	0.50	0.39
	24	7.7	305			9.1			0.41
	30	7.7	470	470	25	12.0	11.7	0.27	0.66
	30	7.7	415			11.5			0.48
	48	7.8	660	660	3	13.1	13.5	....	0.6
	48	8.0	715			13.5			0.7
	72	8.3	715	715	0	....	....	0	0.7
	72	8.2	770			....			0.7

with one loopful of an 18-hour culture of a Park 8 strain of diphtheria bacilli which had been subcultured daily, for several weeks, on bouillon of the same composition. Twenty hours later, a second 0.1 per cent of dextrose was added to the flasks of series IV, using care in mixing the contents of the flasks, after the addition, that the thin, friable membrane at the liquid surface was not disintegrated.

Two flasks were withdrawn from each series, after the incubation intervals recorded in table 1, and placed in the refrigerator for 48 hrs., after the addition of 0.5 per cent phenol. The contents of the flasks were then centrifugated, the sediments of killed diphtheria bacilli washed, partially resuspended in N/10 NaOH, and their nitrogen equivalents determined. Some of the sediments were rejected because of persistent inclusions of crystals containing ammonia. The brilliantly clear, bacteria-free supernatants were used for the determination of P_H, Lf unitage,[19] and the amount of nitrogenous substances precipitable at P_H 3.8.

The outer left hand ordinates in figure 1 represent the total amounts of toxin present in the cultures, and the inside left hand ordinates the amounts of toxin present per cc. The abscissae denote the duration of the incubation intervals. It may be seen that in the absence of proteose, a total of approximately 10 Lf units was produced; in the presence of unenriched proteose, 275 units were produced; after one enrichment with dextrose, 415 units; and after two enrichments with dextrose, 710 units.

The rate of toxin accumulation upon the different mediums is described in figure 4. The ordinates represent the amount of toxin produced per hour and the abscissae the duration of incubation. The values are derived from figure 1 and the relations expressed are, therefore, the same. Toxin was accumulated most rapidly and for the longest time on the sugar-enriched, proteose-containing mediums.

Figure 2 describes the variation in P_H of the different mediums, during the growth period. The P_H values are recorded along the vertical axis. They were little influenced by the presence of proteose, slightly depressed by one sugar addition, and considerably depressed by two additions of sugar. No toxin was accumulated in any of the cultures at a P_H exceeding 8.0 to 8.1, and the greatest amount of toxin was accumulated in those cultures where the alkalinity had been maintained for the longest time at a P_H below this limiting value, by virtue of the sugar additions.*

The amounts of filtrable bacillary substance present in the different cultures could not be determined with sufficient accuracy to permit graphic representation. The approximate values are recorded in column 10 of table 1 and were found to parallel, roughly, the amounts of toxin present.

19. Locke, Main and Miller: J. Infect. Dis., 1927, 41, p. 32.

* We wish to suggest that the second sugar addition is of practical value in the routine production of diphtheria toxin for immunization purposes, since it increases the toxin yield, on this type of medium, by 50%. The optimum time for the second sugar addition is during the interval between the time of minimum P_H and the time when the P_H again reaches 7.8.

The first quantitative studies of bacterial growth were made by Buchner, Longard and Riedlin,[20] who introduced the use of the formula:

$$b = a.2^n \ldots\ldots\ldots\ldots (1)$$

This formula describes a condition of logarithmic increase where a and b represent the bacterial populations at the beginning and end of an interval of observation t, and where the exponent n represents the number of times which the population has doubled during that interval. Since the population can double only by a process of growth and cell division, n may be construed as the average number of individual cell divisions and the quotient t/n taken to represent the average generation time or interval between successive cell divisions.

Each individual organism in a given bacterial culture does not grow and divide at a uniform rate, however. The law of probability requires that the growth energy of the culture be so distributed that some of the organisms grow very rapidly and some very slowly, while the remainder grow at varying intermediate rates. This point is so vital for the proper interpretation of growth studies that we have presented, in figure 7, a pattern analysis of a typical bacterial growth curve drawn from the data reported in table 1 of Chesney's classic study of the population changes in a broth culture of type 2 pneumococcus.[21] These data are incorporated in curve IV, which presents the population changes B during the incubation periods T, as recorded upon the respective vertical and horizontal axes. Curve III presents the number of organisms dB produced per hour as indicated by the contour of curve IV. Curve II records the variation in the average number of organisms dB/B produced per hour per organism and describes the growth activity of the culture. The growth activity appeared to reach its maximum during the fifth hour of incubation, while the population of the culture was still comparatively small, and decreased progressively to a value of zero as the population increased to its maximum. This is shown more clearly in curve I where the growth dB/B per organism per hour is plotted directly, as ordinates, against the population B as abscissae. The remarkable linearity of this curve indicates that growth activity is quantitatively inhibited by population increase according to the relation:

$$dB/B = k(B_{max} - B) = k'(1 - B/B_{max}) \ldots\ldots\ldots\ldots (2)$$

in which k and k′ are proportionality constants and B_{max} the population of the culture at saturation. k′ may represent the maximum average rate at which the organism is capable of growing upon the particular medium employed.

A progressively falling growth rate implies, not that each individual bacillus grows and divides more and more slowly, but that the fraction of the total bacterial population which can grow rapidly becomes progressively smaller and that the fraction which is forced to grow slowly becomes progressively larger.

Let $B - B^2/B_{max}$, from equation (2), represent the proportion of the population growing at the average rate k′. Since k′ represents the maximum average growth rate possible on the given medium, the fraction B^2/B_{max} would, therefore, be growing at a rate approaching zero. Let this latter fraction be B′. Then:

$$B' = B^2/B_{max};\ B'/B = B/B_{max};\ \text{and:}$$

$$dB'/B' = d(B^2/B_{max})/(B^2/B_{max}) = 2dB/B \ldots\ldots\ldots\ldots (3)$$

In other words, the hardly growing fraction B′ increases in concentration, by virtue of the falling growth rate, twice as rapidly as the total bacterial population B

20. Buchner, Longard and Riedlin: Centralbl. f. Bakteriol., 1, O., 1887, 2, p. 1.
21. Chesney: J. Exper. Med., 1916, 24, p. 387.

increases, and bears the proportion to the total population that the total population bears to the population at the growth saturation limit.

Upon this interpretation, growth inhibition is not continuously distributed over the total population but is discontinuously distributed, almost completely inhibiting the growth of the part affected and scarcely affecting the remainder. The phenomenon of lag becomes due simply to the fact that an inoculum of old culture contains a much smaller concentration of growing cells than has been appreciated, the formula $b=a.2^n$, where b and a represent total concentrations of viable, growing and nongrowing cells being inapplicable and the calculated generation times erroneous. The lag phenomenon is not manifested when young, maximally growing cultures are inoculated.[22]

Figure 3 gives the bacillary population of cultures I-IV, in terms of nitrogen equivalents, after the incubation periods recorded along the horizontal axis. It may be noted that the mediums which favored the largest accumulations of toxin likewise favored the largest accumulations of bacilli.

The rate of increase in the bacillary population is presented in figure 5. The rates are seen to have maxima for the sugar-containing, proteose mediums and to diminish to zero as the P_H of the cultures approaches 8.0 to 8.1.

The average rate of growth of the individual bacilli in the different cultures is indicated in figure 6. The curves here are not entirely satisfactory but are essentially correct and demonstrate that the amount of growth per bacillus has diminished progressively as the cultures have approached their growth saturation limits, according to the mathematical relation already discussed. It is interesting that the growth rates had their smallest values for the mediums which supported the largest bacillary populations and permitted the accumulation of the most toxin. Bacillary growth was most rapid upon the simple peptone medium but was unable to persist so long as upon the proteose, sugar-containing mediums.

An effort to correlate the toxin accumulation curves described in figure 1 with the bacillary population curves described in figure 3 was, unexpectedly, entirely successful.* It was found that the toxin concentration had been continuously proportional to the square of the bacillary population and had increased, therefore, twice as rapidly as the bacilli.

The squares of the bacillary population, B, in terms of nitrogen equivalents, are plotted along the right hand margin of figure 1 and it

22. Penfold: J. Hyg., 1914, 14, p. 215.

* A rough interdependence between toxin concentration and bacillary population and between toxin concentration and the concentration of filtrable, acid-precipitable nitrogenous substance has already been reported by Watson and Wallace.[23]

23. Watson and Wallace: J. Path. & Bacteriol., 1924, 27, p. 289.

may be noted that the points obtained were so nearly identical with the points describing the toxin concentration, A, that a single curve was drawn for both. That is:

$$A \propto B^2;\ dA \propto 2B.dB;\ \text{and: } dA/A = 2dB/B \qquad (4)$$

These relations are confirmed in figures 4 and 6. They indicate, since dA and dB necessarily decrease to zero simultaneously, that toxin accumulation stops when growth stops, and that toxin can be produced only by a living, growing bacillus.

It would seem that the concentration of hardly-growing but viable organisms, as given by equation (3), might be used, fairly, as an index of the amount of growth inhibition existing in the culture. It then becomes apparent that the toxin concentration in these cultures increased at the same rate as the growth inhibition, i. e.:

$$dA/A = 2dB/B = dB'/B' \qquad (5)$$

Growth inhibition increases with the square of the population regardless of the elaboration of toxin so that it cannot be concluded from relation (5) that the accumulated toxin is the source of the inhibition or that the inhibition is, in itself, the cause of toxin production. The possibility remains that the clash of growth momentum and growth inhibition may indirectly favor toxin production by accelerating a normal, minute rate of toxin secretion or, perhaps, by increasing the frequency with which the more fragile cells become exploded and dispersed into the culture medium.

The term accumulation has been used in place of production throughout this discussion because of the dynamic natures of the growth and toxin production equilibriums. It should be clear that bacilli and toxin have been continuously destroyed as well as created and that the persistence and accumulation of toxin in each culture has been largely determined by the stability of the toxin under the conditions of growth in that culture. The principal source of destruction lies in the lytic action of extracellular enzymes of the trypsin type.[24]

The quantity of toxin which can be destroyed by a given concentration of extracellular enzyme ought to be greatly reduced by the presence of other substances capable of binding the enzyme[25] and

24. Dernby and Walbum: Biochem. Ztschr., 1923, 138, p. 505.

25. For a discussion of the inhibitory action of high concentrations of protein disintegration products on the further proteolytic activity of pepsin and trypsin-like enzymes, see Northrop: J. Gen. Physiol., 1924, 6, p. 723; 1920, 2, p. 471; Peckelharing and Ringer: Ztschr. f. physiol. Chem., 1911, 75, p. 282.

diverting it from immediate action on the toxin principle. The proportion of proteose to filtrable bacillary protoplasm in mediums II-IV at the ten-hour incubation period was of the order of 100 to 1. Proteoses are avidly bound and disintegrated by enzymes of the trypsin type and it may be seen that in the proteose mediums the chance for survival of the toxin principle was considerably greater than in the simple peptone medium where the proteolytic enzymes were not so well diverted.

The essential condition for the cultivation of an organism from which an unstable, extracellular product is desired is, in our opinion, the presence of a suitable buffer for the extracellular enzyme activities of the culture.

Several theories have been proposed to account for the manner in which toxins are produced in cultures of toxicogenic organisms. The first, suggested by Roux and Yersin,[18] postulated the toxin to be a secretory product, possibly of an enzyme nature. This theory has been given an added interest by the recent work of Jensen and Falk.[26] They have quantitatively correlated toxicogenicity with electrophoretic mobility, not only for different strains of the diphtheria bacillus but for the same strain at different cultural stages and under different cultural conditions. The differences in mobility have been further correlated with differences in cell permeability, through the Donnan equilibrium relation, and the suggestion has been advanced that toxicogenicity is a function of the permeability of the cell wall. They postulate that increased permeability favors increased toxin secretion, but of course increased permeability may also mean increased thinness and fragility of the cell membrane, favoring the occurrence of an explosion mechanism, as has been discussed.

Equations 4-5 imply that the rate of toxin accumulation, dA, is not a function either of the total bacillary population B or of the respective growing and non-growing populations, B-B′ and B′. It is difficult, therefore, to regard toxin as a continuous secretion of a surviving organism. Moreover, the diphtheria bacillus has never been demonstrated to possess an appreciable secretory activity. Such enzymes as find their way into the culture medium appear to result from the disintegration of dead cells[27] rather than from the operation of a secretion mechanism. Diphtheria toxin does, of course, pass certain types of semipermeable membrane[28] and is excreted into the urine of rats and mice,[29] indicating that it may not be too large a molecule or aggregate to permit secretion. Arrhenius has computed that diphtheria toxin may be 100 times smaller in size than its antitoxin,[30] and that its molecular weight may be 15,000, a figure approximately half that usually assumed for the albumin molecule.[31]

Dernby and Walbum[24] have suggested that the toxin may be an intermediate split product of the action of extracellular enzymes on the proteoses. It is difficult to reconcile this hypothesis with the marked antigenic activity of the toxins. The

26. Jensen: Proc. Soc. f. Exper. Biol. and Med., 1926, 23, p. 783.
27. Dernby and Siwe: Biochem. Ztschr., 1922, 134, p. 1.
28. Glenny and Walpole: Biochem. J., 1915, 9, p. 298.
29. Pettit: Ann. de l'Inst. Pasteur, 1914, 28, p. 663.
30. Cited by Wells: Chemical Aspects of Immunity, 1925, p. 98.
31. Du Noüy: Surface Equilibria of Colloids, 1926, p. 106. The approximate size of antibody aggregates is discussed in ref. 57.

proteoses, much less their split products, are not good antigens.[32] Neither this theory nor the similar one of Vaughan[33] accounts satisfactorily for the specificity of the toxin nor for the fact that its isoelectric range is close to that exhibited by extracts of the diphtheria bacillus.[34]

The idea of the toxin as a filtrable form of the parent organism, presumably produced at the time of cell division, has recently been given new impetus by the finding and cultivation of a filtrable phase by Hauduroy.[35] Through some oversight, the investigator did not test the toxicity of the filtrable microphase and no confirmation of his original, preliminary report has been published.

Warden regards diphtheria toxin as being an emulsion of fats derived from the dead diphtheria bacillus, rendered stable and given particulate entity by the proteoses of the broth medium.[36] He does not regard the bacillary proteins as being an integral or necessary part of the toxin principle. Dernby and Walbum[24] have been unable to verify the results of the experiments upon which these conclusions are based.

The hypothesis that diphtheria toxin may be a disintegration or extraction product of the dead bacillus[37] is not only incompatible with the findings herein presented but has also been rendered improbable by the many failures to prepare highly toxic extracts from dead bacilli by artificial disintegration procedures.[1a] Dead, washed diphtheria bacilli are toxic for guinea-pigs but the toxicity per mg. of substance is not of the same order as that of diphtheria toxin and appears not to be neutralized by diphtheria antitoxin.[38]

However, Casper Nelson has succeeded in obtaining true toxin extracts of Cl. botulinum by means of a freezing and thawing procedure.[39] The toxin of this organism appears to be more stable than diphtheria toxin in that it is able to resist autolytic, gastric and intestinal digestion. Purified preparations of botulinus toxin resist a procedure of peptic digestion[39] which entirely destroys diphtheria toxin.[27]

II *

The physiochemical properties and reactions of diphtheria toxin may be examined more critically after the crude toxin filtrates, which are ordinarily less than 1% pure, have been concentrated and partially purified.

Diphtheria toxin was originally concentrated[18, 40] by saturation with ammonium sulfate; the resulting separation of toxin-containing substances rose to the

* A preliminary report of the findings described in this section was presented before the Chicago Pathological Society, May 9, 1927 (Arch. Path. & Lab. Med., 1927, 4, p. 660).

32. Fink: J. Infect. Dis., 1919, 25, p. 97.

33. Vaughan: J. Am. M. A., 1916, 67, p. 1559.

34. von Gröer: Biochem. Ztschr., 1923, 138, p. 13.

35. Hauduroy: Compt. rend. Acad. d. Sc., 1927, 184, p. 409. The virulence and toxicogenicity of diphtheria bacilli were at one time believed to be dependent on the presence of intracellular granules, cf. Megrail: J. Infect. Dis., 1922, 31, p. 393.

36. Warden, Connell and Holly: J. Bact., 1921, 6, p. 103.

37. Gamaleja: Compt. rend. Soc. de Biol., 1892, 44, p. 153. The physicochemical nature and structure of the living bacterial cell and the changes which accompany cellular death are discussed by: Gaidukow, "Dunkelfeldbeleuchtung and Ultramikroscopie in d. Biol. u. Med.," Jena, 1910; Bayliss: Proc. Roy. Soc., 1920, B91, p. 196; Clowes: Science, 1916, 43, p. 750; Seifriz: Am. J. Physiol., 1923, 66, p. 124.

38. Rist: Compt. rend. Soc. de Biol., 1903, 55, p. 978; Cruveilhier: ibid., 1909, 66, p. 1029.

39. Nelson: J. Infect. Dis., 1927, 41, p. 9.

40. Brieger and Frankel: Berl. klin. Wchnschr., 1890, p. 241; Wassermann and Proskauer: Deutsch. med. Wchnschr., 1891, p. 585; Brieger and Boer: Deutsch. med. Wchnschr., 1896, 22, p. 783.

surface, was collected, dried in vacuo, and redissolved in alkali as desired. Toxin is now usually concentrated by a method of acetic acid precipitation originally proposed by Glenny[28] for use with dialysed toxin and recently adapted for use with whole toxin by Watson.[23] The toxin is acidified to 1 or 2% with glacial acetic acid, in the cold; the resulting precipitate is collected by high speed centrifugation, washed with cold distilled water, and redissolved in alkali. The method has yielded preparations with a minimum nitrogen content of about 0.005 mg. per Lf unit.[34, 23, 41]

Acetic acid is an excellent reagent for the precipitation of diphtheria toxin, because the buffering effect of the sodium acetate progressively formed during the acid additions prevents the P_H of the mixture from greatly exceeding the optimum point, 3.8, even when the acid is added in great excess. We have preferred to use 0.035N HCl. The difficulty of obtaining an end-point with this stronger acid has been largely eliminated by recourse to a preliminary titration of the toxin to be precipitated, somewhat as follows:

One-half cc. of the toxin was measured into each of a series of micro test-tubes containing graded volumes of the acid precipitant (0.035N HCl). The contents of the tubes were mixed, left overnight in the refrigerator, and examined next morning for flocculation. The middle tube of the group in which good, complete flocculation had occurred was selected as the indicating tube and the amount of acid required to precipitate a given volume of the toxin calculated accordingly.

For concentration, the toxin was distributed among a sufficient number of 50 cc. glass centrifuge tubes, chilled below 5 C., and precipitated tube by tube with the required volume of chilled acid. After 18 to 24 hours in the refrigerator, the well-separated flocculent precipitates were collected by centrifugation, combined, and washed thoroughly with a minimum volume of cold distilled water. The washed sediment contained from 80 to 100% of the toxin and toxoid present in the original broth filtrate. It varied from a flesh tint to a dark olive in color, depending on the conditions of precipitation and the origin of the broth medium, was markedly cohesive, and dissolved readily in alkali. Its nitrogen content varied from 0.000,8 to 0.006 mg. per corrected Lf unit.

Preparations were also secured by a method of dialysis against 0.1N HCl. The electrodialysis apparatus of Locke and Hirsch[42] was used, excepting that no electrode potential was maintained, and chilled 0.1N HCl was circulated within the membranes in place of distilled water. The apparatus was kept surrounded by a cooling mixture and the toxin stirred continuously. The P_H of the toxin dropped rapidly, approaching 4.5 within 3.5 to 4.0 hours. Shortly after, on cessation of the stirring, a stratum of precipitated toxin substances was visible, creeping downward from the liquid surface. The dialysis was continued until no further change was evident, the suspension was held in the refrigerator overnight, and the precipitate collected and washed by high speed centrifugation as before. The supernatant remained cloudy and the precipitate was found to contain 30 to 50% of the toxin of the original broth filtrate associated with approximately 0.002 mg. of N_2 per corrected Lf unit. The preparations obtained in this way were lighter in color and more rapidly soluble than those obtained by the acid precipitation method.

The presence in diphtheria toxin preparations of precipitinogens derived from the death, disintegration and lysis of diphtheria bacilli

41. Watson and Langstaff Biochem. J., 1926, 20, p. 763; Moloney and Weld: Trans. Roy. Soc. Canada, 1925, 19V, p. 125.

42. Locke and Hirsch: J. Infect. Dis., 1924, 35, p. 519.

prior to filtration is generally recognized [43] and the separability of these precipitinogens from the true toxin principle has been demonstrated by the work of Moloney and Weld [44] and H. Schmidt.[45] The latter investigator mixed diphtheria toxin with an agglutinating serum prepared by immunizing rabbits against washed diphtheria bacilli, separated the resulting flocculent precipitate by centrifugation, and compared the toxicity of the supernatant with that of equally diluted, untreated toxin. No loss in toxicity could be detected in the supernatant and no toxin could be found in the washed voluminous precipitate.

The precipitinogen substances have an isoelectric range within that in which the toxin principle is precipitated from diphtheria toxin broth filtrates and are, therefore, mixed with the toxin in such precipitates. Indeed, the amount of precipitinogen in an ordinary preparation of concentrated toxin is so large that the Ramon flocculation titration method cannot be used, directly,* for the estimation of the amount of toxin present.

Diphtheria antitoxin serum, as ordinarily prepared, contains a considerable proportion of precipitins which produce general flocculation with concentrated toxin preparations with no maxima observable excepting in the tubes containing the largest amounts of serum, as is indicated in table 2. This table describes the flocculation titration of a concentrated toxin preparation before and after partial removal of its nontoxin precipitinogens. After separation of the precipitinogens, the true toxin-antitoxin flocculation became more apparent, whether the separation was accomplished by precipitation with specific precipitin serum or by means of an isoelectric separation procedure described below. The true toxin-antitoxin flocculation occurred more slowly and had a characteristic, well defined maximum indicating a concentration yield of about 80%. Neither of the procedures used for the removal of the precipitinogen reduced the toxicity of the preparations, as measured in MLD, again demonstrating the separability of the toxin and precipitinogen principles.

Table 3 illustrates the procedure used to obtain preparations of the toxin and precipitinogen principles for the purpose of comparing their physical and chemical properties.

43. Cf. Bacteriology of Diphtheria, 1908, p. 226.
44. Moloney and Weld: J. Path. & Bact., 1925, 28, p. 666.
45. Schmidt, H.: Ztschr. f. Immunitätsf. u. exper. Therap., 1926, 48, p. 217.

* The method can, however, be used with an accuracy of 80 ot 85% after the nontoxin precipitinogen content of the preparation is partially removed as described below. The corrected Lf unit, so obtained, would seem to be a better index of the actual toxin and toxoid content of the preparation than the L+, MLD, and MRD units, on account of the variable amount of denaturation inherent in the concentration process.

The antigenic entities were precipitated from toxin broth filtrate isoelectrically, as has been described, suspended in cold, distilled water, and partially redissolved by the addition of N/100 NaOH, using P_H 8.0 as the end point. The suspension was centrifugated until perfectly clear, decanted from an undissolved gelatinous residue, made isotonic, and finally brought just to the flocculation point by the careful addition of N/100 HCl. The precipitated substances flocculated and settled rapidly. They were collected by centrifugation and separated from the opalescent supernatant by decantation. Solution and reprecipitation was then

TABLE 2.—FLOCCULATION TITRATIONS OF A TYPICAL PREPARATION OF CONCENTRATED DIPHTHERIA TOXIN BEFORE AND AFTER PARTIAL REMOVAL OF THE NONTOXIN PRECIPITINOGEN CONTENT

	Apparent Lf Titer of the Undiluted Toxin Preparation							
	Before Treatment with Precipitin			After Treatment with Precipitin			MLD per cc., ±10%	
	200	400	600	80	160	320	Before	After
Solution of crude, unwashed precipitate...	F	FF	FFF	F	FF	F	3300	3300
Solution of the same precipitate after 3 extractions with water.	FF	tr	?	tr	FF	0	3300	....*

* Undetermined.

TABLE 3.—THE SEPARATION, ISOLATION AND PROPERTIES OF THE TOXIN AND PRECIPITINOGEN PRINCIPLES OF A TYPICAL DIPHTHERIA TOXIN BROTH FILTRATE

100 Lf units diphtheria toxin + 0.035N HCl to P_H 3.4 (broth filtrate)
N_2 per Lf unit, 0.44 mg.

Precipitate: 80 to 100 Lf units of toxin, precipitinogen, associated substances. N_2 per Lf unit, 0.0008–.006 mg.

Supernatant: 99% of the nitrogenous substances of the original mixture, rejected

Precipitate dissolved in alkali and fractionated by isoelectric reprecipitation

	P_H 5.0 to 5.2 toxin, associated substances, N_2 per Lf unit, 0.000,6 ± 2 mg. (colored)	P_H 4.6 to 5.0 precipitinogens, toxin, and associated substances (slightly colored)	P_H 4.0 to 4.6 precipitinogens, and associated substances (colorless)
Biuret	+	+	+
Millon	+	+	+
Xanthoproteic	+	+	+
Molisch	0	±	+
Carbohydrate	0	±	+

Alkaline solution diluted to 85% with alcohol and precipitated by slight acidification

Residue, 80% recovery of toxin principle. N_2 per Lf unit same

Supernatant, lipoid solvent extractives rejected

Repetitions of alcohol precipitation resulted in injury and destruction of the toxin principle

repeated until the flocculation supernatants no longer remained opalescent and gave no trace of precipitation on slight acidification. The supernatants were pooled and fractionated in a similar way. Three fractions were finally obtained: a toxin fraction, an intermediate fraction, and a precipitinogen fraction.

The precipitinogen-containing fractions represented approximately 50% of the total nitrogenous substances in the original, washed toxin precipitate. They were not completely free from toxin, nor was the toxin completely free from precipitinogen. The precipitinogen fractions flocculated voluminously with antitoxin serum before but not after precipitation with precipitin serum, excepting in high concentrations. The toxin fraction retained a measure of its capacity to flocculate with precipitin serum and flocculated very poorly with antitoxin. An appreciable amount of antitoxin was found only in the floccules formed from the toxin fraction,* indicating that the precipitinogen had no antitoxin binding power. The toxicity of the toxin fraction, per mg. of nitrogenous substances, was more than 100-fold greater than that of the precipitinogen fraction, when injected subcutaneously into guinea-pigs. Less than 25 to 50% of the toxicity of the original precipitate was recovered in the final toxin fraction but the losses were possibly due to

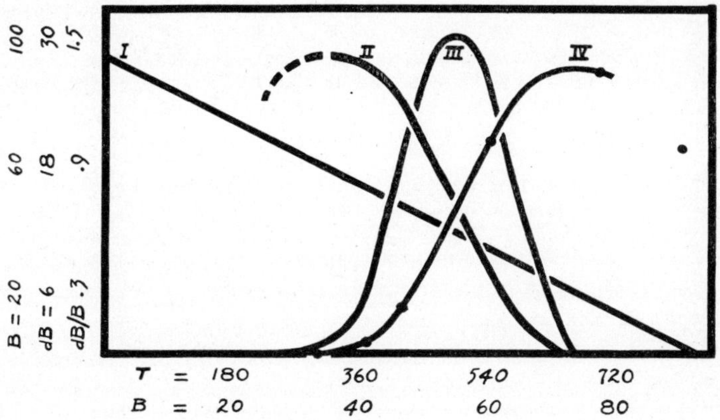

Fig. 7.—Analysis of a typical bacterial growth curve. The figure is explained in the text.

denaturation, since the major part of the antitoxin binding power (Lf units) of the original toxin was conserved in this fraction.

The final toxin fraction by no means represents pure toxin but since it is more nearly pure than any preparation which has been described elsewhere, its properties are reported as follows. The isoelectric range is P_H 5.0 to 5.2 as compared with approximate values of 4.0 to 4.6 for the precipitinogen fractions. The toxin fraction is soluble in acid only in the absence of salt. It is flocculated from slightly alkaline solution by the addition of less than 15% of ammonium sulfate, probable due to the acidity of this reagent. It is not precipitated by the addition of

* The floccules formed by the respective fractions with antitoxin serum were collected, washed, and their antitoxin content recovered by a method which is published elsewhere.[46]

46. Locke and Main: J. Infect. Dis., 1926, 39, p. 484.

Neither of the precipitinogen fractions showed an affinity for antitoxin such as would be expected had they represented, in part, the haptene groups of the original toxin.

85% of alcohol excepting from solutions of a P_H close to the isoelectric point. Boiling causes a slightly alkaline, isotonic solution to become opalescent but causes no coagulation. The color of the Biuret is a mauve, characteristic of whole protein or of plastein rather than of proteose. The Millon and xanthoproteic tests are positive for all of the fractions. The sugar-reduction and Molisch tests are negative for the toxin fraction, faintly positive for the intermediate fraction, and strongly positive for the final precipitinogen fraction.

The more successful toxin fractionations yielded preparations containing about 0.000,6 mg. of N_2 per corrected Lf unit. This N_2 value was found to be little changed after isoelectric extraction with alcohol, although a considerable amount of lipoid extractives was removed. The toxicity and antitoxin-binding power of the preparation seem to be only slightly diminished by a single alcohol treatment, but further extraction injures and finally destroys the toxin.

Chemically, then, there is reason to believe that toxin may be very little different in constitution from the protoplasm of the bacillus in which it has its origin. It seems to contain protein and lipin as integral components, to have an isoelectric range not far removed from that characteristic of bacillary extracts, and to be, like protoplasm, extremely sensitive to denaturation.

The protein-like nature of the bacterial toxins was first indicated by the early work of Brieger and Fränkel and Wassermann and Proskauer.[47] Their analyses and separations were made upon considerably less favorable material than that available to more recent workers but are, nevertheless, classic in their comprehensiveness.

Moloney and Weld [41] and Watson and Langstaff [41] have prepared isoelectric precipitates of toxin broth filtrates which they report to contain 11% of nitrogen—a normal value for material of protoplasmic origin—and which they state give positive biuret, Millon, xanthoproteic, Hopkins-Cole, and reduced sulfur reactions and, occasionally, positive Molisch and phosphorus reactions. Other investigators have, of course, reported purified toxin preparations which have consistently failed to give any of the accepted chemical tests for the presence of protein, but these failures may be attributed to the use of insufficient material. A properly prepared diphtheria toxin culture filtrate contains 1,000,000 or more MRD per cc., associated with 0.15 mg. or less of precipitable substance. Crude toxin precipitate is potentially able, therefore, to elicit a skin reaction in nonimmune guinea-pigs in a protein concentration of less than one part in a billion. One-billionth of a gram is a quantity many thousand times too small to respond to chemical identification.

The isoelectric range of the precipitated toxin material was first critically investigated by von Gröer.[34, 48] He found that all of the toxic principle is not

47. This work is admirably reviewed by Pick in Kraus and Levaditi: Handbuch der Technik und Methodik der Immunitätsf., 1908, 1, p. 489.

48. Michaelis: Biochem. Ztschr., 1923, 144, p. 4.

separated from toxin broth unless the P_H of precipitation lies between 3 and 4; that toxin prepared from synthetic mediums precipitates sharply at P_H 3.3; that the optimum flocculation point of an electrodialysed solution of toxin precipitate lies between P_H 5.3 and 5.5 but may be shifted toward more acid values by the addition of salt; and that the isoelectric point of a well washed alkaline extract of diphtheria bacilli is P_H 4.7 to 5.0. His findings agree more nearly with our own than do the more recent findings of Wallace[49] and Koulikoff and Smirnoff,[50] possibly because the latter workers have used a different type of broth medium for their original cultures.

The physical character, the isoelectric range, and the high sugar content of the precipitinogen fraction suggested that it might consist largely of glucoprotein. There is glucoprotein in nearly all of the known favorable mediums for the production of diphtheria toxin. It occurs as a readily extractable intercellular cement in the muscle tissues that provide the meat infusion and tryptic digests, and in the stomach linings that furnish the peptone. Although it is not a necessary ingredient for toxin production, since it may be partially removed from a broth medium without impairing its toxin producing power, it is not entirely eliminated in the usual methods for the preparation and concentration of toxin broth filtrates. Glucoproteins form an integral part of the bacillary capsule and may be responsible for the cementing together and flotation of the bacilli on the surface of the culture medium.[51] They are, also, probably responsible for the cohesiveness of the floccules obtained in the Ramon toxin-antitoxin titration method. Glucoproteins are not only antigenic in themselves[52] but are the haptenes or specificity carriers of many bacterial antigens,[53] acting, possibly, as aggressins[54] in certain infections. They are not a constituent part of the diphtheria toxin principle because the more highly purified preparations of this agent contain no detectable traces of sugar.

III

The specific properties which characterize a bacterial toxin are: a capacity to combine with susceptible tissues in lethal concentration, a capacity to combine with certain cell receptors or pre-antitoxin substances in such a way as to stimulate the production of an antitoxin, and a capacity to combine with the antitoxin so produced. The common factor of each of these properties is a capacity to combine. The combining capacity of one substance for another is determined by the extent of the mutual avidity which urges that combination. A preparation of toxin which attracts its antitoxin so strongly that combination occurs almost instantaneously is described as highly avid. A preparation which combines with antitoxin only after several days' incubation is regarded as very poorly avid. Avidity has the dimensions of potential energy.[46] It is measured as the product of a quantity factor (the number of combining units) and an intensity factor (the avidity per unit).

49. Wallace: J. Path. and Bact., 1927, 30, p. 667.

50. Koulikoff und Smirnoff: Ann. de l'Inst. Pasteur, 1927, 41, p. 1166; cf. also, De Potter: Bull. Acad. roy. Med. belg., 1923 (5), 3, p. 394.

51. Cf. Bacteriology of Diphtheria, 1908, p. 154.

52. Lewis and Wells: J. Infect. Dis., 1927, 40, p. 316.

53. Avery and Heidelberger: J. Exper. Med., 1925, 42, p. 367.

54. Cf. Felton and Bailey: J. Infect. Dis., 1926, 38, p. 131.

The number of combining units in a toxin preparation is a fairly stable quantity, determined primarily by the amount of toxin substance present, and is measurable in terms of Lf units.[55] The avidity per unit it variable. It is affected by the degree of dispersion of the toxin substance,[56] by the degree of its denaturation, and possibly also by constitutional factors such as we have found to influence the avidity of hemolysin preparations.[57] It is measurable in terms of the time required for one unit of the toxin preparation to become bound by one unit of standard antitoxin.[19, 46]

Figure 8 presents our impression of the distribution of avidity among the individual antigenic aggregates of five typical hypothetical toxin preparations. The distributions were calculated from a formula derived from the law of probability.* The avidities are plotted vertically and

$$P = c/e^{(E/Eav)} \qquad (6)$$

the fractions of the unit of toxin substance which possess avidities in excess of the respective values are plotted horizontally.

We have drawn two horizontal, broken lines, one to represent a high avidity threshold, and the other a minimum one. The curve A represents a practical maximum for the average avidity which a toxin preparation can have, and curve H is very close to the minimum. We have postulated that all of the curves shall represent the same, original toxin preparation; the less avid ones being derived from A by progressive denaturation such as is accomplished by aging, heating, or formolization.

Note that the high avidity level is less stable than the low one. The same amount of denaturation which reduces the per cent of the toxin substance having an avidity in excess of the lower, minimum level by only 18%, reduces the fraction having an avidity in excess of the higher level by 97%.

It is known that a denaturing action which decreases the avidity of a toxin preparation from a flocculation time of less than one minute (the calculated value for A) to a value of more than 4 days (the calculated value for F) practically destroys its toxicity, although the antitoxin-binding power and antigenicity are thereby only slightly reduced.[55] It is upon this principle that the manufacture of "toxoid" is based.

55. Ramon: Compt. rend. Soc. de Biol., 1927, 97, p. 635; Glenny and Okell: J. Path. & Bact., 1924, 27, p. 187.

56. Schmidt, H., and Scholz: Arch. f. Hyg., 1925, 95, p. 308.

57. Locke, Main and Hirsch: J. Infect. Dis., 1926, 39, p. 126.

* Let the average avidity, per antigenic aggregate, be represented by Eav. Let c be a proportionality factor, e the natural logarithm base, and P the fraction of the total toxin concentration which may be expected to have an avidity value equal to or greater than E. Then:

We wish to suggest that the antigenicity, antitoxin combining power, and toxicity of bacterial toxins may be manifestations of one and the same property,[58] their combining avidity. When this avidity is low, due to lack of dispersion, to denaturation incidental to the method of prepara-

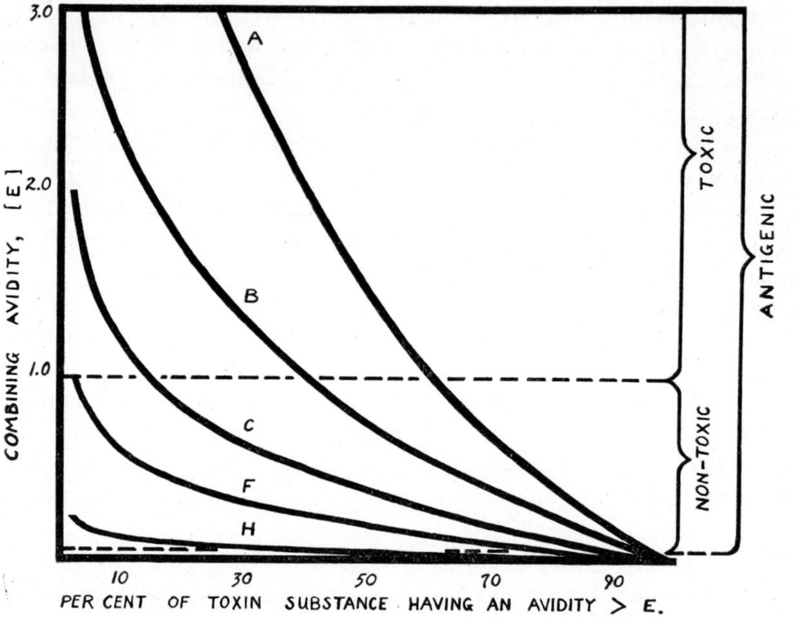

HYPOTHETICAL TOXIN PREPARATION.	PROBABLE FLOCCULATION TIME, HRS.	PROBABLE PERCENT OF TOXIN WHICH IS:	
		TOXIC	ANTIGENIC
A	≠0	60	98
B	.017	40	96
C	5-6	14	90
F	100	2	80
H	1000	0	40

Fig. 8.—The relation of toxicity to combining avidity. The figure is explained in the text.

tion, to postmortem autolytic actions, or to a constitutional structure which does not permit the building up of a high avidity, the preparation may be antigenic and bind its antibody, but it cannot be highly toxic.

58. These properties were originally postulated by Ehrlich to reside in chemically distinct haptophore and toxophore groups. Ehrlich: Deutsch. med. Wchnschr., 1898, 24, p. 597; cf. also, Madsen: Ann. de l'Inst. Pasteur, 1899, 13, p. 576; Arrhenius: Immunochemistry, 1907; Bordet: Ann. de l'Inst. Pasteur, 1903, 17, p. 161.

Only when the combining avidity exceeds an upper, limiting threshold, such as the upper dotted line in figure 8, can the preparation be sufficiently toxic to be lethal in small concentrations.

SUMMARY

A study of the conditions favoring growth and toxin production in differently prepared cultures of a toxicogenic strain of the diphtheria bacillus has indicated that toxin is not accumulated unless there is a definite growth momentum, a concommitant growth inhibition, and unless there are present enzyme-buffers like proteose to protect the toxin from extracellular proteolysis.

The toxin principle has been concentrated and separated from the greater part of the accompanying precipitinogen and nonspecific principles. Preparations have been obtained with a nitrogen equivalent of 0.000,6 $\pm$ 2 mg. per corrected Lf unit, which give intradermal skin reactions in dilutions approaching one part in a billion. These purified preparations have been unmistakably lipoprotein in character and contain no carbohydrate. They have an isoelectric range within that manifested by preparations of the bacillary substance in which they have their origin and they are, like protoplasm extremely sensitive to denaturation.

The theory of the nature and origin of diphtheria toxin has been discussed and the suggestion made that the antigenicity, antitoxin-binding power, and toxicity of bacterial toxins may be manifestations of an identical, more fundamental property—their combining avidity.

COMPARISON OF SEROLOGIC AND PULLORIN TESTS FOR BACILLARY WHITE DIARRHEA

L. D. BUSHNELL

From the Department of Bacteriology Kansas Agricultural Experiment Station, Manhattan

One of the important problems confronting the poultry industry today is the control of bacillary white diarrhea. While the macroscopic agglutination test has proved to be efficient in controlling the disease in flocks tested over a series of years it is so expensive and time consuming as to be a burden to the industry. Since it also seems desirable to use low dilutions of serum in this test in order to eliminate the reactors as rapidly as possible, certain difficulties of technic develop which make the results difficult or impossible to interpret. Under these conditions the reaction may be obscured by a precipitate in the presence of phenol added as a preservative, or, if but small amounts of phenol are added, there are certain phenol-fast organisms which grow in the tests and obscure the results. Such conditions naturally lead to search for cheaper and more accurate methods of testing which may be equally effective in controlling the disease.

In the following discussion we have compared the results of three series of tests. The tube agglutination test with one tube of a 1:25 dilution has been used as a standard. Reactions were marked as positive only when there was complete agglutination. All doubtful reactions were called negative.

The following comparisons have been made: the tube agglutination with complement fixation; the tube agglutination with the "rapid" or "slide" method using dilutions of serum and antigen in the ratio of about 1:25; and the tube agglutination test with the pullorin reaction. In this last group of tests we have used two types of pullorin: pullorin 1 supplied us by a commercial house, and pullorin 2 prepared in our own laboratory.

Cultures.—The cultures used for making the antigens and pullorin were the same except in case of the first series. These cultures were typical throughout of the type A described by Hadley.[1] We have not included a type B culture in this work since we have not found sero-

Received for publication, Dec. 31, 1927.

1. Rhode Island Agric. Exper. Sta. Bull., 1917, 172, p. 1.

logical difference between types A and B. In this we agree with Hendrickson.[2] The cultures were tested frequently for purity and all agglutinated easily with known reactive serums but not with known inactive serum.

The Association Coefficient.—The association coefficient was determined according to the method of Yule.[2a] The results by the two methods X and Y are first tabulated.

		Y positive	Y negative
X	positive	a	b
	negative	c	d

The degree of association, or coefficient of association, is then expressed by the formula $\frac{ad - bc}{ad + bc}$

If ad is equal to bc the coefficient becomes zero, which indicates no correlation. A, + 1 or — 1, indicates a perfect positive or negative correlation in the comparison of any two characters. If a, b, c, or d is zero a more complicated formula is necessary.

TESTS

Comparison of Tube Agglutination and Complement Fixation.—Bushnell and Hudson [3] made a comparison of the results of the tube agglutination and complement fixation tests. In all, 230 tests were made on 98 birds. Of these birds 41 were considered reactive and 57 as not reactive. The comparisons in this series of tests was made of 1 : 50 dilutions of serum. The results are shown in the following tabulation.

230 tests: 98 fowls, 41.9% reactive

Complement fixation positive	: agglutination negative	13	5.6%
	: agglutination positive	95	41.3%
Complement fixation negative	: agglutination negative	113	49.1%
	: agglutination positive	9	3.9%

Coefficient of association 0.97

The two tests vary to about the same extent and in the same direction. The complement fixation test has a serious disadvantage because of the high anticomplementary action of the fowl serum. This cannot be successfully removed by heating since this treatment also reduces the complement fixing substance. We have found that 32% of 400 samples of fowl serum were anticomplementary in 0.05 cc. amounts. This prevents use of low dilutions of the serum in complement fixation tests.

2. J. Am. V. M. A., 1927, 23, n. s., p. 629.
2a. Phil. Trans. Roy. oc. London, Ser. A., V. 194, p. 257, 1900.
3. J. Infect. Dis., 1927, 41, p. 383.

The association coefficient is very high and, while 3.9% of the birds reacting to the agglutination test were considered as negative to the complement fixation test, it must be understood that the tube agglutination test is also subject to a certain amount of error. The complement fixation test is probably as effective in detecting actual carriers as the agglutination test and might be used to replace it except for the anticomplementary action of fowl serum. It is, however, an effective check on the agglutination test in determining reactors and some writers consider it more accurate than the agglutination test in indicating actual infection.

Tube and Rapid Macroscopic Methods.—The rapid method which we used was similar to that described by Runnells, Coon, Farley and Thorp.[4] The antigen used was about 25 or 50 times as concentrated as that used in the tube method. In part of the tests two drops of serum were added to a 50 × antigen and in part one drop of serum was added to a 25 × antigen and mixed immediately.* The tests were warmed by placing the slide above an electric bulb. Readings were made within 5 minutes after mixing the antigen and serum. In some cases there was a fairly typical clumping after standing for some time but these were considered as negative reactions. This is probably incorrect although we have not had enough experience to state definitely. The difference between one and two drops in a 25 × and 50 × antigen appeared to make no difference in the reactions. This is to be expected since there is no difference in the dilution. We believe that a 25 × antigen and one drop of serum gives equally clear cut results and is a saving of antigen.

The following table shows the result of a comparison of the above methods on part of our experimental flock and on serum sent to us from different flocks in the state.

A comparison of the tube with the rapid macroscopic agglutination for 735 birds (48.1% reactive) gave an association coefficient of 0.98. The results are tabulated.

735 fowls, 48.1% reactive

Rapid agglutination positive:	tube agglutination negative	20	2.6%
:	tube agglutination positive	312	42.4%
Rapid agglutination negative:	tube agglutination negative	361	49.3%
:	tube agglutination positive	42	5.7%

Coefficient of association 0.98

4. J. Am. V. M. A., 1927, 23, n. s., p. 660.

* The term 50 × antigen refers to an antigen containing 50 times as many bacterial cells per volume as that used in the macroscopic tube agglutination test, approximately 50 times the turbidity of McFarland's nephelometer tube 1.

By comparing the results obtained in the above tests it is seen that the correlation is high. This method would probably be effective in freeing flocks of the infection in a few tests and is much simpler and more rapid than the tube test. It also avoids the difficulty arising from contamination, as described by Hinshaw and Dunlap.[5]

An analysis was made of the results on those birds showing a positive tube agglutination test and a negative rapid test in an attempt to determine the reason for the difference. In the case of 15 tests the serum was titrated and the limit determined. It was found that 6 of the serums showed a titer limit of 40, 5 a limit of 80, 2 a limit of 160, and 2 a limit of 320. This would indicate that a certain number of highly reactive fowls would be missed by this reaction and the reason for the lack of reaction is not because of a low agglutinin content of the serum but to delayed reaction. This is a point which needs further study.

Tube Agglutination with the Pullorin Reaction.—We do not know from the results of our work the best method of preparing pullorin or of introducing it into the bird. Neither do we know what kind of a reaction to consider as indicating a dangerous carrier of the disease. This should not, however, condemn the method without an exhaustive study.

Pullorin 1 was obtained from a commercial house and has not been given as extensive a trial as pullorin 2. We do not know how the first product was prepared but our own was a dissociation product obtained by washing 18-hour agar cultures of the organism four times in sterile salt solution and centrifugating out most of the cells. The fourth washing of 10 cc. of salt solution for the growth from one Kolle flask was autoclaved for 20 minutes at 15 pounds pressure. The heating precipitates a very fine sediment and the turbidity of the produce used is about one-half of tube 1 of McFarland's nephelometer. This substance does not give any of the ordinary qualitative protein reactions but does cause the formation of agglutinins in birds and rabbits. This product was also found to fix complement in the presence of positive antipullorin serum.[3] Such products have been called "ectoantigens." Several modifications have been tested to a limited extent but we are not ready to report on them at present.

The material was injected intracutaneously in the wattle. The injection was not considered satisfactory unless a small white area of the skin

5. J. Am. V. M. A., 1928, 25, n.s., p. 594.

persisted for a short time. It is impossible to inject a uniform amount into all birds but we attempted to obtain a small lump about the size of a grain of wheat at the point of injection.

Reactions at the end of 24 hours of about the size of the original swelling were read as a one plus reaction, a somewhat larger swelling as a two plus, etc. We have arbitrarily chosen a full one plus as indicating a reactor. Smaller swellings and discolored areas at the point of injection were considered as negative.

Pullorin 1: The following tabulation shows a comparison of the tube method and pullorin 1. These results were obtained on birds from miscellaneous sources and of various ages. Of the 142 fowls tested 61.2% reacted to the tube agglutination test.

142 fowls, 61.2% reactive

Pullorin positive:	tube agglutination negative	17	11.9%
:	tube agglutination positive	63	44.3%
Pullorin negative:	tube agglutination negative	38	26.7%
:	tube agglutination positive	24	16.9%

Coefficient of association 0.71

It may be seen that 11.9% of the birds negative to the agglutination test were positive to the pullorin and 16.9% positive to the agglutination test were negative to pullorin. This makes an agreement of 71.1%. The latter group are of great importance since they contain some very highly reactive and some undoubtedly dangerous carriers.

Pullorin 2: In the following tabulation we have listed the results obtained on three flocks of birds. Flock 1 consisted partly of our own experimental flock and a few birds from miscellaneous sources. These fowls were of all ages and breeds, some having been in our test flock for two or more years. Some were very highly reactive while others were borderline cases and others not reactive. Of the fowls in this group 68.7% reacted consistently to a 1:25 dilution in the tube test.

Flock 1: 170 adult fowls, 68.7% reactive

Pullorin positive:	agglutination negative	13	7.7%
:	agglutination positive	92	54.1%
Pullorin negative:	agglutination negative	40	23.5%
:	agglutination positive	25	14.7%

Coefficient of association 0.83

The pullorin reactions were read as previously described and the agglutination tests after 24 hours at 45 C. No preservative was added in these tests. For flock 1 the results are somewhat better than those obtained with the commercial pullorin.

Flock 2 was a flock of pullets in which severe losses had occurred from the disease a few days after hatching. This flock showed a surprisingly small number of reactive fowls although they had run on infected ground. This flock was tested first when the birds were about 8 months of age and about two months in production and again when they were about 10 months of age. At the time of the second test several other birds had been added. Two of the reactive fowls detected at the time of the first test had died and a fowl negative to the first test became reactive at the time of the second test.

Flock 2: 83 pullets, 3.6% reactive. First test Aug. 2

Pullorin positive:	agglutination negative	14	16.9%
:	agglutination positive	2	2.5%
Pullorin negative:	agglutination negative	66	79.2%
:	agglutination positive	1	1.3%

Coefficient of association 0.81

Flock 2: 87 pullets, 3.4% reactive. Second test Oct. 9

Pullorin positive:	agglutination negative	8	9.2%
:	agglutination positive	1	1.1%
Pullorin negative:	agglutination negative	76	87.4%
:	agglutination positive	2	2.3%

Coefficient of association 0.65

Flock 3 was a flock of hens on the college farm. These birds were considered as entirely negative to the agglutination test on first test, and there was but one reactive hen in the second test. All the chicks which died from this flock, about 7%, were examined bacteriologically and not a single chick was found to have died from bacillary white diarrhea. The one hen which reacted to the agglutination test was negative to the pullorin test. Tabulation of the results follow.

Flock 3: 185 adult hens, 0.0% reactive. First test July 18

Pullorin positive:	agglutination negative	8	4.3%
:	agglutination positive	0	0.0%
Pullorin negative:	agglutination negative	177	95.7%
:	agglutination positive	0	0.0%

Flock 3: 180 adult hens, 0.5% reactive. Second test Oct. 5

Pullorin positive:	agglutination negative	13	7.3%
:	agglutination positive	0	0.0%
Pullorin negative:	agglutination negative	166	92.2%
:	agglutination positive	1	0.5%

A comparison of all the reactions obtained with the agglutination test to those due to the use of pullorin 2 on 705 fowls with 17.5% reactive gave an association coefficient of 0.93. The results are shown in the following tabulation.

705 fowls, 17.5% reactive

Pullorin positive:	agglutination negative	56	7.9%
:	agglutination positive	95	13.4%
Pullorin negative:	agglutination negative	525	74.5%
:	agglutination positive	29	4.1%

Association coefficient 0.93

There was a disagreement on 85 birds in this group or an agreement in both tests of 87.9%.

Hinshaw, Scott and Payne [6] found that 45.7% of the reactive fowls laid infected eggs and 10.4% of the eggs from these birds were infected thus considerably reducing the danger from those which might be missed by the test. We know, however, that in many cases very heavy losses may result from but one or two birds in a flock, or the hatching of a few infected chicks may contaminate the incubator, runs and brooders for hundreds of healthy chicks.

Of the 847 birds which have been tested by the two types of pullorin, 53 which reacted to the agglutination test were missed by the pullorin test. And of those considered negative by the agglutination test 73 were considered positive by the pullorin test. Thus there were 126 or 14.9% disagreement or 85.1% agreement between the two tests. While the above results are favorable enough to encourage further research, we do not feel that we are in position to recommend the test at the present time.

CONCLUSIONS

The results of several years experience have shown that the tube agglutination test has proved effective in detecting and thereby eradicating bacillary white diarrhea and may be used as a basis of comparison for other methods. The complement fixation test cannot be used to advantage because of the difficulties of technic which prevent the use of low dilutions of serum. From our experience we still believe that low dilutions should be used.

The rapid slide macroscopic agglutination test is probably as efficient in detecting reactive fowls as the tube methods and can be used as a substitute for the latter.

The pullorin test, in its present stage of development, cannot be recommended to replace the present agglutination methods for the diagnosis of bacillary white diarrhea. However, it is a promising field for further research in an attempt to cheapen the method.

6. J. Am. V. M. A., 1928, 25, n. s., p. 599.

INFLUENCE OF CARBOHYDRATES ON BACTERIAL DECOMPOSITION OF UREA

Mitsuteru Ishikawa

From the Department of Bacteriology and Public Health, Washington University School of Medicine, St. Louis, Mo., and the Research Department of Bacteriology, Northwestern University Medical School, Chicago

Since Pasteur[1] had observed that urine is subject to bacterial decomposition, a number of investigators studied, from different angles, the disintegration of urea by microorganisms. That urea is broken up into ammonia and carbon dioxide by bacteria was described by Schnitzler.[2] Brodmeier[3] stated that glucose added to the medium prevented the liberation, by B. proteus, of ammonia from urea. According to Laschina[4] no increased urea decomposition could be demonstrated when the culture of B. pasteuri was brought within the field of a solenoid, even if $MgSO_4$ and K_2HPO_4 were added to the culture, as recommended by Jaksch.[5] Gellinger[6] reported that, of his 72 cultures of urea-splitting organisms obtained from soil and manure, four were able to decompose urea in the absence of oxygen. Jacoby[7] observed that glucose added to the urea solution accelerated the decomposition of urea by the proteus bacillus. He[8] also investigated influences of various substances on the urea-splitting action of the organism, and found that the decomposition was increased markedly by dextrose, d-galactose, glycerol, d, l-glyceric aldehyde, dioxyacetone, pyruvic acid and lactic acid, moderately by d-fructose, d-arabinose and l-arabinose, and very slightly by d-mannose, d-sorbose, rhamnose, heptose, saccharose, lactose, raffinose, alpha-methyl glucoside, beta-methyl glucoside, mannitol, dulcitol, sorbitol, erythritol, inositol and prophyl alcohol. Jacoby[9] also obtained a dried preparation of the bacillus, of which urease could be preserved for a long time and was active in the presence of toluol. He[10] stated that leucine was necessary for the formation of bacterial urease but had no effect upon its activity, since the amino acid did not increase the urea decomposition of the dried preparation while it accelerated the urea-splitting action of the organism when added to the culture medium. He[11] further stated that it was necessary to have leucine in the culture medium for the production of urease by B. coli as well as by B. proteus, but, on the other hand, the addition of leucine to the medium containing glucose inhibited the fermentation of the carbohydrate by the bacteria. Takahata[12] found that the optimum reaction of Sörensen's solution for the urea-decomposition of the proteus bacillus was P_H 7.0 and that[13] urease was extracted

Received for publication, Jan. 5, 1928.

1. Ann. de chimie et de physique, 1862, 64, p. 50.
2. Centralbl. f. Bakteriol., 1, O., 1893, 13, p. 68.
3. Ibid., 1895, 18, p. 380.
4. Arch. f. Physiol., 1911, p. 260.
5. Ztschr. f. physiol. Chem., 1881, 5, p. 395.
6. Centralbl. f. Bakteriol., 1, O., 1917, 47, p. 245.
7. Biochem. Ztschr., 1916, 77, p. 405.
8. Ibid., 1917, 79, p. 35.
9. Ibid., 1917, 84, p. 354.
10. Ibid., p. 358.
11. Ibid., 1918, 86, p. 329.
12. Ibid., 1923, 140, p. 166.
13. Ibid., p. 168.

from the dried bacterial preparation by the neutral phosphate solution and its activity was favored by the presence of glycocoll. It was noted by Itano[14] that urease was possessed by Azotobacter beijerinckii. Rubentschik[15] reported that urobacillus psychrocartericus and urosarcina psychrocartericus, urea-splitting organisms isolated by him, grew at temperatures below zero. Lehr[16] concluded that $BeCl_2$ increased the urease activity of B. proteus in the phosphate buffer mixture.

It would seem, as mentioned above, that the finding, in connection with the effect of glucose upon the bacterial decomposition of urea, of Brodmeier[3] and that of Jacoby[7] are not in accord. And yet, so far as the available literature shows, neither of them has been corroborated by other experimentalists. This work has been carried out mainly for the purpose of detecting influences of various carbohydrates on the urea-splitting action of several kinds of bacteria.

EXPERIMENTS WITH BACTERIAL CULTURES

Ammonia from Urea.—In this experiment, the comparison, through which the ability of bacteria to decompose urea could be detected, of the amounts of ammonia produced in plain broth, in broth with urea, and in broth with urea and glucose, was made.

Methods: Broth consisted of peptone 10 gms., sodium chloride 5 gms., meat extract 1 gm., and water 1000 cc.; the reaction was adjusted to P_H 7.0. Into each of clean 100 cc. flasks, 40 cc. of the broth were poured. The top of the flask was covered with a small beaker, instead of being plugged with cotton, and was autoclaved in the proper way. Distilled water, 10% glucose solution and 10% urea solution were held in separate flasks; the first two were sterilized by autoclaving and the urea solution was filtered through a Berkefeld filter. Thus, three flasks of broth were arranged for one organism; with aseptic manipulation, 10 cc. of the distilled water was added to the first flask, 5 cc. of the urea solution and 5 cc. of the distilled water to the second, and 5 cc. of the glucose solution and 5 cc. of the urea solution to the third. One-tenth cc. of a plain broth culture of an organism was inoculated to the flask, and the flasks were kept at 37 C.

Ammonia was determined quantitatively, 1 cc. of the medium from each flask being tested, by the air current method recommended by Kendall.[17] The determination was conducted at different periods of incubation, on the first, third, fifth and seventh days. With proper care of avoiding contamination of the remnant, a small portion of the medium was removed from the flask each time.

Different types of bacteria were examined. B. proteus and B. mesentericus were selected as proteolytic, sugar-splitting bacteria, B. pyocyaneus was chosen as a proteolytic, nonfermenting bacillus, B. pyogenes foetidus as a nonproteolytic, acid-producing organism, and B. alkaligenes

14. Abstr. Bact., 1924, 8, p. 6.
15. Centralbl. f. Bakteriol., 1, O., 1925, 65, p. 166.
16. Biochem. Ztschr., 1926, 168, p. 166.
17. J. Infect. Dis., 1922, 30, p. 211.

as a nonproteolytic, nonfermenting bacillus. The results are shown in table 1.

Bacillus proteus showed that it produced large amounts of ammonia in the mediums containing urea, that the ammonia came chiefly from urea and that glucose increased the production of ammonia. But B. alkaligenes, B. mesentericus and B. pyogenes-foetidus seemed to be unable to attack urea to a noticeable degree; the latter two furnished an example of the protein-sparing action of carbohydrates, of which principle has been established by investigations of Kendall and others. And B. pyocyaneus indicated its ability, though not strong, to yield ammonia from urea.

Table 1.—Ammonia Nitrogen: Mg. per 100 Cc. of Medium

	Day	Broth	Broth, Urea	Broth, Urea, Glucose
Control	1	2.8	2.8	2.8
B. alkaligenes	1	5.6	5.6	5.6
	3	7.0	8.4	8.4
	5	8.4	8.4	14.0
	7	11.2	11.2	14.0
B. mesentericus	1	7.0	5.6	5.6
	3	22.4	22.4	14.0
	5	30.8	30.8	22.4
	7	43.4	44.8	29.4
B. proteus[1]	1	9.8	154.0	240.8
	3	18.2	267.4	313.6
	5	22.4	281.4	355.6
	7	25.2	308.0	378.0
B. pyocyaneus	1	8.4	8.4	9.8
	3	18.2	21.0	46.2
	5	26.6	29.4	88.2
	7	32.2	61.6	119.0
B. pyogenes-foetidus	1	5.6	5.6	5.6
	3	9.8	9.8	8.4
	5	12.6	14.0	8.4
	7	15.4	16.8	11.2

In brief, the results indicated that of the two glucose-fermenting organisms, the urea-splitting organism, as B. proteus, generates more ammonia, chiefly from urea, in glucose broth than in plain broth, while the nonurea-splitting bacterium, as B. mesentericus, produces less ammonia, from nitrogenous substances other than urea, in broth containing glucose.

Other diverse organisms were also tested in the same way, except that ammonia was determined only once on the third or the fourth day. B. anthrax, B. cloacae, B. coli, B. communior, B. dysenteriae (Shiga), B. enteritidis, B. mucosus, B. paratyphosus A and B, B. suipestifer, B. typhosus, and Micrococcus ovalis apparently did not possess the urea-decomposing enzyme. But considerable amounts of ammonia from urea were produced, both in plain and glucose broths, by B. ammoniagenes, B. aerogenes, B. morgani, B. proteus vulgaris and Staphylococcus aureus. Of these organisms, different strains of one bacterium did not yield equal amounts of ammonia under the same condition. For instance, of five strains of B. aerogenes three decomposed urea strikingly but the other two very slightly. It should be recalled that B. ammoniagenes has been described by Cooke and Keith[18] as a nonfermentative, nonproteolytic, urea-splitting organism, although the quantitative study of its ammonia production appears to have never been attempted. Two strains of the bacterium used in this series of experiments were obtained through the courtesy of Dr. Cooke.

It was observed, throughout the experiments which have been described, that the medium containing urea and glucose showed an alkaline reaction to bromthymol blue, when an urea-splitting organism had been cultivated, but an acid reaction when a nonurea-decomposing bacterium had been grown. This phenomenon did not occur, however, if an organism was a non-glucose fermenter, as in the case of B. alkaligenes.

Influence of Carbohydrates.—The result of preceding experiment illustrated that the proteus bacillus liberates more ammonia from urea in the presence of glucose than in the absence of the sugar. It was intended, thereupon, to find out the effect of not only glucose but also lactose, mannitol and sodium formate upon the urea decomposition of several bacteria which have been proved to have a definite urea-splitting action. The experimental procedure was practically the same as in the preceding experiment.

Five flasks, each of which contained 40 cc. of broth, were allotted to an organism, and to each of the flasks 5 cc. of distilled water or of 10% solutions of glucose, lactose, manitol and sodium formate were added. Five cc. of 10% urea solution were also added to all of the flasks. The broth and the solutions were sterilized separately, solutions of urea and sodium formate being sterilized by filtration. Ammonia was determined on the first, third and fifth days. Bacteria employed were B. morgani, B. proteus, Staphylococcus, B. ammoniagenes, and B. aerogenes. Table 2 shows the results.

The results indicate that the liberation of ammonia by B. proteus and B. morgani, which ferment glucose but neither lactose nor manitol, was accelerated noticeably only in the medium containing glucose. B. aerogenes and Staphylococcus, which are able to cleave glucose, lactose and mannitol as well, produced definitely greater amounts of ammonia in the presence of glucose, lactose or mannitol than in the absence of such

18. J. Bact., 1927, 13, p. 315.

carbohydrates. B. ammoniagenes decomposed urea more vigorously in the medium containing glucose than in the mediums with lactose or mannitol or without any additional carbohydrate, though the difference is not so marked. It should be noted, in this connection, that this organism was described by Cooke and Keith [18] as having no fermentative ability, but it gave an indication of acid production in a glucose agar tube after a few days incubation at 37 C., which suggests that it utilizes glucose to some extent. Sodium formate did not exert any noticeable effect on the urea decomposition either by B. aerogenes, B. morgani and B. proteus which are able to split it into hydrogen and carbon dioxide or by B. ammoniagenes and Staphylococcus which apparently do not attack the substance. Although omitted in the table, those bacteria produced

TABLE 2.—AMMONIA NITROGEN: MG. PER 100 CC. OF MEDIUM

	Day	Urea	Urea Glucose	Urea Lactose	Urea Mannitol	Urea Formate
B. proteus [2]	1	28.0	95.2	28.0	30.8	22.4
	3	308.0	345.8	309.4	309.4	294.8
	5	310.8	375.2	313.6	310.8	305.2
B. morgani	1	26.6	115.0	33.6	30.8	28.0
	3	282.8	347.2	284.2	285.6	285.6
	5	284.2	350.0	288.4	285.6	288.4
B. ammoniagenes	1	168.0	205.8	170.8	169.4	168.0
	3	285.6	302.4	282.8	285.6	282.8
	5	287.0	302.4	285.6	287.0	287.0
B. lactis-aerogenes	1	8.4	16.8	81.2	19.6	8.4
	3	33.6	210.0	324.8	236.6	36.4
	5	49.0	355.6	364.0	355.6	47.6
Staphylococcus aureus	1	11.2	169.4	67.2	78.4	14.0
	3	116.4	207.2	168.0	168.0	117.8
	5	210.0	319.2	240.8	252.0	218.4

very small amounts of ammonia in plain broth free from urea, just as in the previous experiments. So, it is reasonable to regard the figures in the table as manifestations of the extents of urea decomposition.

Besides the bacteria shown in the table, other strains of B. ammoniagenes, B. aerogenes, B. proteus and Staphylococcus were tried in the same manner. All of them resulted in showing analogous tendencies to what have been described.

Anaerobic Bacteria.—Apparently very little is known about the urea-splitting action of anaerobic bacteria. An attempt was made, therefore, to get some information concerning the urease activity of anaerobes—B. welchii, B. sporogenes and B. oedimatiens. Two strains of each organism were studied. The bacteria were inoculated heavily into ordinary test tubes containing 10 cc. of plain broth, of 1% urea-broth or of 1% urea-glucose broth, the mediums having been prepared as in the previous experiments. And the tubes were kept in a jar in which the anaerobic condition was secured by means of phosphorus; this method of anaerobic culture has been described by Varney.[19] After the incubation of four days at 37 C., the tubes were tested for ammonia. The bacteria grew fairly well, but failed, in both plain and glucose broths, to show any evidence of their capability of splitting urea to an appreciable degree.

EXPERIMENTS WITH ASSOCIATIVE CULTURES

Investigations of the associative actions of bacteria had been carried out by not a few workers, as pointed out in the previous paper.[20] In the following experiments, it was desired to detect what effect, if any, the association of a fermenting, nonurea-splitting organism has upon the decomposition of urea by an urea-splitting bacterium in plain and carbohydrate mediums. The experimental procedure, in the main, followed that of preceding experiments. Symbiotic bacteria were inoculated simultaneously, 0.1 cc. of broth culture of each organism being used. After two days incubation of the flasks, ammonia was measured.

B. Proteus and B. Coli.—It has been shown that B. proteus decomposes urea more intensively in the presence of glucose, but not of lactose or mannitol, than in plain broth. B. communis, which was used in this series of experiments, liberated practically no ammonia from urea either in plain broth or in broth containing glucose, lactose or mannitol, all of which would be fermented by the organism. These two bacilli were cultivated, singly and symbiotically, in plain, lactose and mannitol broths. The results were as follows.

	Urea	Urea Lactose	Urea Mannitol
B. proteus (1)	350.0	351.4	350.0
B. coli	9.8	8.4	8.4
B. proteus and B. coli	271.6	383.6	365.4

As could be expected in the light of previous experiments, B. proteus alone produced nearly equal amounts of ammonia in plain, lactose and mannitol broths, and B. coli did not generate much ammonia in any of those mediums. A significant fact, however, was unfolded by the symbiotic culture. According to the figures in the table, total amounts of ammonia nitrogen produced by single cultures of B. proteus and B. coli are 359.8 (mg. per 100 cc.), 359.8 and 358.4, while those given by the symbiotic culture are 271.6, 383.6 and 365.4, in plain, lactose and mannitol mediums respectively. By comparing these figures, it will be

19. J. Lab. & Clin. Med., 1926, 11, p. 1183.
20. J. Infect. Dis., 1927, 41, p. 238.

found that the liberation of ammonia nitrogen of the symbiotic culture was less than that of single cultures by 88.2 in plain broth, but greater by 23.8 and 7.0 in lactose and mannitol broths respectively, and that the associative culture yielded more ammonia, by the margin of about 100, in broth containing lactose or mannitol than in plain broth.

The fact that in plain broth a larger amout of ammonia was produced by B. proteus alone than by the association of B. proteus and B. coli may be understood by assuming that the colon bacillus hampered somewhat the growth of the proteus bacillus to make the number of the latter smaller in the mixed culture than in the single culture; this was proved to be the case by plating out the cultures. The reason why the synergic culture brought forth a larger quantity of ammonia than the single culture of B. proteus in the medium with lactose or mannitol, in contrast to the result in plain broth, seems to be that the colon bacillus paved the way for the urea-splitting activity of the proteus bacillus by breaking down such carbohydrates into simpler substances, which accelerated, in some way, the decomposition of urea by the proteus bacillus, this favorable influence overcoming the obstacle for growth. It may be assumed, moreover, that not only glucose but also some other intermediate products of carbohydrates exerted a promoting effect on the urea decomposition of the proteus bacillus, inasmuch as mannitol does not yield a glucose molecule on hydrolysis.

B. Ammoniagenes and B. Coli.—A previous experiment has revealed that the generation of ammonia from urea by B. ammoniagenes, which does not attack any sugar very actively, is but slightly intensified by the presence of glucose. B. ammoniagenes and B. coli were grown, singly and synergically, in plain, glucose and lactose mediums. Results quite different from those of B. proteus and B. coli were obtained, as follows.

	Urea	Urea Glucose	Urea Lactose
B. ammoniagenes	280.0	296.8	282.8
B. coli	11.2	9.8	9.8
B. ammoniagenes and B. coli	81.2	36.4	33.6

The single culture of B. ammoniagenes liberated a slightly larger amount of ammonia in glucose broth than in plain or lactose broth, in conformity to the previous experiment of the organism. Far smaller, by approximately 200 mg. per 100 cc., amounts of ammonia were given off by the associative culture than by B. ammoniagenes alone in plain, glucose and lactose broths, and the symbiotic culture produced a definitely greater amount of ammonia in plain broth than in sugar-containing broths; this is quite contrary to the finding of the experiment with B. proteus and B. coli. As the result seemed to be puzzling, the experiment was repeated, but practically the same result came out.

By plating out the associative culture, it was found that B. coli decisively outnumbered B. ammoniagenes. In addition, Cooke and Keith [18] stated about B. ammoniagenes that "The most rapid development of cultures occurs on media with a reaction of P_H 7.0 to P_H 8.5, while greater degrees of acidity or alkalinity cause a marked inhibition of growth." Therefore, the inhibitory effect of B. coli upon the liberation of ammonia by B. ammoniagenes probably originated in the impedimental influence of the colon bacillus upon the growth of the other. Thus, it would seem, in plain broth the hindrance was not so strong as in sugar broths, because in the latter, as a result of fermentation by B. coli, the reaction became highly acid, which is particularly inimical to the development of B. ammoniagenes; hence a greater amount of ammonia was generated in plain broth than in sugar broths.

After all, in the symbiosis, the colon bacillus appears to have influenced the urea decomposition of the other only unfavorably; products of its fermentation did not give enough accelerating effect, if any, to surpass the inhibitory influence of its acid production upon the growth of the other.

B. Aerogenes and B. Coli.—It is evident, from the result of a previous experiment, that B. aerogenes has the urea-splitting ability which is accelerated by glucose and other utilizable carbohydrates. B. coli was the same strain which had been used in the proceding two experiments. In this experiment, single and associative cultures of the two bacteria in plain, glucose and mannitol mediums were tested. The results shown in the tabulation indicate that the symbiotic culture of B. aerogenes with B. coli produced slightly smaller amounts of ammonia than the single culture of B. lactis aerogenes, in plain broth as well as in glucose or mannitol medium.

	Urea	Urea Glucose	Urea Mannitol
B. aerogenes	156.8	336.0	281.4
B. coli	11.2	9.8	9.8
B. aerogenes and B. coli.......	145.6	324.8	277.2

This result can reasonably be explained by assuming that the fermentation of glucose and mannitol by the colon bacillus was well-nigh ineffective in increasing the urea-decomposing activity of B. aerogenes, which attacks such carbohydrates intensively per se, and that the number of B. aerogenes was smaller in the symbiotic culture than in the pure culture.

Experiments similar to those just described were also carried out, using B. pyogenes-foetidus instead of B. coli. Both B. coli and B. foetidus, it must be recalled, drive practically no ammonia from urea, but, in the process of fermentation of glucose and other carbohydrates, the former produces acid and gas, while the latter yields only acid. The experiments brought very much the same results as obtained with the colon bacillus. Accordingly, it may be concluded that the gas-former and the acid-producer act in the same way, so far as their effect on the urea-decomposition of the symbiotic bacteria is concerned.

It may be stated, in summarizing the results of these experiments of symbiosis, that the associative culture of an urea-splitting organism with a nonurea-splitting, fermentative bacterium liberates more ammonia from urea than the single culture of the former, in the medium containing a carbohydrate which is not attacked by the urea-splitting organism but fermented actively by the other, provided that the fermenter does not hamper the growth of the other to a great extent.

EXPERIMENTS WITH WASHED BACTERIA

That the urea-splitting organism yields more ammonia from urea in a medium containing an utilizable carbohydrate than in a plain medium has been brought out by the previous experimentation. Yet, as bacteria under ordinary circumstances grow better in a medium containing a proper carbohydrate than in a sugar-free medium, it is not unreasonable to suppose that the increase in ammonia production in this case is caused partly, if not entirely, by the increase in bacterial growth.

By means of washed bacteria, an attempt to throw light on this question was made in the following experiments.

Method.—Bacteria were seeded heavily on ordinary plain and 1% glucose agar plates. After incubation for 24 hours at 37 C. the bacteria were scraped off with an aluminium rod which has a flattened, dull-edged end, care being taken not to break the agar. To the mass of bacteria thus collected in a small beaker was added a proper amount of physiological salt solution, and a very dense bacterial suspension was prepared by careful mixing and vigorous stirring. The suspension was then centrifugated at a high speed, the supernatant fluid was poured away, salt solution was added, the bacteria were stirred up thoroughly, and the suspension centrifugated again. The bacteria were washed 5 times by repeating the process. Suspensions of bacteria in physiologic salt solution thus obtained were used. Densities of two kinds of suspensions of an organim, the one being of the bacteria grown on plain agar and the other of the organisms cultured on glucose agar, were matched macroscopically by comparing the shades of suspensions kept in tubes of approximately the same diameter.

Carefully cleansed test tubes were used as the containers of bacteria, urea and carbohydrates. The ratio of the mixture in a tube was: physiologic salt solution 7 cc., bacterial suspension 1 cc., 10% urea solution 1 cc., and 10% carbohydrate solution, or salt solution, 1 cc. The solutions of urea and carbohydrates were prepared originally with physiologic salt solution. Tubes were stopped tightly with rubber stoppers, and kept at 37 C. Ammonia was determined, in the same manner as described before, at different periods of incubation. Results of the experiments with B. ammoniagenes, B. aerogenes, B. proteus and Staphylococcus are shown in table 3.

Ammonia of the control tubes, that is, of the bacterial suspensions and of the urea solution—mixtures of the salt solution 9 cc. with the bacterial suspension 1 cc. and with the urea solution 1 cc. were examined —was nearly zero. And the bacteria, when one loopful of the suspension

Table 3.—Ammonia Nitrogen: Mg. per 100 Cc. of Medium

	Agar Medium	Urea	Urea Glucose	Urea Lactose	Incubation, Hours
B. ammoniagenes..........	Plain...........	305.2	309.4	308.0	4
		326.2	333.2	327.6	20
	Glucose........	308.0	309.4	306.6	4
		326.2	338.8	327.6	20
B. proteus [1]...............	Plain...........	9.8	14.0	11.2	5
		55.2	184.8	56.0	20
	Glucose........	11.2	16.8	11.2	5
		67.2	196.0	70.0	20
B. lactis-aerogenes.........	Plain...........	33.6	166.6	35.0	18
		81.2	305.2	98.0	42
	Glucose........	280.0	313.6	288.4	18
		281.4	333.2	308.0	42
Staphylococcus aureus.....	Plain...........	50.4	104.4	53.2	18
		92.4	278.6	109.2	42
	Glucose........	56.0	198.8	61.6	18
		106.4	324.8	120.4	42

was inoculated into the salt solution containing 1% glucose and 1% urea, did not grow to any noticeable degree. Figures in the table, therefore, would be considered as indicating the amounts of ammonia liberated from urea through the urea-decomposing action of the suspended bacteria; in other words, they would be interpreted as representing a catabolical, apart from an anabolical, phase of bacterial activities.

On the whole, the results show that washed bacteria disintegrated urea definitely, that the disintegration was intensified by the presence of glucose, and that bacteria grown on glucose agar plates seemed to have a stronger urease activity than those cultured on plain agar plates.

By comparing table 2 and table 6, it will be found that there is a discrepancy concerning the effect of carbohydrates. In both tables B. ammoniagenes and B. proteus gave similar results, which illustrates that glucose, but not lactose, exerts, strikingly to B. proteus and slightly to B. ammoniagenes, an accelerating influence on the ammonia production. In table 2 B. aerogenes shows that its urea decomposition is intensified by lactose and mannitol as significantly as by glucose, while in table 6 it indicates that the effect of lactose, in comparison with that of glucose, is almost nil. Staphylococcus also reveals the phenomenon essentially similar to that of B. aerogenes. Moreover, though not shown in the table, the effects of mannitol on B. aerogenes and Staphylococcus was identical to those of lactose.

There is interesting information which seems to provide a sound interpretation to the discrepancy mentioned above. That was brought out by the following experiment:

Four sets of clean test tubes—four tubes for a set—were arranged. Into each of them 8 cc. of physiologic salt solution were poured. And a drop of bromcresol purple indicator was added to all of the tubes. One cc. of distilled water or of 10% solutions of glucose, lactose and mannitol was added to tubes of a set. One cc. of a bacterial suspension was then added to each tube of a set. Suspensions of four kinds of bacteria employed in the main experiment, viz., B. ammoniagenes, B. proteus, B. aerogenes and Staphylococcus were thus made use of. After the incubation of 24 hours at 37 C. reactions of the tubes, as manifested by the change of color, were examined.

All of the control tubes, which did not contain any carbohydrate, remained changeless. B. ammoniagenes produced no change of color in all of the tubes. B. proteus showed a definite acid reaction in the glucose tube but not in the others. B. aerogenes exhibited an acid reaction, distinctly in the glucose tube and slightly in the lactose and mannitol tubes. Staphylococcus indicated the production of acid in the glucose tube, the others remaining practically without change.

Taking the acid reaction as an indication of the cleavage of carbohydrates, the results would be considered as illustrating that the washed bacteria, save B. ammoniagenes which appears to have an extremely feeble fermentative ability, attacked noticeably glucose only.

Then, the reason why lactose and mannitol did not accelerate the liberation of ammonia by suspension of washed B. aerogenes and Staphylococcus would seem to be that these washed bacteria could not cleave the carbohydrates to such an extent as they do glucose or as they can attack lactose and mannitol in the culture medium. This discrepancy of the effect of carbohydrates, on the other hand, seems to intimate that the growth phase of bacteria was practically eliminated in the experiments of washed bacteria, since if bacteria such as B. aerogenes and Staphylococcus had developed, they could have attacked lactose and mannitol markedly.

Influence of Thymol.—Thymol (methyl-isopropyl phenol) is a sparingly soluble substance (0.083 gm. to 100 cc. of water), which is used mostly as an anthelmintic and sometimes as an antiseptic. Influence of this substance on the urea-splitting action of washed bacteria was investigated.

In this experiment, physiologic salt solution, in which thymol has been dissolved by shaking, was used, in place of pure salt solution, as the main part of the mixture of bacterial suspension, urea and glucose. Otherwise, methods were identical to those of the preceding experiments of washed bacteria. All of the bacteria—B. ammoniagenes, B. aerogenes and Staphylococcus—were grown, before being washed, on 1% glucose agar plates. One organism was tested in two ways, that is, in the presence and in the absence of glucose. Ammonia was determined after the incubation of from 18 to 20 hours at 37 C., as shown in the following tabulation.

	Thymol	Urea	Glucose and urea
B. ammoniagenes	Without	351.4	359.6
	With	271.6	294.0
B. aerogenes	Without	274.4	336.0
	With	193.2	296.8
Staphylococcus	Without	190.4	324.8
	With	134.4	235.2

In brief, the results indicate that those washed bacteria were able to split urea in the presence of thymol, though their activity was impaired distinctly by this substance, and that, in the presence of thymol as in its absence, glucose accelerated the urease action of B. aerogenes and Staphylococcus considerably but that of B. ammoniagenes slightly. The mixture of urea and thymol did not liberate ammonia. Nor did the mixture of urea and the filtrate of B. ammoniagenes suspended in the salt solution containing thymol. Thence, it is obvious that the liberation of ammonia shown in the table manifests the activity of washed, suspended bacteria themselves.

The mixtures of glucose with suspensions of B. aerogenes and of Staphylococcus produced an acid reaction in the presence of thymol as definitely as in the absence of it. This finding is to support the previous observation that the accelerating effect of a carbohydrate on the urea decomposition seems to be in consequence of the utilization of the carbohydrate by bacteria.

It may not be useless to note here that an attempt was made to obtain bacterial urease in the filtrate of cultures. Filtrates of cultures of B. ammoniagenes, B. aerogenes and B. proteus in plain and glucose broths were examined at different periods of incubation for evidence of urease, but none of the sterile filtrates had urea-splitting action. Evidently the bacterial urease is an endoenzyme.

DISCUSSION

It has been brought out that not only glucose but other carbohydrates, such as lactose and mannitol, exert a definite accelerating influence on the disintegration of urea by various kinds of bacteria, either when added to the culture medium or when contained in the mixture of washed, suspended bacteria, albeit such substances do not give rise to the urease activity of an organism which is unable to split urea to any extent in the absence of them.

The acceleration seems to depend on the utilization; unless the urea-splitting organism attacks the carbohydrate catabolically, no intensifying effect can be detected. The fact that the presence of an utilizable carbohydrate increases markedly the liberation of ammonia from urea by washed bacteria intimates that the accelerating influence is essentially in a direct connection with the activity rather than the growth of bacteria.

It was revealed in the experiments of symbiosis that an urea-splitting organism can decompose urea more intensively in association with a nonurea-splitting, carbohydrophilic bacterium than it can do alone, in the medium containing a carbohydrate fermentable to the nonurea-splitting organism but not to the other. This phenomenon, on the one hand, can be explained by, and on the other hand, furnishes an evidence in support of, the statement that the acceleration and the utilization of a carbohydrate are in an inseparable relation.

The beneficial effect of carbohydrates on urea decomposition originates, as pointed out before, probably in some intermediate products of fermentation. It is of interest, in this connection, to recall that Jacoby [8] described pyruvic acid and lactic acid as accelerating substances for the urease activity of the proteus bacillus, whereas in this work sodium formate was proved to be almost effectless for various bacteria, some of which are able to decompose formic acid into hydrogen and carbon dioxyde. It is an established fact that formic, lactic and pyruvic acids are produced in the process of fermentation by diverse organisms.

When an organism attacks a carbohydrate catabolically, several kinds of acids, sometimes with gas, are produced which affect the medium. The question arises: does fermentation result in acidifying the medium and consequently stimulate the urea-decomposing action of bacteria? The finding of Takahata,[12] however, that the optimum reaction for the urease activity of B. proteus is at P_H 7.0, and the fact, as observed in this work, that the medium in which a vigorous urea decomposition takes place remains alkaline, even when an utilizable carbohydrate has been added, appear to rule out this question. Just how carbohydrates utilizable to bacteria give such an accelerating influence—by increasing the formation of urease, by simply stimulating the activity of urease, or by both—has not been elucidated. It is impossible at present to formulate precisely the exact relationship between accelerating substances and bacterial urease, owing to the lack of a method which enables the isolation of the enzyme itself.

SUMMARY

B. ammoniagenes, B. aerogenes, B. morgani, B. proteus vulgaris and Staphylococcus aureus actively decompose urea in culture mediums; the washed cells of these bacteria also possess a definite urea-splitting activity.

The presence of an utilizable carbohydrate accelerates the disintegration of urea by these bacteria, cultured and washed. Sodium formate added to the culture medium does not exert any increasing effect.

Thymol has an inhibitory influence on the liberation of ammonia from urea, by cultured or washed organisms, in the presence or absence of glucose.

The symbiosis of an urea-splitting organism with a nonurea-decomposing bacterium, in a medium containing a carbohydrate fermentable by the latter organism but not by the former, increases the generation of ammonia, in comparison with the single culture of the urea-splitting organism.

BEHAVIOR OF BRUCELLA MELITENSIS AND ABORTUS TOWARD GENTIAN VIOLET

I. Forest Huddleson and Elizabeth Abell

From the Department of Bacteriology and Hygiene, Michigan State College, East Lansing

Several years ago, it was pointed out by one of us [1] that Brucella abortus belonged to a group of bacteria, termed according to Churchman,[2] gentian-negative. It was further demonstrated that by incorporating the dye in a dilution of 1 : 250,000 to 1 : 500,000 in a suitable medium, a condition was created which made possible the isolation of Br. abortus from infective material, particularly milk, highly contaminated with gram-positive bacteria.

Recently, in culturing the organs of a group of guinea-pigs inoculated with a porcine strain of the Br. abortus variety, it was discovered that the strain in question failed to grow on a medium containing gentian violet in a 1 : 100,000 dilution, but grew well in the absence of the dye. This observation led us to institute a study of strains of the several varieties of this genus, according to the classification of Evans,[3] to ascertain if such an anomalous behavior toward different dilutions of gentian violet could be detected in other strains. The results of the study are presented in this paper.

Method of Study.—The medium used in the study was beef liver infusion agar prepared according to the formula given in a former paper.[4] A 2% aqueous solution of gentian violet was prepared and added to the medium in sufficient amounts to obtain dilutions of 1 : 50,000, 1 : 100,000 and 1 : 250,000 of the original dye. The three batches of medium were poured into petri dishes, and after jellying, were placed in an incubator over night to evaporate the condensed liquid which had collected on the surface of the medium. The plates were divided into three sections so that three strains could be cultivated on a single plate.

The cultures under study, with the exception of newly isolated ones, were grown aerobically on beef liver infusion agar slants at 37 C. for 72 hours. The newly isolated strains of bovine origin were grown in an increased CO_2 atmosphere. The resulting growth of each culture was suspended in the water of condensation, about 0.4 cc., at the bottom of the slant. A platinum loop (3 mm. diameter) full of the dense suspension was streaked across the surface of plates of the medium containing each of the three dilutions of the dye and also one containing no dye. By using a dense suspension of the organism the question of

Received for publication, Jan. 18, 1928.

1. Huddleson, I. Forest: Tech. Bull. 49, pt. 4, Michigan Agric. Exper. Station, 1920.
2. Churchman, John W.: J. Exper. Med., 1912, 16, p. 221.
3. Evans, Alice C.: Hyg. Lab. Bull. 143, 1925.
4. Huddleson, I. Forest; Hasley, D. E., and Torrey, J. P.: J. Infect. Dis., 1926, 40, p. 352.

the lack of communal activity was obviated in case the growth of a certain strain was inhibited. In addition the piling up of growth on the surface of the medium was avoided. The inoculated plates, excepting those inoculated with newly isolated strains were incubated aerobically at 37 C. for 72 hours. This length of time is considered sufficient for microorganisms of this genus to reach maximum growth, providing there was not complete inhibition. The results were recorded by comparing the amount of growth with that obtained on the medium minus the dye.

The growth behavior of 42 strains of Br. melitensis—paramelitensis of caprine and human origin, 95 strains of Br. abortus—paraabortus of bovine, human and porcine origin from various parts of Europe and the United States has been studied. The strains were furnished us

TABLE 1.—HISTORY OF STRAINS OF BR. MELITENSIS-PARAMELITENSIS AND THEIR GROWTH BEHAVIOR TOWARD GENTIAN VIOLET

Strain	Where Isolated	Received From	Host	Variety	Dilution of Gentian Violet: 1:250,000 and 1:100,000	Dilution of Gentian Violet: 1:50,000
27	Not known	Dr. K. F. Meyer	Caprine	Melitensis	++++	++++
20	Not known	Dr. K. F. Meyer	Not known	Melitensis	++++	++++
3U	Italy	Dr. C. Cerruti	Human	Melitensis	++++	++++
4U	Italy	Dr. C. Cerruti	Human	Melitensis	++++	+++
504	Italy	A. C. Evans	Caprine	Melitensis	++++	+++
462	Texas	A. C. Evans	Human	Melitensis	++++	++++
47	Tunisia	Dr. Et. Burnet	Caprine	Melitensis	++++	++++
Ost	Tunisia	Dr. Et. Burnet	Human	Melitensis	++++	++++
Soria	Tunisia	Dr. Et. Burnet	Human	Melitensis	++++	++
5	Tunisia	Dr. Et. Burnet	Human	Melitensis	++++	++++
10	Tunisia	Dr. Et. Burnet	Caprine	Melitensis	++++	+++
70	Tunisia	Dr. Et. Burnet	Caprine	Melitensis	++++	+++
104	Malta	A. C. Evans	Human	Melitensis B	++++	++++
522	Malta	A. C. Evans	Caprine	Melitensis B	++++	++++
525	Malta	A. C. Evans	Caprine	Melitensis B	++++	++++
520	Malta	A. C. Evans	Human	Melitensis B	++++	+++
521	Malta	A. C. Evans	Caprine	Paramelitensis	++++	++++
509	Tunisia	A. C. Evans	Caprine	Paramelitensis	++++	++++
Alia	Tunisia	Dr. Et. Burnet	Human	Paramelitensis	++++	++++
83	Tunisia	Dr. Et. Burnet	Human	Paramelitensis	++++	++++
92	Tunisia	Dr. Et. Burnet	Human	Paramelitensis	++++	++++

through the kindness of the individuals mentioned. It was considered unnecessary to present data on all of the stains of the genus Brucella in our possession that have been studied. The presentation of data on the dye affinity of a number of strains in each of the varieties should be sufficiently convincing.

In table 1 is recorded the history of 16 strains of Br. melitensis and of 5 strains of Br. paramelitensis and their growth in the presence of gentian violet; in table 2, 21 strains of Br. abortus of bovine origin; in table 3, 19 strains of Br. abortus and one strain of Br. paraabortus of human origin; and in table 4, 12 strains of Br. abortus of porcine origin. The variety to which the strains of Br. melitensis and Br. paramelitensis belonged, with the exception of those obtained from

Drs. Burnet, Cerruti and Meyer, was determined by Evans [3] according to their absorbing capacities. The strains of Br. abortus of bovine, human and porcine origin were classified in the laboratory from whence they were sent, by means of reciprocal agglutinin absorption tests and confirmed by the writers.

EXPERIMENTAL DATA

The growth behavior of the strains of Br. melitensis and Br. paramelitensis is recorded in table 1. It is apparent from the percentages of growth recorded that none of the strains is inhibited by the dye in dilutions of 1 : 250,000 and 1 : 100,000. A few strains are slightly inhibited by a 1 : 50,000 dilution of the dye. The growth behavior

TABLE 2.—HISTORY OF BOVINE STRAINS OF BR. ABORTUS AND THEIR GROWTH BEHAVIOR TOWARD GENTIAN VIOLET

Strain (Abortus Variety)	Where Isolated	Received From	Dilution of Gentian Violet		
			1:250,000	1:100,000	1:50,000
2	Michigan	Mich. State College	++++	++++	++
90	Michigan	Mich. State College	++++	+++	+
920	Michigan	Mich. State College	++++	+++	++
60	Michigan	Mich. State College	++++	+++	+
200	Michigan	Mich. State College	++++	+++	+
B144	Michigan	Mich. State College	++++	+++	+
6	Michigan	Mich. State College	++++	+++	0
216	Michigan	Mich. State College	++++	+++	0
206	Michigan	Mich. State College	++++	+++	++
670	Michigan	Mich. State College	++++	++++	++
A754	Michigan	Mich. State College	++++	+++	+
221	Michigan	Mich. State College	+++	+	0
400	Michigan	Mich. State College	++++	+	0
239	Michigan	Mich. State College	++++	+++	+
B167	Michigan	Mich. State College	++++	++	0
C111	Michigan	Mich. State College	++++	+++	+
H16	Kansas	Dr. Lenheart	++++	+++	++
2509	California	Dr. Traum	++++	+++	++
King	England	Sir. S. Stockman	++++	+++	++
172	England	Sir. S. Stockman	++++	+++	0
80	California	Dr. Carpenter	+	0	0

of the remaining strains in our possession, but not recorded herein, coincides with the results presented in the table.

It is of interest to note in the light of our own findings, that in his first studies on the behavior of bacteria toward gentian violet, Churchman [2] placed a strain 33, of Br. melitensis in the gentian-positive group. This strain was obtained from the American Museum of Natural History. Its origin apparently is unknown.

The effects of the three dilutions of dye on the growth of 21 strains of Br. abortus, bovine origin, are set forth in table 2. It may be observed that, with the exception of strain 80, none of the strains is inhibited by a 1 : 250,000 dilution of the dye, but a 1 : 100,000 dilution does retard the growth of nearly all strains. A dilution of

1 : 50,000 completely inhibited the growth of seven strains and noticeably retarded the growth of the others. The growth of the remaining bovine strains in our laboratory is affected by these dilutions of the dye in a similar degree.

The growth inhibiting action of a 1 : 50,000 dilution of the dye is nearly sufficient to serve as a means of distinguishing this variety of the genus Brucella from the variety Br. melitensis. The inhibition of the growth of strain 80 is interesting in that not another strain of bovine origin in our possession in inhibited to the same degree. In connection with the difference in growth behavior of this strain, it may be said that it reveals no difference from other bovine strains

TABLE 3.—HISTORY OF HUMAN STRAINS OF BR. ABORTUS AND THEIR GROWTH BEHAVIOR TOWARD GENTIAN VIOLET

Strain (Abortus Variety)	Where Isolated	Received From	Dilution of Gentian Violet		
			1:250,000	1:100,000	1:50,000
528	S. Dakota	A. C. Evans	+++	0	0
455	Maryland	A. C. Evans	+++	±	0
534	Utah	A. C. Evans	+++	0	0
533	New York State	A. C. Evans	+++	0	0
531	Connecticut	A. C. Evans	++	0	0
L	New York State	Dr. C. M. Carpenter	++	0	0
W	New York State	Dr. C. M. Carpenter	++	0	0
Wa	New York State	Dr. C. M. Carpenter	+++	±	0
X	New York State	Dr. C. M. Carpenter	+	0	0
K	New York State	Dr. C. M. Carpenter	+++	0	0
44	New York State	Dr. C. M. Carpenter	+++	0	0
Smith II	California	Dr. K. F. Meyer	++++	+++	+
Clark	Indiana	Dr. Girdano	++++	++++	++
Woll	Michigan	Mich. State College	++++	++++	++
Par	Michigan	Mich. State College	++++	+++	+
Dun	Michigan	Mich. State College	++++	++++	+
Bart	Michigan	Mich. State College	++++	+++	+
Du. Rand	Rhodesia, S. A.	Dr. Ross	++++	++	0
Narcee	Rhodesia, S. A.	Dr. Ross	++++	++	0
William	Rhodesia, S. A.	Dr. Ross	++++	++	0
Weldon (para-abortus)	Rhodesia, S. A.	Dr. Ross	++++	++	0

according to reciprocal agglutinin absorption tests. This fact was established by Feusier and Meyer [5] who first studied strain 80 together with other strains of the bovine group. Strain 80 was originally isolated by Meyer in 1920, from certified milk in California.

The growth behavior of the human strains of the abortus variety is presented in table 3. It may be seen at once that there is a wide difference in the growth of the strains of this variety isolated from humans; a difference great enough to classify the strains into two separate groups according to their behavior toward gentian violet, namely group 1 and group 2. Let group 1 include those strains that are inhibited from growing on the medium in the presence of a

5. Ibid., 1920, 27, p. 185.

1 : 100,000 and 1 : 50,000 dilution of the dye and markedly retarded from growing in the presence of a 1 : 250,000 dilution of the dye. Let group 2 include those that are not affected by a 1 : 250,000 dilution of the dye, but are retarded in their growth as the concentration of the dye increases. The strains in group 1 were isolated from human cases of undulant fever in widely distributed sections of the United States. None of the strains in this group came from Michigan. The source of the strains causing the disease in humans was in some cases, traced to porcine origin, in others, to the ingestion of raw milk containing Br. abortus.

The strains falling into group 2 were isolated in Michigan, in Indiana, California and in Rhodesia, South Africa. We have isolated six other strains in Michigan, not recorded in the table, that fall into this group. According to their reaction toward the different dilutions of

TABLE 4.—HISTORY OF PORCINE STRAINS OF BR. ABORTUS AND THEIR GROWTH BEHAVIOR TOWARD GENTIAN VIOLET

Strain (Abortus Variety)	Where Isolated	Received From	Dilution of Gentian Violet 1:250,000	1:100,000 and 1:50,000
Ky	Kentucky	Prof. Good	+++	0
481	Missouri	A. C. Evans	+++	0
H. F. 4	California	Dr. Traum	++	0
2A	California	Dr. Traum	++	0
M18	Missouri	Dr. Connaway	++	0
168	Missouri	Dr. Connaway	+++	0
Jac.	Missouri	Dr. Connaway	+	0
Iw. 5	Iowa	Dr. Buchanan	++	0
2012	Illinois	Dr. Graham	+++	0
4H	Hungary	Royal Vet. College	++	0
5H	Hungary	Royal Vet. College	++	0
7H	Hungary	Royal Vet. College	+++	0

the dye, the human strains falling into group 2 behave very much like the bovine strains, with the exception of strain 80. Group 1 human strains parallel strain 80 in their behavior toward the dye.

The effects of the dilutions of the dye on the growth of 12 porcine strains of the abortus variety are presented in table 4. It is apparent that the strains show an astonishing sensitivity toward the three dilutions of gentian violet in the medium. All fail to show visible growth in the presence of two of the dilutions of the dye, namely 1 : 50,000 and 1 : 100,000 and are retarded markedly in their growth by the presence of a 1 : 250,000 dilution of the dye in the medium. The sensitivity of the porcine strains toward gentian violet parallels the action of group 1 human strains of the abortus variety and also bovine strain, 80.

There is no resemblance between the swine strains and the bovine strains which we have studied, according to their behavior toward gentian violet, in spite of the fact that no difference can be distinguished between them (excepting strain 481) by means of reciprocal agglutinin absorption tests. In other words, a physiological irrelation is possible of detection in strains of the same variety, where no distinguishable antigenic difference appears to exist.

DISCUSSION OF RESULTS

This study was concerned with a genus of microorganisms, separable into two major varieties, namely, abortus and melitensis. Each major variety is divisible into subvarieties. The microorganisms falling into the genus are identical in so far as the cultural, morphological and tinctorial characteristics are concerned.

It has been observed that the major varieties of the genus Brucella differ in their growth activity on a medium containing certain concentrations of gentian violet, and a group of strains in one variety hereto-fore indistinguishable, exhibit, according to their behavior toward the dye, a remarkable difference from others of the same variety. This group is comprised of the porcine strains, several of the human strains and one bovine strain in our possession.

The first observation of the exhibition of gentian violet fastness by a strain of gram-negative species of organisms was made by Churchman.[6] The strain belonged to the Bacillus enteritidis group and was otherwise indistinguishable. Churchman[7] also separated a "strain from within a strain" of Bacillus coli which also failed to grow in the presence of certain dilutions of the dye. He observed, also, that these two gram-negative organisms would not grow even if they were suspended in dilutions of the dye before planting on mediums.

Churchman asserted in a later communication[8] "that in a large number of experiments made with gentian violet and allied dyes, no single exception to this parallelism between the selective behavior of the dye when present in the medium, and its selective behavior when added directly to the bacteria, has ever been encountered; organisms which are 'killed' by exposure to the stain never grow when it is present in the medium on which they are planted unstained; and organisms which are not affected by exposure to the dye grow readily on media containing it."

6. J. Exper. Med., 1912, 16, p. 822.
7. Ibid., 1921, 33, p. 569.
8. Ibid., 1923, 37, p. 543.

When the dye fast strains of the abortus variety were suspended in an aqueous solution of the dye, we were astonished to find that a luxuriant growth occurred when they were planted on a solid medium minus the dye. There was no noticeable inhibition of growth even when they were suspended in a 1 : 10,000 dilution of the dye for 48 hours.

This is apparently the first time a group of strains "within a variety" of a gram-negative organism have been distinguished from others in the same variety by their inability to grow on a medium containing certain concentrations of gentian violet.

The factor or factors that are responsible for the peculiar behavior of a certain group of strains of Br. abortus toward gentian violet, arouses considerable speculation. The dye fastness can neither be explained on the basis of "variants" within a strain since no artificial environmental conditions have been employed to induce the difference, nor as a transient occurrence, since repeated examinations of the strains in question during the past eight months have given the same results. It may be stated, however, that all strains of the genus can be made gentian-positive by increasing the P_H of the medium to 7.2. This observation confirms the experiments of Stearn and Stearn,[9] who have shown that the bacteriostatic action of a dye depends on the P_H of the medium on which a given organism is grown. That is to say, alkalinity increases the bacteriostatic action of a basic dye for an organism whose P_H for optimum growth is on the acid side.

The explanation for the exhibition of bacteriostasis on the part of the strains of Br. abortus in question may be found by studying the sulphur metabolism of the major varieties of the genus, that is to say, the ability of the strains to reduce sulphur containing compounds to hydrogen sulphide. Our studies of the sulphur metabolism, which will be presented in another paper, have revealed that strains differ markedly in hydrogen sulphide production and, further, that a striking relation exists between the amount of hydrogen sulphide produced and the degree of inhibition in growth, or fastness to gentian violet in the medium. In other words, growth inhibition, due to gentian violet, is directly proportional to the amount of hydrogen sulphide produced by a given strain.

The porcine and human strains and one bovine strain of Br. abortus produce an abundance of hydrogen sulphide gas. They are likewise the ones most affected in their growth by the dye. The remaining

9. J. Bact., 1926, 11, p. 345.

bovine and human strains vary in hydrogen sulphide production, and never produce the quantity that the first mentioned ones do. The Br. melitensis and paramelitensis strains in our possession have never been found to produce even a trace of hydrogen sulphide aerobically, if the cystine content of the medium is kept below 0.01 per cent, and likewise are not inhibited in their growth by the dilutions of the dye used in this study. It therefore, appears to us that a chemical combination takes place between the dye and the hydrogen sulphide, of such a nature as to retard or prevent the growth of strains, according to their ability to produce the gas. The difference which we have observed in the porcine strains and several of the human strains as regards their behavior to gentian violet tends to confirm what Smith [10] has said with respect to the difference between porcine and human strains and bovine strains in their pathogenicity for guinea-pigs. It cannot be said with certainty that all gentian fast strains of this genus are the porcine type regardless of origin until more strains from different sources and different parts of the country are studied.

The difference in strains of this genus as manifested by their action toward gentian violet has some practical significance in that it furnishes more light on the source of undulant fever in this country, and should aid in the classification of human strains of the genus already isolated and those which will be isolated in the future. It may prove to be a certain means of determining the variety of the strains already isolated and those which will be isolated in the future.

Recently, we have encountered two other violet-positive stains of Br. abortus of bovine origin.

Further proof of the existence of two groups of the abortus variety has been obtained by using other dyes of the tri-phenol methane series, and thionin. The latter dye inhibits the growth of the bovine abortus variety, but not the porcine or melitensis varieties.

CONCLUSIONS

Varieties, and strains within a variety, of the genus Brucella exhibit a difference in sensitiveness to gentian violet in a medium, expressed in degree of growth. The growth of strains of the Br. melitensis and paramelitensis variety is not inhibited on a medium by the presence of gentian violet in dilutions of 1 : 100,000 and 1 : 250,000. A few of the strains are slightly inhibited by the presence of a 1 : 50,000

10. J. Exper. Med., 1926, 43, p. 207.

dilution of the dye. Strains of the Br. abortus variety may be divided into two groups as regards their ability to grow on a medium in which gentian violet is present, namely, those which are markedly inhibited and those which fail to grow in the presence of 1 : 50,000 and 1 : 100,000 dilution of the dye. The latter group contains one bovine strain, several human strains and all porcine strains in the possession of the writers.

The difference in dye sensitivity may prove to be a means of distinguishing strains of the abortus variety not otherwise distinguishable.

THE ACTION OF PHENOL AND FORMOL ON AEROBIC AND ANAEROBIC ORGANISMS

JOSEPH P. SCOTT

From the Veterinary Department, Kansas State Agricultural Experiment Station, Manhattan

The action of dilute solutions of phenol and formol was studied on cultures of spore-forming and nonspore-forming organisms. The phenol stock solution was made up by adding 5 cc. of melted crystaline phenol c. p. to 95 cc. of water. The 5% formol solution was made by adding 12.5 cc. of commercial 40% formaldehyde to 87.5 cc. of water.

The cultures used were anaerobic spore-forming organisms, Clostridium chauvoei, Cl. septicus, Cl. botulinum A and B., Cl. welchii, Cl. novyi, Cl. tetani, Cl. tertius, Cl. multifermentans, and Cl. histolyticus. The aerobic spore forming organisms were B. anthracis, B. subtilis, B. mycoides and B. megatherium. Nonspore-forming anaerobes were Micrococcus gasogenes and C. fallax. The nonspore-forming aerobes were Escherichia coli, Eberthelia bienstockii, Micrococcus cereus and Staphylococcus aureus. Cultures of all these organisms were transferred to brain liver medium and in the case of the aerobes to liver broth in addition, the amount of medium in each tube being about 18 cc. After 24 to 48 hours incubation 2 to 3 cc. of 5% phenol or 5% formol were added to the tubes, making dilutions of 0.5 and 0.75%. Subcultures from these tubes were made at intervals of 2, 4, 6, 15 and 24 hours, also of 2, 3 and 4 days and after one to 3 or 4 weeks at room temperature and at 37 C.

It was found that phenol in strengths of 0.5% (2 cc. of 5% phenol to 18 cc. culture) did not destroy any of the anaerobes studied during the course of one month either at room temperature or in the incubator. Strengths of 1% had also no affect. Five per cent solutions sterilized some cultures in a few days, others were not affected for ten days. Isolations of Cl. chauvoei and Cl. welchii were made from fresh muscle kept in 2% and 5% phenol solution for four days and from material kept in 1% phenol for ten days. Tubes containing muscle covered with 15 cc. of 1% and 2% phenol developed gas and cloudiness when incubated for 24 hours.

Among the aerobes B. anthracis and B. vulgatus were also resistant to 0.5% phenol for two weeks. B. coli was in some cases still viable after ten days in 0.5% phenol brain liver medium. B. subtilis was also

Received for publication, Jan. 28, 1928.

occasionally found viable after exposure for one week to 0.5% phenol. B. dysenteriae, B. mycoides, and B. megatherium were sterilized in from four to seven days.

The nonspore-forming anaerobes withstood concentrations of 0.5% phenol. The nonspore-forming aerobes, however, were destroyed in from 12 hours to two days.

Formol in strengths of 0.5% (2 cc. of 5% formol to 18 cc. of culture) sterilized all aerobic organisms both spore-forming and non-spore-forming in six to twelve hours.

The saccharolytic anaerobes, Cl. chauvoei, Cl. septicus, Cl. tertius, and Cl. welchii were sterilized in 48 hours. The proteolytic types Cl. tetani, Cl. sporogenes, Cl. botulinum, and Cl. histolyticus were not readily sterilized by this strength of formol. These organisms were sterilized in four days by 0.5% formol which sterilized the other anaerobes in six to twelve hours.

The stricking difference between the action of phenol and formol on anaerobic and aerobic organisms has led to the use of these disinfectants for the elimination of aerobic organisms during the course of isolation of anaerobic cultures. Cultures containing both aerobes and anaerobes are purified by inoculating two tubes of brain liver medium containing 0.5% phenol with one loopful of the mixed culture. One of these tubes is then heated to 65 C. for 15 minutes. These two subcultures are incubated for 24 hours and the process repeated. An agar slant test for aerobes is made each time. After two to five transfers the aerobe will be found to have been eliminated.

It is often possible to hasten the action of phenol or formol by using a 24 to 48 hour culture of the mixture. Two cc. of 5% phenol or 2 cc. of 5% formol is added to the culture medium which is then heated to 75 or 80 C. for five minutes. After cooling subcultures are made to fresh brain liver medium and to agar slants. One such treatment is usually sufficient to eliminate the aerobe.

The older the culture the greater heat can be applied. Leclainche and Vallee [1] find that spores of 24-hour cultures of Cl. chauvoei are killed at 70 C. in one-half hour. Four day old spores resist a temperature of 80 C. for two hours and 95 C. for one-half hour. Dry spores are not killed at 100 to 105 C. for one-half hour. Two-tenths cc. of commercial 40 cc. formol seemed to have a greater efficiency than 2 cc. of 5% formol in the sterilization of anaerobic cultures.

1. Rev. Gen. Med. Vet., 1925, 34, p. 292.

The possibility of pathogenic anaerobes developing in biological products containing 0.5% phenol and causing disease must be guarded against by special care in the production of these products. Anaerobic culture mediums such as brain liver or meat piece mediums should be included in all sterility tests and should be inoculated with from 5 to 10 cc. of the material to be tested. Recent reports of losses in cattle and poultry following the use of biological products have been proved to be due to the presence of pathogenic anaerobes or their toxins in the products used.

SUMMARY

It is shown that phenol in strengths up to 5% acts very slowly on anaerobic organisms, while formaldehyde in dilutions of 0.5 to 0.75% sterilizes anaerobic cultures rapidly.

The greater susceptibility of aerobic spore-forming organisms to these disinfectants make it possible to eliminate aerobic contaminations from anaerobic cultures by the use of 0.5% phenol or formol.

RICKETTSIA OF ROCKY MOUNTAIN SPOTTED FEVER IN THE BRAIN OF THE INFECTED GUINEA-PIG

HOBART A. REIMANN*

From the Pathological Institute of the German University, Prague, Czechoslovakia

From the studies of Wolbach[1] and Nicholson[2] it is evident that Rickettsia associated with Rocky Mountain spotted fever (Dermacentroxenus rickettsi) are invariably found only in tissues showing the characteristic vascular lesions described in the literature. Wolbach states that the central nervous system in animals suffering from Rocky Mountain spotted fever shows no lesions attributable to that disease and one must therefore assume that this tissue contains no parasites. It is known, however, that the brain tissue of infected guinea-pigs serves as good material for the experimental transfer of Rocky Mountain spotted fever from one guinea-pig to another. Breinl[3] has shown by titration experiments that the brain of an infected guinea-pig, and also the testes, contains approximately 100,000 infectious doses. Therefore a tissue which is apparently free from organisms (brain) and a tissue (testes) in which the organisms are present in abundance are equally infectious.

The blood of animals suffering from the disease contains Rickettsia and it is also highly infectious. According to Connor,[4] .001 cc. of blood is often sufficient for infecting another animal. It is, of course, possible that the infectiousness of the brain tissue, as demonstrated by Breinl, is due merely to the organisms in the blood remaining in the vascular system of the brain. The quantity of blood remaining in the brains of the guinea-pigs employed in his experiments was, however, very small, since the animals were killed by exsanguination. The infectiousness of the brain tissue seemed to be far out of proportion to that of the testicular tissue, in view of the abundance of Rickettsia demonstrable in the testes. It appeared to be important, therefore, to determine whether the infectiousness of brain tissue is due to Rickettsia harbored in the nervous tissue, or whether, in spite of the absence of characteristic vas-

Received for publication, Jan. 23, 1928.

* Fellow in Medicine, National Research Council.

1. J. M. Research, 1919, 41, p. 1.
2. J. Exper. Med., 1923, 36, p. 211.
3. Ztschr. f. Immunitätsforsch. u. exper. Therap., 1926, 46, p. 123.
4. J. Infant Diseases, 1924, 35, p. 587.

cular lesions, they are present in the walls of the blood vessels, or, finally, whether they are present in sufficient numbers in the residual blood in the brain to account for the infectiousness of brain tissue.

Material and Methods.—The pathologic material used in this study was obtained from guinea-pigs used by Breinl during a study of another aspect of Rocky Mountain spotted fever. The brains and testes of 8 guinea-pigs were examined. The animals were infected by injecting intraperitoneally an emulsion of the spleen of an infected animal, and they were killed by exsanguination at intervals of from one to eight days after the onset of the characteristic fever. Two animals died spontaneously from the disease on the eighth day of the fever. Necropsies were made immediately after death in all instances, and the tissues at once placed in Zenker's fluid. The brains were cut sagittally or transversely, and several serial sections from four different levels were examined. Sections were prepared and stained with Giemsa's stain, according to the techic described by Wolbach.[1]

Observations.—Careful examination of the brain tissue and cerebral vascular tissue from the 8 guinea-pigs did not reveal the presence of Rickettsia, and no pathological changes attributable to Rocky Mountain spotted fever could be demonstrated in the brains. Evidence of meningo-encephalitis was present in some of the brains examined, but the same changes were also found in several normal control guinea-pigs.

Rickettsia, however, were found in the lumen of a vein in the brain of one guinea-pig which was killed while in a moribund state, on the eighth day after the onset of the fever (10th day after infection). This animal showed characteristic extensive petechial hemorrhages of the skin of the paws, ears and scrotum, with necrosis of the latter. Sections from the skin and testes showed many of the parasites in the vascular lesions, while sections of the brain showed no organisms anywhere in the tissues. Rickettsia were found in only one location, grouped in the blood in the lumen of a rather large tangentially cut vein in the cerebral cortex, as shown in figures 1 and 2. None of the organisms appeared to be located within the erythrocytes, but one cluster seemed to be enclosed within an enthothelial cell. A similar and corresponding area in the same vein, in the next serial section on the same slide was searched for the organisms but none could be found.

Rickettsia present in this small area in the brain, and those present elsewhere in the tissues of the guinea-pigs, did not differ materially in morphology from those described previously in the literature, except

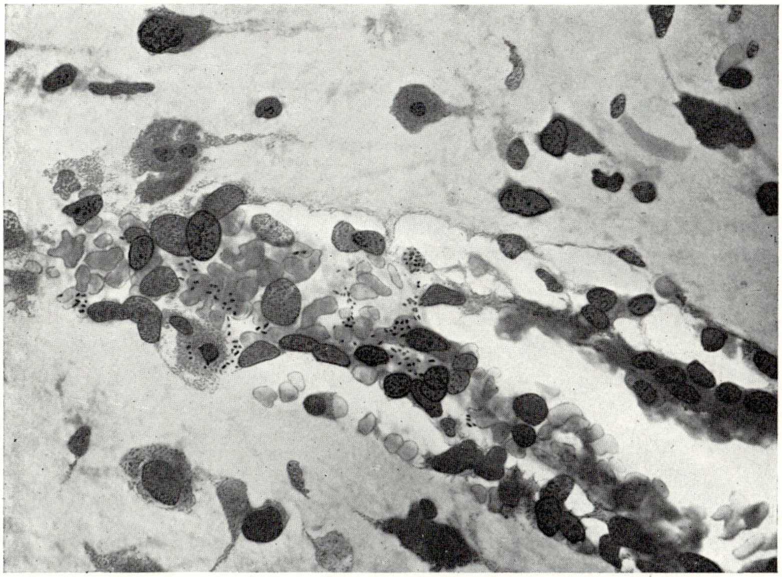

Fig. 1.—Section of vein, cortex of cerebrum, showing Rickettsia in the lumen. Retouched photograph at 950 diameters.

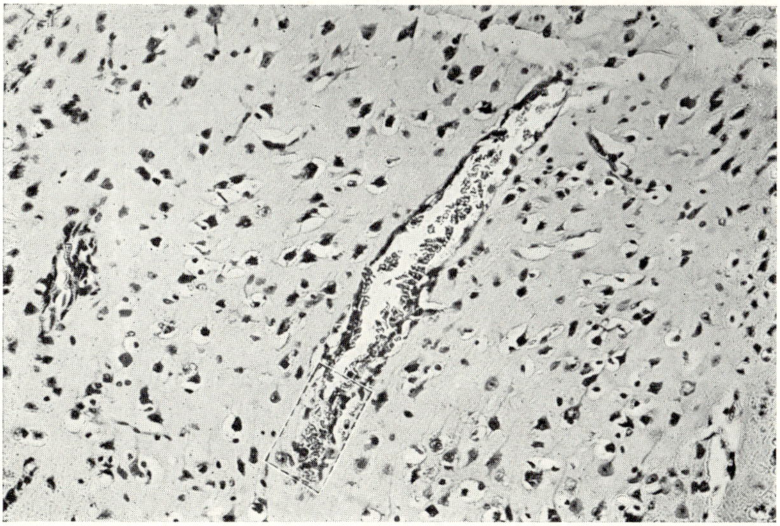

Fig. 2.—Same vein reduced to 110 diametetrs to show the general character of the area containing the organisms.

that, in agreement with Nicholson,[2] and Connor,[4] no definite coccoid or diplococcoid forms were recognized. As shown in figure 1, several Rickettsia seem to represent coccoid forms, but it is likely that these are cross sections or end-on views of the bacillary forms.

Summary.—The reason for the infectiousness of the brain tissue of guinea-pigs has been sought, since previous investigations have not demonstrated Rickettsia of Rocky Mountain spotted fever in the nervous tissue of animals suffering from that disease. In the present study Rickettsia were found in only one of the eight brains examined, and in this instance the organisms were located in the blood in the lumen of a vein in the cerebrum. On the other hand, many Rickettsia were present in the vascular lesions of the testes of all of the animals examined. Considering the apparent scarcity of demonstrable organisms in the tissues of the brain and the abundance of organisms in the testes, and assuming that Rickettsia are the actual cause of the disease, it is still difficult to explain the fact that these two tissues are equally infective. If the presence of Rickettsia in the blood in the brain does account for the infectiousness of that tissue, the number of organisms present in the minute amount of blood remaining in the brains of animals killed by exsanguination, can scarcely account for the arbitrary 100,000 infectious doses, even if .001 cc. of blood is often infectious. It is possible, however, that many more Rickettsia are present in the brain than can be demonstrated with the technic now available. On account of their extremely small size and the fact that Rickettsia as a rule stain less intensely than bacteria and are rapidly decolorized, they may be easily overlooked, especially when the organisms are single and isolated instead of in clumps. Another possibility is that very few organisms suffice for infection, as in other Rickettsial diseases, and that the abundance of the organisms in the testes is superfluous. Until further work indicates otherwise, however, it appears that Rickettsia present in the blood of the brain account for the infectiousness of that tissue.

SURFACE TENSION IN RELATION TO BACTERIAL GROWTH

WITH SPECIAL REFERENCE TO LACTOBACILLUS ACIDOPHILUS AND LACTOBACILLUS BULGARICUS

ALEXANDER ALFRED DAY AND WILLIAM MERRIOTT GIBBS

From the Department of Bacteriology and Patten Research Laboratories, Northwestern University Medical School, Chicago

Interest in surface tension as a factor in bacterial development was aroused by the work of Larson in 1919, and the development of methods of determining surface tension, notably by Fahrenwald and by du Noüy, have given the study an added impetus. As a result of recent investigations there are many conflicting data and the exact relationship of surface tension and bacterial development is a debated question. The physical forces involved in a culture medium are in such close association with the chemical factors that an entire separation is frequently not possible. Surface tension variation without radical chemical change presents a difficult study, and one which has led to much confusion. It is quite a simple matter to vary the surface tension of a culture medium for the development of bacteria, but to do so and at the same time not alter the chemical nature of the medium is a different matter. On the addition of substances designed to reduce surface tension the chemical nature of the depressant frequently is a factor which overbalances the factor of surface tension. In any event the only possible means of determining the effect of surface tension as the variant is to employ a sufficient number of well selected depressants that the chemical effect of each may be recognized. When such procedure is established it may be found that surface tension plays a minor rôle in the results obtained.

There are no two methods of determining the surface tension of a liquid which will give identical values. The film method developed by Fahrenwald is quite simple and yields values in relatively close accord with those obtained by the du Noüy tensiometer. It is readily applicable to bacteriological problems and has the advantage of ready control of temperature and dispersion of depressants, the importance of which was pointed out by Pizarro.

Received for publication, Jan. 14, 1928.

THE LITERATURE

Avery [1] made use of the observation that soaps prevent the growth of certain bacteria and on this principle developed a culture medium for the cultivation of the influenza bacillus. The inhibitory action of the soap was attributed to the chemical action and no suggestion was made that surface tension played a rôle. It has since been suggested that surface tension might have been instrumental in the results obtained, but in the light of more recent experiments it appears that the chemical nature of the soap was the responsible factor and that surface tension had no part in the reaction.

Larson, Cantwell and Hartzell [2] were undoubtedly the first to make a direct study of the effect of surface tension on the growth of bacteria. They studied the effect of lowered surface tension on the growth and characteristics of certain organisms, and concluded that the growth of bacteria in ordinary broth was greatly influenced by the surface tension of the medium. The surface tension was lowered by additions of castor oil soap and measured by the drop weight method. The standard broth employed had a surface tension of 59.0 dynes per cm. B. subtilis did not form a pellicle when the surface tension was reduced to 45 dynes, but grew in the body of the medium. They concluded that all pellicle formers ceased to grow at the surface when the surface tension was below 45 dynes per cm. B. subtilis was found to form spores more slowly in a medium of lowered surface tension.

Some anaerobes, particularly B. tetani, were found to grow aerobically in a medium of lowered surface tension. The authors suggest that the favorable action of the oil seal in anaerobiosis is probably due to the lowered surface tension. They are inclined to believe that the toxicity of the depressant is a factor of more or less importance. In a later report Larson [3] found the surface tension of ordinary broth to be about 59 dynes, and inorganic mediums with glycerol as a source of carbon, 73 dynes. The surface tension was depressed by additions of castor oil soap, giving a range from 32.0 to 73.0 dynes per cm. The growth of pneumococcus and streptococcus was depressed at a surface tension of 50 dynes and lower. The limit of B. anthracis was sharply defined at 46 dynes. The intestinal bacteria grew well at lowered surface tension. The ability of this group to develop in mediums of low surface tension was thought to be related to the resistance of the group to bile, which has a low surface tension. The concentration of the colon-typhoid group of bacteria at the surface of the medium was attributed to the concentration of the surface tension depressants at the surface. Pellicle formers were found to grow throughout the body of the medium when the surface tension was reduced, while non-pellicle formers developed pellicles after long cultivation in mediums of high surface tension. It was suggested that in some cases symbiosis and antibiosis were due to surface tension. Larson and Montauk [4] cultivated tubercle bacilli in a medium containing soap and glycerol and found that the organisms grew in this medium with a diffuse cloudiness, and appeared to have lost all pathogenicity, giving rise merely to local and temporary nodules on injection into guinea-pigs. They ascribe the attenuation to the lowered surface tension.

It is not surprising that interest in surface tension as a factor in bacterial development was aroused by the above statements of Larson and associates. If indeed all these suggestions and theories are true our prospects for productive research of untold interest are most encouraging. It is interesting to note that

[1] J. Am. M. A., 1918, 71, p. 2050.

[2] J. Infect. Dis., 1919, 25, p. 41.

[3] Abstr. Bact., 1921, 5, p. 2.

[4] Proc. Soc. Exper. Biol. & Med., 1923, 20, p. 229.

Larson selected a surface tension reducent which has proven to exert more than ordinary toxic action, and whether the results observed were due to surface tension or to chemical action of depressant is not clearly established

Some of the points touched upon by Larson were studied by Gibbs, Batchelor and Sickels.[5] Ordinary broth was found to have a surface tension of 48 to 50 dynes per cm. when determined by the film method of Fahrenwald. The surface tension was altered by the addition of soaps especially prepared from castor oil, olive oil, cocoanut oil, and palmitic acid. The authors show that these depressants exert varying degrees of surface tension depression, and likewise have toxic action toward bacteria. The soaps vary in their specific toxic action, a given soap being toxic to a certain organism and not toxic to others. Castor oil soap was found to be the most toxic of the depressants employed. By using all four depressants, in varying concentrations of each, it was possible to determine whether the inhibiting action obtained was due to surface tension or due to the chemical nature of the depressant. The organisms studied consisted of Escherichia coli, B. subtilis, Eberthella typhi, Staphylococcus aureus, Azotobacter chroococcum, and 8 different clostridia. Any variation which was noted from applications of the depressants was definitely shown to be due to the chemical nature, or toxic action, of the depressant. No instance was found in which variation from normal could be attributed to surface tension. Anaerobes could not be coaxed into growing aerobically, and the pellicle formers either persisted in forming pellicles or refused to develop. It was further shown that the development of bacteria in the medium greatly alters the surface tension in those instances where depressants have been added, and development is at an entirely different surface tension. It must therefore be born in mind in studying the effect of surface tension on bacterial development that the initial surface tension must be considered as the condition which is to be met by the organism, and any development will produce a change in the surface which varies with the organism, the medium and the depressant.

Ayers, Rupp and Johnson[6] conclude that some species of streptococci are retarded in growth at surface tension of 53 dynes, and suppressed at 45 dynes. Others are retarded at 43 dynes. Still other species are retarded in growth at 43 and suppressed at 40 to 41 dynes. In general 40 to 41 dynes prevented the growth of streptococci. They further state "By depressing the surface tension to the same point with different substances, the same results were not obtained." They employ sodium ricinolate, sodium glycocholate, iso-amyl alcohol, and sodium oleate as depressants. The data shown does not bear out the above conclusions, and we are unable to understand by what reasoning one may impute bacterial inhibition to surface tension when no inhibition is procured at the same surface tension when certain other depressants are employed.

One of the outstanding discrepancies in the literature may be cited here. Ayers and his associates reports inhibition of bacterial growth at surface tension of 53 dynes per cm., while Pizarro found ordinary broth as routinely prepared and containing no depressant to have a surface tension of 50 dynes per cm. These results are therefore not comparable in dynes per cm. and can only be compared by considering the departure from normal. This discrepancy lies in the method of determining surface tension, Ayers and his coworkers employing the drop method, which gives values in general 10 to 12 dynes higher than the film method.

Frobisher[7] studied the effect of surface tension on B. typhosus, B. morgani, B. aerogenes, B. diphtheriae, B. xerosis, Staphylococcus, Streptococcus and Pneu-

[5] J. Bact., 1926, 11, p. 393.
[6] J. Infect. Dis., 1923, 33, p. 202.
[7] Ibid., 1926, 38, p. 66.

mococcus. He criticizes the work of Ayers, Rupp, and Johnson on the grounds that acidity was used as a test for the growth of the organisms. He determined the growth by plate count, or physical appearance. The surface tension was determined by the du Noüy tensiometer. He concluded that by measuring the ability of organisms to grow at low surface tension one may distinguish B. typhosis and B. morgani from B. aerogenes, B. diphtheriae from B. xerosis and B. hofmanni, certain resistant types of streptococci from sensitive types, and pneumococci from streptococci. The data presented do not eliminate the possibility that the inhibiting action is one of toxicity rather than lowered surface tension. In a later report Frobisher [8] pointed out the relationship between surface tension and the action of disinfectants, especially phenol and hexylresorcinol. He found that .1 cc. of 1.0% sodium oleate exerted a protective action for typhoid in the presence of the germicides, and .25 cc. brought about an increased germicidal effect, while .5 cc. again exerted a protective action.

Pizarro [9] studied the influence of surface tension on streptococci, staphylococci, and pneumococci. By using four well chosen depressants in varying concentrations he was able to show that surface tension was not a factor in the results obtained. The depressants inhibited the growth in many instances, but this inhibition could not be ascribed to surface tension.

Albus and Holm [10] studied surface tension in relation to L. acidophilus and L. bulgaricus. The depressants consisted of sodium ricinolate, sodium taurocholate and sodium glycocholate. The surface tension was determined by the drop weight method. The authors found that none of the strains of L. bulgaricus showed evidence of growth after 7 days when the surface tension was depressed by sodium ricinolate to less than 40 dynes, while all L. acidophilus strains grew as low as 36 dynes. The P_H was found to influence the results somewhat. Sodium taurocholate was used in one experiment. The lowest surface tension obtained was 41 dynes at P_H 6.5. Six strains of L. bulgaricus showed growth after six days at the lowest surface tension but nine strains failed to develop, while all strains of L. acidophilus developed. Sodium glycocholate was used in one experiment but did not give satisfactory results. The authors conclude that surface tension may be used as a practical means of differentiating between L. acidophilus and L. bulgaricus, the former developing at a surface tension sufficiently low to inhibit the latter. Sodium oleate did not give the same results as the sodium ricinolate.

Albus [11] in a later study found that the growth of Escherichia coli in 1% peptone solution was affected when the surface tension was lowered by additions of castor oil soap. The effect was one of reduction in number of organisms rather than inhibition of growth and could not at any time be detected by gross appearance. Plate counts revealed the fact that rapid growth occurred in all cultures, both with and without castor oil soap, until the ninth hour after which time there was a slight steady increase in the cultures containing no depressant and a decrease in those containing depressant. The decrease in number of organisms was attributed to decreased surface tension but the possibility of chemical action of depressant and metabolic products is not precluded.

Koppeloff and Beerman [12] presented data which they consider a confirmation of the work of Albus and Holm, and concur in the idea that the two organisms may be differentiated by susceptibility to surface tension. When sodium ricinolate

[8] J. Bact., 1927, 13, p. 163.
[9] Ibid., p. 387.
[10] Ibid., 1926, 12, p. 13.
[11] J. Infect. Dis., 1927, 41, p. 211.
[12] J. Bact., 1927, 13, p. 7.

was used as the depressant a concentration was reached which allowed the development of L. acidophilus but inhibited L. bulgaricus and this occurred when the surface tension was approximately 43 dynes per cm. It was accordingly concluded that the low surface tension was the responsible factor, even though the organism would develop at a lower surface tension in the presence of sodium oleate as depressant. Here again it is difficult to follow the reasoning which led to this conclusion. It is obvious that Albus and Holm, and Kopeloff and Beerman, have not differentiated between the toxicity of sodium ricinolate and surface tension depression. This point will be emphasized later in this discussion.

In a general summary of the outstanding work on surface tension in bacterial development we find: Larson and associates contend that surface tension plays an extremely important rôle in bacterial activity while Gibbs, Batchelor and Sickels perform some of the same experiments with contrary findings. Ayers and associates contend that streptococci may be classified by their ability to develop at certain surface tensions, and that all streptococci studied are inhibited at 40 dynes per cm. Frobisher could not confirm these results and agrees with Pizarro in that the streptococci are not influenced by the surface tension of the medium. Frobisher on the other hand contends that pneumococci, staphylococci and other organisms are greatly affected by surface tension, while this is disputed by Pizarro. Frobisher further maintains that C. diphtheriae and C. xerosis may be differentiated by surface tension susceptibility. Albus and Holm affirm that L. acidophilus and L. bulgaricus may be differentiated by the ability of the former to develop at a surface tension which is prohibitive to the latter, using sodium ricinolate as depressant. This is also supported by Kopeloff and Beerman. Gibbs, Batchelor, and Sickles furnish evidence which shows that this agent is usually more toxic than other depressants and its inhibiting action is not due to surface tension depression.

In this paper data will be presented to throw more light on surface tension as a factor in the development of the aciduric bacteria. It may be safely stated that at the present time there is no adequate and undeniable proof that surface tension plays a rôle in bacterial development. There are data which may be suggestive of this as a fact but on closer inspection it will be found that the chemical properties are intimately associated with the physical and that a sharp differentiation is not always possible.

METHODS OF STUDY

Surface Tension Depressants.—The substances employed for the depression of surface tension consisted of soaps especially prepared and purified as previously described,[5] together with solutions of sodium ricinolate, sodium taurocholate, and sodium oleate. Unless otherwise noted these depressants were prepared in 2% solutions and from these stock solutions the desired amount added to the medium by pipette. In the tables and discussion the amount of depressant is expressed on the basis of dry substance per 100 cc. broth, or percentage. The six depressants gave a wide range in surface tension and made it possible to determine whether the results obtained were due to surface tension depression or chemical action.

Determining Surface Tension.—The surface tension of the medium was determined by the film method as described by Fahrenwald.[13] Approximately 15 cc. of medium were used in each determination. The disc which engaged the solution was platinum, which facilitated the matter of cleaning between each examination. The solution to be tested was cooled to 20 C., poured into a dish, allowed to stand for a few moments, and the surface tension measured. A second reading was then taken and considered correct in the event it checked the first reading. The broth prepared for the work usually had a surface tension of 47 to 50 dynes per cm.

Medium Used.—Several mediums were investigated to determine the value in the cultivation of L. acidophilus and L. bulgaricus. The medium which was finally selected was prepared after the following formula:

Aminoid	5.0 gm.	Lactose	10.0 gm.
Peptone	10.0 gm.	Beef infusion	1,000.0 cc.

The reaction was brought to a PH of 7.1 before sterilization and after sterilization and cooling was found to be approximately PH 7.0.

Strains of L. acidophilus and L. bulgaricus.—A total of eight strains of L. acidophilus and twelve strains of L. bulgaricus were employed. Some of these strains are very well known and there is every reason to believe that all the strains employed are authentic. For convenience the L. acidophilus strains are indicated by the numbers A 1 to A 8 and the L. bulgaricus B 1 to B 12 inclusive. All strains of each organism coagulated milk within 24 to 48 hours, and gave a characteristic smooth gas-free curd.

RESULTS

Effect of Surface Tension on L. acidophilus and L. bulgaricus.—The broth was prepared as previously described, treated with the various pressants, tubed 15 cc. per tube, and sterilized. After cooling they were

[13] J. Opt. Soc. Am. and Rev. Sci. Insts., 1922, 6, p. 722.

incubated 24 to 48 hours at 37 C., cooled to 20 C., and the surface tension determined. They were then inoculated as indicated in table 1 with 0.25 cc. of actively growing broth cultures, and incubated at 37 C. The P_H was determined at 48 hour intervals. It was found that the acidity was in proportion to the apparent growth, and a maximum development was usually reached at the end of four days. The acidity is therefore taken as a criterion of growth. The P_H of the mediums immediately after inoculation was 6.8 to 6.9. Reinoculations were made in the sodium ricinolate series after 48 hours incubation but no further develop-

TABLE 1.—EFFECT OF SURFACE TENSION ON L. ACIDOPHILUS AND L. BULGARICUS

P_H 6.0 and above (in parentheses) indicates no growth, P_H 5.9 and less indicates growth.

			L. bulgaricus				L. acidophilus			
Depressant	Amount per 100 Cc. Broth, Gm.	Surface Tension, Dynes per Cm.	B 1 P_H	B 5 P_H	B 6 P_H	B 9 P_H	A 1 P_H	A 2 P_H	A 3 P_H	A 4 P_H
None	0	47.3	4.70	4.66	4.75	4.74	4.94	5.42	5.28	5.47
Sodium oleate	.02	34.6	4.6	4.7	4.7	4.5	4.7	4.7	4.7	4.6
	.06	30.2	4.6	4.7	4.7	4.5	4.7	4.7	4.7	4.6
	.10	28.4	4.6	4.7	4.9	4.6	4.7	4.7	4.7	4.6
Sodium taurocholate	.02	40.3	4.8	4.7	5.1	4.8	4.7	4.7	4.8	4.8
	.06	36.0	5.3	4.8	5.6	(6.3)	4.7	4.9	4.9	5.2
	.10	32.5	5.9	4.9	5.9	(6.3)	5.0	5.1	5.1	5.4
Sodium ricinolate	.02	33.3	(6.5)	5.1	(6.3)	(6.4)	5.0	(6.5)	(6.5)	(6.6)
	.06	32.4	(6.5)	(6.7)	(6.5)	(6.3)	(6.5)	(6.5)	(6.5)	(6.5)
	.10	31.5	(6.5)	(6.7)	(6.4)	(6.5)	(6.5)	(6.5)	(6.5)	(6.6)
Cocoanut soap	.02	36.4	(6.4)	5.6	(6.5)	(6.5)	5.5	5.5	5.5	(6.0)
	.06	27.3	(6.3)	(6.5)	(6.6)	(6.6)	(6.5)	(6.5)	(6.5)	(6.5)
	.10	26.4	(6.6)	(6.7)	(6.6)	(6.7)	(6.3)	(6.5)	(6.6)	(6.5)
Palmitic soap	.02	37.6	5.1	4.6	4.9	5.1	4.7	4.7	4.7	4.5
	.06	32.3	5.9	4.8	5.2	(6.4)	4.7	4.8	4.7	4.8
	.10	30.9	(6.3)	4.9	5.2	(6.4)	4.7	4.8	4.7	5.3
Olive soap	.02	36.9	(6.0)	4.7	4.7	(6.1)	4.7	4.7	4.7	4.7
	.06	32.3	(6.3)	4.7	5.0	(6.3)	4.7	4.7	4.7	4.7
	.10	31.6	(6.3)	4.8	5.0	(6.3)	4.7	4.7	4.7	4.7

ment of the organisms was obtained, although the added inoculum brought a slight decrease in P_H. The control tubes received no depressant but were inoculated and incubated in the manner above described.

It will be observed in table 1 that all P_H values of 6.0 and above are in parentheses in order to make them more easily observed. A P_H of 6.0 and above was regarded as no growth, while 5.9 and below was considered growth. A P_H of 6.0 represents a drop of approximately 0.8.

It will be seen from the data that the surface tension varied from 26.4 to 47.3 dynes per cm. The lowest surface tension obtained was 26.4 dynes in the case of 5% cocoanut soap. All strains of both L. acidophilus and L. bulgaricus developed in each concentration of sodium oleate, in fact the acidity produced by the acidophili was greater than in the controls, indicating a favorable action of the depressant. Referring to the sodium taurocholate column it will be observed that all strains of L. acidophilus developed as well as in the control tubes, but that the B 9 strain of L. bulgaricus failed to develop in two concentrations, and strains B 6 and B 1 gave poor growth in the higher concentrations. It is quite obvious that this is not due to surface tension because excellent growth occurred at a lower surface tension obtained by use of sodium oleate. In the sodium ricinolate column a marked toxicity is noted. In only two instances is growth obtained, one in the case of L. bulgaricus B 5, the other in L. acidophilus A 1, and it must be remembered that this series was reinoculated after 48 hours in an effort to obtain growth. It is obvious that this lack of development is not due to surface tension because growth is present at a lower surface tension in the case of sodium oleate, palmitic soap and olive soap. Cocoanut soap is also toxic, both L. acidophilus and L. bulgaricus developing in only the 0.02% concentrations. It is apparent that this is not due to surface tension because more vigorous growth has occurred at a lower surface tension in the case of sodium oleate, palmitic soap and olive soap. The findings in the palmitic column show two strains of L. bulgaricus inhibited in the higher concentrations with all strains of L. acidophilus developing. The same may be said for the olive soap column. That this is not due to surface tension is made clear by a comparison with the sodium oleate column.

In general summary it may be set forth that the various depressants either retarded the development of the organisms or produced a stimulation. This stimulation was noted in L. acidophilus strains but not in the L. bulgaricus strains, and occurred in the presence of all depressants except cocoanut soap and sodium ricinolate. The two latter depressants were toxic to both L. acidophilus and L. bulgaricus, and the toxic action cannot be attributed to surface tension. Palmitic soap, olive soap, and sodium taurocholate exerted toxic or inhibitive action toward the L. bulgaricus strains, but this again cannot be ascribed to surface tension.

These results point rather conclusively to the fact that surface tension, within the limits of these experiments, has played no part in the development of the organisms under study. The inhibition noted by Albus and Holm and by Kopeloff and Beerman is due to the chemical action of the depressant and not to the fact that the surface tension is lowered. If surface tension is the prime factor then we could not expect to obtain growth of the organisms at a lower surface tension with the other depressants.

Effect of Sodium Ricinolate on L. acidophilus and L. bulgaricus.—Insofar as sodium ricinolate proved the most toxic of the depressants employed it was desirable to determine if a concentration could be found which would permit the development of L. acidophilus and at the same time inhibit the development of L. bulgaricus, thus affecting a means of separation and identification on the basis of toxicity. Accordingly the standard broth was treated with amounts of sodium ricinolate varying from 0.008% to 0.04%, tubed, incubated for 24 hours, then inoculated with an actively growing milk culture, the surface tension determined,

TABLE 2.—EFFECT OF SODIUM RICINOLATE ON L. ACIDOPHILUS AND L. BULGARICUS
P_H 6.0 and above (in parentheses) indicate no growth.

		Grams Depressant per 100 Cc. Broth				
	Control 0	.008	.016	.024	.032	.04
Surface tension............	50.8 dynes	43.1 dynes	39.8 dynes	37.1 dynes	35.8 dynes	34.4 dynes
	P_H	P_H	P_H	P_H	P_H	P_H
L. acidophilus						
A 1..................	4.7	4.7	4.7	4.7	4.8	4.8
A 2..................	5.1	5.2	5.3	(6.2)	(7.0)	(7.0)
A 3..................	5.0	4.7	4.8	4.8	4.6	5.3
A 4..................	5.1	5.4	(6.4)	(6.4)	(7.0)	(7.0)
A 5..................	4.9	4.9	4.6	5.0	(6.7)	(7.0)
A 6..................	4.9	4.8	4.6	4.7	4.7	(6.7)
A 7..................	5.1	4.9	4.6	4.6	4.6	4.6
A 8..................	5.0	4.8	4.9	4.6	4.6	4.6
% showing growth...	100	100	87.5	75.0	62.5	50.0
L. bulgaricus						
B 1..................	4.6	5.0	5.2	(6.3)	(6.8)	(6.8)
B 2..................	5.9	5.9	(6.9)	(7.0)	(7.0)	(7.0)
B 4..................	4.4	4.7	4.8	4.8	5.0	4.8
B 5..................	4.5	4.5	4.7	4.6	4.6	4.5
B 6..................	4.5	4.8	5.3	5.7	5.8	(6.7)
B 7..................	4.5	4.9	4.7	4.7	4.8	4.8
B 8..................	4.4	4.7	4.6	4.6	4.6	5.8
B 9..................	4.4	5.1	5.7	(6.0)	(6.3)	(6.6)
B 10..................	5.9	(7.0)	(7.0)	(7.0)	(7.0)	(7.0)
B 11..................	4.6	5.1	(7.0)	(7.0)	(7.0)	(7.0)
B 12..................	4.5	4.8	4.4	4.6	4.7	4.7
% showing growth...	100	90.9	72.7	54.5	54.5	36.2

and then incubated at 37 C. These tubes were prepared and inoculated in duplicate. The hydrogen-ion concentration was determined and growth observed at intervals of 3, 5, and 10 days. The results are shown in table 2. A P_H of 6.0 and above was considered as no growth and all such cases are in parentheses in order that they may be more readily seen.

The data in table 2 show that the bulgaricus strains were slightly more susceptible to the unfavorable action of the sodium ricinolate than were the acidophilus strains. Five of the 11 L. bulgaricus strains, 45%, developed in the highest concentration of ricinolate employed, while 4 of the 8 acidophilus strains, 50%, developed in this concentration. It is obvious from a study of these data that these strains cannot be separated by the use of sodium ricinolate. It is apparent from the data in table 2 that some of the strains, both L. acidophilus and L. bulgaricus, developed through the highest concentration of the ricinolate, whereas in table 1 all strains were either retarded or completely inhibited at a lower concentration. This variation is due to the inoculum and was a factor of importance throughout the work. It was found that the size and the source of the inoculum had a profound influence on the development of the organism, and frequently was the factor which determined whether growth would or would not result. A concentrated inoculum of actively growing organisms would overcome unfavorable conditions and growth

TABLE 3.—SUGAR FERMENTATION BY L. ACIDOPHILUS AND L. BULGARICUS

Organism	Maltose	Sucrose	Levulose
L. bulgaricus			
B 1	+	±	±
B 2	0	0	0
B 3	0	0	0
B 4	+	+	+
B 5	+	+	+
B 6	+	+	+
B 7	+	+	+
B 8	+	+	+
B 9	+	+	+
B 10	0	0	0
B 11	+	+	+
B 12	+	+	+
L. acidophilus			
A 1	+	+	+
A 2	+	+	+
A 3	+	+	+
A 4	+	+	+
A 5	+	±	+
A 6	+	±	±
A 7	+	+	+
A 8	+	+	±

+ indicates growth with acidity, 0 indicates no growth nor acidity.

result, whereas failure would result from a smaller less active inoculum. Actively growing cultures in milk offered the best inoculum, and not less than 0.1 cc. was used as inoculum. The inoculum in the tubes presented in table 2 was from milk while that in table 1 was from broth. In all set-ups the inoculum was the same as that used with other strains in order that the results would be comparable.

Sugar Reaction of Strains Under Study.—Broths were prepared after the formula used throughout the work, omitting the lactose and adding 1% Andrade indicator. After sterilization the sugars were added by pipet from Berkefeld filtered solutions in such amount that the final concentration in the broth was 1%. All tubes were then incubated at 37 C. for 24 hours before use. Maltose, sucrose, and levulose broth tubes were inoculated in triplicate from each culture. The results are presented in table 3, + signifying growth with acidity produced, — indicating no growth and no acidity.

According to the classification of Rahe [14] all strains of L. acidophilus ferment maltose while no strains of L. bulgaricus may ferment this sugar. Following this classification nine of our L. bulgaricus strains would be designated L. acidophilus. Kulp and Rettger [15] classify the organisms by their reaction toward maltose, sucrose and levulose, L. acidophilus fermenting all three while typical L. bulgaricus ferments none. Yet, out of a very small group of authentic strains tested they found two bulgaricus strains which fermented maltose and one which fermented sucrose.

It will be seen in table 3 that out of 12 strains of L. bulgaricus, 9 fermented maltose, 8 fermented sucrose, and 8 fermented levulose. Of the 8 strains of L. acidophilus all fermented maltose, 6 definitely fermented sucrose, and 6 definitely fermented levulose. It is obvious that the sugar reactions cannot be relied upon to identify the strains.

SUMMARY

The effect of lowered surface tension on the development of L. acidophilus and L. bulgaricus was studied. The surface tension was depressed by applications of four soaps, together with sodium ricinolate, sodium oleate, and sodium taurocholate. No instance was found in which inhibition of growth could be attributed to lowered surface tension.

Sodium ricinolate exerted a toxic action toward both L. acidophilus and L. bulgaricus, but this action could not be employed as a means of identifying the two organisms.

The fermentation of maltose, sucrose, and levulose does not offer a means of differentiating L. acidophilus from L. bulgaricus.

[14] J. Infect. Dis., 1914, 15, p. 141.
[15] J. Bact., 1924, 9, p. 357.

MONILIA FROM OSTEOMYELITIS

Charles L. Connor

From the Pathological Laboratories of the Montreal General Hospital and the Department of Pathology, Harvard Medical School, Boston

In spite of the numerous attempts to classify the pathogenic fungi and the voluminous literature concerning them (or perhaps because of these things) the organisms known variously as blastomycetes, oïdia, monilia, cryptococci, etc., remain a source of confusion to the pathologist who comes across them in the performance of routine duties. However, it is a duty to report such organisms when found, along with their peculiarities as to source, cultivation and pathogenicity in order that in the future some rational method of classifying them may be worked out.

The organism reported here was encountered in pus from an abscess of the buttock. The patient, a girl of 19, had had osteomyelitis of the humerus for about four years. This had begun in the shaft, had healed, only to recur in the same bone, but slightly below the original lesion. She entered W. L. Barlow's service at the Montreal General Hospital with several draining sinuses above the elbow.* Later she developed abscesses of the buttock which communicated with the ilium of the left innominate bone. There had been no history of a previous skin lesion, or of internal (visceral) infection. Except for these foci of infection the patient was in excellent health. There was no fever and no leukocytosis.

Tissue from the lesion of the humerus was obtained, and tissue from the abscess of the buttock. The tissues showed the same histological picture, namely, a very cellular granulation tissue made up mostly of macrophages, many of them very large and vacuolated, but without the multinucleate form of the Langhans type of giant cell. The pus consisted of polymorphonuclear cells and macrophages. No tubercles were present, and there was little fibrosis within the acute areas, though the sinus and abscess walls were densely fibrous in nature. Large rounded organisms, some in process of budding, were present in tissue and smears from the pus.

Pus from the abscess was smeared and stained by Gram's method and for tubercle bacilli; aerobic cultures were made on Saboraud's medium, dextrose agar, blood agar, dextrose broth, and Löffler's

Received for publication, Jan. 30, 1928.

* The clinical aspects of the case are to be reported in full by Dr. Barlow.

medium; similar mediums were used in making anaerobic cultures by the pyrogallic acid method; and two guinea-pigs received injections intraperitoneally and subcutaneously, and intraperitoneally, respectively, with the exudate.

In the gram-stained smears numerous large encapsulated bodies were found. The bodies were gram-positive; the capsules took the red counter stain. They varied considerably in size, from 4 to 20 microns in diameter, and many were budding. Some of the larger organisms contained a granular material, but most were densely stained, and showed no internal structure. No thread forms were seen. The organisms did not retain the carbol-fuchsin stain after treatment with acid alcohol, and stained very poorly with the methylene blue counter stain. They were differentiated with difficulty from mononuclear blood cells in these smears. No tubercle bacilli were found, and no other organisms.

Cultural Characteristics.—Growth on mediums was noticed first three days after planting. Very small colonies, almost transparent, looking like small drops of mucus appeared on the blood agar slants. Growth appeared on Saboraud's acid agar in four days. Here the colonies were small, white, and pasty, at first isolated; but they soon coalesced. Stained smears from blood agar and Saboraud's tubes showed a budding organism with less irregularity as to size and a great deal less capsular material than were present in smears of the pus. Organisms from the blood agar tubes consistently contained more capsular material than those from other mediums. No mycelia were present in early cultures.

On further cultivation the yeast grew abundantly on dextrose agar, and on almost any other medium. The blood agar cultures never grew beyond small isolated colonies, although they appeared first on this medium. It grew poorly at first in liquid mediums, but later grew out in 24 hours in all sugar mediums. No growth occurred in the anaerobic cultures, and these were discarded after three weeks.

Except on the mediums containing blood or serum the organisms on all solid mediums produced much the same type of growth; a white pasty raised colony with rounded outline, the colonies joining eventually to form smooth sheets with roughly crenated edges. After a few weeks the white turned to a slightly more transparent gray, and these remained stationary. After two months on Saboraud's medium a few short filaments were noted penetrating the medium from above. No aerial hyphae were formed, and no surface mycelium.

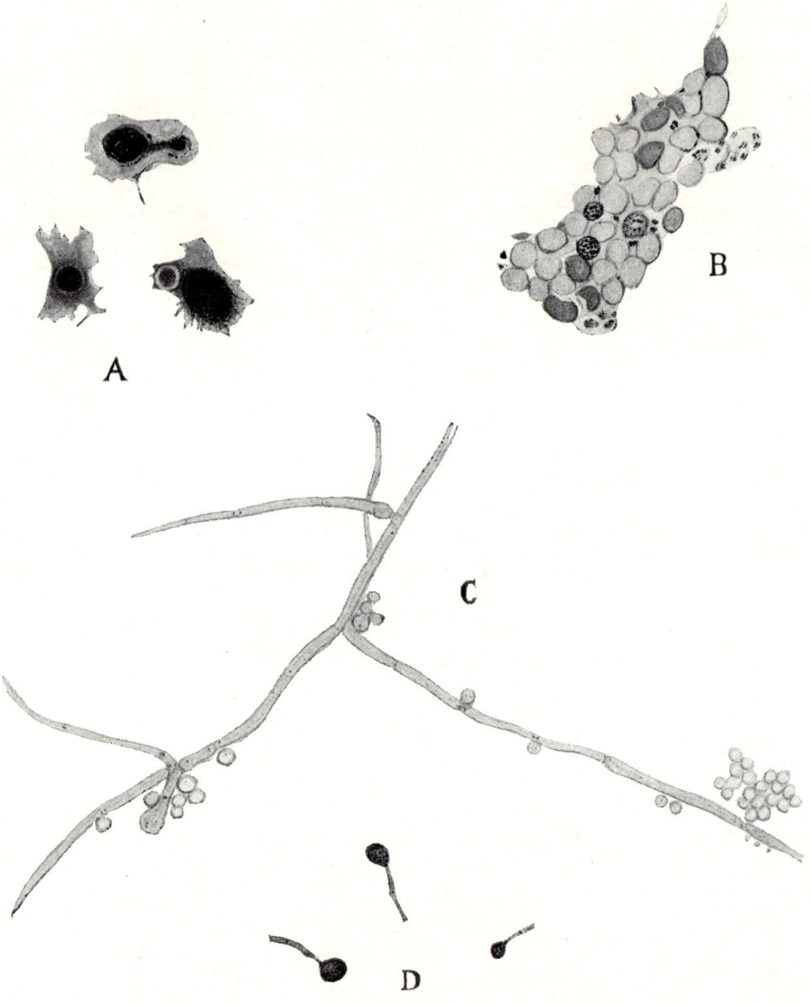

Fig. 1.—A: drawing of organisms in smear preparations. The densely staining cell bodies are surrounded by a mass of capsular material. One is in a large mononuclear cell. B: the typical yeast network, from Saboraud culture. C: short septate mycelium with lateral and terminal conidia, from dextrose broth culture. D: rounded terminal bud which somewhat resembles a sporangium.

In liquid mediums growth is first at the bottom of the tubes, but later a thin pellicle forms on the surface. Mycelia are formed which continued to reproduce by budding only. Lateral and terminal conidia were formed, but no sporangia or ascospores. At the end of many mycelia there formed a rounded bud somewhat larger than the usual lateral conidia, separated from the adjacent segment by a thin wall. This superficially resembled a sporangium, and an effort was made to force the organism to sporulate. Cultures were transplanted to carrot, to filter paper which had been moistened and placed over a slice of carrot in a Petri dish, and to filter paper in a Petri dish containing a few drops of salt solution or distilled water. No spores were formed, however. The rounded end bud reproduced other buds in all ways similar to the lateral conidia.

The mycelia were septate, each segment made up of an elongated organism. Very short branches were present, arising anywhere along the mycelium, but consisting of only two or three slightly elongate buds.

On gelatin growth was very slow, only a thin grayish layer forming on the surface at first. Later (in about eight weeks) the inverted pine tree appearance is duplicated along the line of stab. In this relatively unfavorable medium the organism grows in very small pairs or in slightly elongate ellipsoidal bacillary form. Some of the pairs are no larger than staphylococci, and the elongate forms superficially resemble large bacilli. The filaments radiating out from the stab do not form chains of spores as in Oïdia.

The structure consisted of a doubly refractive membrane which in unstained preparations treated with weak acetic acid showed numerous radiating lines between the two layers of membrane. With Giemsa's stain the cytoplasm is clear except for a small bit of rounded material which takes the basic stain and has the appearance of a nucleus. Two of these are present in many of the elongated forms, one at each end, and in some four are present, a pair at each end. Some contain minute vacuoles which stain red with Scharlach R. Some of the cells from one plate which had been partly flooded with a dilute solution of neutral red contained red bodies after 24 hours.

The organism forms acid and gas in dextrose, maltose, and levulose, and acid only in sucrose, lactose, galactose and xylose. Other substances which were tested and which were negative were mannitol, rhamnose, l-arabinose, inulin, dextrin, salicin and glycerol. Litmus milk became slightly acid, but did not clot in 10 days. It did not liquify gelatin. The gas formed was shown to be CO_2. Alcohol was formed from levulose. No indol or hydrogen sulphide was formed. The organism grows well at any temperature between 20 and 37.5 C. It is killed by heat at 60 C. in ten minutes.

The guinea-pig which had been given injections intraperitoneally died in two days of peritonitis. No yeasts could be separated from the rank postmortem growth which had occurred. The second guinea-pig was killed 18 days after the subcutaneous and intraperitoneal injections. There was no peritonitis and no gross lesions of the omentum, liver, spleen, lungs, or lymph nodes. Smears from the peritoneum contained elongate bodies resembling the elongate cells which make up segments of a mycelium, with the same basic staining dots present, one at each end, or a pair at each end. Very small budding forms were also present. Cultures from the peritoneum contained these same forms, which appeared after eight days on dextrose agar. These form, i. e., the slightly elongate bacillary forms, and the very small (1.5 to 5 microns) diplococcoid forms seem to represent a pleomorphic stage which forms under unfavorable conditions and are similar to the forms appearing on gelatin, filter paper, and in certain liquid mediums (hormone broth). They were shown not to be true spores.

Four other guinea-pigs which received intraperitoneal or subcutaneous injections of pure cultures remained well. When killed four and six weeks later one had an adhesion between the abdominal wall and several loops of bowel, and a small granulomatous lesion of the tunica vaginalis on one side. These lesions had the histologic structure of a tubercle but with more fibrous tissue proliferation and no caseation. The organsms were seen in some of the macrophages. The other guinea-pigs had no lesions.

Four mice were injected intraperitoneally with 0.2 cc. of an emulsion of the live organisms in salt solution. Two of these mice received also 0.2 cc. and 0.4 cc. respectively of serum from the patient. Because of circumstances, these had to be killed in two weeks. The two which received no serum, and the mouse which received 0.2 cc. of serum contained one or two small tubercular lesions of the liver or omentum from which Monilia were recovered. The fourth mouse which had received 0.4 cc. of serum contained no lesion. It was not possible to repeat this experiment.

No antibodies could be demonstrated in the patient's serum by in vitro experiments. It did not agglutinate the organism in any dilution. The serum of a rabbit into which were injected 41 cc. of a heat-killed vaccine in six doses over a period of six weeks showed doubtful agglutinating properties in high concentration (positive in 1:20; some controls also positive). Intraperitoneal injection of live organisms into rabbits caused small, slowly growing lesions; intravenous injection killed a rabbit in four days, with multiple abscesses of the kidneys, liver, spleen, lungs, and pericardium. The "immunized" rabbit after intravenous injection of live organism died also in four days, with somewhat different lesions. In the nonimmunized rabbit the abscesses were small and numerous, with necrotic centers in which the polymorphonuclear cell predominated. Large mononuclear cells containing Monilia were present in the periphery of the lesions. In the vaccinated animal there were no frank abscesses; rather small acute tubercle-like lesions were the rule, with the large mononuclear cell as the common invader. Small giant cells were numerous in lymph node and kidney lesions. Whether this difference in types of reactions was caused by the vaccine is hard to say, but it is thought that a slight relative immunity might be expressed in this way.

The organism, from these experiments, seems to be almost inert so far as pathogenicity and antigenic properties are concerned. It does not produce progressive lesions in the guinea-pig, as does the organism of blastomycetic dermatitis. Except when injected intravenously, it behaves as a foreign body, soon destroyed. Even the lesions from intravenous injection have been shown by Nye, Zerfas, and Cornwell [1] to depend on dosage, and the death of animals after injections to be due to organ insufficiency (kidneys, liver, etc.) because of the amount of tissue affected, rather than to the virulence and multiplication of the organism. Why such an organism should be capable of initiating a lesion in the human is difficult to answer. The abscess from which the cultures were obtained had begun in the deep tissues, not in the skin, and had not ruptured. There seems to be no doubt that this organism did, however mysteriously, initiate the lesion.

Classification.—It is impossible in a short report to enumerate all the characteristics by which a classification of this group of organisms is attempted. Blastomycosis is a general term under which all affections caused by yeast-like organisms which reproduce only by budding are designated. But there is no botanical group which may be called Blastomycetes, and no two classifications agree as to their position. In general they are regarded as altered yeast forms, having lost the properties of forming spores in sacs (ascospores), and of sexual reproduc-

1. Am. J. M. Sc., 1928, in press.

tion. They are designated Fungi imperfecti because of this, and for the same reason (i. e., that they represent accessary fruit forms of the ascomycetales [2] they are sometimes classed under ascomycetes. This last group of true yeasts, is divided into Saccharomyces and Nonsaccharomyces by Guilliermond,[3] though most authorities do not include them here; they are most often placed in a group entirely separate from Ascomycetes (e. g. Harshberger [2]). The saccharomyces are unicellular fungi which multiply by budding, sometimes by partition, and form asci, these arising in a cell (ascosporangium) which may be formed sexually or asexually. The nonsaccharomyces of Guilliermond (Fungi imperfecti, Hyphomyces, of other authors), represent those budding yeasts which form no asci. They may or may not form a mycelium: those which do not are classified as Torula by some authors,[4] or Cryptococcus by others,[5] and those which do form a mycelium are variously classified as Oïdia,[6] Blastomyces,[7] Oospora,[8] or Monilia,[9] although an occasional torula may form short filaments (T. lactis [10]), Blastomyces, Oospora, and Monilia may form chains of spores which property is supposed to characterize the oïdia, and an oospore is a sexually produced spore.

Fermentation tests may form a basis for separating genera or families but are notoriously unreliable in separating species. Different strains of what appear to be the same organisms frequently give different fermentation reactions, and the same organism under different conditions may change its fermentation reactions. Smith [11] lists 21 strains of Monilia psilosis, Ashford, all with slightly different sugar reactions, and Castellani and Chalmers list 40 Monilia, no two of which have exactly the same zymogenic properties. Ashford's [12] M. psilosis always produces acid and gas in dextrose, maltose, and levulose, and occasionally in sucrose and galactose. Castellani [13] more recently reduced his number of species of Monilia to 12 on a basis of gas

2. Harshberger, J. W.: Textbook of Mycology and Plant Pathology, 1917.

3. The Yeasts (translation by Tanner), 1920.

4. Stoddard, J. L., and Cutler, E. C.: Torula Infection in Man. Monograph 6, Rockefeller Inst. for Med. Res., 1916; also Guilliermond.[3]

5. Castellani and Chalmers: Manual of Tropical Medicine, 1919.

6. Ricketts, H. T.: J. M. Res., 1901, 6, p. 374.

7. Gilchrist, T. C.: Bull. Johns Hopkins Hosp., 1896, 1, p. 269.

8. Attributed to Saccardo, P. A.: Syllage fungorum, 1895, by Castellani.

9. Monilia was created by Persoon, according to Guilliermond.[3]

10. Heinze, B., and Cohen, E.: Ztschr. f. Hyg., 1908, 46, p. 286.

11. J. Am. M. A., 1924, 83, p. 1549.

12. J. Am. M. A., 1915, 64, p. 810, 1893; Am. J. M. Sci., 1915, 150, p. 680; 1916, 151, p. 520; 1917, 154, p. 157.

13. Castellani, A.: Arch. Derm. & Syph., 1927, 16, pp. 383, 511, 714.

formation in certain sugars, but he points out that "many Monilias after a few transplantations lose some of their fermentation characters or these are altered."

Acid formation without gas is even more unreliable. Still, as a result of persistent attempts to classify these organisms by their fermentation reactions nearly every new fungus described is called a new species, or even a new genus.

On a morphological basis there seems to be only one outstanding characteristic separating this group; they do or do not form a mycelium. Those which do may be roughly divided into: (a) a group which forms mycelia reluctantly, and (b) those which form abundant mycelia. This is the method of classification used by Ricketts [6] in 1901. Or the mycelia-forming group may be divided, as Zinsser [14] does, into fermenting and nonfermenting groups. Anderson [15] has arranged a classification which is much simpler than the more recent one of Castellani, ignoring fermentation reactions altogether. His groups are Mycoderma *—forms a heavy dry pellicle on liquid mediums; Parasaccharomyces (Monilia)—vegetative cells reproducing mostly by budding, but forming mycelia under certain conditions (this includes Blastomyces, Oïdia, Oospora, and Monilia); and a group in which no mycelia are formed, which are subdivided according to the shapes of the cells into three genera. Here belong (a) Torula or Cryptococcus, which are the same, and are typically yeast-like; (b) an apiculate form, and (c) an elongate non-septate form.

Nye, Zerfas, and Cornwell [1] have used Anderson's classification in a study of fungi from the gastrointestinal tract, and found it the most satisfactory. They have reported a most painstaking study of this group of organisms, and were able to classify the strains found under Anderson's headings, with minor variations manifested chiefly by different sugar reactions.

The present organism could be called Monilia, Oïdia, Blastomyces, or Parasaccharomyces. It is similar also to Saccardi's Oospora. If the fermentation reactions were considered, it would be a new species, as it corresponds exactly with none of Castellani and Chalmers named species, nor with Smith's 21 strains of M. psilosis, nor with the reported strains of Nye, Ashford, or Guilliermond. It falls into the group of Monilia

14. Hiss and Zinsser: Textbook of bacteriology, 1927.

15. J. Infect. Dis., 1917, 21, p. 341.

* Mycoderma, Persoon (Guilliermond [3]), usually oval cells without mycelia, forming a folded scum containing bubbles of air. Various species produce undesirable tastes in beers and wines. They are probably asporogenic forms of a group of Saccharomycetes; do not cause alcoholic fermentation.

studied by Ashford and by Smith most closely, and with Parasaccharomyces A of Nye. It should therefore be classified with (or as) M. psilosis, or, which is the same thing, as a strain of Parasaccharomyces, Anderson.

SUMMARY

A budding yeast-like organism forming reluctantly a mycelium in certain culture mediums, and otherwise behaving as Monilia was isolated from an abscess of the buttock which communicated with the iliac bone. There had been a long-standing osteomyelitis of the humerus, and the organisms were seen in tissues from this lesion also. This strain of Monilia corresponds with no described species so far as fermentation tests are concerned, but it is pointed out that such tests are unreliable as a means of differentiating the group of organisms variously called Torula, Cryptococcus, Blastomyces, Oïdia, Monilia, or Oospora. A review of the characters by which these organisms are classified shows that they do not differ sufficiently to be given different names; that, in fact, they represent only two different types, namely, a mycelia-forming group (Blastomyces, Oïdia, Monilia, Oospora, all classified as Parasaccharomyces by Anderson), and a nonmycelia-forming group (Torula or Cryptococcus). These two groups with a third, Mycoderma, provide for all those yeast-like organisms known as Fungi imperfecti. The nature of these organisms does not permit at present of a more elaborate classification.

CHANGES IN BLOOD DEXTROSE IN RABBITS AFTER INTRAVENOUS INJECTIONS OF HISTAMINE

Maud L. Menten and Helen M. Krugh

From the Pathological Laboratories, University of Pittsburgh, Pittsburgh, Pa.

The present work was undertaken with the tentative assumption that the toxic principle of the enteritidis-paratyphoid B group may be related to the poisonous amines. Of these, histamine has been most widely studied biologically. Among the changes developing in the blood in response to intravenous injections of histamine, hyperglycemia (which is a fair index of the glycolysis taking place) can be readily followed. The hyperglycemia varies in the laboratory animals already studied. Chambers and Thompson [1] report in the dog a 200% increase in blood dextrose 30 minutes after intravenous injections of 3 mgm. of histamine per kg. of body weight. LaBarre [2] found that injections of 0.25 mgm. per kg. into the jugular vein of guinea-pigs caused little reaction while 0.5 or 1 mgm. resulted in convulsions with death in two to three minutes. Twenty seconds after entrance into the circulation there was a rapid rise in blood sugar followed by a return to normal or by an appreciable hypoglycemia in one minute. The varying susceptibility of these two animals, as shown by chemical changes, is paralleled by the difference in vascular response which Dale and his coworkers have observed in rodents and carnivora.

The close similarity between the rapidly developing histamine hyperglycemia observed in guinea-pigs and that reported by Zeckwer and Goodell [3] in anaphylactic shock following immunization of the rabbit to organisms of the coli-typhi group suggested testing whether the histamine response in rabbits, which so frequently carry spontaneous paratyphoid infections, might simulate that of the guinea-pig. The rabbits used were as far as possible of the same stock and only those weighing between 2400 and 2700 grams were selected. They were fasted 20 to 24 hours previous to the experiment. One cc. of histamine hydrochloride (Pfanstiehl) in aqueous solution was rapidly injected

Received for publication, Jan. 25, 1928.

1. J. Infect. Dis., 1925, 37, p. 229.
2. Compt. rend. Soc. de biol., 1926, 94, p. 779.
3. J. Exper. Med., 1925, 42, p. 57.

into the lateral ear vein from which blood was also withdrawn for sugar estimations. These latter were made according to the Folin and Wu [4] procedure. From the sugar values tabulated in table 1 it will be seen that while there is a considerable difference in the susceptibility of individual animals the reactions fall into two main groups. One of these, with a maximal rise at 30 minutes followed by gradual return to normal, is similar to that of the dog and the other showing terminal convulsions and death resembles that of the guinea-pig. Unlike the guinea-pig, however, all rabbits immediately succumbing to the histamine do not have a hyperglycemia. The wide variation in agonal blood dextrose might conceivably be due either to differences in the concentration of hepatic glycogen or to a more permeable condition of the cells in the

TABLE 1.—SHOWING CHANGES IN MGS. OF DEXTROSE PER 100 CC. OF BLOOD FOLLOWING INTRAVENOUS INJECTIONS OF HISTAMINE

Number of Rabbit	Dose in Mg. per Kg.	Hours after Injection 0	¼	½	1	2	3	4	5
1...........	1.0	86	96	102	108	102	97	97	
2, 3, 4, 5.....	2.5	92‡	102	111	100	97	105	93	99
6...........	2.5	102	105 (3 min.)*						
7, 8.........	3.3	97‡	109	132	119	102	120	101	100
9...........	1.0	92	133	160	107	102	102	98	95
9, 5 hours after previous injection.......	3.3	103	356 (3 min.)*						
10...........	3.0	99	351 (8 min.)*						
11...........	4.0	105	133	178	156	124	131	122	113
12...........	4.0	76	102 (10 min.)*						
13...........	4.0	102	227 (3 min.)*						

* The number of minutes in parentheses indicates the time after injection that convulsions and death occurred.

‡ These series of figures represent average values.

liver permitting the glycogen to be more readily released by glycolytic agents.

As indicated by Zeckwer and Goodell's [3] experiments, allergy induced by the coli-typhi group apparently so increases the permeability of the liver to these specific antigens that in anaphylactic shock a maximal increase of blood dextrose occurs within ten minutes after injection. Studies were made with a view to determining whether previous immunization to B. paratyphosus B (of animal origin) and B. enteritidis would increase in a similar manner the hyperglycemic response to histamine injected during the anaphylactic periods. At no time have we been able to produce an active agglutinating serum against the strain of B. paratyphosus B isolated by us from guinea-pigs.[5] Immunizing doses of B. enteritidis were, therefore, continued until an agglutination

4. J. Biol. Chem., 1920, 41, p. 367.
5. J. Infect. Dis., 1925, 37, p. 400.

titer of 1:1600 was obtained and a similar number of injections of B. paratyphosus B were given for a comparable period to another series of rabbits. Twenty-one days after the last dose each animal was injected with histamine. The results of these experiments, seen in the first half of table 2, indicate that any modifications in the tissue which may have been induced by injections of bacterial suspensions do not appreciably influence the degree of the hyperglycemia induced by the rapid introduction of histamine into the blood stream. In fact, such animals appear slightly more resistant to histamine than normal rabbits. It may, of course, be questioned whether all or any of the animals used in these experiments were anaphylactic. Of three control rabbits immunized with a suspension of killed B. enteritidis, only one developed

TABLE 2.—CHANGES IN MGS. OF DEXTROSE PER 100 CC. OF BLOOD OF IMMUNIZED RABBITS FOLLOWING INJECTIONS OF HISTAMINE AND WITTE'S PEPTONE

No. of Rabbit	Substance Injected per Kg.	Bacteria Used in Immunization	Hours after Injection					
			0	¼	½	1	2	3
14, 15, 16	0.4 mgs. histamine	B. paratyphosus B	117†	117	120	120	119	108
17, 18	0.4 mgs. histamine	B. paratyphosus B	102†	129	163	119	121	107
19	0.45 mgs. histamine	B. paratyphosus B	125	177 (3 min.)*				
20	0.5 mgs. histamine	B. paratyphosus B	87	154 (3 min.)				
21	0.5 mgs. histamine	B. paratyphosus B	90	95 (3 min.)				
22, 23, 24‡	0.35 mgs. histamine	B. enteritidis	90‡	97	103	105	100	
25	0.35 mgs. histamine	B. enteritidis	100	125 (3 min.)				
26, 27	0.25 mgs. histamine	B. enteritidis	108†	116 (3 min.)				
28	0.8 gms. Witte's peptone	B. paratyphosus B	133	131	125	132	136	121
29	0.8 gms. Witte's peptone	B. enteritidis	125	330 (10 min.)				
30	0.8 gms. Witte's peptone	B. enteritidis	92	335 (7 min.)				
31	0.8 gms. Witte's peptone	B. enteritidis	87	417 (10 min.)				

* Number of minutes in parentheses indicates the time after injection that convulsions and death occurred.

† These series of figures represent average values.

‡ One of these animals had prostration and convulsions for 10 minutes after injection and recovered in 30 minutes.

anaphylactic shock when injected with enteritidis antigen 21 days after the last dose. But that such immunized animals do react differently from normal rabbits is demonstrated by the figures appearing in the latter part of table 2. When injections of aqueous Witte's peptone were substituted for those of histamine the rabbits previously treated with B. enteritidis died with convulsions and anaphylactic shock in from 7 to 10 minutes and the blood showed a maximal hyperglycemia. As previously reported [6] with a single dose of a similar amount of this peptone (sample 3) it has been impossible either to cause the death of the animal or to produce more than a moderate rise in blood dextrose. There is, of course, the possibility of passive nonspecific immunization, similar to that recorded by Olitsky and Denzer,[7] by the transfer of

6. J. Biol. Chem., 1927, 72, p. 255.
7. J.Infect. Dis., 1917, 20, p. 145.

small amounts of peptone from the agar slants on which the antigenic organisms were grown. This seems unlikely since an analogous procedure with B. paratyphosus B gave negative results. One concludes, therefore, that allergy, induced by organisms of the enteritidis-paratyphoid B group is not a modifying factor in determining variations occurring in the blood dextrose following lethal or sublethal injections of histamine. Furthermore, the experiments reported here give no clue to the explanation of these differences. That the sample of Witte's peptone used contained among its many hydrolytic constituents an antigen analogous to that of B. enteritidis would appear likely and suggests that the toxic substance found in B. enteritidis filtrates, which gives a hyperglycemia, is due to a disintegration product of the bacteria, but that this toxic product is not histamine.

CONCLUSIONS

The convulsions and anaphylactic shock produced by lethal doses of histamine in the rabbit may be accompanied either by no appreciable change in the blood dextrose or by a maximal hyperglycemia.

The experiments reported indicate that allergy is not a factor in the production of agonal hyperglycemia.

INSULIN CONTENT OF THE PANCREAS FOLLOWING INTOXICATION OF RABBITS WITH PARATHYPHOID B FILTRATE AND DYSENTERY BACILLI

Maud L. Menten and Helen M. Krugh

From the Pathological Laboratories, University of Pittsburgh, Pittsburgh, Pa.

The presence of hydropic degeneration in the cells of the islets of Langerhans of rabbits and guinea-pigs, suffering from spontaneous infections or subjected to injections of organisms of the enteritidis-paratyphosus B group and the coincidence of these lesions with disturbances in the dextrose content of the blood suggested that the lesion in the islets might be associated with a diminished concentration of insulin in that tissue.

The ease with which insulin can be extracted from pancreatic tissue and the comparative accuracy of its biological assay by injection of this extract into rabbits offer an acceptable means of testing this assumption. A modification made in the standard method of assay was in the use of rabbits weighing about 1000 grams instead of the customary two kilos. Animals of this weight were chosen because a few preliminary experiments indicated that the insulin content of the pancreas of the normal rabbit averaged one-half unit of "Lilly" insulin. Attempts to use white rats and guinea-pigs were unsatisfactory because of the difficulties experienced in making repeated heart punctures.

The hypoglycemic response of half grown rabbits, weighing between 750 and 1200 grams to a known amount of commercial insulin was determined and this was compared with the hypoglycemia produced by the insulin extracted from the pancreas of a normal full grown rabbit. After a week's interim the reaction of the same test rabbit to the insulin obtained from a treated animal was determined. In this way a graphic comparison was made of the reaction of 11 test rabbits to one-half unit of "Lilly" insulin, to the insulin from a normal rabbit, as well as to the insulin content of the pancreas of one or more animals, which had been subjected to the toxic effects of bacteria or their products. In each case a small fragment of pancreas was removed before extraction for microscopic examination.

Received for publication, Jan. 25, 1928.

The extraction of the insulin was carried out in a manner similar to that used by Macleod [1] in obtaining the insulin from the principal islets of teleost fish. The pancreas, removed immediately after the rabbit was killed, was placed in 60% alcohol containing 0.1% HCl and kept for several days in the refrigerator. The supernatant fluid was decanted and filtered, and the residue was then repeatedly ground in a mortar with additional acid alcohol. After each grinding the super-

TABLE 1.—CHANGES IN MGS. OF DEXTROSE FOLLOWING INJECTION OF INSULIN FROM PANCREAS OF NORMAL RABBITS AND OF THOSE TREATED WITH PARATYPHOID B FILTRATE

Number and Weight of Test Rabbit	Hours After Injection 0	½	1	2	3	Source of Insulin
1	101		59	47*		One-half unit "Lilly" insulin
1000 gm.	117		62	50*		Pancreas of normal rabbit (2200 grams)
	118		73	62	46*	Pancreas of rabbit (2630 grams) 5 cc. dose,** 97% blood dextrose increase, killed in 3 hours
2	86	59	56	63	82	One-half unit "Lilly" insulin
1000 gm.	79		58	50	40*	Pancreas of normal rabbit (2375 grams)
	108		53	56	40*	Pancreas of rabbit (2560 grams) 4 cc. dose, 118% blood dextrose increase, killed in 5 hours
3	93	78	53	64	89	One-half unit "Lilly" insulin
950 gm.	99	78	52	76	61	Pancreas of normal rabbit (2360 grams)
	108	125?	67	55	56	Pancreas of rabbit (2475 grams) 5 cc. dose, 158% blood dextrose increase, killed in 5 hours
4	107	95	55	67	102	One-half unit "Lilly" insulin
930 gm.	94		68	57	53*	Pancreas of normal rabbit (2100 grams)
	104		50	39	33*	Pancreas of rabbit (1650 grams) 3 cc. dose, 214% blood dextrose increase, killed in 3½ hrs.
	83		46	43	62	Pancreas of rabbit (2050 grams) 3 cc. dose, 191% blood dextrose increase, killed in 3 hours
5	107		75	103	105	One-half unit "Lilly" insulin
920 gm.	95		73	76	86	Pancreas of rabbit (2360 grams) 2 cc. dose, 3 times at 5 day intervals, 20% blood dextrose increase, killed in 4 hours after last dose
6	131	75	76	66	82	One-half unit "Lilly" insulin
1180 gm.	119		62	62	38*	Pancreas of normal rabbit (2190 grams)
	105		118	131	140?	Pancreas of rabbit (2300 grams) 6.5 cc. dose, 300% blood dextrose increase, killed in 3 hours

* Convulsions occurred a short time after withdrawal of blood.
** Dose throughout table signifies amount of paratyphoid B filtrate injected intravenously.

natant fluid was filtered, the various filtrates were added together and then evaporated to dryness by means of an electric fan. The dried residue was taken up in 2 cc. of water and the fat removed by shaking out with ether a couple of times in a separatory funnel. The aqueous solution was then immediately injected into a test rabbit whose hypoglycemic response to insulin had been previously determined. An interval of at least a week was allowed between the various injections into the test rabbit.

1. Macleod, J. J. R.: J. Metab. Res., 1922, 2, p. 149.

In the first series, in which paratyphoid B filtrates were used as the toxic agents, the induced hyperglycemia was estimated hourly for 3 or 4 hours. The potency of the filtrate was indicated by the production of a characteristic curve,[2] with a maximal dextrose rise in ½ to 1 hour

TABLE 2.—CHANGES IN MGS. OF DEXTROSE FOLLOWING INJECTION OF INSULIN FROM PANCREAS OF NORMAL RABBITS AND OF THOSE TREATED WITH B. DYSENTERIAE (SHIGA)

Number and Weight of Test Rabbit	Hours After Injection 0	1	2	3	4	Source of Insulin
7 1000 gm.	105	49*				One-half unit "Lilly" insulin
	107	60*				Pancreas of normal rabbit (2570 grams)
	92	56	53	60	64	Pancreas of rabbit given ½ cc. dose,** died in 2 days
	118	91	87	96	112	Pancreas of rabbit given ½ cc. dose,** died in 2 days
8 800 gm.	105	50*				One-half unit "Lilly" insulin
	97	53*				Pancreas of normal rabbit (2650 grams)
	101	69	63	74	87	Pancreas of rabbit given ½ cc. dose,** died in 2 days
	107	68	60	56	89	Pancreas of rabbit given ½ cc. dose,** died in 2 days
9 950 gm.	110	52*				One-half unit "Lilly" insulin
	113	60	45*			Pancreas of normal rabbit (2500 grams)
	130	100	100	90	85	Pancreas of rabbit given ½ cc. dose,** died in 2 days
	110	98	105	117	112	Pancreas of rabbit (2550 grams): injection† 2 consecutive days, 75% blood dextrose increase, dying in 4 days, killed
10 875 gm.	112	48*				One-half unit "Lilly" insulin
	75	92	71	52*		Pancreas of normal rabbit (2690 grams)
	89	69	87	95	102	Pancreas of rabbit (2200 grams); injection† 2 consecutive days, 300% blood dextrose increase, dying in 3 days, killed
	95	53	63	71	93	Pancreas of rabbit (2700 grams): injection† 2 consecutive days, 60% blood dextrose increase, dying in 3 days, killed
11 1200 gm.	107	59*				One-half unit "Lilly" insulin
	112	63	46*			Pancreas of normal rabbit (2450 grams)
	98	72	80	90	100	Pancreas of rabbit (2370 grams): injection† 260% blood dextrose increase, dying in 4 days, killed
	93	84	76	97	101	Pancreas of rabbit (2400 grams): Injection† 83% blood dextrose increase, dying in 24 days, killed
	118	113	113	104	120	Pancreas of rabbit (2620 grams): injection† 172% blood dextrose increase, dying in 6 days, killed

* Convulsions occurred a short time after last withdrawal of blood.

** "One-half cc. dose" indicates that this amount of a killed suspension of B. dysenteriae (Shiga) was injected, intravenously.

† "Injection" indicates the intravenous injection of a suspension of killed B. dysenteriae (Shiga) containing 1,500,000,000 bacteria.

and a return to normal in 3 or 4 hours when the animal was killed. A brief survey of table 1 which records the results obtained demonstrates that single sublethal doses of paratyphoid B filtrates do not materially alter the insulin content of the islets. No appreciable difference (within the limits of the method) between the insulin content of

2. Menten, M. L.: J. Infect. Dis., 1926, 38, p 354

the pancreas of normal and treated rabbits was discernible. Furthermore, no striking pathological changes were observed in sections from these pancreases. In both only an occasional karyorrhexis or pyknosis was to be found.

While the work with the paratyphoid B filtrate was in progress there became available for study the pancreases of rabbits which had been given lethal doses of killed Shiga dysentery bacilli. As a result of these bacterial injections the rabbits became exceedingly ill, developed a marked diarrhea and paralysis of the hind limbs and died in two days from toxemia and exhaustion. Unfortunately the exact weight (roughly between 2 and 3 kilos) of these rabbits, which were full grown, were not recorded and no estimations were made on the blood sugar changes developing. However, some of the pancreatic extracts, e. g., from the second rabbit used with test 6 gave sufficient evidence of lowered insulin content, as indicated by the altered hypoglycemia response, seen in table 2, to warrant a continuance of the experiments. The increased number of nuclear degenerations found on microscopic examination gave added support to the conviction that prolonged toxemia due to dysentery toxins was not without effect on the islets of Langerhans.

The subsequent experiments with rabbits of controlled weight and in which the permanent and continuously increasing toxic hyperglycemia was followed are tabulated in the latter half of table 2. These reports confirm the preliminary findings that a small but appreciable diminution of the insulin content of the pancreas coincident with nuclear changes in the islets of Langerhans occurs with fatal dysentery intoxications. The islet tissue showed more or less chromatolysis with a considerable number of pyknotic nuclei. This occurred chiefly in the beta cells. Little hydropic degeneration, or even swelling of the cells, was observed.

Whether the phenomenon described is referable to the direct action of the toxin on the islet cells, or to an increased stimulation of these cells by induced hyperglycemia to a greater output of insulin, or to an interference with sympathetic or parasympathetic nerve control, or to a general exhaustion or finally to a combination of various factors, is not clear. In view of the fact that one of us (Menten) has produced destruction of principal islet tissue in selected species of teleost fish by sublethal intraperitoneal injections of paratyphoid B filtrates, it would seem that cellular degeneration due to direct toxic effect can not be excluded.

CONCLUSIONS

Single intravenous sublethal injections of paratyphoid B filtrates do not appreciably alter the insulin content of the pancreas as demonstrated by comparative biological assays in test rabbits.

The hypoglycemic potency of the insulin extract of the pancreas from rabbits in which injections of B. dysenteriae (Shiga) had caused a prolonged fatal toxemia and hyperglycemia was slightly diminished

BACTERIAL ADAPTATION TO ACRIFLAVINE

VICTOR BURKE, CATHERINE ULRICH
AND
DON HENDRIE

From the Bacteriological Laboratories State College of Washington, Pullman

The power of adaptation is to a greater or less degree characteristic of all living cells. In general the more highly specialized a cell the less its power of adaptation. As a class the bacteria are primitive forms of life. However, some are very highly specialized. Undoubtedly the power of adaptation to different factors will be found to vary among both the individuals and the species. Bacteria may become modified both morphologically and physiologically as the result of an exposure to a new environment. The change in the organism may be temporary or permanent, an adaptation, a mutation or a change in the life cycle. This article describes experiments bearing on the rate, specificity and permanence of bacterial adaptation to the antiseptic dyes.

Exper. 1.—To determine how quickly Staphylococcus albus will adapt itself to neutral acriflavine.

Duplicate series of 6 tubes each of neutral acriflavine agar slants were prepared as follows: to 6 tubes of melted extract agar titrated to P_H 7.4 was added sufficient 1% neutral acriflavine to make dilutions of 1:4,000,000; 1:3,000,000; 1:2,000,000; 1:1,000,000; 1:900,000; 1:800,000. After thorough mixing the half of each tube was poured into an empty tube. A tube of dye broth was prepared by adding to a tube of plain broth titrated to P_H 7.4 sufficient neutral acriflavine to make a dilution of 1:3,000,000. This tube of dye broth and a tube of dye free broth were inoculated with Staphylococcus albus from a 9-hour culture. At the end of 8 hours one of the series of dye agar slants was inoculated from the dye broth culture and the other series from the dye free broth culture. The cultures were examined at intervals of 24 and 36 hours. The results, given in the table indicate that within a period of 8 hours Staphylococcus albus can increase its tolerance for acriflavine.

The experiment was repeated with various modifications. A slight increase in dye tolerance was noted after exposure for 6 hours. When exposed to a much weaker concentration of the dye in broth the organisms adapt themselves more slowly or not at all. When exposed to a stronger concentration of dye in broth the organisms are injured so that they do not grow as rapidly or on as great a concentration of the dye as the control. The favorable concentration of dye in broth

Received for publication, Jan. 28, 1928.

for demonstrating rate of adaptation varies with the P_H and other factors affecting the strength of antiseptics.

When an organism is placed under unfavorable conditions such as dye agar it may die, remain dormant, remain dormant for a period and then grow at a normal rate, or it may grow steadily from the beginning at a reduced rate. In order to determine whether this delayed growth occurred as the result of a change in the environment or an increased tolerance on the part of the organism the following experiment was made.

Exper. 2.—To determine whether delayed growth of Staphylococcus albus when grown on dye agar occurs as the result of the organisms developing increased tolerance for the dye or is due to a decrease in the antiseptic action of the dye:

Dye agar slants were prepared by adding sufficient 1% acriflavine to melted agar titrated to P_H 7.4 to make a dilution of 1:250,000. One of these slants and a slant of dye free agar was inoculated with Staphylococcus albus. The dye free agar showed heavy growth in 24 hours. The dye agar showed a faint growth in 72 hours. When transplants were made from this culture to a similar tube of dye agar growth was visible in 24 hours. The tube of dye agar on which growth occurred in 72 hours was sterilized by placing in boiling water for 10 minutes and reslanted. This was then reinoculated from the stock culture. Faint growth was visible at 72 hours. This was repeated and growth was visible at 24 hours.

COMPARISON OF GROWTHS OF STAPHYLOCOCCUS ALBUS FROM PLAIN BROTH AND FROM DYE BROTH DILUTIONS OF ACRIFLAVINE IN AGAR SUBCULTURE

Hours	Organism	1:4,000,000	1:3,000,000	1:2,000,000	1:1,000,000	1:900,000	1:800,000
24	control	+	+	0	0	0	0
24	dye exposed	+	+	+	+	0	0
36	control	+	+	+	+	0	0
36	dye exposed	+	+	+	+	+	0

The results obtained indicate that when Staphylococcus albus is exposed to acriflavine and growth is much delayed, the organisms are able to grow as the result of an increase in dye tolerance. The organisms become adapted and then grow. Growth may be rapid or slow, depending on the concentration of the dye. There may also be some change in the dye immediately surrounding the organisms. The growth of Staphylococcus caused the agar to become slightly more alkaline. The hydrogen-ion concentration was determined before and after the organisms had grown on the agar. No change occurred in control tubes. With an increase in alkalinity there is at first an increase the dye to decompose with a loss of bacteriostatic action. The experi-
in the bacteriostatic action of the dye. However, alkali later causes

ment failed to demonstrate any reduction in the action of the dye as the result of the growth of the organism within 6 days but it does not eliminate that possibility. With repeated and prolonged growth of the organism there is an evident reduction in the action of the dye. This is apparently due to the action of the organism and not to the repeated heating or standing. Tubes of dye agar heated a number of times and left standing for days inhibited growth to the same extent as when fresh.

Exper. 3.—To determine the specificity of increased dye tolerance:

Staphylococcus albus was plated out on agar containing concentrations of neutral acriflavine from 1 : 50,000 to 1 : 400,000. Two colonies appeared on the agar containing the dye in 1 : 180,000 dilution. These colonies arose from the two most dye tolerant cells of all those added to that agar. No colonies developed on the plates containing greater concentrations of the dye. More than two colonies appeared on the plates having weaker concentrations of the dye. One of the colonies on the agar plate containing 1 : 180,000 neutral acriflavine was transferred to agar containing a slightly greater concentration of the dye. This process was repeated as the organism acquired greater tolerance for the dye.

After a number of transfers the organism acquired sufficient tolerance for the dye to grow in a concentration of 1 : 1500 neutral acriflavine in agar with a reaction of P_H 7.4. This appeared to be the limit of adaptability of this strain of Staphylococcus albus for neutral acriflavine. After repeated transplants on agar with this concentration of the dye the organism failed to grow when the concentration of dye was increased.

In order to determine whether the increase in tolerance for neutral acriflavine was specific, the tolerance for gentian violet of the dye resistant strain and the stock culture was investigated. The stock culture grew in a 1 : 1,000,000 concentration and the acriflavine resistant strain grew in a 1 : 500,000 concentration of gentian violet in agar. The stock culture and the acriflavine tolerant culture were grown on gentian violet agar until the limit of tolerance for gentian violet was acquired. The limit was found to be 1 : 200,000 gentian violet in agar. The stock culture which had acquired the ability to grow in 1 : 200,000 gentian violet was now grown on acriflavine and found to grow in 1 : 12,000. By exposure to acriflavine it acquired sufficient tolerance to grow in a 1 : 3,000 concentration.

The results obtained indicate that the increased dye tolerance of Staphylococcus albus upon exposure to the antiseptic dyes is not entirely specific. With an increase in tolerance for one dye there is also an increase in tolerance for other dyes. However, the adaptation is specific to some degree because the tolerance for the other dye may be further increased by exposure to that dye.

Exper. 4.—To determine whether the increased dye tolerance represents a permanent change in the organism.

The Staphylococcus albus organisms used in experiment 3 that developed sufficient dye tolerance to grow in a 1 : 1,500 concentration of neutral acriflavine were grown for a number of generations on dye free agar. At the end of this period they had lost much of the increased dye tolerance and would not grow in a greater concentration of neutral acriflavine than 1 : 6,000. After 2 years growth they grew only in 1 : 200,000. The increased dye tolerance was lost.

The results indicate that the adaptation to the dye was only temporary and disappeared when the factor that stimulated its development was removed. The change in the organisms does not represent a mutation. These results agree with those reported for Rhizobium radicicolum by Burke and Burkey.[1]

The dye resistant organisms were originally selected from one of two colonies that appeared on a dye agar plate containing a 1 : 180,000 concentration of neutral acriflavine. This colony came from one of the two most resistant cells in the large number introduced into the agar. We have shown that these organisms increased their tolerance for acriflavine when exposed to the dye but that this increase was lost when the organisms were grown in dye free agar. These organisms as originally selected had more resistance to the dye than the average cells of the stock culture. In order to determine whether this difference was permanent, the dye resistant organisms were grown for a number of generations extending over a period of two years on dye free agar. Repeated tests indicated that the organisms retained superior dye tolerance. At the end of two years the dye resistant organisms grew in a concentration of 1 : 200,000 and the stock culture in a concentration of 1 : 400,000 acriflavine. The experiment indicates that it is possible by a process of selection to separate Staphylococcus into at least two strains as regards dye tolerance and that this dye tolerance can be further increased by the process of exposure and selection.

DISCUSSION

The rate of bacterial adaptation is a factor effecting the treatment of infections with antiseptics. Since an organism develops resistance

1. Soil Science, 1925, 20, p. 143.

or becomes "fast" in such a short period of time, some advantage may be gained by changing the antiseptic with each application. With repeated application of the same antiseptic, failure may result from the organism acquiring resistance.

The degree of bacterial adaptation is a factor in the rise and severity of epidemics. The morbidity and mortality curves will vary with the power of adaptation of the strain. However, if an organism has reached the limits of acquired tolerance due to exposures in a carrier, then an epidemic will not be affected by an increase in virulence. This explains the results obtained by Smith and Nelson,[2] and Webster.[3] in studying spontaneous epidemics in laboratory animals.

Adaptation is a factor in the testing of antiseptics. Dakin and Dunham [4] in working with the antiseptic dyes found that "after some hours the organisms grew unchecked"—and concluded that "the dyes in question are readily inactivated." The results obtained by them may also be explained on the basis of the organisms acquiring tolerance and then growing.

The rate of adaptation undoubtedly affects the length of the incubation period. An organism with a rapid rate of adaptation will require a shorter period of time to overcome the natural resistance of the host than an organism that adapts itself more slowly. The incubation period in Staphylococcus infections and in cocci infections in general is comparatively short.

CONCLUSIONS

Staphylococcus albus shows increased tolerance for the antiseptic dyes after six to eight hours exposure. This adaptation to the dyes is temporary and disappears when the organism is grown on dye free agar. Delayed growth of the organism in the presence of the dye is due in part at least to the process of adaptation of the organism to the dye. The increased tolerance of the organism for the dye is partially specific. Staphylococcus albus can be separated into two strains which differ in their ability to tolerate neutral acriflavine.

2. J. Exper. Med., 1927, 45, p. 365.
3. Ibid., p. 529.
4. Handbook of Antiseptics, 1918, p. 91.

CHOICE OF ANTISEPTIC DYE IN MIXED INFECTIONS

VICTOR BURKE, M. P. JESSUP AND SMITH PHILIPS

From the Bacteriological Laboratories of the State College of Washington, Pullman

The comparative value of the three most commonly used antiseptic dyes, gentian violet, mercurochrome-220, and acriflavine, has never been satisfactorily determined. Which of the dyes will give the best results under a given set of conditions is problematical. The dyes appear somewhat specific to certain bacteria. On this account Graham-Smith suggested using a mixture of two or more dyes in the treatment of mixed infection such as are commonly found in wounds.[1] Churchman has also suggested the advisability of combining two dyes, one active against the gram-positive organisms and the other active against the gram-negative organisms. As the result of Churchman's work a commercial concern has put forth a mixed dye product, acriviolet. This is a mixture of acriflavine and gentian violet. It was assumed that the acriflavine would be effective against the gram-negative organisms and the gentian violet against the gram-positive. Burke and Skinner [2] have suggested the possibility of enhancing dye therapy by rotating the dyes rather than mixing them. Their suggestion was based upon the belief that any dye which will destroy the gram-negative organisms in a mixed infection will also destroy the gram-positive. Furthermore, since bacteria acquire tolerance for antiseptics on exposure to a non-bactericidal solution they considered it more desirable to use a different dye for the second application. The present article describes experiments to determine the comparative bactericidal action of gentian violet, acriflavine and acriviolet for the gram-positive and gram-negative pyogenic organisms commonly found in wounds.

Exper. 1.—To determine the comparative resistance to dyes * of a mixture of gram-negative and gram-positive bacteria:

Salt solution suspensions of 24-hour cultures of Staphylococcus albus, Staphylococcus tetragenous, Corynebacterium xerosis, Bacterium coli, Bacterium proteus and Bacterium lactis-aerogenes were prepared. One cc. of each suspension were placed in a test tube and mixed. 1 : 10,000 solutions of the three dyes were prepared

Received for publication, Jan. 28, 1928.

1. J. Hyg., 1919, 18, p. 1.
2. J. Exper. Med., 1925, 12, p. 471.

* All dyes used were the product of the National Aniline and Chemical Co.

in distilled water. One cc. of the mixture of organisms was placed in 9 cc. of each of the dye solutions. At intervals up to 3 hours the dye-organism mixture was plated out by the loop method, two plates being used. Not enough dye reached the second plate to inhibit growth. A control, in which physiologic sodium chloride solution was used in place of dye, was run.

In all cases the gram-positive organisms were killed before the gram-negative. The experiment failed to indicate any selective action by acriflavine for the gram-negative organisms, or any superiority of the acriviolet over the dyes in pure state.

Exper. 2.—To determine the comparative bactericidal action of gentian violet, acriviolet and neutral acriflavine for Bact. coli and Staphylococcus albus:

Dye solutions were prepared as in experiment 1. Physiologic sodium chloride suspensions of 24 hour cultures of Bact. coli and Staph. albus were made. One cc. of each suspension was placed in 9 cc. of each dye solution. At intervals up to 3 hours the dye-organism mixtures were plated out by the loop method, two plates being used for each mixture. The plates were incubated for 48 hours.

Table 1.—Comparative Bactericidal Action of Gentian Violet, Acriviolet and Neutral Acriflavine for Bacterium Coli and Staphylocococcus Albus

		Period of Exposure to Dye (Minutes)				
Dye	Organism	20	45	75	120	180
Acriflavine..................	Bact. coli	++++*	+++	++	++	+
Acriviolet....................	Bact. coli	++++	+++	++	++	+
Gentian violet..............	Bact. coli	++++	+++	++	+	+ less
Acriflavine..................	Staph. albus	++++	++	++	+	0
Acriviolet....................	Staph. albus	++++	++	++	+	0
Gentian violet..............	Staph. albus	++++	+	+	0	0

* The plus sign indicates growth. Four of these signs indicates growth equal to control.

The results are shown in table 1. Gentian violet shows greater bactericidal action than acriflavine or acriviolet for both Staphylococcus albus and Bact. coli. Obviously there is no advantage in combining acriflavine and gentian violet for the treatment of mixed infections with organisms of these types. Acriflavine has been described as having increased action in the presence of serum and in this respect differing from the other antiseptic dyes. Experiment 3 was made to determine the effect of blood on the bactericidal action of neutral acriflavine, acriviolet and gentian violet.

Exper. 3.—To determine the effect of blood on the bactericidal action of gentian violet, acriviolet and neutral acriflavine:

A suspension of a 24-hour culture of Bact. pyocyaneum in physiological sodium chloride solution was prepared. Blood was drawn from the jugular of a horse and defibrinated by shaking with glass beads. This was placed on ice in a cotton stoppered flask. The blood when used in the experiments was less than 24 hours old. A 1 : 1,000 dilution of dye was prepared by adding 5 cc. of the defibrinated blood to an equal volume of a 1 : 500 dilution of dye in distilled water. One cc. of the Bact. pocyaneum suspension was added. At intervals up to 3 hours the mixture was plated out as in the preceding experiments.

The results are given in table 2. The experiment was repeated with Staph, albus and Bact. coli. A 1 : 10,000 dilution of the dye was used. Comparable results were obtained. In all cases blood reduced the bactericidal action of the three dyes for both gram positive and gram negative bacteria. And in all cases gentian violet had greater bactericidal action than neutral acriflavine for both gram-negative and gram-positive bacteria.

After this work was completed a paper by Eggerth appeared in which he describes experiments indicating greater bactericidal action

TABLE 2.—EFFECT OF BLOOD ON THE BACTERICIDAL ACTION OF GENTIAN VIOLET, ACRIVIOLET AND NEUTRAL ACRIFLAVINE AGAINST B. PYOCYANEUS

		Period of Exposure to Dye (Minutes)				
Dye	Solvent	20	45	75	120	180
Acriflavine	Water + blood	+++*	++	+	+	0
Acriviolet	Water + blood	+++	++	+	+	0
Gentian violet	Water + blood	+++	++	+	+ less	0
Acriflavine	Water	+	0	0	0	0
Acriviolet	Water	++	+	0	0	0
Gentian violet	Water	+ less	0	0	0	0
Controls						
Blood	......	++++	++++	++++	++++	++++
Blood	Water	++++	+++	+++	+++	+++
Blood	Broth	++++	+++	+++	+++	+++

* The plus signs indicate the degree of growth; 0 = no growth.

of acriflavine in serum than in broth.[3] He believes that the increase in bactericidal action of acriflavine in serum is due to the increase in alkalinity. Serum becomes alkaline on standing due to loss of CO_2 According to Eggerth, if the loss of CO_2 is prevented, the serum does not cause an increase in the bactericidal action of acriflavine. He found the acriflavine titer in such serum equal to that in infusion broth. Since broth causes a reduction in the bactericidal action of acriflavine we may conclude that Eggerth's experiments indicate a reduction in the bactericidal action of acriflavine upon the addition of serum when the loss of CO_2 is prevented. Whether the increase in bactericidal action on the addition of serum from which CO_2 has been lost is real or not is questionable. Eggerth does not give the acriflavine titer in water or physiologic sodium chloride, the usual solvent for the dye. In our opinion a comparison between acriflavine in water or physiologic sodium

3. J. Infect. Dis., 1926, 38, p. 440.

chloride, and in serum would indicate a loss of bactericidal action in the presence of the serum regardless of the loss of CO_2, or of increase in alkalinity. In other words, the loss of bactericidal action due to the organic matter is greater than the increase due to the changes in P_H occurring in the serum. In this connection it should be noted that there is an increase in the bactericidal action of gentian violet with an increase in alkalinity. However, no one has recorded an increase in the bactericidal action of this dye upon the addition of serum.

In our experiments we used defibrinated blood in place of serum. Such blood may not become as alkaline as serum. No attempt was made to control the loss of CO_2. The effect of the P_H is important and has been reviewed by Burke and Grieve.[4] The P_H of the various body fluids varies in health and disease. It is doubtful if the dyes are as effective in those patients suffering with acidosis. This has suggested alkalinization of such patients.

It has been well established that bacteria can increase their tolerance for the antiseptic dyes and grow in concentrations that inhibit the original culture.[5] More recently Meader and Fierer have shown that bacteria may acquire increased tolerance for other germicides.[6] The power of cellular adaptation in the animal and plant kingdom is largely universal. The rate at which organisms increase their resistance to dyes has not been well established but experiments in this laboratory suggest that an increase in tolerance may begin in 6 to 8 hours. The possibility of bacteria increasing their tolerance to the dyes in the body deserves consideration. The dyes can not be applied in sufficient strength or do not penetrate sufficiently to kill bacteria in the blood stream or in deep tissues. If such organisms increase their resistance to the dye a second application is less likely than the first one to be effective. If an increase in tolerance for one dye is not accompanied by an increase in tolerance for other dyes, then the application of a second dye may be more effective than a second application of the first dye.

Exper. 4.—To determine the comparative bactericidal action of different makes of acriflavine:

Three samples of acriflavine were obtained from manufacturer A and two from manufacturer B. The bactericidal strength of the five samples was determined for Staphylococcus albus. The organisms were added to 1 : 500,000 dilutions of the

4. Am. J. M. Sc., 1924, 198, p. 98.
5. Burke, V., and Skinner, H.: J. Exper. Med., 1925, 12, p. 471; Burke, V., and Burkey, Lloyd: Soil Science, 1925, 20, p. 143; Saelhof, C. C.: J. Am. M. A., 1925, 84, p. 1267.
6. J. Infect. Dis., 1926, 39, p. 237.

samples of dyes. Transplants were made on agar at 5-minute intervals. The organisms in the solutions made from the dye samples from manufacturer A died in from 105 to 120 minutes and those in the solutions made from the dye samples obtained from manufacturer B in from 70 to 85 minutes. There was practically no variation between the samples from one manufacturer.

It is evident that the bactericidal strength of acriflavine varies with the manufacturer. Whether the toxicity also varies was not determined. Before the comparative therapeutic value of the acriflavine produced by the two manufacturers can be determined it will be necessary to investigate the comparative toxicity. The samples for intravenous use had the same bactericidal strength as those for external use only. The comparative toxicity was not determined.

The experiment was repeated with Bacterium coli. A 1 : 10,000 dilution of each of the dye samples was made. Transplants to determine viability were made at 5-minute intervals. The experiment was repeated a number of times, but failed to demonstrate a material difference in the bactericidal strength of the five samples of acriflavine for Bacterium coli.

DISCUSSION

The results of our experiments indicate that gentian violet has greater bactericidal action in vitro than neutral acriflavine for both gram-positive and gram-negative bacteria and in the presence or absence of blood. The results of others indicate that it is also superior to mercurochrome. Tinker and Sutton report neutral acriflavine in blood as more effective than mercurochrome against a number of organisms commonly found in wounds.[7] Stearns and Stearns [8] have presented evidence indicating that gentian violet in blood has greater bactericidal action than mercurochrome for both gram-positive and gram-negative bacteria.

The superiority of one dye over the others depends not only on its superior bactericidal action in blood and pus but also on the toxicity for the tissues. In open wounds the difference in toxicity of the three antiseptic dyes is too slight to have a bearing on their comparative value. In subcutaneous injections, however, the acriflavine causes more necrosis than gentian violet. Our rabbits that received repeated intravenous injections of neutral acriflavine in the ear vein invariably lost part or all of the ear by sloughing. A cow developed a large and permanent edema about the point of injection in the jugular. The

7. Tinker, M. B., and Sutton, H. B.: J. Am. M. A., 1926, 87, p. 1347.
8. Am. J. Pub. Health, 1926, 16, p. 1003.

rabbits that received intravenous injections of gentian violet developed no necrosis at the site of injection.

The dye most effective for the treatment of mixed infections in open wounds may not be superior for intravenous therapy. Gentian violet is more toxic than neutral acriflavine intravenously. However, its greater bacteriostatic action in blood may compensate. At least twice as much acriflavine as gentian violet is required to make the blood bacteriostatic.

The selective action of the antiseptic dyes has been recorded by a number of workers. Whether this selective action justifies the combining of the dyes as has been done in the production of acriviolet is problematical. The most resistant organisms commonly found in wounds with the exception of spores are gram-negative Bacterium pyocyaneum and the gram-positive streptococci. Gentian violet is more effective than acriflavine against these organisms. Combining the dyes reduces the action. Acriviolet is less effective for these organisms than gentian violet.

The spore bearers in wounds are practically all gram-positive and more susceptible to gentian violet than to acriflavine.

CONCLUSIONS

Gentian violet is more bactericidal than neutral acriflavine for both the gram-positive and the gram-negative organisms commonly found in wounds. Blood reduces the bactericidal action of both dyes. No advantage is gained by mixing the two dyes. The dye most effective against the most resistant organism in the wound should be used.

Since bacteria acquire specific dye tolerance in a few hours rotation of dyes in the treatment of infections may be beneficial.

The bactericidal strength of neutral acriflavine varies with the manufacturer. Different samples from the same manufacturer are nearly uniform in bactericidal action.

THE PRODUCTION OF POTENT ANTIPNEUMOCOCCIC SERUM IN RABBITS *

B. L. FREEDLANDER

From the George Williams Hooper Foundation for Medical Research, University of California Medical School, San Francisco

The cultivation of pneumococci in artificial mediums is not comparable to conditions as they exist in the tissues of an infected host. The in vitro growth may result in alterations in structure of the bacteria, or in the formation of bacterial metabolic products which may interfere with their antigenic properties. In order to circumvent this possibility an antigen was prepared by extracting the tissues of animals infected with pneumococci.

Ross [1] has demonstrated that an active immunity can be produced in rats by feeding them tissues of animals dead from pneumococcic infection. He was of the opinion that such tissues contained a toxin, which when fed to a healthy animal might result in the production of an antitoxin. However, Ross found later that the feeding of live pneumococci from an artificial culture gave almost as good an immunity. Zinsser and Grinnell [2] attempted the immunization of horses by means of the blood-clot method. Their purpose was to obtain a localized growth of pneumococci within the animal body. It was thought that, by this method, a serum might be obtained which would have antitoxic properties, rather than purely antibacterial effects.

The procedure described below combines some of the theoretical advantages of both the above methods. In the following experiments, rabbits were immunized by the inoculation of infected animal tissues, which had been previously ground, extracted, and treated with various antiseptics, in order to kill or attenuate the pneumococci present. The blood of the rabbits was finally tested for protective action against pneumococcic infection in white mice. The inoculation, rather than the feeding, of infected tissue extracts has a double advantage: it is a more favorable method, in general, for the production of immune bodies; it also precludes the possibility of the destruction of any toxin in the intestinal tract.

Received for publication, Jan. 18, 1928.

* Edith Claypole Memorial Fellowship.

1. J. Immunol., 1926, 12, pp. 219, 237.
2. Proc. Soc. Exper. Biol. & Med., 1925, 23, p. 205.

Procedure.—The substance used as antigen was prepared as follows. Rabbits were infected intravenously with one to two lethal doses of a broth culture of pneumococci. Just prior to the death of the animals from the infection or within one hour after death, the liver, heart, lungs, spleen, and kidneys were removed with sterile precautions. These organs were passed through a meat grinder, then ground with sand. Twenty cubic centimeters of normal salt solution was added to each set of rabbit organs. The mixture was centrifugalized at moderate speed for one-half hour, and the faintly turbid supernatant fluid pipetted off. This liquid was used as antigen after the following treatment.

It was found necessary to treat the organ extract with antiseptics before use. Although a large number of the pneumococci had been removed by centrifugalization, a small dose (0.1 to 0.2 cc.) was sufficient to kill a rabbit. This was probably due to the presence of an aggressin-like substance in the organ extract. Several antiseptics were tried, including rivanol 1:2000, trikresol 1:1000, potassium permanganate 1 : 3000, chinosol 1 : 5000, and ether. The trikresol, chinosol, and potassium permanganate were found to be the least effective and were discarded. Pneumococci were still viable in the potassium permanganate mixture even after 25 days. Ether was effective as an antiseptic but removed or altered the antigenic potency of the organ extract. The antigen treated with rivanol was found to be the most practical. The rivanol was left in contact with the antigenic substance for 10 hours at room temperature, then kept in the ice box. After 24 hours, a loopful of the mixture plated, revealed a heavy growth of pneumococci; each subsequent day showed a decrease in the number of viable organisms, and by the eighth day the fluid was usually sterile. It is probable that this relatively slow antiseptic action is due to certain physical or chemical properties of the tissue extract, which may not allow intimate contact between antiseptic and organisms.

Rabbits were immunized with gradually increasing doses of the antigen subcutaneously and intraperitoneally. The following procedure was found to be the most favorable method of immunization: first injection, 0.3 to 0.5 cc. of a 5-day old antigen subcutaneously; second injection, 0.5 to 1.0 cc. of an antigen three to four days old, intraperitoneally; third injection, 1.0 to 2.0 cc. of a two to three day old antigen intraperitoneally. If subsequent inoculations were given an antigen one to two days old was used. The injections were best given at five to seven day intervals. It was found advisable to prepare a new antigen once a week. The majority of the rabbits did not show any symptoms; in general, there was no loss of weight. Some of the rabbits became sick for a few days following the first inoculation; occasionally one would die of a pneumococci septicemia, if the first immunizing dose was too high.

The rabbits were bled 8 to 12 days after the last injection. The protective properties of the serums were tested by intraperitoneal inoculation in white mice, simultaneously with graduated doses of pneumococci. The mice were kept under observation for seven days following therapy.

The three fixed types of pneumococci were used. The type 1 strain was received from the New York State board of health; the type 2 from O. T. Avery; the type 3 from I. S. Falk. All strains were very virulent for mice, less so for rabbits. The type 3 pneumococcus strain was only slightly virulent for rabbits, the fatal dose being 5.0 to 8.0 cc. intravenously.

Protective Action of Immune Serum Against Type 1 Pneumococci. —Six rabbits were immunized (table 1). The protective titer of the serums was between 1,000,000 to 10,000,000 MLD. Several of the rabbits were bled after three or four immunizing injections, the protective titer being at its maximum (10,000,000 MLD). The mobilization of immune bodies is apparently very rapid by this method. Normal rabbit serum controls gave no protection, neither did the serum of rabbits inoculated with uninfected (normal) rabbit organ extract treated with rivanol.

Protective Action of Immune Serum Against Type 2 Pneumococci.— Eight rabbits were immunized (table 2). The protective titer ran from

TABLE 1.—PROTECTIVE ACTION OF IMMUNE RABBIT SERUMS AGAINST TYPE 1 PNEUMOCOCCIC INFECTIONS IN MICE

Rabbit Serums		Pneumococcus Culture, Type 1		Number of Mice Used	Result	
Number	Dose, Cc.	Dose, Cc.	Number of MLD		Lived	Died
94	0.1	0.01	1,000,000	3	3	0
94	0.1	0.1	10,000,000	6	6	0
93	0.2	0.1	10,000,000	3	3	0
95	0.2	0.01	1,000,000	2	2	0
95	0.2	0.1	10,000,000	2	2	0
95	0.1	0.1	10,000,000	3	0	3
199	0.1	0.01	1,000,000	2	2	0
199	0.2	0.1	10,000,000	2	0	2
98	0.2	0.01	1,000,000	2	2	0
98	0.2	0.1	10,000,000	5	0	5
96	0.2	0.1	10,000,000	3	3	0
Controls	0	0.00000001	1	6	0	6 (died 36-48 hours)
Normal rabbit serum	0.1	0.0000001	10	6	0	6
Serum of rabbits immunized with uninfected rabbit organ extract	0.1	0.0000001	10	4	0	4

10,000 to 1,000,000 MLD, compared with a protection of 100 MLD for normal rabbit serum. An average of four to seven immunizing injections were given to the rabbits. The protection, on the whole, was less than that of the type 1 immune serum.

Protective Action of Immune Serum Against Type 3 Pneumococci.— Two rabbits were given as many as nine inoculations, intraperitoneally, of a type 3 organ extract antigen. The maximum dose was as high as 10 cc. The serums of these rabbits afforded no protection to mice against the homologous type of pneumococcus. This lack of protection against type 3 infections may be due to the low virulence of these organisms for rabbits; or possibly to the same factors which prevent a potent type 3 antiserum from being obtained in horses. Experiments are in progress, using a strain of type 3 pneumococci, which is highly virulent for rabbits.

Comparison Between the Protective Action of Type 1 Immune Rabbit Serum and Antipneumococcic Horse Serum.—The antipneumococcic horse serum was received from the New York State department of health. In as much as both the type 1 antipneumococcic horse serum and the type 1 immune rabbit serum protected as high as 10,000,000

TABLE 2.—PROTECTIVE ACTION OF IMMUNE RABBIT SERUMS AGAINST TYPE 2 PNEUMOCOCCIC INFECTIONS IN MICE

Rabbit Serums		Pneumococcus Culture, Type 2		Number of Mice	Result	
Number	Dose, Cc.	Dose, Cc.	Number of MLD	Used	Lived	Died
70	0.1	0.001	100,000	5	5	0
70	0.3	0.01	1,000,000	3	3	0
70	0.1	0.1	10,000,000	3	0	3
71	0.1	0.001	100,000	3	3	0
71	0.1	0.01	1,000,000	3	0	3
73	0.1	0.001	100,000	5	5	0
73	0.1	0.01	1,000,000	5	4	1
72	0.1	0.0001	10,000	3	3	0
72	0.1	0.001	100,000	3	1	2
75	0.1	0.0001	10,000	2	2	0
75	0.1	0.001	100,000	2	0	2
R-2	0.1	0.0001	10,000	5	4	1
R-2	0.1	0.001	100,000	3	0	3
R-3	0.1	0.0001	10,000	3	3	0
77	0.1	0.0001	10,000	3	3	0
Controls	0	0.00000001	1	4	0	4 (died 24-36 hours)
Normal rabbit serum	0.1	0.000001	100	3	3	0
Normal rabbit serum	0.1	0.00001	1,000	3	0	3

TABLE 3.—DELAYED THERAPY. COMPARISON BETWEEN PROTECTIVE ACTION OF IMMUNE BABBIT SERUM AND ANTIPNEUMOCOCCIC HORSE SERUM

Serum	Dose Serum, Cc.	Therapy Hours after Infection	Number of Mice Inoculated	Result	
				Lived	Died (Hours)
Immune rabbit serum	0.2	4	8	8	0
	0.5	8	7	7	0
	0.5	12	8	5	3
	0.5	15	8	2	6
Anti-pneumococcic horse serum	0.2	4	8	7	1 (72)
	0.5	8	7	6	1
	0.5	12	8	4	4 (56, 120, 96, 24 respectively)
	0.5	15	8	1	7

All mice were infected with 100,000 MLD of type 1 pneumococcus culture. Controls (no therapy) were dead within 24 hours.

MLD in mice, it was thought that by delaying the therapy in mice after infection, a quantitative differentiation in their protective actions could be obtained. Mice were inoculated with 100,000 MLD of pneumococci; therapy was given 4, 8, 12, and 15 hours later. The mice gave a positive blood culture within three hours and were sick within twelve hours after infection. The results (table 3) indicate approximately the same degree of protection between the antipneumococcic horse serum and the immune rabbit serum.

Properties of the Immune Rabbit Serum.—Agglutinins: The sera from two of the six rabbits immunized with type 1 antigen exhibited agglutination with the homologous organism (table 4). In no case was the reaction as high as that with antipneumococcic horse serum. The serum from one of the eight rabbits immunized with type 2 antigen showed agglutination with type 2 organisms.

TABLE 4.—AGGLUTINATION TESTS WITH IMMUNE RABBIT SERUMS

	Tube Number	Serum Number	Serum Dilution	Agglutination
Type 1 antigen plus type 1 immune rabbit serums*	1	94	Undiluted	+++
	2	94	1:5	0
	3	93	Undiluted	+++
	4	93	1:5	0
	5	95	Undiluted	0
	6	95	1:5	0
	7	98	Undiluted	0
	8	98	1:5	0
	9	96	Undiluted	0
	10	96	1:5	0
	11	199	Undiluted	0
	12	199	1:5	0
Type 1 antigen plus type 1 antipneumococcic horse serum	13	199	Undiluted	+++
	14	199	1:5	++
	15	199	1:10	+
Type 2 antigen plus type 2 immune rabbit serums*	16	73	Undiluted	0
	17	72	Undiluted	0
	18	71	Undiluted	+
	19	70	Undiluted	0
	20	R-1	Undiluted	0
	21	R-2	Undiluted	0
	22	R-3	Undiluted	0
	23	77	Undiluted	0
Type 2 antigen plus type 2 antipneumococcic horse serum*	24	77	Undiluted	+++
	25	77	1:10	+

* 0.3 cc. pneumococcus antigen + 0.3 cc. serum in each tube.

Precipitins: No precipitins were found with any of the protective serums, types 1 or 2.

Opsonins: No appreciable increase was observed in the phagocytic properties of leukocytes in the presence of the protective serums (table 5).

Bactericidal Action: The homologous organisms were left in contact with the immune rabbit serum for ¾ hour, plates were poured and counts made. No diminution in the viability of the pneumococci was obtained with bacteria in contact with the immune serum over that of normal rabbit serum.

Type Specificity of Protective Serum: The type 1 protective serums were tested against type 2 and type 3 pneumococci for protection in mice inoculated simultaneously with the heterologous type of organism. No protection was obtained with as small an infection as 10 MLD. Likewise, the type 2 protective serums were tested against types 1 and 3 pneumococcic infections in mice, and gave no protection.

Strain Specificity of Protective Serum: In order to determine whether the action of the protective serum was specific for the strain of pneumococci used in immunization, the protective action was tested against different strains of pneumococci but of the homologous types. The protection of both the type 1 and the type 2 immune serums was found to be as great for the heterologous strains as for the original strain.

TABLE 5.—OPSONINS IN IMMUNE RABBIT SERUMS

Rabbit Serum		Type of Pneumococcus	% Leukocytes Exhibiting Phagocytosis
Number	Dilution		
71	Undiluted	2	7
72	Undiluted	2	8
70	Undiluted	2	4
R-2	Undiluted	2	12
— (normal)	Undiluted	2	8
94	1:10	1	14
93	1:10	1	22
199	1:10	1	16
— (normal)	Undiluted	1	14
— (normal)	Undiluted	Avirulent type 4, to test viability of leukocytes	56

Homologous and Heterologous Animal Organs as Source of Antigen.—An attempt was made to determine whether mouse infected organs could be used as antigen for the immunization of rabbits.

Procedure.—The technic was essentially the same as for the rabbit organ extract-antigen, except that it was found necessary to use a greater amount of salt solution proportional to the volume of the mouse organs as compared with the rabbit organs, as rabbits inoculated subcutaneously with 0.1 cc. to 0.2 cc. of the mouse organ extract would die of pneumococcic septicemia. The organs of four mice, dead of type 1 pneumococcic infection, were removed and ground; to the mixture was added 10 cc. of normal salt solution, then the rivanol solution in the proportion of 1:2000. Immunization of two rabbits was carried out as follows: the first injection of 0.3 cc. of the antigenic mixture was given subcutaneously to each rabbit; a second injection of 1.0 cc. subcutaneously; and a third or final injection of 1.0 cc. intraperitoneally. The rabbits were bled nine days following the last inoculation (or three weeks following the first inoculation).

The protective action of these serums is given in table 6. The protection runs from 1,000,000 to 10,000,000 MLD. It would therefore appear that homologous animal organs are not necessary for the immunization of rabbits.

An attempt was made also to immunize a goat with the organ extract of a rabbit previously infected with type 2 pneumococci. Eight inoculations of the antigenic substance were given to the goat over a period of ten weeks, the largest dose being 60 cc. intraperitoneally. No protective properties were found in the goat's serum when tested in mice with type 2 pneumococcic infection. It is possible that a goat is not a susceptible animal for this method of immunization.

TABLE 6.—PROTECTIVE ACTION OF SERUMS OF RABBITS IMMUNIZED WITH INFECTED MOUSE ORGAN EXTRACT

Rabbit Serum		Pneumococcus Culture Type 1		Number of Mice	Result	
Number	Dose, Cc.	Dose, Cc.	Number of MLD	Inoculated	Lived	Died
140	0.3	0.01	1,000,000	3	2	1
140	0.2	0.1	10,000,000	5	2	3
141	0.3	0.01	1,000,000	3	3	0
141	0.2	0.1	10,000,000	2	2	0
141	0.1	0.1	10,000,000	3	0	3
Controls	0	0.00000001	1	4	0	4 (died 36-48 hours)

DISCUSSION

The tissue-extract mixture, used as antigen, contains many substances, including live pneumococci, dead pneumococci, pneumococci killed by rivanol, dissociation and metabolic products of the bacteria, tissue juices changed or unchanged by the growth of pneumococci in them, and possibly a toxin. It is impossible to state whether one, or all the above components, are responsible for the rapidity of immunization of the rabbits. It is possible that pneumococci derived directly from the animal body possess greater immunizing properties than those obtained by artificial culture, as it is known that the body fluids represent the most favorable conditions for the development and preservation of the capsule.

Another hypothesis is that certain of the substances present in the antigenic mixture act as haptenes in the presence of the pneumococci or their dissolution products, in this way increasing the antibody response.

It is quite possible that rabbits immunized by this method suffer from a low grade pneumococcic infection; a generalized fatal infection being prevented by the action of the rivanol on the pneumococci The mobilization of antibodies may be enhanced by the injection of the foreign protein present in the antigenic mixture.

The fact that the immune rabbit serum has such a high protective titer against type 1 infections, and yet contains only slight agglutinating properties, no demonstrable precipitins, no appreciable opsonins, and no bactericidal properties, would suggest the possibility that other immune bodies may be present, which are not contained in antipneumococcic horse serum. Whether or not these are of the nature of an antitoxin, cannot be definitely stated.

Inasmuch as rabbits are difficult to immunize by the usual methods of producing antipneumococcus serum, but were found to respond rapidly to the method described in this paper, it is not unlikely that higher animals, such as horses, might respond even more favorably in producing an immune serum.

SUMMARY

A method for the rapid production of an antipneumococcic serum in rabbits by injections of extracts of infected rabbit tissue, is described. The type 1 antipneumococcic serum affords the highest protection; the type 2 serum protects to a lesser degree; the type 3 serum gives no protection. The immune serums are type specific, but not strain specific, in their protective action; by in vitro tests they show few agglutinins, no precipitins, no remarkable opsonic powers, and no direct bactericidal action. The antipneumococcic rabbit serum is as effective as a sample of antipneumococcic horse serum in protecting mice against type 1 infections.

The tissues of an homologous animal are not necessary for the production of the antigen.

STUDIES ON BOTULINUS TOXIN

2. FURTHER PURIFICATION BY ADSORPTION ON COLLOIDS

H. Sommer and P. Tessmer Snipe

From the George Williams Hooper Foundation for Medical Research, University of California Medical School, San Francisco

In the first paper of this series [1] experiments which dealt with the isolation of botulinus toxin (parabotulinus strain, type A) by means of colloids were reported. Since the solid products secured in these preliminary studies showed variable degrees of toxicity, protein reactions and enzyme activities it was deemed advisable to make a more carefui analysis of the different steps involved in the process of purification. Special attention was paid to the adsorption and elution at varying P_H values and at different time intervals. An improved method which gives uniform and generally more potent dry products was thus developed.

Different mediums were used as sources for the toxin. They consisted either of commercial peptone or peptic digest, to which in some cases veal infusion, in others beef heart extract was added; some samples contained gelatine. Cl. parabotulinum, type A were cultivated in these substrates for 10 days or longer. These cultures were either used immediately after removal from the incubator, while others were stored for from 1 to 12 months. The potency ranged from $1x10^{-4}$ to $1x10^{-5}$ cc. per MLD. for a 20 gm. mouse after 48 hours. Although extreme care was taken at the beginning to use uniform samples for the same experiment, experience has subsequently shown that mediums of different ages and of varying compositions are similar in their behavior towards the adsorbing and eluting agents. The culture fluids were decanted from the sediments and centrifugated or filtered through paper. In order to remove the organisms as completely as possible and to effect a preliminary purification 5 gm. of kaolin suspended finely in distilled water were mixed with each liter of toxin and the solution filtered through paper. As a rule this treatment removes very little toxin when the solutions are kept at approximate neutrality. The "kaolin filtrate" served as a stock solution for future experiments. When kept on ice it proved stable.

The colloidal preparations and toxin tests, etc., which were used in the studies to be reported were the same as described in the first paper of this series. In these as well as in the former experiments the γ variant of the alumina suspension [2] was used. The hydrogen ion concentration of the solutions was determined colorimetrically. Toluene was added as a preservative.

Adsorption of Botulinus Toxin at Different P_H *Values.*—Fifty cc. samples of "kaolin filtrate" were adjusted to different Sörensen values with 10% H_3PO_4 or N/10 NH_4OH. Experience had shown that adsorption of toxin from mediums rich in proteins was more complete

Received for publication, Jan. 28, 1928.

1. J. Infect. Dis., 1926, 39, p. 345.
2. Ber. d. deutsch. chem. Gesellsch., 1925, 58, p. 2448.

after a preliminary treatment with a small amount of aluminum-hydroxide. One and five-tenths cc. of alumina were therefore added to the 50 cc. samples. This small amount of colloid removed some of the pigments and the odoriferous substances without impairing the toxicity. It is unnecessary to leave the alumina and the toxin in contact for 30 minutes as previously reported. The adsorption equilibrium is established immediately and the homogeneous mixture can be filtered or centrifugated at once. The potency of the different specimens of toxin treated at various P_H values after centrifugating is shown in table 1 (Al-filtrate 1). The filtrates were then thoroughly mixed with 20 cc. of alumina each and centrifugated (Al-filtrate 2 in table 1). The degree of adsorption which took place is expressed by the difference in potency of the two filtrates. As a check the amount of adsorbed

TABLE 1.—ADSORPTION OF BOTULINUS TOXIN ON ALUMINA AT DIFFERENT PH VALUES

	Toxicity of Al-Filtrate 1		Toxicity of Al-Filtrate 2		Toxicity of Al-Suspension		Adsorption of Toxin
P_H	Cc.	Hours	Cc.	Hours	Cc.	Hours	%
3.0	1×10^{-4}	43	1×10^{-3}	68	1×10^{-4}	27	90
3.8	1×10^{-4}	43	1×10^{-3}	S.	1×10^{-4}	43	95
4.5	1×10^{-4}	21	1×10^{-2}	22	1×10^{-4}	24	99
5.0	1×10^{-4}	18	1×10^{-3}	20	1×10^{-4}	18	90
5.7	1×10^{-4}	22	1×10^{-4}	31	1×10^{-4}	24	60
6.2	1×10^{-4}	18	1×10^{-4}	23	1×10^{-4}	23	50
7.0	1×10^{-4}	20	1×10^{-3}	20	1×10^{-4}	20	90
7.5	1×10^{-4}	<20	1×10^{-4}	31	1×10^{-4}	20	60

The hours indicate time of death of mouse after injection. S = showed symptoms, but survived.

toxin was determined directly. For this purpose the alumina toxin precipitate was washed in 50 cc. of a 1% $(NH_4)H_2PO_4$ solution and centrifugated; no toxin was lost in the course of this procedure. The precipitate resuspended in 50 cc. of distilled water was tested for its potency. It goes without saying that a control injection of 1 cc. alumina suspension was made and invariably proved entirely harmless for mice. Numerous tests have shown that alumina does not influence the pharmacological effect of the toxin and the reliability of the MLD determination is in no way impaired. From data presented in table 1 the approximate degree of adsorption was calculated and expressed in percentages of the total amount of toxin present in the Al-filtrate 1. In this connection it must be emphasized that figures are of relative value, since the absolute toxin titers have not been determined. The adsorption curve (fig. 1) which is based on the tests in table 1 is of practical value. Its general trend has been confirmed by numerous adsorption experiments with culture fluids of different origins. The adsorption of the botulinus toxin at a P_H of approximately 4.5 is nearly complete, it is fair at neutrality, but distinctly lower between a P_H of 5 and 7.

At this stage of toxin purification it is inadvisable to attempt any theoretical conclusions as to the electrical charge of the toxin particle. In the light of later experiments, however, the maximum adsorption at P_H 4 to 4.5 is of interest. It will be shown (paper 3 of this series)[3] that at this degree of acidity the toxin is precipitated either as such, or adsorbed to an atoxic precipitate. This flocculation is greatly aided by the addition of aluminum hydroxide. The precipitation is thus

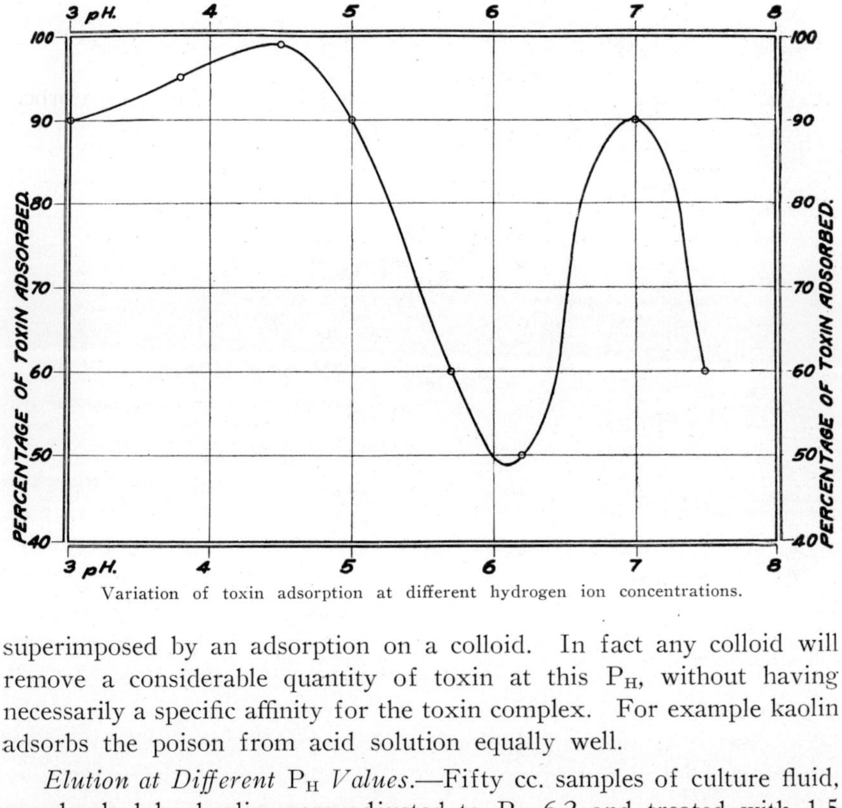

Variation of toxin adsorption at different hydrogen ion concentrations.

superimposed by an adsorption on a colloid. In fact any colloid will remove a considerable quantity of toxin at this P_H, without having necessarily a specific affinity for the toxin complex. For example kaolin adsorbs the poison from acid solution equally well.

Elution at Different P_H *Values.*—Fifty cc. samples of culture fluid, preadsorbed by kaolin were adjusted to P_H 6.2 and treated with 1.5 cc. alumina. The clear centrifugate was brought to P_H 4.5 and detoxified by 20 cc. aluminum hydroxide. The adsorbate was thoroughly washed free from mother liquor with water and its toxicity tested; for this purpose the precipitate was evenly distributed in a known

3. J. Infect. Dis., 1928, 43, pp. 146, 154.

volume of water and dilutions made in salt solution from this suspension. Fifty cc. of 1% solutions of ammonium phosphate at Sörensen values of 4.3, 6.2 and 7.8 were used for elutions. One drop of glycerine was added and the temperature raised to 30 C. One sample of each suspension at different P_H values was centrifugated after standing for 10 and 30 minutes and then after several hours. The results of the toxin determinations as summarized in table 2 indicate an optimum elution effect at slight alkalinity (P_H 7.8). On the other hand this experiment shows that the alumina can be washed with primary ammonium phosphate (P_H 4.3) without any loss of toxin. By fractional elution at the P_H values of 4.3 and 7.8 most of the brown pigment and possibly other impurities can be removed.

TABLE 2.—ELUTION OF BOTULINUS TOXIN FROM ALUMINA AT DIFFERENT PH VALUES

Toxicity of Suspension	1 x 10^{-4} Cc.					
P_H of elution........	4.3		6.2		7.8	
Time of elution.....	10 minutes	2 hours	30 minutes	20 hours (o.n.)	10 minutes	2 hours
Toxicity of elution..	1 cc.	1x10^{-1} cc.	1x10^{-2} cc.	0.5x10^{-2} cc.	1x10^{-4} cc.	1x10^{-3} cc.

Temperature = 30C. (o.n.) = over night at room temperature.

TABLE 3.—ELUTION AT PH 7.8 FOR DIFFERENT LENGTHS OF TIME

	Suspension	Elution				Suspension
Time	0	10 Minutes	45 Minutes	2 Hours	4 Hours	4 Hours
Toxicity......	1x10^{-4} cc. D.	1x10^{-4} cc. D.	1x10^{-4} cc. S. 1x10^{-3} cc. D.	1x10^{-3} cc. D.	1x10^{-3} cc. D.	1x10^{-3} cc. D.

D = death; S = symptoms, survived

Elution as a Function of Time.—In a further experiment the time factor was more closely investigated. Fifty cc. of toxin were worked up as stated in the tests mentioned above and the elution started with a 1% solution of secondary ammonium phosphate (P_H 7.8). After various intervals of time the mixture was centrifugated, 1 cc. withdrawn for toxin tests and the rest thoroughly mixed again. From the results shown in table 3 it is evident that elution longer than 10 minutes is not necessary and even destructive. In this time interval most of the toxin can be brought into solution, while standing for several hours in a weakly alkaline medium causes a deterioration of the larger part of the poison. A parallel experiment was run in which the toxin was adsorbed at neutrality and eluted with alkaline phosphate as above. The same time curve was obtained for the elution as in table 3.

Dialysis.—In order to determine the degree of purification achieved by the adsorption-elution process it was necessary to dialyze the solutions salt-free and to determine the dry weight of the end products.

In the light of the results in table 3 it is advisable to neutralize the alkaline eluate at once and to let the dialysis proceed at ice box temperature (5 C.). Collodion impregnated fish bladders were used (paper 4 of this series).[4] In order to make the dialysis of the salts and amino acids complete it was found necessary to change the outside water twice daily for 4 to 6 days, the relative volumes of in- and outside being approximately 1 : 4. Evaporation in vacuo yields the dry product.

SUMMARY OF PURIFICATION PROCESS

The above experiments lead to a process by which relatively uniform and potent dry toxins have been procured. The procedure is as follows. The supernatant toxic culture fluid of Cl. botulinum—preferably two or more liters—is adsorbed with 5 gms. of kaolin (for 1 liter of fluid) and filtered. After adjusting the reaction to P_H 6.0 to 6.2 with HCl or H_3PO_4 a preliminary adsorption with 30 cc. of aluminum cream per liter is made in order to remove some non toxic substances. The filtrate is brought to a Sörensen value of 4.4 and the toxin adsorbed on 400 cc. alumina per liter. The precipitate is filtered off by suction and thoroughly washed with several portions of 1% $(NH_4)\ H_2PO_4$ solution until the wash water is colorless. The elution is effected with a 1% solution of secondary ammonium phosphate, the volume being about one-half of that of the original culture fluid. The phosphate solution is previously warmed to approximately 30 C. and the mixture kept at that temperature for not longer than 10 minutes. The alumina is then filtered off and discarded although it still contains an appreciable amount of toxin (approximately 10%). The solution is practically without color and odor; it contains as a rule $1 \times 10^{+4}$ MLDs. per cc. When neutralized and stored in a cool and dark place this solution will keep for several months and may with advantage be used for any experiments in which a purified botulinus toxin is needed. For the preparation of a dry product the solution is dialyzed against distilled water for 4 to 6 days; during this process a considerable loss of potency is unavoidable. By evaporation to dryness in vacuo at 40 to 45 C. the solid toxin is secured.

Properties of the Solid Toxin Preparations.—By the method just outlined three isolations were undertaken with two liters of culture fluid in each experiment; 180, 103 * and 80 mg.† of dry substance

4. J. Infect. Dis., 1928, 43, p. 163.

* Some substance was lost by foaming during evaporation.

† A slight modification was introduced in the preparation of this 3rd product. The final solution after evaporation in vacuo to a small volume was again dialyzed for 3 x 12 hours and then the evaporation completed. This procedure resulted in a loss of of toxicity as well as in total yield.

respectively were recovered. During evaporation the solutions turned slightly colored and the solid substances are dark brown amorphous flakes. They are readily soluble in water to collodial solutions; in the strength of 0.1% a slight turbidity is still perceptible. Of the protein color reactions previously enumerated (paper 1), only the biuret test is persistently positive. All products give a slight Molisch reaction. Considering the high sensitivity of the test a positive reaction is of little significance. On addition of acetic acid, heavy metal salts or Millon's reagent to a toxin solution a white flocculent precipitate occurs. From the chemical properties as well as the mode of preparation of the dry toxins the colloidal character of the end products is evident.

The toxicity of the three preparations was tested as dilutions made in saline from the 0.1% solution in water. The MLD in all cases was found to be approximately 1 cc. of the 1:10,000 dilution, thus

TABLE 4.—TOXICITY OF THREE DRY TOXIN PREPARATIONS

1		2		3	
$1/3 \times 10^{-7}$ gm., (two mice)	S. 24 hours D. 24 hours			1×10^{-7} gm.,	S. 26 hours
1×10^{-7} gm.,	D. 24 hours	1×10^{-7} gm.,	D. 22-40 hours (over night)	1×10^{-6} gm.,	D. 26 hours

D = death; S = symptoms, survived.

representing 1×10^{-7} gm. of solid substance. Table 4 shows the details of the toxin tests.

The total yield of the number of MLD originally present in the toxic broth and finally recovered in the purification process is small, 6% and 2.5% in sample 1 and 2 respectively. It is, however, not unlikely that atoxic substances contained in the culture fluid may have had an enhancing action on the potency or on the absorption of the fluid toxin in the animal body, so that the total yield based on the MLD content could not be accurately calculated. On the other hand the degree of purification can be estimated by comparing the amount of solid substance per MLD in the original and the final toxin. For instance the "kaolin filtrate" which yielded toxin 2 showed a potency of $\frac{1}{2} \times 10^{-4}$ cc. per MLD and contained roughly 5% solid substance determined by evaporation and drying of a sample. One MLD is thus contained in 2.5×10^{-6} gm., which compared with the final product (1×10^{-7} gm.) gives a degree of purification of approximately 25.

It was of interest to compare these results with those of a dry toxin secured without specific adsorption. For this purpose one liter of culture fluid was filtered through a Berkefeld candle and dialyzed for eight times 12 hours. During dialysis the toxin titer dropped from 1×10^{-4} cc. to 3×10^{-3} cc. After evaporation in vacuo 1.007 gm. solid substance were obtained having a MLD of 1×10^{-6} gm. Assuming roughly a 5% content of solids in the Berkefeld filtrate, the degree of purification equals 5; the yield in total number of MLD being 10%. The results show that by specific absorption a considerably more concentrated and possibly purer toxic product may be obtained.

In comparing the toxicity of these preparations with those of the former procedure [1] a noteworthy increase in potency is clearly indicated. This may be regarded as the result of a more definite knowledge of the behavior of the toxin and of its accompanying substances towards the adsorptive colloids. Furthermore a thorough dialysis of the salts is of definite advantage, if solid toxins are prepared by evaporation. It has been found repeatedly that concentrated salt solutions are harmful to the poison.

In the former publication the fact was mentioned that the solid toxins exhibit enzymatic activities. "Gelatinase" and a peptidase has generally been found. Contrary to those observations the new products contain only gelatinase. In which step of the purification process the peptidase is eliminated was not determined. Likewise the presence of other enzymes than proteinases was not investigated. The strength of gelatinase activity in the three products described varies considerably. In order to liquefy completely 10 cc. of a 2.5% gelatine solution at 37 C. approximately 1,000, 10,000 and 500 MLD of the preparations 1 to 3 respectively were necessary. Peptidase was tested for in 20 cc. of a 4% Witte peptone solution and titrated according to Sörensen's method with N/20 NaOH. With 50,000 MLD of substance 1, differences smaller than 0.05 cc. as compared with the control were noted. Dry toxin prepared by mere dialysis contains both enzymes.

A simple procedure which yields preparations of high potency and devoid of proteinases will be described in paper 3 of this series.

SUMMARY

The behavior of botulinus toxin towards colloidal alumina, especially the rôle of the P_H, the time in the adsorption and elution processes are described and an improved procedure for the preparation of toxins in solid form is outlined. The products secured by this method have a toxicity of 3×10^{-7} to 3×10^{-8} gm. per MLD for the mouse. They give the biuret test, a slight Molisch reaction, and contain a small amount of gelatinase.

STUDIES ON BOTULINUS TOXIN

3. ACID PRECIPITATION OF BOTULINUS TOXIN

P. Tessmer Snipe and H. Sommer

From the George Williams Hooper Foundation for Medical Research, University of California Medical School, San Francisco

Experiments on botulinus toxin at different hydrogen ion concentrations [1] led necessarily to a closer study of the relationship between toxicity and P_H. There prevails a close agreement among the workers in this field, that botulinus toxin is injured by weak alkalies (P_H 8.0, Bronfenbrenner [2] and observations in this laboratory), but is not harmed by relatively strong acids (acidity of the stomach, Bronfenbrenner [2]). The earlier literature on this subject is reviewed by Bengtson.[3] One outstanding observation, however, has been published by Bronfenbrenner and Schlesinger.[4] These workers reported on an enormous increase in potency on acidification of toxin to P_H 4.0. Young culture fluids could thus be enhanced in their toxicity from a MLD for the mouse of 3×10^{-6} cc. to 3×10^{-18} cc. and occasionally to 3×10^{-21} cc. Geiger and Gouwens [5] and several workers in this laboratory (unpublished observations) were unable to substantiate these findings. On the other hand, Bengtson [3] reported on a 5 and 32 fold increase in two type A culture fluids on acidification to P_H 4.0. In a later discussion of the question Bronfenbrenner [6] states that: "the degree of this increase probably is not as great as some of our findings seem to indicate. We suspect that there may occur an ultramicroscopic * precipitation of the toxin-carrying portion of the medium. If the minute particles of such a precipitate should possess particularly high adsorption power, they could be carried from dilution to dilution and thus vitiate the accuracy of the calculation," and furthermore: "we are preparing detailed protocols of the experiments to date which we hope to publish in the near future." Although the experimental records have not been pub-

Received for publication, Jan. 28, 1928.

1. J. Infect. Dis., 1928, 42, p. ?? (later).
2. J. Exper. Med., 1924, 39, p. 509.
3. Hyg. Lab. Bull. 136, 1924, p. 62.
4. Proc. Soc. Exper. Biol. & Med., 1921, 19, p. 1; J. Am. M. A., 1922, 78, p. 1519.
5. Pub. Health Rep. 39, 1923, 38, p. 2249.
6. Science, 1922, 56, p. 280.

* Original text reads "ultramiscropic."

lished by Bronfenbrenner to this date, a short presentation of the findings in this laboratory seemed justified.

EXPERIMENTAL

After numerous earlier experiments had failed to demonstrate an enhanced potency of acidified toxin, more recent tests seemed to substantiate Bronfenbrenner's findings. Type A culture filtrates with a potency of 1×10^{-4} to 1×10^{-5} cc. per MLD could be increased 10 to 100,000 times by adjusting the toxin to a P_H of 4.0 to 4.6. The statements of Bronfenbrenner and Schlesinger concerning the differences in culture fluids of various ages, toxins of different purity, etc., could be confirmed. It was, however, soon discovered that the increase in potency was due to an experimental error. In diluting the original culture fluid in saline only one pipet had been used for one set of dilutions. Whereas at neutrality this simplified procedure gives dependable results and only occasionally a small positive error, it is inapplicable with solutions of a P_H lower than 5.0. The highly dispersed toxic precipitate which occurs on acidification of a botulinum culture fluid adheres firmly to the glass and is carried over with the pipet into the higher dilution tubes. The positive error which thus arises is variable to a large degree and depends mainly on the personal technic used in making the dilutions. More careful and repeated rinsing of the pipet in the saline gives rise to a larger error. One worker (Snipe) using the same method did not find an increased potency on acidification. If a fresh pipet is taken for each transfer of toxin into the next tube of salt solution the error is avoided, and the same potency was found in acid and neutral culture fluids. The small variations in potency which have occasionally been observed in toxins adjusted to different P_H values were inconsistent and within the limit of error in animal experimentation.

In a more recent publication [1] Bronfenbrenner and Schlesinger report on a slightly increased potency of acidified toxin in two cases. The result in table 1, p. 513 of their paper, however, does not necessarily substantiate this assumption. As all the tubes containing the toxin at different acidities were incubated for 24 hours at 37 C. an apparent maximum potency at P_H 4.1 to 5.0 may merely mean an optimum stability at this acidity, the samples at the remaining P_H values being injured in their potency to various degrees. The findings in table 2 would indicate an increase in toxicity at a P_H of 3.0; but since the observations on the unadjusted control toxin (according to the text on page 514 incubated at 37 C.) are not tabulated, it is doubtful if this actually occurred. It is a well known fact that toxin at a P_H of 7.0 gradually decreases on incubation at 37 C. In fact the decline runs a similar course as shown in table 2 for tubes 4 and 5. Probably the same deterioration took place in tube 1, but no record is made of this fact.

The numerous observations made in this laboratory do not furnish any evidence for an enhanced potency of acid botulinus toxin.

PREPARATION OF DRY TOXIN BY ACID PRECIPITATION

The fact that acidification of Cl. botulinum culture fluid yields a toxic precipitate made it possible to arrive at solid toxin preparations

TABLE 1.—PRECIPITATION OF BOTULINUS TOXIN AT DIFFERENT P_H VALUES

Drops of HCl (conc.)	P_H	Turbidity in Fluid	Precipitate	Toxicity of Supernatant Cc.
1	6.3	—	—	1×10^{-4}
2	5.1	±	—	1×10^{-4}
3	4.2	+	++	1×10^{-4}
4	3.3	—	+++	$> 1 \times 10^{-3}$
5	2.4	—	+++	$> 1 \times 10^{-3}$ *
6	1.8	+	+++	$> 1 \times 10^{-3}$ *
7	1.2	++	++	$> 1 \times 10^{-2}$ *
8	< 1.2	++	++	—
9	< 1.2	++	+	—
10	< 1.2	+	+	—

* Determined after roughly neutralizing the excess acid. The tests show, that botulinus toxin is not completely destroyed at very low P_H values.

by a simple procedure. In order to obtain a relatively pure product it was necessary to employ a medium which contains no acid precipitable constituents. Four per cent peptone (an equal mixture of Difco and Berna peptone) with or without addition of phosphates served the purpose. Three strains, all type A, were used. Hydrochloric, phosphoric and acetic acids in concentrated or dilute solutions can be employed for precipitation equally well; concentrated hydrochloric acid was generally used. All P_H values reported in this paper were determined colorimetrically.

In order to ascertain the optimum P_H for precipitation increasing amounts of HCl conc. were added to 10 cc. samples of culture fluid. The precipitate is usually not visible at first, but becomes apparent as a light flocculum on standing. The tubes were therefore put in the ice chest for 24 hours and were then centrifuged for 10 minutes. In table 1 the approximate turbidity and amount of precipitate at the various P_H values are recorded. The results indicate a wide range of flocculation with an optimum precipitation at a P_H of approximately 3.0. Different results are obtained with culture fluids freed from electrolytes by dialysis and with products that were purified by repeated precipitation and dissolution. In these instances a narrow zone of flocculation around a P_H of 4.4 (determined with bromphenol blue) was found. It is probable that the electrolytes present in the culture fluid shift the isoelectric point of the substance to the acid side. At various times acidification of salt free toxins to P_H values of 4.3 and 4.5 only produced a turbidity throughout the solution without flocculation. On subsequent careful adjustment to P_H 4.4 the substance often settled in a few minutes.

TABLE 2.—RELATION OF AGE OF CULTURE TO TOXICITY AND PRECIPITABLE PROTEIN

Length of Growth Period	40 Hours	64 Hours	108 Hours	156 Hours	288 Hours
Toxicity of culture fluid					
Before acidification..........	1×10^{-4} S 1×10^{-3} D	1×10^{-5} S 1×10^{-4} D	1×10^{-4} D	1×10^{-4} D	1×10^{-4} D
After acidification............	1×10^{-4} S 1×10^{-3} D	1×10^{-4} D	1×10^{-4} S 1×10^{-3} D	1×10^{-4} D	1×10^{-4} S 1×10^{-3} D
Weight of precipitate mg........	15.4	24.0	40.5	30.8	48.5
Toxicity of precipitate 1×10^{-6} gm.	0.5	0.5	0.2	0.2	0.2
M L Ds recovered: % of total number	1	0.5	3.3	2.5	4

D = death, S = symptoms, survived

A set of experiments was then undertaken to ascertain at which stage of growth the maximum toxicity and the largest amount of acid precipitable material is produced.

Five flasks containing 600 cc. of medium each were inoculated with an equal amount of heated spores of strain 62 and incubated for varying periods. The cultures were then centrifugated for one hour and filtered through Berkefeld candles. The clear fluids on being adjusted to P_H 3.0 became turbid and after standing on ice for several days yielded a flocculent sediment. The supernatant solutions were siphoned off, the precipitate collected by centrifugalization, washed with 20 cc. of distilled water, dried in vacuum and weighed. The toxicity of the culture fluids before and after precipitation, the yield of the dry substances and their potency was determined; the results are tabulated in table 2.

Considering the possible differences of growth in the various flasks, the probable adsorption of toxic precipitate by the filter candles and other uncontrollable factors the results given in table 2 cannot be considered quantitative. They suggest, however, that the amount of precipitable substance increases during the growth of the organisms and that a product of higher potency and a greater yield can be obtained after the fourth day of growth. Furthermore, the maximum toxicity of the culture fluid does not coincide with the largest amount of precipitable substance which can be secured.

From the data in tables 1 and 2 it is evident that only a small part of the total potency of a botulinum culture fluid is precipitated by acid, a fact which Bronfenbrenner and Reichert [7] have emphasized in a recent publication. There is, however, a possibility that the precipitable substance is partially held in solution by some constituent of the culture fluid. Subsequent experiments confirmed this assumption. If the electrolytes and possibly other substances are removed by dialysis a precipitate with considerably greater potency is formed. The following experiment illustrates this statement. Six hundred cubic centimeters of a culture fluid with a potency of 1×10^{-4} cc. was adjusted to P_H 3.0

TABLE 3.—ACID PRECIPITATION BEFORE AND AFTER DIALYSIS OF CULTURE FLUID

Fraction	Amount	Toxicity	Per Cent of Total Potency
Culture fluid neutral.....	600 cc.	1×10^{-4} cc. D 68 hours 1×10^{-3} cc. D 18 hours (o. n.)	100
Filtrate P_H 3.0 after precipitation	610 cc.	1×10^{-4} cc. D 65 hours 1×10^{-3} cc. D 16 hours (o. n.)	Approximately 100
Precipitate 1 before dialysis	123.5 mg.	0.0001 mg. S 0.001 mg. D 24 hours	Approximately 4
Filtrate after dialysis....	350 cc.	1×10^{-3} cc. S. 1×10^{-2} cc. D 27 hours	2 (corrected for 600 cc.)
Precipitate 2 after dialysis	7.0 mg. (12 mg. per 600 cc.)	0.00001 mg. D 66 hours 0.0001 mg. D 19 hours (o. n.)	20 (corrected for 600 cc.)

D = dead, S = symptoms, survived, (o. n.) = over night

with 12 cc. of concentrated hydrochloric acid. The precipitate settled over night in the ice chest, was collected by centrifuging, washed with water and dried in vacuo. It represented approximately 4% of the potency originally present. The supernatant fluid, tested after filtration through paper, was practically undiminished in its potency. Three hundred and fifty cubic centimeters of it were then placed in a membrane and dialyzed against distilled water for six days, the outside fluid being changed twice daily. After 45 hours a flocculent precipitate was noticed inside the membrane. Upon completion of dialysis the sediment was separated from the fluid, washed and dried. Its weight amounted to 7.0 mg. and its potency to 0.00001 mg. per MLD. The final filtrate had lost most of its toxicity; it contained only 2% of the numbers of MLD originally present. The tabulation of the results in table 3

7. J. Exper. Med., 1926, 44, p. 553.

reveals that the largest part of the potency is recovered in the precipitate 2, after dialysis of the salts.

For the practical purpose of toxin preparation it is evidently unnecessary to separate precipitate 1 and 2 as in the foregoing experiment. A fair amount of solid substance with a considerable toxicity may be obtained by the simple procedure of dialyzing an acidified culture fluid regardless of the precipitate it contains. After diffusion of the salts is complete the sediment is collected, washed and dried as in the previous experiments. For comparison three samples of a culture fluid having a toxicity of 3×10^{-5} cc. were adjusted to the P_H values 1.8, 3.0 and 4.4 and treated in the manner described. The results as presented in table 4, suggest an optimum yield at P_H 3.0. It is not unlikely that different results may be obtained with culture fluids of variant compositions; the three products are merely cited as actual examples of the yields obtained.

TABLE 4.—YIELD OF TOXIC PRECIPITATE IN DIALYSIS AT DIFFERENT PH VALUES

PH of Toxin	Yield of Solid Substance Mg. per Liter	Approximate MLD	Yield in % of Total Toxicity
1.8	72	3×10^{-8} gm.	8.0
3.0	171	2×10^{-8} gm.	28.5
4.4	91	2×10^{-8} gm.	15.2

PROPERTIES OF THE ACID PRECIPITATE

The freshly precipitated substance from a Cl. botulinum culture fluid under its supernatant liquid is practically white, on washing with water and exposure to air it usually turns gray. After drying in the vacuum desiccator it appears as a brown or black amorphous powder. The substance is insoluble in water and acids; it can be brought into solution with alkalies and forms a stable, slightly turbid colloidal suspension. For toxin tests it is triturated to a fine powder and suspended in a 1 per cent sodium phosphate solution of P_H 7.0. The excess of undissolved material is centrifugated off and suspended in fresh phosphate mixture and the process is usually repeated until dissolution is complete. A saturated phosphate solution contains approximately 0.1% solid substance. Attempts to purify the acid precipitable substance by repeated dissolution at neutrality and reprecipitation at P_H 4.4 were temporarily discontinued as most of the toxicity is lost during this procedure. A closer chemical analysis of the products has therefore not been undertaken. The crude compound, dissolved in alkali gives a positive biuret reaction. Four different samples, after destruction with boiling concentrated acid, yielded a small amount of phosphoric acid These properties as well as the fact that the substance is insoluble in an excess of acid tend to show that the compound belongs to the group of nucleoproteins.

From tables 2, 3 and 4 the high toxicity of the substances isolated is evident. It will be seen also that the products obtained by acid precipitation alone show a lower potency than those procured by dialysis. Fifteen samples prepared by acid precipitation showed toxicities of 5×10^{-7} to 1×10^{-7} gm. (one sample 5×10^{-8} gm.) per MLD. The yield averaged 0.5 to 4% of the total amount of toxin present in the original culture fluid. If precipitation was aided by dialysis the minimum lethal doses were lowered to 3×10^{-8} to 1×10^{-8} gm. (tables 3 and 4), with an increase in yield to 8.0 to 28.5% of the initial potency. These latter products likewise show a higher enzyme content than the former ones. Gelatinase, peptidase and lipase were tested for as described in paper 2 [1] of this series. With several products prepared by precipitation alone no enzyme action could be detected when tested with 1 cc. samples containing 10,000 MLD. Dialyzed acid culture filtrates were generally found to be devoid of most of the toxic as well as enzymatic activities.

In view of the recent experiments of Nelson [8] the action of pepsin on the nucleoprotein was investigated in a preliminary test. A large part of the acid precipitate disappeared on incubation with pepsin for 21 hours at 37 C. but the toxicity remained equal to the potency in the control tube.

DISCUSSION

Since the culture medium used in these experiments contained no acid precipitable substances, it is evident that the products isolated originated through bacterial activity. It is not unlikely that they arise through autolysis of the bacterial bodies. Further chemical and immunological examinations are under way to ascertain the nature of the substance. Analogies of these findings with experiments recently published by Nelson [8] suggest, however, that the "nucleoprotein" may be identical with the substance called "globulin" by Nelson. The question as to the identity of acid precipitate and toxin is naturally of primary importance. Most of the results tend to show that the nucleoprotein is pharmacologically inert and that the toxin and the

8. J. Infect. Dis., 1927, 41, p. 9.

enzymes of the culture fluid are merely adsorbed to it. Specially in salt-free solutions the adsorption can become practically quantitative. Furthermore, the fact that pepsin partially dissolves the precipitate leaving the toxin intact, adds considerable weight to this assumption. On the other hand there is a bare possibility that the precipitate represents a mixture of toxin and inactivated toxin (toxoid or anatoxin) which cannot be differentiated by the crude chemical methods employed. In this way the widely variant potencies of the chemically identical precipitates could be explained.

The resemblances of this work with studies on diphtheria toxin are evident. Glenny and Walpole[9] were the first to employ acid precipitation of dialyzed culture fluids for the practical preparation of concentrated toxins. In detailed studies on the precipitation of "diphtherin" with hydrochloride acid v. Groer[10] showed a similar influence of the salt content on the P_H range of the flocculation as recorded in our experiments. A noteworthy difference between botulinus and diphtheria culture fluids, however, is the high yield of toxin which may be obtained when the latter is treated with acids; for example v. Groer[10] and Sedallion and Gaumont[11] found a quantitative precipitation, while Watson and Wallace[12] reported a 60-70% yield from dialyzed as well as undialyzed toxins. According to Predtechenskiy and Schevyakova the isoelectric point of the active protein from the diphtheria culture is given as P_H 4.2 to 4.6.[13]

Long and Seibert[14] have precipitated part of the tuberculin from cultures of the tubercle bacillus at P_H 4.0 with the aid of acetic acid. They have found the precipitation to be very incomplete. In view of the findings presented here dialysis might possibly increase the yield considerably. The authors prefer ammonium sulfate for the precipitation of tuberculin, because the acting substances could be removed quantitatively from the culture fluid. It is, however, not evident from the experiments if the reacting substance is concentrated in the precipitate quantitatively, as part of the tuberculin might be destroyed by the concentrated salt solution. In the case of botulinus toxin only a small percentage of the poison can be recovered in the ammonium sulfate precipitate; the largest part (at least 90%) is destroyed and the super-

9. Biochem. J., 1915, 9, p. 298.
10. Biochem. Ztschr., 1923, 138, p. 13.
11. Compt. rend. Soc. de biol., 1927, 97, p. 93.
12. J. Path. & Bacteriol., 1924, 27, p. 271.
13. Mikrobiol, J., Leningrad, 1926, 3, p. 109; abstr. J. Am. M. A., 1926, 87, p. 2042.
14. Am. Rev. Tuberc., 1926, 13, p. 398.

natant fluid is completely atoxic. Furthermore, the precipitate often contains lower protein derivatives. The reasons why acid precipitation has been preferred to the salting out of botulinus toxin are therefore apparent. Watson and Langstaff[15] also have obtained purer products in the preparation of diphtheria toxoid by precipitation with acid in place of ammonium sulfate.

Bronfenbrenner and Reichert[7] have recently investigated the Ramon flocculation test with botulinus toxin and have found that the substance responsible for the flocculation is the acid precipitable protein of the culture fluid. After its "removal" with acid no flocculation with antitoxin occurred. Since it is shown here that the protein cannot be completely removed by acidification the experiment does not necessarily substantiate the conclusions drawn by the authors. The identity of toxin and "nucleoprotein" is not disproved, since some electrolytes in the acid culture fluid hold part of the "nucleoprotein" in solution. Separation of proteins in the presence of salts is necessarily not complete (in the case of serum proteins see for instance Ettisch and Beck[16]). It is also quite probable that the electrolytes have a dissolving action on the flocculum of toxin and antitoxin, and that dialyzed toxin samples might give different results on titrating according to Ramon's technic.

SUMMARY

The potency of impure or of purified botulinus toxin cannot be increased by acidification. The data presented in the literature can be explained on a different basis.

By acidification of botulinum (type A) culture fluids toxic substances were isolated representing 0.5 to 4% of the total potency and having a toxicity of 5×10^{-7} to 5×10^{-8} gm. per MLD.

By dialysis of acidified culture fluids 8 to 28% of the original number of MLD can be recovered with a toxicity of $3 \times 10^{-8} — 1 \times 10^{-8}$ gm. per MLD.

The preparations give the biuret reaction, contain a small amount of phosphorus and exhibit slight enzymatic actions.

15. Biochem. J., 1927, 21, p. 426.
16. Biochem. Ztschr., 1926, 172, p. 1.

STUDIES ON BOTULINUS TOXIN

4. DIALYSIS EXPERIMENTS

H. Sommer, P. J. Nealon and P. Tessmer Snipe

From the George Williams Hooper Foundation for Medical Research, University of California Medical School, San Francisco

A casual review of the literature discloses only a few statements regarding the dialysis of botulinus toxin through semi-permeable membranes. Bronfenbrenner and Schlesinger [1] found the neutral toxin to dialyze "with a comparative ease," whereas the acidified toxin (P_H 4) remained "quantitatively inside the parchment thimble." Schübel [2] states that the poison dialyzes very readily through parchment and collodium membranes.

In the course of purification experiments (papers 2 and 3 [3] of this series) it was necessary to separate the botulinus toxin from the salts and amino acids. For this purpose dialysis through fish bladders was found convenient. It has repeatedly been noted by numerous workers e.g.[4] that the commercial fish bladders are unsuitable for prolonged dialysis. Their permeability increases on continuous contact with water. Eventually small leaks will develop which may cause a loss of active material. It has been found, however, that these hazards can be avoided to a large extent by impregnating the membranes with a dilute collodium solution. No attempts were made to work out a standardized method; the following empirical procedure, however, gave satisfactory results.

The dry fish bladders were immersed for 5 to 10 minutes in a dilute solution of collodium (Parlodion du Pont) in equal parts of alcohol and ether. (One sample of a solution used for this purpose showed a collodium content of 0.7%). The membranes were then drained and washed with alcohol and ether consecutively in order to remove any excess of nitrocellulose. Although these bladders cannot be distinguished by their outer appearance from the untreated ones, their durability is considerably increased. They may be used for dialysis in a watery medium for several weeks without any appreciable change in their permeability.

EXPERIMENTAL

It has been shown in the second paper [3] of this series that repeated dialyses (8 to 12 times) against distilled water which was renewed every

Received for publication, Jan. 28, 1928.

1. Proc. Soc. Exper. Biol. & Med., 1922, 19, p. 299.
2. Arch. f. exper. Path. u. Pharmakol., 1923, 96, p. 248.
3. J. Infect. Dis., 1928, 43, pp. 146, 154.
4. Seibert, F. B., and Long, E. R.: Am. Rev. Tuberc., 1926, 13, p. 404.

12 hours at icebox temperature usually removed the salts and amino acid from the culture fluid. It has likewise been stated that a large part of the poison is irreversibly destroyed during dialysis, and that only a small amount of toxin can be accounted for in the outside fluid. The following experiment is a typical example.

One liter of an aged type A culture fluid of a $P_H = 7.3$ was filled into three collodium coated fish bladders and dialyzed against distilled water, the outside fluid being renewed mornings and evenings for four consecutive days. The inside fluid was then evaporated in vacuo and the residue weighed. The toxin tests before and after dialysis as shown in table 1 reveal a loss of 90% of the active material.

Table 2 of paper 3[3] of this series shows similar results when dialysis was carried out at P_H values of 1.8 to 4.4. The yields were 8 to 28% and the maximum amount of toxin was recovered at P_H 3.0.

In a second set of experiments the diffusion of botulinus toxin through various membranes at different P_H values was investigated.

TABLE 1.—DIALYSIS THROUGH FISH BLADDERS AT NEUTRALITY

	Amount	MLD	% of Total Potency
Before dialysis	1000 cc.	1×10^{-4} cc. D 3×10^{-5} cc. S	100
After dialysis	Slightly increased; not determined	3×10^{-2} cc. D 1×10^{-3} cc. S	Approximately 4
Dry residue	1007 mg.	0.001 mg.	10

D = death, S = symptoms, survived.

Different lots of culture fluid ranging in toxicity from 1×10^{-4} to 2×10^{-5} cc., but samples of the same lot were used for one set of experiments. The general procedure was as follows:

A membrane was filled with a measured amount of toxin and immersed to equal levels in a known volume of distilled water or salt solution. Dialysis was allowed to proceed at icebox temperature until enough poison had accumulated in the outer fluid to be detected by injection of 1 cc. into a mouse. From time to time the dialyzing thimble had to be lowered in order to equalize the inside and outside levels. Furthermore, in order to avoid irregularities the same membrane was used for one set of experiments only, care being taken to wash it free from toxin with warm water after each test. Any defects in the dialyzing sacs could readily be ascertained by testing their permeability for toxin at P_H 4.4, since it was noticed that the rate of diffusion at this P_H was very slow.

Collodium impregnated fish bladders were first tested. Three samples of 250 cc. of toxin each adjusted to a different P_H value were dialyzed against 750 cc. of distilled water in membranes which were tightly closed by means of a pair of tongue depressors. After 24 hours 1 cc. of each of the outside fluids was injected. At the P_H values 6.9

and 1.8 part of the toxin had passed the membranes, whereas no poison could be detected in the outside fluid at P_H 4.4. Repetition of the tests by interchanging the membranes gave analogous results. The highest toxin titers encountered in the outside solution were 0.1 cc. at P_H 6.9 and 0.01 cc. at P_H 1.8. In one experiment at P_H 4.4 the mouse showed slight symptoms. In the culture fluids of P_H 4.4 a precipitate formed readily while at a P_H of 1.8 only a slight turbidity was noticed after standing for 24 hours.

The results of the foregoing experiments can hardly be considered conclusive on account of the difference in osmotic pressure which may have developed at the various degrees of acidity in the closed membranes. The tests were therefore repeated in open dialyzing sacks. Only the neutral toxin dialyzed to a certain degree during the first 24 hours, while the outside fluids at P_H 1.8 and 4.4 were atoxic.

TABLE 2.—DIALYSIS THROUGH PARCHMENT PAPER

	Days							
	Inside 120 cc. of toxin; outside 230 cc. of distilled water; progress of dialysis							
P_H	1	2	3	4	5	6	7	8
2.0	+		+					
3.0		+ (1:10 —)						
4.0	—						+	
4.5	—				S	—	S	S
5.0	S	S	S		S			
6.1	+							
8.0	S		+	+				+ (1:10 +)

+ = death of mouse, S = symptoms, survived, and — = no symptoms, in all tables.

Preliminary experiments with an open dialyzing thimble of parchment paper (A. H. Thomas, No. 4463) confirmed the results obtained with fish bladders; toxin having a P_H of approximately 4.4 showed the slightest diffusion. A set of tests with this membrane was then performed to obtain data on intermediate P_H values. The progress of the diffusion was measured by injecting 0.5 cc. of the outside fluid at various time intervals. The results recorded in table 2 substantiate the fact that the diffusion of botulinus toxin is at a minimum between P_H 4.0 and 5.0.

In order to rule out as much as possible any specific influence of the membrane material on the process of diffusion, other dialyzing sacks of different chemical composition were employed. A set of experiments with a "cellophane" membrane (candy wrapping material) is represented in table 3. From the data it is evident that the presence of phosphates in the outer solution increased the permeability of this membrane for the toxin.

The collodium sacks which were employed in the subsequent studies were prepared from Parlodion du Pont in an analogous manner as described by Looney.[5] Their permeability was slightly less than that of the membranes previously employed. Regardless of the P_H of the culture fluid, dialysis for 48 hours was required in most instances before a lethal amount of toxin had accumulated in 1 cc. of the diffusate. The general observation of a decreased permeability at P_H 4.4 could again be substantiated in a qualitative way. In several experiments the toxin was dialyzed against a 1% sodium chloride solution. A slight increase in the diffusion of the poison at all P_H values tested (2.0, 4.4, 7.0) was again recorded.

TABLE 3.—DIALYSIS THROUGH "CELLOPHANE" AGAINST WATER AND PHOSPHATE SOLUTIONS

P_H	Cc. of Toxin Inside	Outside	Days 1	2	3	
2.0	20	80 cc. H_2O	+	+	+	
4.5	20	80 cc. H_2O	—	S	S	— 4th to 9th day
7.3	20	80 cc. H_2O	—	+	+	+ 4th and 9th days
4.4	40	200 cc. of a 1% $(NH_4)H_2PO_4$ solution	—		+	
7.0	40	200 cc. of a 1% ammonium phosphate solution, P_H 7.0	+		+	

TABLE 4.—DIALYSIS THROUGH ALCOHOL TREATED COLLODIUM MEMBRANES AGAINST WATER AND SALT SOLUTION

P_H	Inside	Outside	Days 1	2	3
6.9	30 cc., toxin	82 cc. NaCl solution 1%	1:10+	1:100+ 1:1000 S	
4.4	30 cc., toxin	82 cc. NaCl solution 1%	+	1:100+	
4.4	30 cc., toxin	82 cc. H_2O	+	+	1:10—
2.0	30 cc., toxin	82 cc. NaCl solution 1%	+	1:10+	

Brown[6] has succeeded in preparing collodium membranes of increased permeability by soaking the air dry thimbles in alcohol water mixtures of different concentrations. Membranes prepared according to the method of Looney were treated with 50% alcohol as described by Brown. The increase in permeability was at once apparent. Table 4 illustrates the results of the tests in which distilled water and 1% sodium chloride solution were used as outside fluids. It may be inferred that a combination of the two factors—presence of salts in the diffusate and treatment of the collodium thimbles with alcohol—enables the toxin to permeate the membrane quite rapidly. It is not unlikely that this procedure may permit the separation of the active principle from the

5. J. Biol. Chem., 1922, 50, p. 1.
6. Biochem. J., 1915, 9, p. 591.

larger inactive molecules of the toxic culture fluid. An interesting phenomenon observed was the decreased diffusability of the brown pigment through these modified collodium sacks. While dialysis through all other membranes resulted in an equal distribution of color between inside and outside fluid within a few days, no coloration of the diffusate was perceptible in the same length of time when alcohol treated collodium membranes were used.

DISCUSSION

It would be premature at this stage of the experimental work to draw any far reaching conclusions as to the molecular weight and the charge of the toxin molecule from the data presented in this paper. Many secondary factors may influence the accuracy of the determinations. The adsorption of the toxin on the different membranes for instance has not been investigated. Considering the results of adsorption experiments in paper 2 [3] of this series, it is not unlikely that the P_H of 4.4 may represent an adsorption maximum for the toxin on the membranes and thus explain the minimum diffusion at that P_H. Selective adsorption at other P_H values, however, is naturally a possibility. Furthermore, it is very probable that the toxic precipitate which forms in an acidified culture fluid influences to various degrees the dialysis at different hydrogen ion concentrations. It has been mentioned in paper 3 that a P_H of approximately 3.0 represents the optimum for the precipitation of the whole culture fluid, while by dialysis of the electrolytes the isoelectric point of the precipitable protein is shifted to P_H 4.4. Maximum flocculation would be expected to coincide with minimum diffusability. On the other hand final conclusions as to the actual amount of toxin passing through the membranes cannot be drawn without consideration of the spontaneous and irreversible inactivation of the poison which takes place on storage especially of a diluted culture fluid. Whether spontaneous hydrolysis or oxydation are responsible for the disappearance of the potency, or if enzymatic reactions are involved, is as yet unknown. From the experiments of Bronfenbrenner and Schlesinger [7] and numerous observations in this laboratory it is, however, quite certain that a P_H of 4.0 to 5.0 represents the optimum stability for the poison. Furthermore, investigations similar to those conducted by Sbarsky and Nikolaeff [8] on tetanus and diphtheria toxin have not yet been undertaken with the botulinus poison. These authors found a reversible inactivation

7. J. Exper. Med., 1924, 39, p. 509.
8. Biochem. Ztschr., 1927, 183, p. 419.

of the toxins on addition of certain amino acids. They have subsequently noticed that these protein split products abundantly present in the diffusate of the dialysis test may mask the poisonous properties, so that less toxin can be demonstrated in the outside fluid than is actually present.

In spite of these secondary factors which may influence the results in a quantitative way the experiments of this and the two previous papers are believed to have a bearing on the explanation of the clinical findings. Since the botulinus toxin exerts its action when taken by mouth and must be absorbed in the alimentary tract, precipitation, dialysis and adsorption at different P_H values seem of primary importance if conclusions from in vitro tests to phenomena in vivo are justified. Further experiments, especially of pharmacological nature are planned to correlate these findings with in vivo observations.

SUMMARY

The durability of fish bladders for dialysis can be greatly improved by impregnation with a dilute collodium solution.

Botulinus toxin can be separated from the electrolytes of the culture fluid by prolonged dialysis; 8 to 28% of the total potency present can be recovered inside the membrane after this procedure. A small fraction of the active material can be accounted for in the diffusate, while the largest part of the toxin is irreversibly inactivated.

Measurable amounts of the poison pass through fish bladder, parchment, collodium and cellophane membranes. Presence of salts in the outside solution increases the permeability of these membranes for the botulinus toxin.

The rate of diffusion of the toxin is slow at a P_H of approximately 4.4 and the amount of poison may become immeasurable at that acidity. On the alkaline as well as the acid side of this P_H the toxin diffuses more rapidly.

Some secondary factors influencing the dialysis of the toxic substance are discussed.

A METHOD OF INOCULATING BLOOD PLATES FOR THE IDENTIFICATION OF HEMOLYTIC STREPTOCOCCI

EUGENIA VALENTINE

From the George Williams Hooper Foundation for Medical Research, University of California Medical School, San Francisco

The identification of beta hemolytic streptococci is based on the appearance of deep colonies in blood agar pour plates. It may happen occasionally that the making of pour plates is impossible and instead, the material is streaked on the surface of a blood plate previously poured. In the majority of instances this method is satisfactory since it gives definite evidence of hemolysis. A few strains of hemolytic streptococci however, have been encountered, the surface colonies of which are sursounded by a narrow, translucent zone which may appear greenish by transmitted light. Even after incubation for 48 hours hemolysis about the colony is not distinct. It is the occasional occurrence of such strains which makes the more convenient method of surface streaked mediums unreliable.

The following procedure for inoculating surface blood agar is suggested as an aid in diagnosis whenever the making of pour plates is not feasible. The procedure is based on an observation which was made during a study of middle ear infections. It was customary to streak the material from the ear and from the throat on the surface of blood plates in duplicate, one for aerobic and the other for anaerobic incubation. Blood agar pour plates (10 cc. of veal infusion agar, P_H 7.4, containing 1% Witte peptone plus 1 cc. defibrinated sheep blood) were made also and incubated aerobically. Specimens from three different patients were encountered in which the anaerobically grown surface colonies were surrounded by wide, clear zones of hemolysis, while the surface colonies on the duplicate plates incubated aerobically for 48 hours showed no definite hemolysis, but exhibited a greenish zone. In the pour plates typical hemolytic colonies developed, having a 3 to 4 mm. clear zone with no blood cells remaining intact. Pure cultures were fished from the greenish colonies on the surface plate and replated immediately. They still failed to hemolyze the blood when grown on

Received for publication, Jan. 28, 1928.

the surface, but when plated again after 2 weeks cultivation on artificial mediums the surface colonies were surrounded by clear hemolyzed zones. Eighteen-hour broth cultures of these strains in cultivation for 2 weeks, completely hemolyzed 3% washed sheep cells in one-half hour when 0.5 cc. of culture was incubated with 1 cc. of cell suspension.

The observation that the strains produced definite zones of hemolysis when free access of oxygen was excluded, but failed to do so under aerobic conditions of growth suggested the following procedure in inoculating surface blood plates. The material or culture is taken on a moderately heavy loop, smeared over a small area of the blood plate, then pushed under the surface and moved around in a small section. The loop is then removed and surface streakings are made over the remainder of the plate. If the material contains hemolytic streptococci, a distinct zone of hemolysis develops, after incubation for 24 hours, in the portion of the plate where the culture has grown within or under the blood agar, whereas the surface colonies may not be definitely hemolytic. When pure cultures of green (alpha) or alpha prime [1] streptococci are inoculated in the same manner the growth is readily distinguished from that of the beta hemolytic strains by the absence of the clear hemolyzed area. Even when the inoculum consists of a mixture of hemolytic and green streptococci, the clearing of the red cells in the cut section of the agar indicates the presence of the hemolytic type. All hemolytic streptococci tested in this way have shown a clearer zone of hemolysis when cut into the agar than around the surface growth of individual or crowded colonies.

Recently, a hemolytic streptococcus having the same peculiar characteristics described above was encountered in the blood culture of a fatal case of sepsis which had been treated for a number of days by intravenous injections of polyvalent antistreptococcic serum. Although the blood culture broth showed hemolysis, the colonies which grew on the surface blood plates were not hemolytic but appeared greenish in transmitted light. In blood agar pour plates, typical hemolytic colonies developed. When the cultures had been in cultivation on blood streaked agar for six days, surface plating revealed colonies which were less hemolytic than deep colonies although they did not have the nonhemolytic, greenish appearance noted at the time of the first plating.

An experiment was carried out in an endeavor to determine whether the action of the antistreptococcic serum was a factor in the atypical

1. Rockefeller Inst. for M. Res., Monograph 9, 1919.

growth of the strain when first isolated, and furthermore, if the culture could be made to revert to its original growth characteristic when passed through the peritoneal cavity of mice. In the first experiment the mouse which received 0.5 cc. of the 18-hour broth culture intraperitoneally died in 20 hours, while the animal which was given an injection of 0.5 cc. of culture plus 0.5 cc. of antistreptococcic serum simultaneously, died in 48 hours. Samples of the peritoneal exudate of both mice were removed at intervals of 2, 6, and 18 hours. Surface platings from this material as well as from the peritoneal fluid and heart blood at necropsy revealed typical hemolytic colonies. The same result was obtained when the culture was grown for 24 to 48 hours in beef broth to which had been added varying dilutions of the antistreptococcic serum. Mouse passage or growth in antistreptococcic serum had apparently failed to induce the development of variants.

References to hemolytic streptococci having somewhat similar characteristics are found in the literature. The streptococcus isolated by Davis [2] from epidemic sore throat was described as having a "faint greenish tint on transmitted light with a zone of hemolysis relatively narrow." Krumwiede and Valentine,[3] also studying septic sore throat, noted that "typical hemolysis may not be present on surface streaked blood plates although it may develop after longer incubation." With regard to the growth of a strain of B. hemolytic streptococcus (epidemicus) on veal infusion agar containing Difco peptone, Brown [1] states "if on this medium surface colonies only were observed macroscopically the organism might readily be called streptococcus viridans." Fisk and Burky [4] described an unusual hemolytic streptococcus as follows: "A typical hemolytic colony grew in the depths but on the surface there appeared a wrinkled 2 to 3 mm. colony surrounded by a greenish zone which looked like neither green nor hemolytic hemolysis, but more like a green pigmentation independent of the blood itself." Whether the growth characteristic on surface streaked plates changed after prolonged artificial cultivation is not stated. Reference to the influence of anaerobiosis on the growth of streptococci is found in Brown's [1] monograph on streptococci. He observed that "hemolytic strains grew equally well anaerobically as aerobically" but noted, in respect to B. hemolytic streptococcus (epidemicus), that aerobic surface colonies on blood agar made with Difco peptone were slightly greenish

2. J. Am. M. A., 1912, 58, p. 1852.
3. J. M. Res., 1915, 33, p. 231.
4. J. Infect. Dis., 1922, 30, p. 128.

by transmitted light but when grown anaerobically the surface colonies were "whitish and transparent."

The marked difference in the growth characteristic of the strains described above when grown anaerobically and aerobically on the surface of blood plates suggests that, in the absence of free oxygen, the hemolytic agent acts more completely on the red blood cells in the blood agar. The advantage of blood agar pour plates over surface streaked plates for observing the hemolytic capacity of all beta hemolytic streptococci may be ascribed, in part at least, to the partial anaerobiosis resulting in the deep colonies. Another factor, however, may be the greater surface of blood agar exposed to the growing streptococci with the result that the hemolysin diffuses through the entire depth of the agar and produces more perfectly hemolyzed areas. The same factors are doubtless involved in the formation of the clearer area of hemolysis in the section of the blood agar which has been cut by the loop according to the procedure described in this article.

The reason for the failure of these strains to hemolyze the blood cells after growth on surface plates when first recovered from the body, and the change after artificial cultivation requires further study. The observations of Schnitzer and Munter [5] and of Morgenroth, Schnitzer and Berger [6] may have some bearing on this subject. These authors noted that hemolytic streptococci, after growth for 1 hour in the peritoneal cavity of a mouse or after being in contact with varying dilutions of rivanol * in the presence of red blood cells, would lose their ability to hemolyze and become green. A preliminary experiment was carried out to test this observation. In two experiments with mice, hemolytic colonies only were recovered from the mouse peritoneum. In two out of four experiments with rivanol and washed red blood cells, surface platings from the tubes containing the largest amounts of rivanol revealed a high percentage of colonies which were not definitely hemolytic but which had the same greenish appearance noted above with the otitis media strains. Only hemolytic colonies grew in the blood agar pour plates made from the same rivanol tubes and from individual isolations of the greenish colonies, thus showing that no permanent change in the colony characteristics had occurred. It is interesting to speculate whether some bactericidal or other property of the body cells, immune serum, or blood cells in the presence of

5. Ztschr. f. Hyg. u. Infectionskrankh., 1923, 99, p. 366.
6. Klin. Wchnschr., 1923, 2, p. 1633.
* Diaminooxyethylacridin.

rivanol may be capable of exerting some temporary inhibitory action on the hemolysin or ferments of certain strains of beta hemolytic streptococci.

SUMMARY

A method is described of inoculating surface blood plates by cutting the agar with the infected loop, and then moving the loop under the agar in a small section of the plate prior to the surface streaking. After 18 hours growth a hemolytic zone is produced where the organism has grown under the agar, although colonies on the surface of the plate may not be definitely hemolytic even after 48 hours incubation. The greater ability of streptococci to hemolyze red blood cells when inoculated under the agar or when grown in blood agar pour plates is ascribed, in part, to the partial anaerobiosis.

Four strains of beta hemolytic streptococcus are described which, when first cultured from the human source, failed to show hemolysis on surface-streaked plates but appeared greenish by transmitted light.

INCIDENCE OF CLOUDY REACTIONS IN AGGLUTINATION TESTS FOR SALMONELLA PULLORUM INFECTION

G. S. Schilling and S. J. Schilling

From the Experiment Station, College of Agriculture, University of Arkansas, Fayetteville

In 1899, Rettger[1] isolated the causative agent of bacillary white diarrhea of chicks, Salmonella pullorum, or Bacterium pullorum, as it was formerly designated. Rettger and Stoneburn[2] in 1909 determined that the original source of the infection is the hen, that the organism is contained in the yolks of eggs from infected hens, and that chicks produced from infected eggs may have the disease when hatched. These findings served to focus attention on the carrier problem, and Jones[3] adapted the agglutination test to the identification of adult birds infected with Salmonella pullorum. Since that time large numbers of birds have been tested in various states of this country in an effort toward the suppression of bacillary white diarrhea.

One of the difficulties encountered early in use of the agglutination test for detecting S. pullorum infection was that a nonspecific precipitation frequently appeared when chicken serum was added to the test fluid, and interfered with a proper reading of the results of the test. This nonspecific precipitation has been spoken of in the literature as a "cloudy reaction," which for want of a more convenient term will also be used in this paper. The study here presented relates to the incidence of the cloudy reaction and is a partial report of an investigation aimed at finding the cause of, and a means of inhibiting such nonspecific precipitations.

The nonspecific reaction known as the "cloudy reaction" presents considerable variability in the modifications of the test fluid which may be encountered. Essentially this reaction consists of a nonspecific precipitation. The precipitating material may manifest itself in floccules floating at the surface, by being in suspension throughout the medium, by forming a flocculent sediment at the bottom of the tube, by being in a minutely divided and evenly dispersed state throughout the medium, or by appearing as some combination of these states; these states probably are all manifestations of the same phenomenon differing only in the degree of aggregation or dispersion of the precipitates. A floating precipitate will commonly settle out when the equilibrium is disturbed as by jarring. The precipitate may begin to settle down in the form of long strands or as floccules of variable size. A diffuse clouding probably is due to a dispersion of extremely minute particles of the precipitate in the test fluid. All diffuse increases in turbidity of the agglutination antigen as well as all flaky precipitations varying distinctly from clumping and settling of organisms as in the true agglutination reaction are here regarded as instances of the cloudy reaction.

Received for publication, Feb. 3, 1928.
Research Paper No. 76, Journal Series, University of Arkansas.

1. New York M. J., 1900, 71, p. 803.
2. Storrs Agric. Exper. Sta. Bull. 60, 1909.
3. J. M. Research, 1913, 27, p. 481.

In this work, blood samples which had been submitted to this laboratory were used, and the source of the samples, the sex and age of birds, the breeds represented, and the condition of the serum were recorded. The samples were used in the routine diagnostic tests for bacillary white diarrhea by the agglutination method; and cloudy reactions as well as positive specific reactions entered separately into permanent records. These data thus became available for a study to determine whether correlations exist between the factors mentioned and the appearance of the cloudy reaction. Some of the early tests pertained to the relative time of appearance of the agglutination reaction and of the cloudy reaction.

A number of studies designed to find means of inhibiting the cloudy reaction by modification of the agglutination antigen have been published.[4] Data have been gathered in this laboratory to test the efficacy of the various means of avoiding clouding which have been suggested and will shortly be published. Here, however, our interest is confined to the incidence of the cloudy reaction when the agglutination antigen is prepared and used in a manner comparable to that employed in the agglutination test of the sera of other species of animals against various bacteria. For in many laboratories the problem of avoiding the cloudy reaction is still considered unsolved, the means suggested for avoiding this reaction have a more or less tentative acceptance and for routine testing an unmodified antigen is still in use.

Mathews [5] found that as high as 75% of the birds of some flocks may give the cloudy reaction. Taking into account the possibility that a cloudy reaction may mask or prevent the agglutination reaction the committee on poultry diseases of the U. S. Live Stock Sanitary Association [6] has recommended that all birds giving a cloudy reaction be condemned unless retested. Thus, it is quite apparent that the interference of this nonspecific precipitation is a matter of serious consequence.

A number of influences such as age and sex of the birds, season of year, and that of a period of starvation preceding the taking of blood samples have been correlated with the occurrence of cloudy reactions. Following the work of Warner and Edmond [7] who showed that the blood of older birds does not contain as much fat as that of pullets,

4. Hektoen, L.: J. Infect. Dis., 1918, 22, p. 561; Beach, J. R., and Ter-Michaelian, S.: Hilgardia, 1927, 2, p. 545; Mathews, F. P.: J. Immunol., 1926, 11, p. 499; Mallman, W. S.: J. Am. Vet. M. A., 1927, 61, p. 600.

5. J. Immunol., 1926, 11, p. 499.

6. J. M. Vet. M. A., 1927, 70, p. 922.

7. J. Biol. Chem., 1917, 31, p. 281.

Hitchner [8] tried the practice of starving the birds 36 hours before bleeding; this he found eliminated part of the interference. Stafseth [9] showed that starvation prior to bleeding reduces the number of samples giving cloudy reactions, although the type of ration which the birds received appeared to be without influence.[10] He further found that fewer cloudy reactions are encountered in October, November, and December and that this reaction did not occur with the blood of male birds. Moreover, he concluded [9] that hens only should be selected for breeding purposes to avoid the frequent cloudy reactions encountered among pullets in heavy lay. That clouding may be predicted by noting the appearance of chicken serum at the time of setting up the test has been suggested by Mathews.[5] This investigator further states that by examining a quantity of samples of blood serum one may select those which may be expected to yield the cloudy reaction and he recommends using such serums with antigen containing sodium hydroxide.

Procedure.—The antigen employed in this work was made by cultivating five strains of S. pullorum separately on standard agar. In 48 hours when approximately maximum growth had occurred, the cultures were washed off with physiologic salt solution containing 0.5% phenol. They were combined into one composite suspension of organisms, filtered through glass wool, and heated at 60 C. for 30 minutes. The composite suspension was placed in refrigeration, and as needed, portions were removed and diluted with phenolized salt solution so that the turbidity was reduced to be comparable with tube one of the McFarland nephelometer; the dilutions thus secured from the composite suspension served as the antigen. Each serum was set up in two dilutions, 1:50 and 1:100 by placing respectively 0.02 and 0.01 mils of serum in each of two tubes. The 1:50 dilution, however, was used as the criterion for charting positive specific reactions, or the nonspecific cloudy reactions. Thorough mixing of serum and antigen was obtained by shaking each tube immediately after the blood serum had been introduced. The tubes were then incubated at 37 C. Except when specifically stated to the contrary, final readings were made at 48 hours.

Time of Appearance.—In a group of 834 serums readings of the agglutination test were made after incubation for 2, 12, 24, as well as 48 hours. The object was to determine the relative time of appearance of the specific and the cloudy reaction, and the most favorable time at which to read the tests for purely diagnostic purposes, i. e., the length of incubation least apt to yield cloudy reactions which mask or inhibit agglutination.

The results are given in figure 1 in graphic form. It should be noted that of the tubes which showed clouding at 2 hours, a considerable

8. J. Am. Vet. M. A., 1923, 63, p. 759.
9. Michigan Agric. Exper. Sta. Report, 1925, p. 196.
10. Ibid., 1924, p. 186.

number became cloudy immediately after the addition of the serum, and before being incubated. At the expiration of two hours then, 175 tubes showed the cloudy reaction, at 12 hours 207, at 24 hours 235, and at 48 hours such tubes totaled 239. Agglutination reactions on the other hand lagged behind, there being 6, 61, 87, and 117 complete and 8, 17, 15, and 35 partial agglutination reactions noted at the same respective periods of observation. The data clearly show that the cloudy reaction tends to appear earlier than the agglutination reaction. Since this is

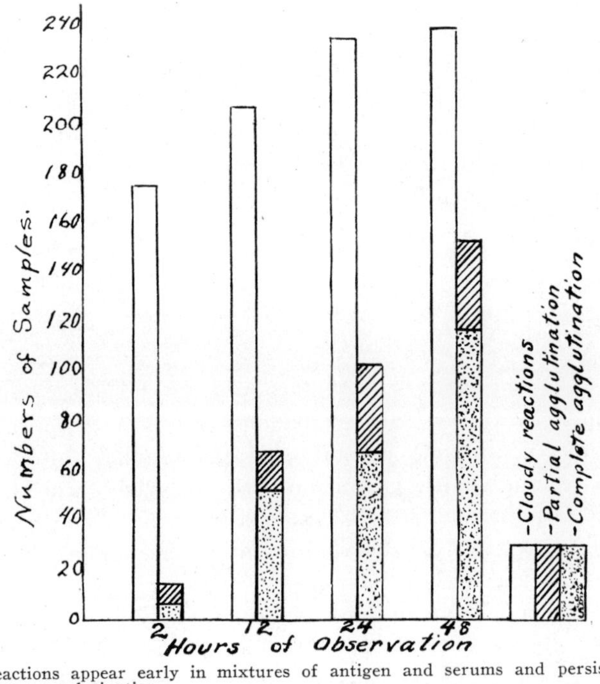

Cloudy reactions appear early in mixtures of antigen and serums and persist through the time of maximum agglutination.

the case, and since the cloudy reaction when once it has appeared tends to persist, a selection of the time of reading does not offer a means of escape from the interference of this nonspecific precipitation.

Condition of Serum as Related to Clouding.—The interesting statement by Mathews,[5] that cloudy reactions can be predicted by the appearance of the serum and that adding sodium hydroxide to the antigen to be used with serums giving such evidence of clouding is a means of preventing interference, led to the compilation of data on the possibility of a relationship between the appearance of precipitates or other changes of the whole blood serum, and the occurrence of the cloudy reaction when the serum is set up in the agglutination test.

In the classification of whole blood serums a multiplicity of designations which might lead to confusion was avoided and three designations were adopted: clear serum, a clear serum of a pale straw color; roily serum, a serum opalescent to milky in appearance, but which does not contain aggregations of suspended precipitates; and precipitated serum, which has definite precipitates and a curded appearance, whether the precipitate was floating as a layer at the top of the tube, was suspended in the serum, or had settled out in the tube. In each case after centrifugation and at the time when the agglutination test was set up the condition of each sample of serum was recorded under one of the foregoing classes. Then at the end of 48 hours incubation at 37 C. the tests were read and all cloudy reactions were recorded.

TABLE 1.—INFLUENCE OF CONDITION OF SERUM ON CLOUDING IN ANTIGEN. 1,013 SAMPLES

Condition	Number of Serums	Cloudy Reactions	
		Number	%
Clear	911	323	35.4
Roily	46	26	56.5
Precipitated	56	17	30.3
Totals	1,013	366	36.1

In Table 1 are presented the tabulated results on serums from five different flocks comprising a total of 1,013 samples. For this comparison, no serums showing laking of red corpuscles were considered. An inspection of the table shows that relatively the percentages of clear and precipitated serums which cloud in antigen are about equal. Of the roily serums, the chances are about equal that such serums will produce clouding or remain clear in the agglutination system. Of 911 clear serums 323 (35.4%) produced clouding, of 56 precipitated serums 17 (30.3%) produced clouding, and of the 46 roily serums 26 (56.5%) produced clouding in the antigen.

Our attention was especially drawn to the behavior of one group of samples comprising 179 serums. These were all clear with the exception of four, which were roily when received at the laboratory, 48 hours after they had been collected. The roily serums did not produce clouding while 136 of the clear serums did. When these serums were examined again, after refrigeration for one week, no further roily serums had appeared, nor had any of the clear serums changed in character so far as could be determined by visual inspection. After two weeks of refrigeration, inspection of this lot showed seven additional roily serums all of which had originally clouded the antigenic suspension; there also appeared at this time 42 precipitated serums. The entire lot was then placed at room temperature for 30 hours at which time the condition of the serums were again noted. Six additional samples showed precipitation and of these, four had not clouded antigen. These observations indicate importance of the time factor in determining whether or not changes in the blood serum may be noted by the operator but lead to no association of a roily or precipitated condition of the serum with the cloudy reaction.

It was concluded that the condition of the serum is no reliable criterion by which to predict whether or not a given serum will produce a cloudy reaction in the agglutination system. The time of appearance of precipitates in the blood serum of fowls is highly variable and no correlation was found as between the presence of precipitates in the serum and the appearance of a cloudy reaction.

Data were gathered on 217 serums to determine the effect of hemolysis on clouding, and to learn whether clouding serums which are hemolyzed offer greater handicaps for accurate diagnostic work than slight hemolysis or clouding alone. Without presentation of extensive detailed data it may be stated that 43% of clear, roily, and precipitated hemolyzed serums yielded the cloudy reaction while in similar but unhemolyzed serums from the same flocks clouding was encountered in only 13.1% of the tests. It is generally recognized that laked serums and those giving the cloudy reaction are not satisfactory for an accurate reading of agglutination. The factors causing interference apparently tend to reinforce each other when both are present, and thus tend to intensify the interference each would separately cause.

Relationship of Sex.—In the literature only one investigator, Stafseth,[9] has reported observations on the relationship of the sex of the bird to the appearance of the cloudy reaction; this investigator did not encounter any cloudy reactions with blood from male birds. Obviously, relatively few male birds are kept in breeding flocks, and thus in a season's testing observations for males must be based on smaller numbers than are observations of females. However, 243 male birds became available for purposes of observation of the occurrence of the cloudy reaction as against 2,981 females in a total of 3,224 birds. Fifteen (6.1%) of the blood serums of the cocks gave the cloudy reaction against 694 or 21.5% of the serums from hens. The records were gathered from tests which were made prior to the breeding season. Thus at this time in many of the flocks, the male birds were not kept with the females and on somewhat different rations. The influence of a possible variation in the type or quantity of feed thus prevents drawing conclusions on the influence of the sex factor per se in leading to cloudy reactions. That the cloudy reaction may be found, however, in tests on serum from males is established, and it is further to be noted that in one group, 20% of 50 males and only 15% of the 323 females gave cloudy reactions. A number of flocks were found in which the serum of none of the males produced the cloudy reaction which was contrary to what might have been expected in view of the percentage of such reactions encountered with serum from females in the same flock. The influence of feed above referred to may have been accountable for this difference.

Sex is not a controlling influence in determining the incidence of the cloudy reaction.

Percentage of Cloudy Reactions for Different Flocks: Influence of Breed.—The statement has previously been made that other workers have found as high as 75% of the birds of some flocks give the cloudy reaction, and that this reaction may cause such serious interference with diagnosis by means of the agglutination test, that it has been recommended to condemn birds giving cloudy reactions (unless retested, in which event, the possibilities are, according to Stafseth [9] that such birds will continue to give the cloudy nonspecific reaction), as well as those giving the positive specific reaction. Records presented here in table 3 are of interest in this connection. There are also presented in the table records which show the incidence of the cloudy reaction in the serums of different breeds. Both sexes are included.

The highest percentage of clouding encountered was 75.5% which corresponds with the values reported by Mathews. The lowest percentage encountered was 1.6%, and the average for all birds of the 16 groups was 24.8%. It would appear then that so drastic a recommendation as advising the condemnation of birds giving a cloudy reaction might in many instances cause a severe hardship for certain flock owners, and undoubtedly would alienate many poultrymen from support of a system of control of bacillary white diarrhea based on the elimination of carriers of S. pullorum infection as indicated by the agglutination test. The success of any plan for the control of bacillary white diarrhea by elimination of infected adults depends of course on the accuracy of the diagnostic procedure, or rather its reliability in not leaving infected birds in the flock. It depends also, however, on the ability of the plan to secure and maintain popularity with the flock owner by not causing excessive inconvenience or inflicting excessive losses.

The accompanying table presents records on a few breeds only. Blood samples from birds of breeds which are not represented, were not obtained. While 36.1% of samples from birds of the light breeds and 13.5% of birds of the heavy breeds gave the cloudy reaction, no clearcut differences as between breeds can be made, for flock L of brown leghorns yielded 13.1% and flock D of white wyandottes yielded 22.4% cloudy reactions.

The conclusion is that the incidence of the cloudy reaction is quite variable as between blood samples of different flocks. In some instances, it may rarely occur (or be absent) and in others be as high as 75.5%. The breed of birds was not found clearly to influence the incidence of the

TABLE 2.—COMPARISON OF CLOUDY REACTIONS FOR DIFFERENT FLOCKS AND BREEDS

Flock	Number Tested	Cloudy Reactions		Breed
		Number	%	
A	182	3	1.6	White plymouth rock
B	101	36	15.6	White wyanodtte
C	86	15	18.4	White leghorn
D	223	50	22.4	White wyandotte
E	373	66	17.6	Barred rock
F	193	17	8.8	Barred rock
G	180	136	75.5	White leghorn
H	221	8	3.6	White plymouth rock
I	317	174	54.8	White leghorn
J	181	5	2.7	Barred rock
K	100	28	28.0	White wyandotte
L	99	13	13.1	Brown leghorn
M	133	18	13.5	Barred rock
N	519	84	16.1	White leghorn
O	349	82	23.4	White leghorn
P	147	110	74.8	White leghorn
Totals				
Light breeds	1697	614	36.1	
Heavy breeds	1707	231	13.5	
All breeds	3404	845	24.8	

cloudy reaction, although on the whole, light breeds in the work here presented yielded higher percentages of cloudy reactions.

Comparison of Pullets and Hens.—Opportunity was afforded to make a limited number of observations regarding the relative frequency with which the cloudy reaction may be observed as between samples of blood obtained from pullets and those obtained from hens. An implication from the literature by Stafseth [8] to the effect that according to his experience a higher percentage of cloudy reactions occurs with blood from pullets than with hens' blood, has previously been noted. No other statement on the point in question seems to appear.

Table 3 presents data on three groups of blood samples from a total of 673 birds, 283 hens and 390 pullets. These samples originated from three flocks, pullets and hens being kept in each of them. In running tests on 283 bloods from hens the cloudy reaction was encountered in 30.3% of them. The percentage of cloudy reactors from 390 pullets was 39.7 which is but slightly higher; and most of this difference is accounted for by samples included in group C in the table originating in a flock where many of the hens and pullets were kept separately and on different rations. In this latter flock where hens and pullets were kept in one pen and were fed together the percentages of cloudy reactions of hens and pullets were 88.0 and 91.8, respectively. This close accordance is also borne out by records from the other two flocks reported on in the table.

The percentage of cloudy reactions among the bloods of pullets appeared to approximate that observed in the bloods of hens so closely that the age of the bird cannot be regarded as a controlling factor.

TABLE 3.—COMPARISON OF FREQUENCY OF OCCURRENCE OF CLOUDY REACTION AS BETWEEN BLOODS OF HENS AND PULLETS

		Samples from Hens			Samples from Pullets		
			Cloudy			Cloudy	
Group	Number Samples	Number	Number	%	Number	Number	%
A	296	90	20	22.2	206	47	22.2
B	199	114	21	18.4	85	19	20.0
C	178	79	45	56.9	99	89	89.8
C_1*	62	25	22	88.0	37	38	91.8
Total	673	283	86	30.3	390	155	39.7

* Samples from 62 birds of group C housed in a single pen and fed together.

SUMMARY

In testing the bloods of birds for carriers of Salmonella pullorum by the agglutination method the cloudy reaction tends to appear as early or earlier than the agglutination reaction. Moreover, the cloudy reaction tends to persist, thus a selection of the time of reading does not offer a means of escape from the interference of this nonspecific precipitation.

The condition of the serum at the time of setting up the agglutination test is no reliable criterion as to whether or not a given serum will produce a cloudy reaction. When hemolysis is present in addition to varying amounts of precipitates in the blood serums, the frequency of nonspecific reactions is increased. Neither sex nor age is the controlling factor in determining the incidence of the cloudy reaction which is quite variable for blood samples of different flocks, being in some instances absent or low, and in others as high as 75.5%. Although on the whole the light breeds in the work here presented yielded higher percentages of cloudy reactions, conclusive evidence as to the influence of breed was not obtained.

PROTEUS AMMONIAE

Thomas B. Magath

From the Section on Clinical Pathology, Mayo Clinic, Rochester, Minnesota

In 1925 Hager and I [1] described an organism which we believed to be the etiologic agent in incrusted cystitis in cases in which the urine was alkaline. In 1926 Hager [2] found the same organism in a case of calcerous pyelonephritis and later we [3] found the organism in certain cases in which urinary calculi were present. We demonstrated that this organism could be implanted in the urinary bladder of rabbits and of guinea-pigs following trauma, the traumatic agent being a dilute solution of salicylic acid. Under proper experimental conditions the organism caused incrusted cystitis and in a relatively large percentage of cases the incrustation became dislodged and formed free stones composed of alkaline earthy metallic salts. The condition is quite comparable to that found in human beings suffering from incrusted cystitis and vesical calculi of this type. The organism was demonstrated to have the ability to transform quickly urinary urea into ammonia. The resulting alkaline condition of the urine was responsible for the precipitation of the salts. Incrustations and stones conceivably can form in the bladder on any already existing lesion.

The organism was originally described under the name Salmonella ammoniae. At this time we had two strains; these did not liquefy gelatin and did not grow with ameboid colonies. Since the organism did not ferment sucrose and since it evidently was not very different from Salmonella foetida, the name Salmonella ammoniae seemed proper. Since then, however, many strains have been studied, and in 1926 we concluded that the organism belonged to the genus Proteus in spite of certain apparent incompatibilities. I shall describe here 18 cultures, which taken in comparison with many other cultures, present the following characteristics of Proteus ammoniae.

The organism is gram-negative, from 1 to 3.5 microns long and about 0.5 micron in diameter. It usually occurs singly, does not form spores and is motile. It produces white colonies on Endo's medium. It

Received for publication, February 6, 1928.

1. J. Am. M. A., 1925, 85, p. 1352.
2. J. Urol., 1926, 15, p. 133.
3. Med. Clin. N. Amer., 1926, 10, p. 693; J. Am. M. A., 1928, 90, p. 266.

forms glistening, moist, sticky, bluish-gray colonies on agar. All but six of the strains produce ameboid colonies on agar. Milk is rendered at first acid, then strongly alkaline with quick peptonization. All but three strains form indol but none forms acetyl-methyl-carbinol. Maltose, lactose, sucrose, mannitol, dulcitol, insulin, inositol, salicin, arabinose, rhamnose and dextrin were not fermented. Acid was produced in glycerol, and acid and gas in glucose, galactose, xylose and trehalose. Occasionally acid was produced in certain samples of levulose; however, this was

REACTIONS OF CULTURES OF PROTEUS AMMONIAE

Culture	Sucrose, Incubation for 4 Days, P_H* (Bromthymol Blue)	Levulose, Incubation for 4 Days, P_H (Bromthymol Blue)	Ameboid Colonies, Incubation for 7 Days	Gelatin		Indol Production, Incubation 4 Days
				Liquefied	Incubation, Days	
1		6.5	+	+	2	+
2†	6.0	6.5**	+	+	2	+
3		6.5	0	+	5	+
4		6.5	0	0	14	+
5		6.5	+	+	2	+
6		6.5	+	+	2	+
7		6.5	+	+	5	0
8	6.5	6.5	+	+	14	+
9	6.5	6.5	0	0	14	+
10		6.5	+	0	14	0
11		6.5	+	+	9	+
12		6.5	+	+	2	+
13	6.5	7.0	0	+	2	+
14		6.5	+	+	2	+
15		6.5	0	+	2	+
16		6.5**	+	+	2	0
17	6.5	6.5**	0	+	5	+
18		6.5	+	+	2	+

* No signs of acid or gas.

** A small bubble of gas appeared at the end of two days, and was absorbed by the end of four days.

† Culture 2 was tested in different batches of sucrose; it was incubated in 3 tubes with original P_H 7.0 for 7 days, with resulting P_H 6.0, 6.5 and 7.0 respectively. The hydrogen-ion concentration in 10 tubes had increased from P_H 7.2 to P_H 7.6 at the end of 7 days. The gelatin was incubated at 37.5 C. and cooled in the icebox.

regarded as due to impurities in the particular sample of sugar. Its action on sucrose was studied particularly and the production of acid or of acid and gas was not encountered in any of the cultures. In ten cultures gelatin was liquefied in two days, in three cultures after 5 days, in one after 9 days, and in one after 14 days; in four there was no liquefaction after 14 days. The tabulation gives the details of the experiments.

From the foregoing characteristics it would seem that the organism should be considered a member of the genus Proteus but a modification of the characteristics of the genus will have to be made to include it. I therefore suggest that the generic description be so modified as to indicate that sucrose is not always fermented by members of the genus Proteus.

Shaw [4] in 1927, described an organism which he called Proteus henricensis and which he obtained from putrefying material. The description of the organism is so much like that of Proteus ammoniae as to cause one to question the former's identity. It would be extremely interesting to know if Proteus ammoniae is present in putrefying material as this would offer some clue as to its origin in the bladder. In most cases of incrusted cystitis and in many cases of carbonate-phosphate stone formation there is a history of trauma following treatment, catheterization or childbirth so that it seems quite likely that this organism is introduced by chance.

The presence of bacilli of the genus Proteus is by no means uncommon in cultures of urine. Unfortunately there are practically no detailed studies of these organisms in the literature and most of the references refer to Proteus vulgaris. It is quite likely that this organism has in the past usually been identified by its ability to liquefy gelatin, by the spreading type of the colonies and by the putrid odor, but if Proteus vulgaris was identified correctly, it must have been on the basis of its fermentation of sucrose. If this is true the organism usually described in literature is not Proteus ammoniae but its prevalence in alkaline urine is so common as to make one suspect that it has been encountered many times in the past and has been incorrectly identified as Proteus vulgaris. Fresh urine with a hydrogen-ion concentration of more than P_H 7, is not common and in most cases in which it is found and we have studied the condition, we have been able to culture Proteus ammoniae; also in these cases incrusted cystitis or calculi are often noted. It is not possible that the high alkalinity we have encountered can be produced by Bacillus coli and a consideration of this Proteus species is very important.

SUMMARY

Detailed description is given of eighteen cultures of Proteus ammoniae from urine. Since the organism does not ferment sucrose it is proposed to modify the generic characterization of the genus Proteus.

4. Science, 1927, 65, p. 477.

SEROLOGIC TYPES OF CLOSTRIDIUM TETANI

From the George Williams Hooper Foundation for Medical Research, University of California Medical School, San Francisco

GEORGE E. COLEMAN AND JANET B. GUNNISON

Based on the specificity of the agglutination reaction numerous microbic species have been differentiated into various types or groups. While the clinical picture of the disease caused by the different types of a given bacterial species may be the same, or very similar, this differentiation of the causative organism into types has been of inestimable value in the study of the etiology and epidemiology of the disease and particularly of its vaccinal or serum prophylaxis and therapeusis.

With this idea in mind Tulloch [1] during the World War began anew the study of the bacteriology and serology of Cl. tetani. He was able to differentiate the organism into four serologic types. He furthermore investigated the proportion of the different types in the war wounds of those receiving prophylactic serum injections and concluded that future successful serological prophylaxis probably would be dependent on a greater extension of the knowledge of types which he had thus far gained.

The serological investigation of Cl. tetani has since been continued by several workers, notably by Fildes,[2] Bauer,[3] TenBroeck and Bauer,[4] Bauer and Meyer [5] and Coleman and Meyer.[6] These studies have had to do largely with the determination of the proportion of the various types of Cl. tetani isolated from various sources, principally from the feces of man and the agglutinating titer of the different types found in normal human serums. Owing to the importance of this question it would seem that a brief historical review of the sources and the proportion of the various types thus far isolated in different parts of the world and of those used at present in our studies in this laboratory would not be without interest.

After the isolation by Tulloch of four types from war wounds in France a strain of Cl. tetani was sent to him from France which would not agglutinate in any of his four serums. This type was found only once. Cultures of these five

Received for publication, Jan. 28, 1928.

1. J. Hyg., 1919, 18, p. 103.
2. Brit. J. Exper. Path., 1925, 6, p. 91.
3. Proc. Soc. Exper. Biol. & Med., 1924, 21, p. 265.
4. Ibid., 1925, 22, p. 562.
5. J. Infect. Dis., 1926, 38, p. 295.
6. Ibid., 39, p. 332.

types were sent by him to Bauer and TenBroeck in China in 1921 and 1923. Type 1 was labeled "U. S. A. II" and was the strain used in the United States in the production of antiserum. Type 2 was labeled "T. 67," type 3, "T. h. 22 d.," and type 4, "118 Nogouchi." The strain which Tulloch received originally from France was named type 5 by TenBroeck and Bauer. This proved to be the predominant type found by these workers in China. They also isolated strains of two new types from human and guinea-pig stools and named them 6-227 and 6-167 and 7-309 and 7-128. Cultures of all of these strains except that of type 5 have been received by us through the courtesy of these workers.

During a survey by Bauer and Meyer of human carriers of Cl. tetani in California, three strains were isolated which will not agglutinate with any of the seven type serums prepared from the cultures mentioned and which we have named type 8 (3, 41, 43). The cultural characteristics of these three strains were studied by Coleman and Meyer[7] comparatively with two type 1 cultures and no essential differences were found between any of them.

Recently one of us isolated from the hillside soil on the site of this institution a strain of Cl. tetani which is agglutinated to full titer by none of our eight serums and with which we have prepared an agglutinating serum. We have marked this strain "IX E" and consider it to be a type 9. The strain is motile,

TABLE 1.—AGGLUTINATION REACTIONS

Antigen	Serum 1	Serum 2	Serum 3	Serum 4	Serum 5	Serum 6	Serum 7	Serum 8	Serum 9
1	1:3,200+	—	—	—	—	—	1:800+	—	—
2	—	1:6,400+	—	—	—	—	—	—	—
3	—	—	1:12,800+	—	—	—	—	—	—
4	—	—	—	1:1,600+	—	—	—	—	—
5	—	—	—	—	1:12,800+	—	—	—	1:200+
6	—	—	—	—	—	1:3,200+	—	—	—
7	1:400+	—	—	—	—	—	1:3,200+	—	—
8	—	—	—	—	—	—	—	1:3,200+	—
9	—	—	—	—	1:1,600+	—	—	—	1:1,600+

Serums 1 to 5 prepared by Dr. J. Bauer, serums 6 to 9 prepared by Miss J. B. Gunnison.

liquefies gelatin but does not produce indol and is an average toxin producer as are all of the above mentioned strains.

With the exception of type 5 which was isolated from a patient (feces ?) with beriberi in China these are the type cultures used by us in the preparation of antigens for our type determinations. We have typed several other strains isolated in this laboratory from feces, post operative cases, wounds, etc.

In order to study their serologic relationship agglutination tests have been carried out using serums and antigens prepared from each of the nine type strains. The results of these tests are given in table 1.

It will be seen that in only two instances does cross agglutination between our types occur. TenBroeck has observed (personal communication) a marked cross reaction between types 1 and 7 which our results confirm. Our type 9 strain reacts with type 5. Tulloch[1] stated that there was no cross reaction between types 1, 2, 3 and 4 and this was confirmed by Bauer.[3] Fildes,[2] however, noted cross agglutination between types 2 and 3 and between types 4 and 5. It seems possible

7. J. Infect. Dis., 1926, 39, p. 328.

that in some instances the occurrence of cross reactions might be due to the presence in the cultures of more than one type.

Absorption tests were made with the strains showing cross reactions and by this method the types were proven to be distinct (table 2). Reciprocal absorption tests were also carried out with two of the strains designated type 8, since by this method alone can strains be positively identified. It was found that absorption of the serum agglutinins of either type 8 strain, with the antigen of either, removed the agglutinins for both; thus proving them to be identical.

Bauer [3] and Fildes [2] have referred to the spontaneous agglutinability of type 3. We have worked with several strains of this type and have never observed the slightest tendency of this or any other type

TABLE 2.—ABSORPTION REACTIONS

TYPE 1 AND TYPE 7

Antigen Tested	Type 1 Serum Absorbed with		Type 7 Serum Absorbed with		Unabsorbed Control Serums	
	Type 1	Type 7 (309)	Type 1	Type 7 (309)	Type 1	Type 7 (309)
1	1:80+ 1:160—	1:3,200+	—	1:400+	1:3,200+	1:800+
7 (309)	1:400+	—	1:3,200+	1:80+ 1:160—	1:400+	1:3,200+
7 (128)	1:400+	—	1:3,200+	—	1:800+	1:3,200+

TYPE 5 AND TYPE 9

Antigen Tested	Type 5 Serum Absorbed with		Type 9 Serum Absorbed with		Unabsorbed Control Serums	
	Type 5	Type 9	Type 5	Type 9	Type 5	Type 9
5	1:160+ 1:320—	1:12,800+	—	1:100+	1:12,800+	1:200+
9	1:1,600+	—	1:1,600+	—	1:1,600+	1:1,600+

to agglutinate spontaneously. Young cultures of certain strains may flocculate slightly while growing in broth but saline suspensions prepared from such growths do not clump spontaneously. This is in marked contrast to the observation of Fildes [2] and of Bauer [3] that young broth cultures showed less tendency toward spontaneous agglutination than did saline suspensions.

Regarding the known types of Cl. tetani it may be of interest to resume in tabulated form the proportion of the various types found by the workers previously cited (table 3).

In Tulloch's early work with the war wounded in France, with the exception of finding type 5 once, he was able to include all of the strains isolated within four groups. In England, according to Fildes, type 5 predominates. In China seven types have been isolated and thus far

Table 3.—Types of Cl. Tetani Found by Various Workers

Results Obtained by	1		2		3		4		5		6		7		8		9		Number of Strains Studied
	Times Found	%	Times Found	%	Times Found	%	Times Found	%	Times Found	%	Times Found	%	Times Found	%	Times Found	%	Times Found	%	
Tulloch from war wounds in France	60	47.2	25	19.7	35	27.5	5	3.9	1	0.8	0	0	0	0	0	0	0	0	127
Tulloch: fecal cultures in England	9	75	2	16.6	1	8.3	0	0	0	0	0	0	0	0	0	0	0	0	12
Fildes: feces of man and horses, soil, wounds, cases of tetanus, etc., in England	13	17.3	6	8	14	18.6	3	4	39	52	0	0	0	0	0	0	0	0	75
Bauer, Tang, Yü and TenBroeck*: cultures of feces of man and domesticated animals in China	21	8	17	6.5	52	19.9	1	0.4	155	59.3	10	3.8	5	1.9	0	0	0	0	261
Bauer and Meyer in California	78	65	9	7.5	21	17.5	3	2.5	6	5	0	0	0	0	3	2.5	0	0	120
Coleman and Meyer †: agglutinations at 1:40 or higher of 104 normal human serums in California	4	3.8	5	4.8	0	0	0	0	11	10.5	0	0	0	0	0	0	0	0	104
Coleman: isolated once from soil	0	0	0	0	0	0	0	0	0	0	0	0	0	0	0	0	1	100	1
Stock cultures in this laboratory collected by Heller[8] from different laboratories in the United States were typed by Bauer and Meyer. These cultures have been isolated in this country from sources other than feces and are used in some institutions for the production of commercial antitoxin	18	90	0	0	2	10	0	0	0	0	0	0	0	0	0	0	0	0	20

* These and preceding data are cited by Bauer and Meyer.

† These results are given as being of interest on the assumption that the individuals furnishing these serums at one time probably harbored tetanus spores. Of these 104 serums 80% showed agglutinins at 1:10 or higher. One serum agglutinated as many as 5 types. Many of them 2 or more types. 35.5% of all agglutinations were of type 2 and 46.7% type 5. Type 8 was found 4 times at 1:10 dilution. No serum tests were made for type 6 and 7 as they were not found in stools. Forty-four of these serums were tested for antitoxin with negative results.

[8] J. Infect. Dis., 1922, 30, p. 18.

in California the same number (types 6 and 7 have not been found). Whether other types exist we do not know but in all probability a complete survey in this and in other countries of the types obtained from wounds, feces and soils will disclose other types. That this survey should be made for various regions is of the utmost importance if, as we are tentatively assuming, the control of the tetanus problem should ultimately depend upon a more extensive knowledge of as many types as possible. Added weight will be given to this suggestion when it is remembered that type 5 was found only once in France and appears to be the predominating type in China and in England.

CONCLUSION

Evidence is given that there are at least nine distinct serologic types of Clostridium tetani.

THE TREATMENT OF TYPHOID FEVER WITH DETOXICATED VACCINE

W. B. Wherry, T. J. LeBlanc, L. Foshay and R. Thomas

From the Department of Bacteriology and Preventive Medicine, Medical College, University of Cincinnati

One obvious objection to the treatment of acute infections by the inoculation of specific antigens is that one may add to an already existing toxemia. The demonstration by Ramon that the toxicity of certain bacterial, vegetable and reptilian poisons could be destroyed by formaldehyde without effecting their antigenic properties make it appear hopeful that one may actively immunize a patient acutely ill of an infection. Following the work of Wherry and Bowen [1] on the detoxication of B. dysenteriae (Shiga) and B. typhosus, these workers in 1926 treated thirteen patients with typhoid fever with vaccine. As the patients did so well under this treatment it was deemed advisable to treat a sufficient number of patients and then analyze the data statistically. While we have not succeeded in treating a sufficient number of patients we feel that the results obtained are significant enough to warrant this preliminary note and we hope that other workers will add to the data presented here. Obviously the efficacy of therapeutic inoculation may be judged by a shortening of the course of the disease, or by a reduction of mortality. Since the latter method would entail the treatment of a very large number of cases, we chose the former. Although we had a number of cases in which the clinical diagnosis was typhoid fever and in which the patients did well under the treatment, we have excluded from this report all cases which were not confirmed by a bacteriologic examination of the blood, stool, urine, or a positive Widal obtained within the first two weeks of the disease. The majority were diagnosed by inoculating bile with blood taken early in the course of the disease.

Preparation of the Vaccine.—Nearly all the patients treated in Cincinnati were inoculated with vaccine prepared from a domestic strain of B. typhosus; all of those treated in Mexico with a Mexican strain, and a few were treated in Cincinnati, after our return from Mexico, with the Mexican strain. We have not sufficient data to determine whether the question of strain plays any rôle or not.

Received for publication, Feb. 24, 1928.

1. J. Infect. Dis., 1925, 37, p. 520.

The vaccine was prepared by suspending three agar slant cultures in 9 cc. of 0.9% sterile sodium chloride solution and adding to this 1 cc. of a 1:100 dilution of a 40% aqueous solution of formaldehyde. The tube was corked with a sterile rubber stopper and incubated for three weeks at 37 C. The germs were then washed three times with sterile salt solution and enough carbolic acid added to make 0.5%. This dense suspension was diluted 1:9 with carbolized salt solution for treatment.

A rough attempt to introduce uniformity into the procedure was made by growing the germs on + 1 * meat infusion agar slants occupying three-fourths of the length of 150 x 15 mm. test tubes. While counts made by plating out dilutions of the suspension varied a great deal we believe that the diluted suspension contained about 100 million bacilli in each 0.1 cc.—the daily dose used most often in therapeutic inoculation. The optical density of the suspension of organisms treated with formaldehyde and the number of bacteria used for treatment in Mexico (which was made to correspond in density with the suspension previously used in Cincinnati) was determined for me by C. T. Butterfield of the U. S. Stream Pollution Laboratory. This corresponds to 230 parts per million of the silica standard adopted by the U. S. Geological Survey. Direct counts in a Petroff-Häuser counting chamber showed that the vaccine used for inoculation contained 825,000,000 cells per cc. The cells were well defined and showed no signs of lysis. Therefore it may be presumed that the therapeutic daily dose of 0.1 cc. contained about 82,000,000 bacilli. Often twice this dose was used. It may be mentioned here that the optical density of a formalinized suspension is greater than that of a heated suspension.

Dosage of the Vaccine.—The treatment above described does not completely detoxicate the typhoid bacillus. However we have injected healthy human beings with about 500 million bacilli every other day with no more than local tenderness and slight malaise. However in immunizing healthy adults we injected subcutaneously, as a rule, about 100 millions bacilli daily for a week or ten days. This dose produces only slight local congestion and tenderness, no constitutional symptoms, and the reaction usually subsides in 24 to 36 hours. There are slight individual variations.

Effects of the Vaccine.—We have little information concerning the antibodies produced. The blood serum of healthy human beings collected five days after receiving 12 doses of 0.1 cc. had agglutination titers varying from 1:300 to 1:500. One person received 3.5 cc. of the vaccine in gradually increasing doses, and the serum had an agglutination titer of 1:5000. None of these persons had had typhoid.

Some of our early patients were treated by injecting the antigen intradermally sometimes once a day and sometimes twice daily, however, when we found that the daily subcutaneous doses were borne without discomfort by the patients, and without any aggravation of the symp-

* + 1 indicates 1% acid to phenolphthalein.

toms, we adopted the subcutaneous route in all cases thereafter. We have given such inoculations to markedly toxic cases of typhoid late in the disease and to a few cases with relapse and toxemia, without further aggravating their condition, and with what looked like favorable results. One effect of the vaccine which we consider as significant is that one can almost certainly predict that after the seventh or eighth daily dose the temperature will begin to break in an irregular lysis (chart 1).

General Results.—Part 1 of the table shows the apparent effect of the treatment in the 28 cases we have chosen because they were proven to be typhoid fever soon after the onset and the inoculations were begun probably within the first two weeks of the disease. In the Mexican

	Number Cases	Blood Positive	Widal Positive	Stool Positive	Deaths Number	Deaths %	Average Duration Fever, Days	Average Hospital Stay, Days	Complications Number	Complications %
1. Effect of Treatment in 28 Cases										
Mexico	14	10	3	1	0	0	20.6	27.9	2	14.3
United States	14	11	3	0	0	0	34.4	51.3	0	0
Total	28	21	6	1	0	0	27.5	39.6	2	7.1
2.—Control Cases of Typhoid Fever										
Mexico	41	16	24	1	5	12.2	37.6	56.2	18	43.9
United States	27	16	11	0	2	7.4	40.9	52.8	7	25.9
Total	68	32	35	1	7	10.3	39.0	54.8	25	36.8
3.—Cases Treated Before and After 9th Day										
Treatment before 9th day	Mex. 9, U. S. 5				0	0	21.6	31.4	1	7.1
Treatment after 9th day	Mex. 5, U. S. 9				0	0	33.3	47.8	1	7.1

series we did not wait for the results of the blood culture but commenced the inoculations at once (chart 1). This often enabled us to give several doses of the vaccine sooner than otherwise and may account for the shorter average duration of the fever in this set. Along with this shortening of the course of the disease it was noted by the physicians in charge that the patients came through in fine physical condition and made a rapid convalescence.

By "duration of fever" we mean the interval between the time of the probable date of the onset, as far as we could determine it, and the time when the temperature fell to normal and remained there for four days without any significant or subsequent rise. The data of part 3 of the table point to the advisability of giving the vaccine early in the disease.

The 68 control cases (part 2) which likewise were all proven to be typhoid include 27 cases in which the patients were treated by the

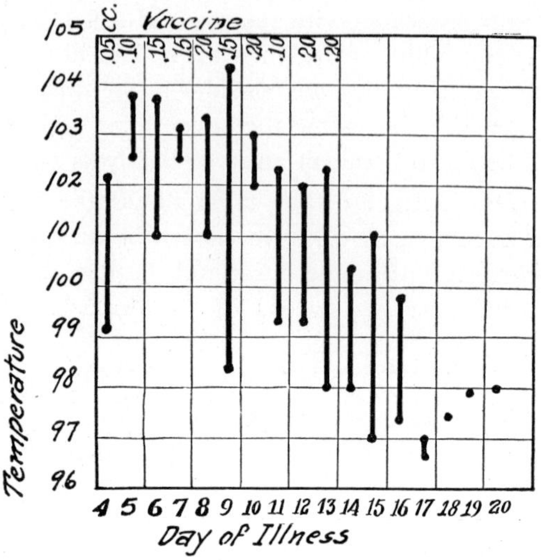

Chart 1.—Average maximum and minimum daily temperature of patient during treatment. Blood culture on 4th day of fever yielded B. typhosus. First two doses of vaccine mixed typhoid and paratyphoid A and B. No complications. Rapid convalescence.

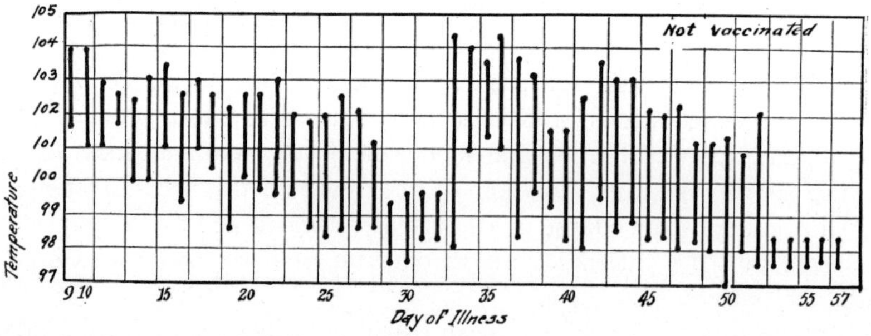

Chart 2.—Average maximum and minimum daily temperature of unvaccinated patient in which fever was of somewhat more than average duration. Blood culture on November 7, two days before first charted temperature yielded B. typhosus. Total duration 76 days. Recovered. Intestinal hemorrhages on November 11 and 12.

ordinary methods in Cincinnati during a period of two years (the year before, and the year following, the year in which vaccine was used), and 41 cases which during a two year period before the vaccine was used in Mexico City—had been diagnosed bacteriologically by H. Mooser, pathologist to The American Hospital and the Cowdray Sanatorium.

Typhoid Pyelitis.—Two cases in which there was high fever were encountered among those not treated with vaccine. One patient had been in the hospital for 123 days. Increasing doses of the vaccine were given for 10 days, the last dose being 1.0 cc. The patient was discharged on the 149th day after the urine had been free of typhoid bacilli for 16 days. In the second case the diagnosis was made on the 32nd day of the disease. Under similar vaccine treatment the urine became clear on the 46th day of the disease, but the vaccine was continued until the discharge of the patient on the 57th day.

SUMMARY

B. typhosus antigen can be detoxicated to a considerable degree by treating it with formaldehyde according to Ramon's method. About 82 to 164 million treated bacilli may be injected subcutaneously, and daily, into a patient with typhoid fever, irrespective of the apparent severity of the disease, without any harm. Twenty-eight patients with typhoid fever (bacteriological diagnosis) were treated in this manner in Cincinnati and in Mexico City by daily subcutaneous inoculations with 82 to 164 million formalinized bacilli. The results of this treatment along with data collected from 68 control cases seems to show that the course of the disease is shortened, the temperature uniformly showing a tendency to drop to normal after the 7th or 8th dose and then coming to normal by irregular lysis. The average duration of the fever in the treated cases was 27.5 days, while that in the controls was 39 days. The incidence of complications seems decreased: 7% in the treated, and 36% in the untreated. Convalescence is shortened for those patients treated early in the course of the disease. The death rate is decreased from 10% for the untreated to zero for the treated. We hope that others will help to collect enough data to make a rigid statistical analysis possible.

REPLACEMENT OF POTASSIUM BY OTHER ELEMENTS IN CULTURE MEDIUMS

C. H. BOISSEVAIN

From the Colorado Foundation for Research in Tuberculosis, at Colorado College, Colorado Springs

Naegeli [1] and Beneke [2] were the first to replace potassium in synthetic culture mediums by other elements. They found that caesium and rubidium could take its place in the cultivation of aspergillus. Their experiments were discredited by Fermi [3] who showed that aspergillus grows in metal containers with only distilled water and ammonium lactate. Cache [4] and Zunz and Gyorgyi [5] demonstrated that bacterium typhosus and bacterium coli can grow in potassium-free medium. This is not the case for all microorganisms; Besançon, Philibert and Boudin [6] state that the tubercle bacillus needs phosphorus, magnesium and potassium in addition to carbon and nitrogen, and I [7] have shown that the potassium may be replaced by rubidium but not by caesium or lithium.

A good deal of interest attaches to the substitution of radioactive elements for potassium. Zwaardemaker [8] states that the action of potassium and rubidium in the perfusion-fluid of the surviving heart is due to the emission of β rays by these elements and that a fluid containing an equo-radioactive amount of any radioactive element may take the place of potassium in Ringer's fluid. Clark [9] who experimented not only with the heart but with several other organs, agrees that rubidium is a perfect substitute for potassium, but adds that caesium is an imperfect substitute. He is of the opinion that uranium and thorium are irritants for the heart but may not be considered as substitutes for potassium. R. F. Loeb [10] and J. Loeb [11] find that both rubidium and caesium may be substituted for potassium in the artificial fertilization of sea-urchin eggs.

Received for publication, Feb. 20, 1927.

1. Untersuchungen über niedere Pilze, 1882.
2. Jahrb. f. wissenschaftl. Botanik, 1895, 28, p. 487.
3. Centralbl. f. Bakteriol., 1. O., 1901, 29, p. 473.
4. Ibid., 1905, 40, p. 255.
5. J. Bact., 1, p. 627.
6. Soc. d'Etud. s. l. Tubercul., 1913, 3, p. 1.
7. Am. Rev. Tuberc., 1926, 14, p. 172.
8. Versl. Kon. Akad. v. Wetensch. Amsterdam, 1916, 25, p. 517.
9. J. Pharm. & Exper. Therap., 1921-1922, 18, p. 425.
10. J. gen. Physiol., 1920-1921, 3, p. 229.
11. Ibid., p. 237.

The original potassium content of animal tissues constitutes an important source of error in these experiments; the heart still contains 0.1% potassium after 6 hours perfusion with a potassium-free fluid (Clark.)[9] This error can be avoided in experiments with bacteria, through the use of serial transplants; the potassium content of the original loopful is diluted many million times in the succeeding transplants. The present paper deals with the substitution of rubidium, caesium, lithium, and radioactive preparations for potassium in the culture of mycobacterium tuberculosis (hominis), mycobacterium leprae, mycobacterium ranae, mycobacterium smegmatis, and a not previously described gram-positive soil-organism.

Methods.—The medium used is a modification of Long's medium and contains:

asparagin	0.5 gm.	$MgSO_4$	0.1 gm.
ammonium citrate	0.5 gm.	glycerol	4.0 gm.
Na_2HPO_4	0.4 gm.	water	100. gm.

Chlorides of the alkali metals or radioactive preparations are added to this medium in the different experiments.

The flame spectrum of commercial rubidium chloride showed a faint line at 404.4$\mu\mu$, probably due to potassium. Determination of the solubility of the chloroplatinate gave a calculated potassium chloride content of 0.21%. The rubidium chloride was purified by recrystallization of its chloroplatinate until the potassium line disappeared from the spectrum.

Experiments.—All acidfast bacteria examined grow well on synthetic medium. Maximum growth is obtained on a suitable medium after three weeks when a thick veil covers the surface. Erlemeyer flasks containing 100 cc. of the standard medium were inoculated with the different acidfast bacteria and the growth compared with that in similar flasks that contained, in addition to 100 cc. of the standard medium, 200 mg. potassium chloride, 200 mg. rubidium chloride, 200 mg. caesium chloride, 200 mg lithium chloride, 50 mg. uranyl nitrate or 10^{-5} mg. radium chloride. These quantities of uranyl nitrate and radium chloride are according to Zwaardemaker[12] physiologically equivalent to 200 mg. potassium chloride. The bacteria were filtered off after three weeks, dried over sulphuric acid and weighed. Only the flasks containing potassium or rubidium chloride showed an appreciable difference from

12. Arch. neerl. de Physiol., 1921, 5, p. 285.

the control flasks (table 1). The leprosy bacillus and the bacillus of frog tuberculosis form a much thinner veil than the smegma bacillus and the human tubercle bacillus, but the relative difference between the growth on the control medium and on that containing potassium or rubidium chloride was the same in all cases.

The bacteria can be transplanted indefinitely on the media containing potassium or rubidium chloride. The human tubercle bacillus had not lost its virulence for guinea-pigs after ten successive transplants on the medium containing rubidium chloride. Some growth usually occurs on the media without either potassium or rubidium and the bacilli may be transplanted through two or three generations before dying out.

TABLE 1.—DRY WEIGHT OF BACILLI AFTER 3 WEEKS' GROWTH

Addition to 100 Cc. of Standard Medium	Mg.	Mycobact. tuberculosis hominis Mg.	Mycobact. leprae Mg.	Mycobact. ranae Mg.	Mycobact. smegmatis Mg.
KCl	200	530	11.8	50	440
RbCl	200	480	10	40	500
CsCl	200	4	< 0.1	< 0.1	9
LiCl	200	3	< 0.1	< 0.1	8
Uranyl nitrate	50	4	< 0.1	< 0.1	12
Radium chloride	10^{-5}	2	< 0.1	< 0.1	8
No addition		2	< 0.1	< 0.1	8

TABLE 2.—DRY WEIGHT OF HUMAN TUBERCLE BACILLI AFTER THREE WEEKS' GROWTH ON 100 CC. OF MEDIUM CONTAINING VARYING AMOUNTS OF KCL OR RBCL

KCl or RbCl %	0.1	0.05	0.01	0.005	0.002	0.001	0.0005
Weights, mg.							
From KCl medium	520	468	312	304	74	30	4
From RbCl medium	480	465	204	214	30	4	3

The weight of the growth after three weeks is proportional to the concentration of potassium or rubidium (table 2). The weight of 4 mg., which is the same as that from the control medium, is produced by a medium with a potassium chloride concentration of 0.001%, or with 0.002% rubidium chloride. Taking into account the higher molecular weight of rubidium chloride, it appears that one molecule of rubidium chloride has exactly the same effect on the growth of the tubercle bacillus as one molecule of potassium chloride, although rubidium produces 3 to 7 times more β rays than potassium.

Caesium is chemically very similar to rubidium but does not have the same favorable effect on bacterial growth. It seemed possible that the combination of an element chemically similar to rubidium or potassium and a radioactive element is necessary for bacterial growth. This was tested by growing the smegma bacillus on medium containing both caesium chloride and radium chloride, but no difference was found between the growth on this medium and on a medium containing only caesium, as the tabulation shows.

Added to 100 Cc. Standard Medium	Caesium Chloride 200 mg.	Radium Chloride 10^{-5} mg.	Caesium Chloride 200 mg. + Radium Chloride 10^{-5} mg.	(Nothing) ..
Dry weight of 3 weeks growth of smegma bacilli	12 mg.	10 mg.	8 mg.	9 mg.

If a flask containing a culture medium is exposed to roentgen rays, the absorbed rays cause the emission of photo-electrons entirely similar to β rays, although of lower velocity. A flask containing 100 cc. standard medium was inoculated with smegma bacilli and exposed continuously during 168 hours to a bundle of roentgen rays. An oil-cooled Coolidge universal tube was used with a target distance of 25 cm.; the current was 3 milliamperes and the potential 80 kilovolts. No growth was observed although a flask containing potassium chloride showed abundant growth of the smegma bacillus in the same length of time and under the same conditions. Roentgen rays are apparently without any effect, favorable or unfavorable on the growth of the smegma bacillus.

Nothing in these experiments indicates that radioactive substances are necessary for bacterial growth. Zwaardemaker [13] states, however, that α rays and β rays have an antagonistic action. Uranyl nitrate and radium chloride emit both α and β rays. It is possible to make a uranium preparation which emits only β rays.[14] This transformation product, uranium XI that emits β rays only has a half period of 24.6 days and is continuously transformed into uranium II, which emits α rays. It is accordingly necessary to use a fast growing organism to determine the effect of uranium XI on bacterial growth. Bacterium coli and bacterium paratyphosus B amongst the gram negative organisms grow well on synthetic medium but do not need potassium. None of the common gram-positive organisms grows well on our medium; even Bacillus subtilis shows only a very scanty growth. A fast growing gram-positive soil bacillus was finally isolated which grows abundantly on our medium when potassium or rubidium have been added to it.

This bacillus has the following characteristics: gram-positive rods 4-6 μ long, terminal spores, rods not swollen at sporulation, nonmotile; round or lobulate colonies on agar, broth cloudy with surface pellicle and sediment, abundant growth on synthetic mediums, stratiform lique-

13. Proc. Roy. Acad. Sc., Amsterdam, 1922, 25, p. 152.
14. Rutherford: Radioactive substances and their radiations, 1913.

faction of gelatin, serum liquefied, litmus milk reduced, indol not formed, nitrates reduced to nitrites.

This bacillus grows on the standard medium only when rubidium or potassium chloride have been added. The minimum concentration of these salts necessary to promote growth is the same as for the acid-fast bacteria. Addition of a preparation of uranium X_I, corresponding to 50 mg. uranyl nitrate in radioactive equilibrium, was without any effect on the growth in 24 hours (tabulation).

Addition to 100 Cc. standard medium (mg.)	KCl 200	RbCl 200	CeCl 200	LiCl 200	Uranium X_I equivalent 50 mg. uranyl nitrate	Radium chloride 10^{-5} mg.	(Nothing)
Growth as shown by cloudy broth, surface pellicle and sediment	++++	++++	0	0	0	0	0

DISCUSSION

These experiments show conclusively that only rubidium can replace potassium in the nutrition of bacteria. The fact that approximately equimolecular quantities of potassium or rubidium chloride are needed to support growth excludes the possibility that the effect of rubidium chloride is produced by some undetected contamination with potassium chloride. Replacement of potassium by radioactive elements or by the other alkali metals or by combinations of the two has no favorable effect on the growth of bacteria. Uranium salts sometimes seem to stimulate the growth of acidfast bacteria; the medium containing the uranium salt may be covered after a few days with a thin veil of bacteria, while in the control flasks only a small part of the surface is covered. When the bacteria are dried and weighed, however, it appears invariably that there has been no increase in weight; only a spreading of the bacteria over the surface instead of real growth takes place. This is confirmed by the fact that it is impossible to keep the bacteria alive through successive transplants on the uranium medium.

All acidfast bacteria, even obligate parasites like the tubercle bacillus grow freely on the synthetic medium and need potassium or rubidium for their growth. At least the majority of the pathogenic gram-negative organisms do not grow on the synthetic medium, and those that grow do not need potassium or rubidium. The gram-positive organisms have an intermediate position: the majority do not grow on the synthetic medium, and the only gram-positive organism that grows freely on the synthetic medium needs potassium or rubidium. It seems possible that the difference in staining properties between these different classes of organisms corresponds to a real biological difference.

SUMMARY

The acidfast bacteria that were tested grew well on a simple synthetic medium. All needed potassium or rubidium for their growth; the minimum concentrations were 0.001% KCl, and 0.002% RbCl.

Caesium, sodium, lithium, or the radioactive elements or combinations of the two cannot replace potassium in synthetic culture mediums.

Continuous exposure to roentgen rays for 168 hours does not kill smegma bacilli and does not favor their growth.

Among the gram-positive organisms, only a soil bacillus not previously described grew freely on the synthetic medium; it needed the same amount of potassium as the acidfast bacteria.

Among the gram-negative organisms examined, Bacterium coli and Bacterium paratyphosus B grew freely on the synthetic medium; they did not need potassium.

"FILTRABLE FORMS" OF THE TUBERCLE BACILLUS

A CRITICAL REVIEW AND PERSONAL OBSERVATIONS

FRANK B. COOPER AND S. A. PETROFF

From the Research and Clinical Laboratory of the Trudeau Sanatorium, Trudeau, N. Y.

Fontes, studying the Much granules in 1910, made the following observations: Berkefeld filtrates prepared from tuberculous pus and inoculated into guinea-pigs gave rise to induration and hypertrophy of the lymph nodes. At necropsy the animals presented an atypical picture not comparable to that of tuberculosis.* The lymph nodes and spleen were enlarged and contained small granules. Typical acidfast organisms were found in the lymph nodes and in the lungs after the second passage. This suspected material after trituration and injection again into guinea-pigs produced no pathologic changes.

Interest in this almost forgotten observation of Fontes [1] has been renewed by intensive study, chiefly in France, in connection with the Chamberland filter-passing form of the tubercle bacillus, with the object of settling the question of congenital tuberculosis which has occupied the minds of students of tuberculosis since Baumgarten's time.

At the present time the problem has been attacked from two angles. Tuberculous material prepared and filtered through the Chamberland filter has been cultivated on culture medium and inoculated into animals. In other studies, the material has been inoculated into pregnant animals and the offspring have been studied.

REVIEW

CULTIVATION AND ANIMAL INOCULATION WITH THE FILTRATES

For twelve years no investigation, to our knowledge, has been reported along this line until the appearance of Vaudremer's [2] work on the filtrable form of the tubercle bacillus. This author observed that the small granules pointed out by Much can be cultivated in glycerolated potato broth and gentian-violet medium and that these granules can pass through Chamberland L 3 filters. The growth, however, was atypical morphologically, consisting of mycelial-like bodies with multiple granules small enough to pass through Chamberland filters.

Received for publication, March 3, 1928.

* In the recent literature this author's experiment with animals has been misquoted. In no instance did Fontes obtain a typical visceral tuberculosis in animals even after the second passage.

1. Mem. do Inst. Oswaldo Cruz, 1910, 2, p. 186.

2. Compt. rend. Soc. de Biol., 1922, 85, p. 10; 1923, 89, p. 80; Presse Med., 1923, 47, p. 534.

Hauduroy and Vaudremer[3] used tubercle bacilli cultivated on solid potato medium, the suspension being made in salt solution and filtered through Chamberland L 3 filters. The filtrate could be cultivated on 2% peptonized, glycerolated water, in which medium the granules developed in bacillus forms.

Valtis and Calmette[4] autolyzed positive sputum at 37 C. for three days. Five cc. of this autolysate were emulsified in 45 cc. of salt solution, filtered through paper covered with diatomaceous earth and then through the Chamberland L 3 filter. Guinea-pigs inoculated subcutaneously with 5 cc. of this filtrate and killed 94 to 96 days later presented a generalized glandular enlargement. The lungs contained granulations surrounded by a zone of hepatization and purulent cavities. Typical tubercle bacilli could be demonstrated. The filtrate did not grow on gentian-violet medium. Another guinea-pig inoculated with 10 cc. of the filtrate died in 60 days with slight tumefaction of the inguinal lymph nodes and a zone of hepatization in the upper lobe of the right lung with a small cavity containing purulent fluid with long granular forms of tubercle bacilli.

Sergent, Durand and Vaudremer[5] triturated pus from an abscess with sand, diluted it to twice the original volume and filtered this suspension through Chamberland L 3 filters. The filtrate was concentrated in vacuum to the original volume and injected into the peritoneal cavity of two guinea-pigs. After 60 days the male guinea-pig developed orchitis with enlarged inguinal glands. The orchitis later broke down and the pus contained a large number of typical acidfast organisms. They further used a culture of tubercle bacilli which was triturated and filtered through the Chamberland filter. The filtrate was inoculated intraperitoneally. Three months later there was swelling of the inguinal lymph nodes. At the end of the fourth month the node was opened and the pus was found to contain many typical tubercle bacilli. One cc. of this was inoculated into two other guinea-pigs. These last two animals presented typical tuberculosis at the point of inoculation. Durand,[6] more recently, was able to cultivate typical tubercle bacilli from these filtrates on Dorset's egg medium.

Arloing and Dufourt,[7] in four out of five cases of infantile tuberculosis, obtained a filtrable form of tubercle bacilli, which did not cause apparent lesions in guinea-pigs of the local caseous type in the viscera or in the lymph nodes. It produced a discrete lymphatic infection followed by a regular progression from the regional lymph nodes to the submaxillary nodes in cases of inguinal inoculation. The bacilli found in the lymphatic system had the morphological and staining characteristics of normal tubercle bacilli. They obtained only one positive culture of the filtrate on gentian-violet medium. Like results[8] were obtained with filtrates obtained from pulmonary lesions, subcutaneous gummata, granules in the lung, noncaseous tracheobronchial lymph nodes and from the spinal fluid in tuberculous meningitis. It was not present in old cultures on glycerolated broth and potato, but organisms cultivated on gentian-violet medium, even at the sixth week of development, presented this filtrable form. Animals inoculated with this filtrate and killed two and one-half months later showed generalized glandular tuberculosis, but no caseation. Tubercle bacilli could not be cultivated.

Durand and Cherchanski[9] prepared filtrates from the fluid of serofibrinous pleurisy. A guinea-pig inoculated with 1 cc. of such a filtrate, three weeks later

3. Compt. rend. Soc. de Biol., 1923, 89, p. 1276.
4. Ibid., 1924, 90, p. 19.
5. Ibid., p. 916.
6. Ibid., 91, p. 11.
7. Reunion Biol. de Lyon, June 15, 1925 (reviewed in La Presse Medicale, 1925, 33, p. 898).
8. Arloing, F., and Dufourt, A.: Compt. rend. Soc. de Biol., 1925, 93, p. 165.
9. Ibid., p. 499.

showed a caseous and juxtasplenic adenitis containing typical tubercle bacilli. The filtrate could not be cultivated on Dorset's egg medium. The experience of Bezançon and Philibert[10] was very similar.

Calmette and Valtis[11] were able to demonstrate typical acidfast organisms in the spleen and the lymph nodes not only in guinea-pigs but also in rabbits, twelve days after the injection of the filtrate prepared from cultures of tubercle bacilli. The injections were intravenous.

Schlossmann[12] attempted to demonstrate the filtrable form of the tubercle bacillus by using collodion sacks. A pressure of 150 cm. was used in filtration. After a large series of experiments this author came to the conclusion that in the filtrates from the sputum and tuberculous material there exists a form of tubercle bacilli which may give rise in guinea-pigs to tuberculous lesions containing typical tubercle bacilli. The work of Fabry[13] seems to suggest the possibility of the filtrable form of the tubercle bacillus.

There is considerable disagreement as to the nature of this filtrable form of the tubercle bacillus in regard to its acidfast properties. Vaudremer[14] believes that the filtrable form is present in the mycelial type of organisms, which form can develop outside of the body. Certain elements of this mycelium pass through the filter in an isolated granulated form, which is nonacidfast. After passing into the animal this nonacidfast form develops into a typical form of the tubercle bacillus. Others believe them to be typical acidfast granules. On the other hand, there are experimental data which deny the existence of such a filtrable form of the tubercle bacillus. Dessy[15] was unable to detect any such form. Eight guinea-pigs into which filtrates had been injected, showed no evidence of macroscopic or microscopic tuberculosis and the tuberculin reaction in all these animals was negative. Cultures on gentian-violet, glycerol bouillon and potato medium were sterile.

The same has been the experience of Frans de Potter.[16] Using nonpathogenic acidfast organisms which could be easily cultivated outside of the body, this author attempted to repeat some of the positive results obtained, filtering the suspension of the organisms through Chamberland filters. None of the filtrates grew on mediums. Montemartini[17] was another investigator who failed to confirm the possibility of the filtrable form of the tubercle bacillus. In guinea-pigs he could not produce tuberculous lesions with the exception of enlargement of the lymph nodes which did not contain any tubercle bacilli.

Fessler[18] in no instance was able to cultivate a filtrable form of the tubercle bacillus from filtrates, nor did he succeed in infecting animals.

Mellon and Jost,[19] in the United States, inoculated 21 guinea-pigs with Berkefeld filtrates from tuberculous material. Twelve animals died up to the time of the study published. In three of the twelve animals acidfast bacilli could be demonstrated by direct method in the lungs, inguinal and tracheobronchial lymph nodes. Two of these three animals had definite tuberculosis, while in the other no evidence of tuberculosis could be demonstrated by histological methods. They

10. Soc. d'études de la tuberculose, March 12, 1914, p. 32.
11. Ann. de Med., 1926, 19, p. 553.
12. Bull. de l'Union internat. contre la Tuberc., 1926, 3, no. 3, p. 2.
13. Bruxelles-Medical, 1927, 7, p. 596.
14. Bull. de l'Acad. de Med., Paris, 1926, 95, p. 440.
15. Boll. Ist. Sieroterap., 1926, 5, p. 41.
16. Compt. rend. Soc. de Biol., 1924, 91, p. 922.
17. Boll. Ist. Sieroterap., 1925, 4, p. 1.
18. Centralbl. f. Bakteriol., 1. O., 1926, 98, p. 148.
19. Proc. Soc. Exper. Biol. & Med., 1927, 24, p. 743.

showed a small punctate area of granulomatous, endothelioid hyperplasia non-specific for tuberculosis. The lesions did not differ from those examined in twelve normal control animals.

THE TRANSMISSIBILITY OF THE FILTRABLE FORM OF THE TUBERCLE BACILLUS FROM MOTHER TO OFFSPRING

The recent studies with the filtrable form of the tubercle bacillus have paved the way for investigations of congenital-hereditary tuberculosis. The importance of such investigations is obvious. If such a form of microorganisms does exist, then what will prevent the passing of the virus through the placenta into the fetus, setting up an infection? If infection does occur under such conditions we may find a true congenital type of disease with well organized anatomical changes or it may be of a latent type. In the latter case the infant may not present any traces of tuberculosis but in due time a hematogenous spread may take place with a definite tuberculosis. The experimental and clinical data up to the present have shown that tubercle bacilli are transmitted very rarely from mother to offspring, when the placenta is perfectly normal and free from tuberculosis.

Péhu and Chalier [20] and Whitman and Greene [21] report 130 cases of supposedly congenital tuberculosis. However, the possibility of the infection taking place at birth had not been controlled in these cases.

Kuhle [22] reports a mother with far advanced tuberculosis who died 24 hours after delivery by forceps. At that time there was no tuberculous person at the hospital. The infant was isolated and never came in contact with any of the relatives. At birth the Pirquet test was negative, becoming positive at the eighth week and followed by temperature. At the ninth week there was evidence of bronchopneumonia, at the eleventh week miliary tuberculosis, and death occurred in the twelfth week. Necropsy revealed miliary tuberculosis of the lung, liver and spleen, tuberculous ulceration of the intestines and caseous lymph nodes of the hilum and the mesentery. The author, however, states that this case in all probability is not a congenital tuberculosis. The bacilli may have entered the mixture of maternal and fetal blood at birth from the placenta.

Arloing and Dufourt [23] present a case of a mother with advanced pulmonary tuberculosis giving birth to a child weighing 1,310 grams. The child was immediately removed from the mother and placed in an incubator. Temperature was 34.2 to 35 C. No tuberculosis was detected by physical examination. Ten days after birth the temperature rose to 37 C. and remained so until death which occurred 56 days after birth. At necropsy no tuberculosis was found. The mesenteric lymph nodes were hypertrophied but not caseous. Microscopic examination revealed some suspicious acidfast rods. These lymph nodes were triturated and suspended in salt solution, filtered through Chamberland filters and the filtrate

20. Arch. d. med. d. enf., 1908, 11, no. 1, p. 100; 1914, 17, p. 921.
21. Arch. Int. Med., 1922, 29, p. 261.
22. Deutsch. med. Wchnschr., 1924, 50, pt. 1, p. 796.
23. Presse Med., 1927, 35, p. 17.

inoculated into a guinea-pig which became emaciated. At necropsy many apparently acidfast organisms were found in the lymph nodes of this animal.

Calmette, Valtis and M. Lacomme[24] claim that this filtrable form is ultramicroscopic but when inoculated into guinea-pigs before or during gestation it is capable of traversing the placenta, thus infesting the fetus and producing tuberculous lesions from which nonfiltrable, acidfast forms of the tubercle bacillus can be recovered. These authors attempted to correlate this with clinical observation on 99 tuberculous pregnant women and their offspring. Of 21 dead infants 10 were subjected to postmortem examination. In three out of four stillborn infants bacilli were found by direct examination in the groundup material from the lymph nodes. Inoculations of the pulp from these glands were positive in four cases and the filtrates of the gland extracts from three of the infants gave positive results when inoculated into animals. Two infants dead without apparent cause, the organs and glands appearing normal and showing no tubercle bacilli on direct examination, also gave positive results by inoculation of the ground-up organs. Thus, out of a total of nine infants or fetuses which had no contact with their tuberculous mothers after birth, it has been possible in three to find bacilli by direct examination and when such material was inoculated into guinea-pigs generalized tuberculosis was the result. Bacillary forms were few in number after prolonged examination. Filtrates of the organs from four of these infants proved virulent and the inoculation of the fluid from the mesenteric lymph nodes of one of them produced a single visible lesion after a period of six months. These authors concluded that transmission from the mother to the unborn child is much more frequent than has been supposed up to the present. Furthermore, they think transplacental tuberculous infection is often due to an ultramicroscopic virus which passes the Chamberland filters and is pathogenic for guinea-pigs.

Couvelaire,[25] studying the fate of the infants of tuberculous mothers concluded that transplacental transmission of a filtrable tuberculous virus without specific anatomical lesions is less rare than true intrauterine tuberculosis with specific lesions.

Debré and Lelong[26] were led to believe that congenital tuberculosis is only a hypothesis and lacks confirmatory facts. They believe that such a state may exist but that it is very rare. When it occurs it is usually from placental infection and is rapidly fatal. Generally death of the fetus takes place in the uterus but if the infant survives, death follows in a few weeks. Therefore, its occurrence is probably due to accidental contamination.

The same authors studied large numbers of cases at the Laennec Hospital which were later removed to the country, dividing the cases into two groups, viz., those that lived and those that died. In the small group that died during the early weeks without apparent cause, 15 painstaking necropsies revealed no trace of tuberculosis. Both gross and microscopic examinations were made from all the organs. Tissues from each body were inoculated into a number of guinea-pigs. At necropsy, in no case was there evidence of tuberculosis in the guinea-pigs. Still later these authors studying 433 cases of mothers with far advanced tuberculosis showed that if protected from tuberculous infection from birth, the skin reaction remained negative indefinitely as long as the infants were kept away from contaminating surroundings. They state there is no inheritance of infection, except very rarely and when it occurs it is due to accidental contamination and

24. Compt. rend Acad. des sci., 1926, 183, p. 835.
25. Presse Med., 1927, 35, p. 225.
26. Ann. de Med., 1925, 17, p. 209; 1925, 18, p. 256.

that the theories of latent congenital-hereditary tuberculosis are founded on impressions which are not substantiated by facts.

Arloing and Dufourt,[23] in a recent communication reviewing hereditary tuberculosis, draw some very sweeping conclusions. These authors considered the question apparently settled, basing such conclusions on animal experimentation. A pregnant guinea-pig was inoculated subcutaneously with filtrates prepared from the caseous lymph nodes of a child. Just before the term the animal was killed and in the lumbar lymph nodes of the fetus acidfast organisms were found. Other guinea-pigs inoculated with various filtrates of tuberculous material from children became very much emaciated and after death tubercle bacilli were found in the hypertrophied but noncaseous lymph nodes.

Analyzing the results obtained by animal experimentation, they called attention to three types of experimental disease which are found in adult guinea-pigs inoculated with this filtrate of tuberculous material, viz., A, the caseous form; B, the cachetic form, and C, the transient curable form. The A form is the rarest. In the majority of cases the B form, i. e., fatal cachexia with enlargement of the lymph nodes containing acidfast organisms, is the commonest found by practically all investigators. In the last form, C, in which recovery is made after inoculations, the skin test may be positive in various degrees but gradually it disappears after several months. Similar results were reported by Calmette, Valtis, Negré and Boquet.[27] How correct they are in this matter time alone will tell. The experimental data presented dealing with this problem so far, with the exception of a few animals, is open to severe criticisms. There are still many questions which are very difficult to answer.

Rabinowitsch[28] inoculated 51 animals with filtrates obtained from cultures, human and animal organs, feces and pus. The filtrates were obtained by two methods, using Zsigmondy-Bachmann membrane and Chamberland filters. Of the 25 guinea-pigs inoculated with membrane filtrates seven developed progressive tuberculosis. The author considered this to be due to imperfection of the membranes. Of the remaining 26 animals inoculated with the filtrate from the Chamberland candle not a single one developed any trace of tuberculosis. No definite lesions were found in the 73 offspring from mothers inoculated with filtrates, although acidfast organisms were demonstrated in some of the inguinal lymph nodes. Negative results were also obtained in an animal which had been injected with suspected lymph nodes from these offsprings. In a large number of the animals the intracutaneous test was positive but not the typical reaction obtained as in tuberculous animals. Cachexia was also present in many of the inoculated animals. Of the animals which survived and were under observation from one to four months, not a single case presented evidence of tuberculosis at necropsy. This author reports one positive result obtained, when a pregnant rabbit was inoculated five days before term with the filtrate of tuberculous material, the lymph nodes of the offspring, when subinoculated, producing tuberculosis in the guinea-pig. In the face of almost complete negative evidence with one exception, this author still believes that there is a filtrable form of the tubercle bacillus.

EXPERIMENTAL WORK

Our method used in the studies about to be reported, with the exception of a few instances, was in many details similar to that employed by several workers reported in the preceding review.

27. Compt. rend. Acad. des sci., 1925, 181, p. 491.
28. Deutsch. med. Wchnschr., 1927, no. 47, p. 1982.

Great care was taken in eliminating any possibility of contamination with acidfast organisms. Test tubes, micro-slides and mortars for triturating the suspected tissue were treated for several hours either with chromic or nitric acid. Berkefeld candles, types V, N and W were used. Whether the Berkefeld candles had been used before or not, they were cleaned with 0.5% potassium permanganate followed with sodium bisulphite, washed with 1,000 cc. of distilled water, and all were sterilized at 15 pounds pressure (121.3 C.) for one-half hour.

The filtrates of two different fluid culture mediums were studied. We used the potato broth described by one of the authors and a synthetic medium similar to that employed at the Koch Institute in the preparation of albumose-free tuberculin.

Sixty-five day cultures of the tubercle bacillus H 37 in potato broth were filtered first through filter paper until fairly clear. This was followed by filtration through a Berkefeld filter V, applying a vacuum of 22 inches. Half of this V filtrate, which represented approximately 250 cc., was again filtered through candle W. From each filtration we had 200 cc. of the filtrates, to which 0.5 cc. of 5% freshly prepared tannic acid was added. A flocculent precipitate formed which could be easily separated by centrifugation, the object of this procedure being that such a precipitate carries down any organisms which may be in the filtrates. The supernatant fluid was discarded and the sediment was redissolved in 2 cc. of 0.85% sodium chloride. Portion of this sediment was inoculated on several slants of egg medium. On January 6, 1927 four guinea-pigs * were inoculated intratesticularly with 0.25 cc. of the sediments, two animals (1 and 2) with V filtrates and two (3 and 4) with V and W filtrates. Smears were also perpared from this sediment using Cooper's (Modified Ziehl-Neelsen) stain and occasional typical acidfast granules could be seen. None of the four guinea-pigs, after the 202nd day, developed any trace of tuberculosis microscopically or macroscopically with the exception of acidfast rods in triturated lymph nodes in animals 2, 3 and 4. The intracutaneous test was done at various times and in no instance was a typical tuberculin reaction observed.

The second medium, a synthetic, was treated approximately the same as the one already described. Filtrates of human tubercle bacilli, H 37, of various ages ranging from 3 to 4 weeks to several months, were mixed and filtered as in the preceding experiment. On February 18, 1927, five cc. of this filtrate were injected into guinea-pigs 5, 6 and 7 The animals were killed on the 186th and 187th days. No macroscopic evidence of tuberculosis could be found at necropsy. The lymph nodes

* All animals were first tested intracutaneously with 5% old tuberculin.

were triturated and smears prepared and in two of the three animals a few atypical acidfast rods were seen. The intracutaneous reaction proved repeatedly to be atypical.

It has been pointed out by many investigators that the medium in which the organisms are suspended plays a very important part in filtration, i.e., a medium of low surface tension may facilitate the passage of the microorganisms. In a few instances we have employed sodium ricinoleate, which is one of the best surface tension depressants, with the hope that by changing the surface tension and the soap acting as a lubricant, the tubercle bacilli might be allowed to pass through our Berkefeld filter W.

Filtrates were prepared by this method and precipitated as in the preceding experiments with 5% tannic acid. The sediment was inoculated into guinea-pig 8. Before the inoculations were made smears showed typical acidfast granules and one showed one typical acidfast rod. This animal was killed on the 150th day and no macroscopic or microscopic evidence of tuberculosis could be found, except from the pool of all the lymph nodes, in which 5 typical acidfast organisms were found.

SPUTUM AUTOLYSATES

We have attempted to repeat in a small number of animals the experiment of Valtis and Calmette with the filtrates of autolyzed positive sputum. Sputum specimens were collected in wide-mouthed bottles for three days. One part of sputum was diluted with 9 parts of 0.85% sodium chloride and incubated at 37.5 C. for 72 hours. This autolyzed sputum was filtered through filter paper and then through various Berkefeld candles V, N and W. The filtrates obtained on February 10, 1927, were inoculated subcutaneously into 10 guinea-pigs (9, 10, 11, 12, 13, 14, 15, 16, 17 and 18), the amount varying from 9 to 10 cc.

One of the ten animals (18) died on the 156th day of generalized tuberculosis. Guinea-pig 10 died on the 82nd day of intercurrent disease with no macroscopic evidence of tuberculosis. The lymph nodes of this animal were triturated with salt solution and typical acidfast organisms were found after long search. A portion of the suspected material was inoculated (May 3, 1927) in two guinea-pigs (19 and 20). These animals were tested intracutaneously at various times with 5% O.T. and failed to react. On the 115th day they were killed and no trace of tuberculosis was found. No acidfast rods were found in the lymph nodes of these animals.

The remaining eight animals were killed between the 179th and 187th days. There was no trace of tuberculosis in any of them, although the intracutaneous skin reaction from two weeks after the inoculations up to the time of death, was very atypical. Smears from the submaxillary and other lymph nodes showed acidfast organisms. In four typical acidfast organisms were found, and in the others atypical.

A small amount of these sputum filtrates was planted on gentian-violet, plain egg medium and also in 2% peptone. All cultures were negative at the end of the fifth month.

Specimens from three other patients with bacilli (Gaffky's Scale of V, VI, and VII) were autolyzed as above, filtered through new Berkefeld filters, W, V and N respectively and precipitated with tannic acid. Duplicate smears were made from each precipitate and each smear was examined for one and one-half hours. One smear from N filtrate, Gaffky VI specimen, showed two typical acidfast bacilli of the same morphology as in the unfiltered sputum in one field, while the others were negative. Cultures on plain egg and gentian-violet medium were sterile four months later.

In another instance, pus from the lymph nodes of a guinea-pig inoculated intratesticularly with tubercle bacilli and presenting visceral lesions, was treated in the same way as the sputum and inoculated subcutaneously into two guinea-pigs (21 and 22). These two animals lived for 110 and 192 days respectively, and both were free from tuberculosis.

In the limited number of filtered specimens of positive sputum we demonstrated in but two instances typical acidfast organisms passing through the filter. We must always keep in mind that imperfect filters may allow intact organisms of typical morphology to pass and in order to demonstrate them some method of concentration must be used. Bronfenbrenner and Muckenfuss [29] believe that any growth of bacteria which may appear in the Berkefeld filtrate is due not to a special filtrable form of organism, but to intact organisms which occasionally pass through the Berkefeld candles. Whether or not these are the filter-passing organisms mentioned by the French observers, we shall reserve our opinion at present.

TRANSPLACENTAL PASSAGE

The transmissibility of filtrable forms of tubercle bacilli from the mother to the offspring was studied with 16 young which were born from 17, 15, 5, 12, 11, 10 and 22. These young guinea-pigs were killed

29. Proc. Soc. Exper. Biol. & Med., 1927, 24, p. 371.

at various times, some at birth, others after 126 days. The tuberculin test was uniformly negative. No gross pathologic changes were seen with the exception of slight enlargement of the tracheobronchial lymph nodes, bronchial, axillary and inguinal nodes and in each case these abnormal lymph nodes were triturated in a porcelain mortar which previously had been treated with a solution of chromic acid, washed well and sterilized. The triturated material was centrifugated and the sediment was studied microscopically. In 12 out of 16 young guinea-pigs acidfast granules could be demonstrated in the lymph nodes, but in no instance could a typical acidfast rod be demonstrated. The nature of these granules at present is unknown. Up to the present we have failed to demonstrate these granules in adult guinea-pigs.

OCCURRENCE OF ACIDFAST ORGANISMS IN APPARENTLY NORMAL GUINEA-PIGS

The finding of acidfast bacilli in some animals inoculated with various filtrates, without reacting to tuberculin and exhibiting no abnormalities at necropsy with the exception of enlargement of the lymph nodes, caused us to question the nature of these particles. When a new shipment of animals that had been in the quarantine room of our animal house since arrival, began dying of intercurrent diseases after the seventh day, an opportunity was offered to study the question of acidfast organisms in apparently normal animals not reacting to 0.2 cc. of 10% old tuberculin intracutaneously. The technique used in necropsies of these animals and in making and examining smears was identical with that used in the whole filter-passing group.

Of the 15 animals so examined, 5 showed the same type of acidfast rods and the same distribution of them on the slides as was found in the series receiving filtrates from tuberculous material. The morphological and staining characteristics of these organisms were in no way different from those found in tuberculous material.

In findings of this nature one must remember that smears were made from highly concentrated material, and that no examination was considered complete until one hour had been spent on each of the two slides from each animal unless, of course, bacilli were discovered sooner. Nevertheless, it is our opinion that these findings throw a new light on the methods used in examining diagnostic animals and we are in favor of placing more importance on the intracutaneous tuberculin reaction than on the finding of acidfast bacilli, especially in the absence of definite lesions.

Cultivation.—An attempt has been made to cultivate the acidfast bacilli found in the normal animals. The glands were removed as in the previous series, ground, suspended in sterile distilled water, an equal volume of 4.0% NaOH added and incubated at 37.5 C. for one-half hour. The digested material was centrifugated, the supernatant layer discarded, the residue brought to P_H 7.0 with $\frac{N}{10}$ HCl and planted on gentian-violet plates.

Cultures from a series of seven animals gave no acidfast organisms; three grew gram-positive bacilli and four remained sterile. So far we have not been able to cultivate any of these organisms.

DISCUSSION

The mass of experimental data on the subject is very confusing. In the majority of instances where an attempt has been made to cultivate a filtrable form of the tubercle bacillus, the results have been negative with the exception of Vaudremer and Arloing and Dufourt. In our own experience we have also failed to cultivate any organism from the filtrates so far studied. The positive results reported have been based on the presence of acidfast bodies in the lymph nodes of the animals inoculated with these filtrates. As we have already pointed out, acidfast organisms were demonstrated in the lymph nodes in 33% of normal guinea-pigs and 36% of those inoculated with tuberculous filtrates excluding the two animals with a definite visceral lesion. As the percentage of findings is about the same in the two series, we are inclined to believe that in all probability the finding of acidfast organisms in the lymph nodes of animals inoculated with tuberculous filtrates is not due to the regeneration of a filtrable form of the tubercle bacillus but to frequent occurrence of acidfast organisms in supposedly normal guinea-pigs. Could it not be possible that some organism like the Timothy bacillus, which is present in hay, the main food of the animal, may enter the body of the guinea-pig through the mouth and be entrapped in some of these lymph nodes? A further study of this problem is suggested.

Furthermore, in the studies reported where the intracutaneous test was done, no mention is made as to the types of the reaction. This test has caused more confusion than any other measure in studying tuberculous infection. A reaction of 2 to 3 mm. or even 5 mm., with slight induration and erythema, using 5% O.T., we believe should be considered as nonspecific and should be recorded as a questionable or negative reaction. There are many references in the literature in which a positive skin test similar to that just described is reported. If an organism like coli communis, staphylococcus, etc., is used for sensitization, after several weeks guinea-pigs may develop a hypersensitive state giving an atypical tuberculin reaction with pale erythema and no necrosis. A positive skin reaction we consider to be a definite induration at least 8 to 10 mm., the erythema not being pale, but a deep red with probably a small whitish center and still better a necrotic center which may vary from 2 to 5 mm. The nonspecific reaction above mentioned, is very often found in animals previously injected with a large amount of old tuberculin (O.T.) and other tubercle bacillus derivatives. In our experience in the past we have considered a mild reaction as described above as nonspecific in experimental animals and especially in the guinea-pig.

Another important point upon which much stress has been laid, is the cachexia which is so commonly present in animals after the inoculation of filtrates. It is not an uncommon observation that inoculation of large amounts of foreign protein, either peritoneally or subcutaneously, may cause a cachetic state in animals. Those who have worked with various antiserums have noticed it. Taken by itself it is not of any significance as a sign of tuberculous infection. Several years ago [30] we pointed out that even when dead tubercle bacilli were inoculated intraperitoneally in guinea-pigs a drop in the weight of the animal took place after each inoculation.

We must also consider the intercurrent diseases which are so common in the guinea-pig as being very often responsible for the cachetic state. In all probability many of the reports which are found in the literature where the principal finding has been cachexia, the animal died probably from intercurrent disease. At necropsy a culture from the heart blood should be made and the sinuses in the head and the middle ear should be examined. Branch,[31] in this laboratory, has shown that a large number of guinea-pigs which show no apparent visceral lesions at necropsy, may have infection of the middle ear or the sinuses and in some instances the culture of the heart blood is positive.

Sweany,[32] recently discussing the filtrable form of the tubercle bacillus, called attention to one guinea-pig inoculated with filtrates where the blood culture gave a growth of motile organisms which he considered probably an early stage of development of the tubercle bacillus. We are inclined to believe that these organisms were not tubercle bacilli, first

30. Am. Rev. Tuberc., 1923, 7, p. 412.
31. J. Infect. Dis., 1927, 40, p. 533.
32. Amer. Rev. Tuberc., 1928, 17, p. 77.

because of their motility, a property which hitherto no one has been able to demonstrate, nor have flagella been found.

In the majority of instances where the guinea-pig died of cachexia the only significant feature has been the presence of the acidfast organism in some of the lymph nodes, but there is no positive evidence that anyone has been able to cultivate this organism and from the more recent work of Rabinowitsch it appears that no one has been able in the past to reinoculate these lymph nodes and obtain the cardinal picture of extensive visceral tuberculosis in the guinea-pig.

As the transplacental passage of a filtrable form of the tubercle bacillus, the evidence is not sufficient to uphold the theory that such a passage is due to an actual special filtrable form of the organism. The cases reported by Calmette, Valtis and Lacomme where the positive results were obtained from stillborn infants, are not necessarily due to a filter-passing microorganism. Studying 433 cases similar to those mentioned by the above authors, Debré and Lelong [33] did not find any trace of tuberculosis in a single infant or stillborn baby. Formerly it was believed that placental tuberculosis was a rare occurrence but Warthin [34] and Weller [35] have pointed out that placental tuberculosis may be present in unsuspected individuals. They cite cases in which miliary placental tuberculosis was present without pulmonary symptoms. Schmorl and Geipel [36] collected 19 cases and were able to demonstrate lesions in nine of these cases. They believe that tuberculosis of the placenta is much more frequent than is generally believed. Norris,[37] studying 111 placentas, was able to demonstrate tuberculosis in four by histological examination, and in a few other instances without histological evidence he was able to demontrate virulent tubercle bacilli by animal inoculation. This author believes that infection of the placenta may take place through the blood stream following an acute exacerbation of the diseased lung. Aschoff [38] believes that placental tuberculosis is common (70 to 85%) in tuberculous mothers probably of advanced type. The figures given by him seem to be rather high.

With other organisms we find that the same thing may take place. Regan, Litvak and Regan [39] reported a case of anthrax infection of the

33. Ann. de Med., 1925, 18, p. 347.
34. J. Am. M. A., 1913, 61, p. 1951.
35. Arch. Int. Med., 1916, 17, p. 509.
36. München. med. Wchnschr., 1904, 51, p. 1676.
37. Penn. M. J., 1916, 9, p. 328; Am. J. Obst., 1916, 73, p. 997.
38. Pathological Anatomy, 1923, 2, p. 638.
39. J. Am. M. A., 1923, 80, p. 1769.

face in a pregnant woman who died of bacillemia, and anthrax bacilli were isolated from the heart blood of the fetus. Bedier and Leger [40] also were able to demonstrate organisms in the heart blood of the fetus whose mother died from Spirochaeta crocidurae. In malaria infections, reports of finding the plasmodium in the fetus and newborn babies are conflicting. Blacklock and Gordon [41] failed to demonstrate the parasite in the babies born of mothers having malaria, although they found infected placentas more common. These same authors consider a congenital malaria to be a very rare occurrence. Buckingham,[42] on the other hand, reports the finding of the plasmodium in the blood of babies immediately after delivery.

In clinically active tuberculosis, in all probability the permeability of the blood vessel wall may be considerably altered and the intact whole organisms may escape into the fetal blood circulation without even leaving a trace. If the placenta is tuberculous, the organisms may more readily enter the circulation of the fetus. Very unfortunately, we have not been able to study the problems in human beings.

With this mass of experimental evidence we are still in the dark and are forced to believe that such a thing as congenital tuberculosis is a rare occurrence and when it occurs in all probability the infection which takes place in the fetus is due to tuberculous placenta or to the alteration of the permeability of the blood vessels of the placenta. Experimentally up to the present we have failed to demonstrate this transplacental infection. Our experience with many thousands of guinea-pigs which have been inoculated with virulent tubercle bacilli has been that tuberculosis did not occur in any of the offspring. In two of the offspring, we have demonstrated tuberculosis after birth but the mother of these two guinea-pigs was inoculated in the mammary glands with virulent tubercle bacilli. The organism was also demonstrated in the milk.

We know that complement-fixing antibodies (Cooke,[43] Ribadeau-Dumas,[44] Debré and Lelong,[45] and others) which are colloids, may be present in the offspring at birth and they may remain so in the infant for three months after birth. Are these antibodies due to a latent disease which heals or to transplacental passage of antibodies? It is not likely

40. Compt. rend. Soc. de Biol., 1922, 87, p. 949.
41. Ann. Trop. Med. & Paras., 1925, 19, p. 37.
42. China M. J., 1925, 39, p. 1140.
43. Am. J. Dis. Child., 1921, 21, p. 78.
44. Nourrisson, 1924, 12, p. 175.
45. Ann. de Med., 1925, 17, p. 610.

that they are due to a latent disease. Therefore, they must pass through the placenta. Such being the case, if one colloidal particle may pass we believe others may do the same. Years ago Zinsser[46] obtained positive skin hypersensitiveness with a nucleoprotein fraction of the tubercle bacillus. This was later confirmed by one of the authors. The conclusion drawn was that this hypersensitiveness was not due to the soluble fraction of the organisms but to fragments of the pulverized insoluble material of the tubercle bacillus.

We know but little of the life cycle of the tubercle bacillus. If Sweany's observation is correct that after the second and third animal passage the virulence of the so-called filtrable forms of the tubercle bacillus is increased and that typical forms develop from it, and if this is confirmed by others, then we may look for some new development in the behavior of this organism. By such a procedure as that described by Sweany and others, we may look forward to transformation of bacterial species, with special reference to virulence. The fact that we have not been able so far to demonstrate such a filtrable form is of small moment. However, we can be cautious in accepting any discoveries until we have a satisfactory scientific evidence, yet we must be open-minded.

SUMMARY

We have failed to obtain growth from Berkefeld filtrates prepared from pure cultures of tubercle bacilli or from sputums which contain large numbers of this organism, and we have failed to observe any demonstrable tuberculosis leading to a progressive disease either in the mothers inoculated with such filtrates or in the offspring. We have been able, however, to demonstrate acidfast granules in such offspring, and typical acidfast organisms were found in about 36% of the full grown guinea-pigs which had received filtrates. However, we have also found these acidfast organisms in the lymph nodes of 33% of our apparently normal animals which have never been inoculated with this material. The positive results reported by others in all probability may be due to organisms which occasionally can pass through the Berkefeld filter. Several factors may play a part in such passage, as follows: imperfect filters; the pressure used for such filtration; the medium employed, and the electro-charge of the candle.

46. J. Exper. Med., 1921, 34, p. 495.

CHRONIC LOCALIZED STREPTOCOCCUS INFECTIONS IN DOGS

EXPERIMENTAL FOCAL INFECTION

From the Pathological Laboratories of the Presbyterian Hospital and the Norman Bridge Pathological Laboratory of Rush Medical College of the University of Chicago

G. Bernice Rhodes and Carl W. Apfelbach

The increasing importance attached to focal infections in their etiological relationship to many acute and chronic diseases has resulted in the development of experimental methods that simulate natural focal infection in man. Rosenow and Meisser [1] infect devitalized teeth. Intravenous inoculation of bacteria is perhaps the most commonly used method in attempts to reproduce infectious diseases. Collodion sacs containing cultures of bacteria have been buried in tissues. We believe that the method of producing focal infections herein described is a novel one because it is not mentioned in the literature so far reviewed, and because several investigators in this field, with whom we have consulted, are not cognizant of its previous use. The two premises on which our method is based are as follows: The majority of focal infections are suppurating, localized inflammations that may persist for months to years and that may undergo alternating periods of quiescence and activity; and infected foreign bodies and bony sequestra frequently prevent the healing of infections.

The focal infections are produced by implanting infected bone in the body. The ends of long bones of dogs are cut into rectangular pieces approximately 10 by 5 by 5 mm., each piece composed of cancellous and compact bone. Sterilization is accomplished in an autoclave. The fragment of bone is then immersed in ascitic dextrose broth which is inoculated with bacteria. After 24 or 48 hours the bone is implanted in an animal. We have used the spleen and sacrospinalis muscles as sites for implantation. When the spleen is used, this organ is delivered through a midline laparotomy incision and walled off by sterile gauze. The arteries of the second and third divisions to one pole are ligated. An incision about 2 cm. long is made through the capsule of this part

Received for publication, March 22, 1928.

1. Arch. Int. Med., 1923, 31, p. 807.

of the spleen and the splenic pulp separated by a hemostat. The profuse bleeding usually diminishes markedly in one or two minutes, during which time sutures are placed in the upper and lower ends of the incision ready to be tied over the bone after it is introduced into the opening. The wound is then covered with a gauze sponge for several minutes. The blood-soaked gauze surrounding the spleen is replaced by new gauze, and when bleeding has stopped, the spleen is reintroduced into the peritoneal cavity, wrapped in the omentum.

Subsequent to implantation of the infected bone, the animals usually develop a rise of temperature of 2 to 4 degrees F., malaise and polymorphonuclear leucocytosis, averaging about 30,000 white blood cells per c.mm. This period of acute infection may last from a few days to a few weeks. Following the acute period, many of the animals recover so that they are quite active. Such periods of improvement then alternate with periods of slight fever and polymorphonuclear leucocytosis. In a few animals, after three or four infected pieces of bone had been implanted during six to seven months, the animals having gone through several severe febrile periods, the pieces of bone were found at necropsy to be encapsulated, some of them with purulent fluid about them and all of them still containing viable bacteria of the type originally implanted. Bacteremia was never demonstrated by blood culture, and in none of the animals were metastatic abscesses found at postmortem examination.

Streptococcus scarlatina was the organism used in most instances, and on one occasion Staphylococcus aureus was inoculated. Only one animal in a group of fifteen died spontaneously, and this was due to infection and renal insufficiency from an acute interstitial nephritis like that which is characteristic of scarlet fever. The only alterations so far noted in animals with chronic infections with Streptococcus scarlatina have been emaciation, hyperplasia of the bone marrow and, during the acute febrile periods, cloudy swelling of the kidneys (associated during life with moderate albuminuria and varying numbers of granular casts). In two dogs iridocyclitis developed and in one of these, in addition, a corneal ulcer.

SUMMARY

Chronic abscesses were produced in the spleen and the sacrospinalis muscles of dogs by imbedding pieces of dead bone infected with Streptococcus scarlatinae; and in one instance with Staphylococcus aureus.

These focal infections resemble those occurring in human beings in so far as chronicity and alternating active and quiescent periods of infection are concerned. Few complications like those occurring in human beings have so far been observed, although one dog had acute interstitial nephritis and two had iridocyclitis. We believe that this method is adaptable in many instances where attempts are made to reproduce infectious diseases experimentally in animals.

DÖDERLEIN'S BACILLUS: LACTOBACILLUS ACIDOPHILUS

STANLEY THOMAS

From the Department of Biology, Lehigh University, Bethlehem, Pa.

In a paper entitled "Concerning the Vaginal Secretions and Vaginal Bacteria," read before the 4th Congress of the German Gynecological Society at Bonn in May, 1891, Albert Döderlein [1] described the cultural and physiological characters of the organism which has since borne his name. From Döderlein's description and from those of subsequent workers we may, for convenience, consider this organism morphologically as a gram-positive, nonspore-forming rod, sometimes quite long and slender, with square or very slightly tapering ends, occurring singly or in chains. Although written as a bacteriological study, the author drew certain conclusions as to the relation of vaginal secretions to puerperal fever. This phase of the study immediately created a widespread interest which gradually developed into one of the great scientific debates in modern surgery. In the controversy as to whether the germs of childbirth fever were to be found in the vaginas of sepsis cases or whether they were introduced by obstetrical examinations—a quite natural bone of contention at the time of the "antiseptic" versus "aseptic" debate—the bacteriological aspects of Döderlein's work received only minor consideration. However, a number of studies of the relative prevalence and cultivation of this organism have been contributed to the literature. Of these the articles by Kruse,[2] Basten,[3] Lowi,[4] Joetten [5] and Solomon [6] are of especial interest. A recent article by Lash and Kaplan [7] fails to take into account the suggestions of Joetten as to nomenclature and offers a specific name Lactobacillus vaginae (n. sp.) to a member of this group. This does not seem justified in the light of the present work.

Owing probably to the initial impetus of Döderlein's assertions and the resulting conflict of opinion, practically all of the studies of this bacterium have been on pregnant women. The present study had its

Received for published, March 31, 1928.

1. Verhandl. d. deutsch. Gesellsch. f. Gynäkol., 1892, p. 35.
2. Allgemeine Mikrobiologie, 1910, chapt. 6, p. 97.
3. Ztschr. f. Hyg. u. Infektionskr., 1914, 77, p. 282.
4. Wien. klin. Wchnschr., 1920, 33, p. 730.
5. Archiv. f. Hyg., 1922, 91, p. 143.
6. Ztschr. f. Geburtsh. u. Gynäkol., 1922-3, 85, p. 554.
7. J. Infect. Dis., 1926, 38, p. 333.

inception in an entirely different field of inquiry. In an investigation of the problem of the diagnosis of gonorrhea in women, the author was struck by the fact that where bacteriological findings showed the gonococci in direct vaginal or cervical smears, Döderlein's bacillus was always absent. This observation gave rise to a number of theoretical questions which the present work attempts to answer.

Inasmuch as the literature from 1892 to 1900 abounds in conflicting findings of the bacterial flora of pregnant women it would seem that if there were such an organism as a vaginal bacillus, using the term in the same sense as we use the term the colon bacillus, and which seems to be Döderlein's idea, then the proper field for study would be in children below the age of puberty. For ease in handling the cases and in order to work with a definite age group, children between the ages of 6 and 12 were used exclusively in this study.

The technic used for obtaining smears and cultures was somewhat similar to that described by Harris and Brown [8] except that a modification of the Menge tube was employed. It did not seem that the disadvantages of the tube pointed out by Fricke [9] applied to the type of case under consideration. The swab-tube consists of a small, tightly wound applicator with the cotton end inserted midway into a straight glass tube very slightly drawn out at one end. Both ends of the tube are plugged with cotton and the apparatus inserted into a testtube which in turn is plugged with cotton. The entire outfit is then sterilized.

The following instructions were drawn up and were used as the standard procedure in collecting all vaginal specimens for culture and direct smear.

Technic for Culture and Smear of Vaginal Secretion.—Materials: Tray, green soap, sponges, sterile water, mercuric chloride 1 : 2,000, sterile towels, package of sterile sponges, sterile drapings, and a bag for discarded sponges; and sterile swabs, petri dish plates of whey agar, clean microscopic slides.

Procedure: The nurse will provide all materials except swabs, petri plates and slides, and will screen and drape the patient. Children between 6 and 12 years (both inclusive) will be examined. The operator will scrub his hands thoroughly with green soap and water, paying particular attention to finger nails. Immerse hands in mercuric chloride 1 : 2,000, dry hands on a sterile towel, powder and put on sterile gloves. Sterile drapings will be laid over the other drapings. The labia are separated with the thumb and first finger of the left hand, until the procedure is over. The vaginal introitus is washed with green soap and water (suds) using four sponges with a downward stroke and not using the same

8. Am. J. Obst. & Gynecol., 1926, 11, p. 4.
9. Cited in Williams: Obstetrics, 1924, p. 997.

sponge twice. Follow with sterile water using three sterile sponges, then mercuric chloride using 6 sterile sponges, and then again with sterile water using 4 sterile sponges, always washing from above downward and discarding the sponge at once.

A sterile swab is inserted into the vagina and the vagina is thoroughly swabbed with a circulatory movement. The swab is then removed and immediately spread over two whey agar plates, and then over a slide for the smear. The inoculated plates are placed immediately into a container held in a water bath at 40 C., and transferred as soon as possible to the laboratory where one set was placed directly in the incubator (aerobically) and the other into a vaccum jar and, after drawing a vacuum, into the 37 C. incubator. In the early part of the work pyrogallic acid and sodium hydroxid were placed in the vacuum jar immediately before drawing the vacuum but later this procedure was abandoned. Both sets of plates were incubated for 48 hours. Fishings were made and the organisms isolated were classified.

In all, 107 smears and plate cultures were made from normal vaginas. Subcultures were made from all different colonies on both aerobic and anaerobic plates in the first 50 cases, after that only the organisms resembling Döderlein's bacillus were subcultured. This procedure accounts for the apparent discrepancy between the microscopic and cultural findings.

In most of the cases from which it was isolated Döderlein's bacillus was found growing in the anaerobic plates only, in one case it was found in the aerobic plate only. In 12 cases it was apparent in direct smear but could not be isolated culturally. Although it might appear from the table that there were a large number of organisms present in smears and cultures this was not the case. In 11 cases no organisms were found either in direct smear or culture, in 18 cases the plates were sterile. In practically every case only a few organisms of each kind listed were found. In general the findings agree most closely with those of Williams [10] except that the Döderlein bacillus does not appear in children as frequently as he found it in adults.

For determining the reaction of the vagina a small glass distillation bulb equipped with a rubber bulb and containing about 5 cc. of sterile distilled water was used. The bulb was inserted into the vagina immediately after the withdrawal of the swab tube and the water forced into the vagina with some little pressure. The rubber bulb was then allowed to expand withdrawing the water back into the glass bulb. The reaction of this washing was determined. In every case where Döderlein's bacillus was found the reaction approached P_H 6.0 (5.6 to 6.2). In cases where Döderlein's bacillus was not found the reaction was

10. Am. J. Obst., 1898, 38, pp. 449 and 807.

around P_H 6.8 (6.7 to 6.9). In two cases only, both of vulvovaginitis and not recorded in table 1 (normal vaginas), was the reaction above P_H 7.0 (7.2 to 7.3).

Various mediums were used in the early part of the work for subculturing Döderlein's bacillus. Huntoon's hormone agar, 3% glycerol agar, 0.5% and 1.0% lactose agar, blood agar, whey agar, whey agar fortified with 1% galactose, trypsin digest agar and liquid media of the same compositions without the agar were all tried without any showing a striking advantage. For the routine carrying of the cultures milk and 1% galactose whey were finally decided upon. Both of these media seem to support the growth of the organism equally well and they have the advantage over solid media in not drying readily, an environmental factor to which the organism is very susceptible.

TABLE 1.—MICROSCOPIC AND CULTURAL FINDINGS FOR 107 SPECIMENS FROM NORMAL VAGINAS

	Smears	Cultures
Döderlein's bacillus	20	8*
Staphylococci	96	49
Diphtheroids	78	30
B. coli (group)	91	48
Streptococci	40	20
Sarcina	10	5

* In a preliminary tabulation of the cultures isolated all were referred by notation to the individual cases examined. As such a table would be too cumbersome for the purpose of this paper, the Döderlein strains are simply called D1, D2, D3, etc. in the time order of their isolation.

For the first few transplants the organism grew much better under anaerobic conditions. Now, after carrying them for over a year, they grow very well under slightly lowered oxygen tension, and some strains grow well aerobically. The reaction of the medium within rather large limits does not have much influence on the growth of Döderlein's organism. In taking the same lot of whey, and dividing it into several lots and adjusting the reaction between P_H 4.8 and P_H 7.6 with lactic acid we obtained a good growth of the bacillus in all tubes. Tubes planted with B. coli and Staphylococcus aureus failed to show growth below P_H 5.3. The alkaline point P_H 7.6 was not exceeded in attempting to show the organism's tolerance for alkalinity as this point is well above that met with in any vaginal reaction.

The power of acid production and the rate of acid production of the organism varies slightly with different strains. Table 2 shows the average end points of acid production in various lots of whey, milk and trysin digest, bouillon, all fortified with the same amount (1%) of lactose.

There seems to be some relationship between the morphology of the cell and the colony formation. Both of these characteristics show a decided tendency to change, even when subcultured into the same medium. Upon original isolation three different morphological types were recorded. Three of our strains were slender rods 0.5μ in diameter and from 3 to 6μ in length, occasionally appearing in short chains of three to six members. Three strains were of about the same shape and size as those above but they showed a rather noticeable palisade formation. Two of our strains were heavy rods, 0.7 to 1μ in diameter and 10 to 15μ in length. They formed long filaments. All

TABLE 2.—ACID PRODUCTION BY DÖDERLEIN'S BACILLUS (D), LACTOBACILLUS ACIDOPHILUS (A) AND BULGARICUS (B)

Medium	Organisms	P_H
Milk	D 1, 2, 4, and 5; A 1 and 2; B 1 and 2	3.5
	D 7	3.6
	D 6	3.7
	D 3	3.9
	D 8	5.5
Whey	D 1, 2, and 6	3.5
	D 3; A 1 and 2	3.8
	D 4, 5, and 7; B 1	3.9
	B 2	4.3
	D 8	5.4
Trypsin	D 7	3.8
	D 1, 2, 3, 4, and 5	3.9
	A 1	4.0
	B 2	4.1
	D 8; B 1	5.0

D 1, D 2, etc. indicate the eight different strains of Döderlein's bacillus isolated, B 1 and B 2 are two strains of Lactobacillus bulgaricus, and A 1 and A 2 are two strains of Lactobacillus acidophilus used as controls in this experiment.

strains were uniformly gram-positive with square ends. All were nonmotile and nonspore-forming.

The colonies on the first plates also divided themselves into three groups. The first was smooth, circular, convex, entire, amorphous and translucent. The second was rough, rhizoid, contoured, flat, and lacerate, resembling a typical Bulgaricus colony but not as irregular. The third type was something in between the two. Six of our colonies were of the first group and one of each the latter two. With the exception of one organism, D2, every one of these strains has changed during the past eighteen months both in cell morphology and in colony formation. An exhaustive study of these changes, with camera lucida drawings and photomicrographs of colonies and colony impressions has been made and is still in progress. Space, however, forbids a further record of our findings here.

As to temperature requirements all strains grow best at 37.5 C. or slightly higher. Below 35 C. there is practically no growth, and none of the strains grow at all at 20 C.

All of our strains are facultative anaerobes. All grow better in a partial (10%) carbon dioxide atmosphere, or in an atmosphere in which the oxygen is further diluted with nitrogen gas. When air instead of CO_2 or N_2 was bubbled through a liquid substratum no better growths were obtained, indicating that an excess of moisture could not account for the increased growth in the presence of these gases.

Good growth was obtained with every strain of Doderlein's bacillus when the surface tension was reduced to 40 dynes, using sodium ricinoleate as a depressant. Controls with Lactobacillus acidophilus grew in the same depressed medium while controls with Lactobacillus bulgaricus did not. None of our strains produced any growth on potato, none produced indol from a tryptophane broth, and all reduced nitrates to nitrites.

In sugar fermentations different strains of Döderlein's bacillus acted differently. The medium used was Huntoon's hormone broth fermented for 48 hours with B. coli. To this sugar-free broth was added 1% of the different carbohydrates. Table 2 shows our results, with cultures of Lactobacillus acidophilus and Lactobacillus bulgaricus as controls. The strains D6, D8, do not always ferment maltose equally well, at times producing only a slight acidity. D1 at times does not ferment sucrose, D4 ferments sucrose usually but not always. D6 is variable on mannitol. D1, D3, D4, sometimes ferment levulose very slightly. None of the strains produces gas in any of the carbohydrate media. In the ability to ferment maltose all of our Döderlein strains correspond to the classical description of Lactobacillus acidophilus. Two of our strains, however, while producing acid from this sugar only form a slight amount at times. The other irregularities noted seem to signify that Döderlein's bacillus forms a heterogeneous group in fermenting powers, not falling into Rahe's groups with any constancy.

In milk some differences have occurred in the type of coagulum but these have not been constant with any strains and may depend on the rate of acid production formed, that is, in overcoming the lag. As a rule the coagulum was soft.

Strains of Döderlein's bacillus were inoculated into rabbits for cross agglutination studies. Strains of Lactobacillus acidophilus and Lactobacillus bulgaricus were used as controls. Table 4 summarizes the results obtained. The serums agglutinated their homologous antigens in every case at a dilution of 1 : 5000 or over. Bulgaricus serum did not agglutinate any of the other antigens and none of the other serums agglutinated L. bulgaricus antigen. The group agglutinins ran to approximately 1 : 160. This point was taken as the group agglutination point. The plus (+) and zero (0) signs in the table indicate whether or not agglutination took place above that dilution. It will be noted that there is no grouping of strains possible by the agglutination test. This fact was borne out by agglutinin absorption tests.

Every strain of our Döderlein's bacillus has been reisolated from feces of human beings after feeding. Organisms for this purpose were fed in a 48-hour incubated milk (1 pint) culture. Approximately two ounces of lactose were added to each bottle of milk just before using.

TABLE 3.—FERMENTATION REACTION WITH DÖDERLEIN'S BACILLUS, LACTOBACILLUS ACIDOPHILUS AND BULGARICUS

Organism	Monosaccharides						Disaccharides			Trisaccharides	Polysaccharides	Alcohols	
	Dextrose	Levulose	Galactose	Xylose	Arabinose	Mannose	Maltose	Lactose	Ducrose	Raffinose	Inulin, Dextrin, Salicin (glucoside)	Mannitol	Dulcitol
D 1	+	0	+	0	0	+	+	+	+	+	0	+	0
D 2	+	+	+	0	0	+	+	+	0	0	0	+	0
D 3	+	0	+	0	0	+	+	+	+	0	0	0	0
D 4	+	0	+	0	0	+	+	+	+	0	0	0	0
D 5	+	+	+	0	0	+	+	+	0	0	0	0	0
D 6	+	+	+	0	+	+	+	+	0	0	0	+	+
D 7	+	+	+	0	0	+	+	+	0	0	0	0	0
D 8	+	+	+	0	0	+	+	+	+	0	0	0	0
A 1	+	+	+	0	0	+	+	+	+	0	0	+	0
A 2	+	+	+	0	0	0	+	+	0	0	0	0	0
B 1	+	+	+	0	0	+	0	+	+	+	0	+	0
B 2	+	+	+	0	0	+	0	+	+	0	0	+	0

From the morphologic, cultural and physiologic characteristics of Döderlein's bacillus there is no doubt but that we are dealing with Lactobacillus acidophilus. However, we are convinced that the name Lactobacillus acidophilus either characterizes a group of related species or that, if it is a single biologic species, this species undergoes transformations, maybe "dissociations" which are in truth remarkable. In every mark which recent workers have distinguished Lactobacillus acidophilus from Lactobacillus bulgaricus this organism agrees with the former. Until, therefore, we know more about Lactobacillus acidophilus no new specific names for the vaginal bacillus are justified.

Assuming then that Döderlein's bacillus is Lactobacillus acidophilus, the question naturally arises, "How does Lactobacillus acidophilus get into the human vagina?" Theoretically the answer seems to lie with its bacterial associates in the vagina. B. coli, diphtheroids and staphylococci are usually present in the vagina. Staphylococci are present on all surfaces of the body but B. coli and the diphtheroids are normal inhabitants of the extremely close body orifice—the rectum. By pure deduction therefore it would seem that Lactobacillus acidophilus gets into the vagina from the intestinal tract.

Two experiments were carried out to sustain this thesis. One was to examine the fecal contents of individuals showing the organism in the vagina, and the other to attempt to plant Lactobacillus acidophilus in the vagina by way of the digestive tract. Out of six cases examined in which this organism was found by smear to be in the vagina, the organism appeared in direct fecal smear in five. In one case the organism was found in the vagina but not in the feces. Two

TABLE 4.—CROSS AGGLUTINATIONS WITH SPECIFIC DÖDERLEIN'S BACILLUS ANTISERUMS AND ANTIGENS

Anti-	Antigens									
serums	D 1	D 2	D 3	D 4	D 5	D 6	D 7	D 8	A 1	B 1
D 1	+	+	0	+	+	0	+	+	+	0
D 2	+	+	0	+	+	0	+	+	0	0
O 3	0	0	+	0	+	0	+	+	+	0
D 4	+	+	0	+	+	+	0	0	0	0
D 5	+	+	+	+	+	0	0	0	+	0
D 6	0	0	0	+	0	+	0	0	+	0
D 7	+	+	+	0	0	0	+	+	+	0
D 8	+	+	+	0	0	0	+	+	+	0
A 1	+	0	+	0	+	+	+	+	+	0
B 1	0	0	0	0	0	0	0	0	0	+

children who did not show Lactobacillus acidophilus in their feces or vagina were fed the organism strain D1 in milk. In both of these cases the organism was reisolated from the feces and from the vagina. Acidophilus feeding was stopped and examinations continued. In one case the organism disappeared from the feces within two weeks and from the vagina within three weeks. In the other case the organism persisted in the feces and in the vagina for more than three months. It then disappeared from the feces but remained in the vagina for at least three months longer when the case was lost to us.

This brings up the question of what the organism lives on in the vagina and from what it produces its acid. There are two possibilities. First that unfermented fecal matter is mechanically transferred from the anus to the vagina in sufficient amount for it to maintain its existence, and second that it finds a nutrient material in the vagina. The first of these alternatives is hard to eliminate. Extracts of normal feces contained fermentable substances. Meconium extracts did not. On the other hand, normal sterilized vaginal washings had material which was fermentable by all of our strains isolated and artificially purified mucus from the mouth was fermentable. Even when no acidophilus is found in the vagina the vaginal washings are slightly acid which seems to indicate that there is a secretion in this organ not wholly derived from the cervix as the secretions from the racemous glands in the cervix are alkaline. It would seem that the vaginal fluid is serous in character and contains a fermentable mucin.

A study of the intestinal contents of children from birth showed the change in flora follows that described by Tissier.[11] The meconium is sterile. On the second day gram-positive rods appear which prove to be B. bifidus. This organism continues dominant in breast fed children for from one to four weeks. Other organisms such as the enterococcus appear soon and in the case of bottle fed babies, Lactobacillus acidophilus. B. coli gradually appears in all cases but remains in the minority. As far as we could determine the changes in the early intestinal flora have no effect on the vaginal flora. In no case did we find Lactobacillus in vaginal smears from the thirteen infants whose intestinal flora we studied.

Having studied the morphologic, physiologic and cultural characters of Döderlein's bacillus and classified it as Lactobacillus acidophilus, having attempted to find out its relative incidence in the human vagina, its source and mode of entrance and on what it lives and produces acid in the vagina, we again returned to our original question, "What is the significance of this organism in gonorrheal infections?" The adult vagina is so exposed to external conditions it seemed that the problem could best be attacked with the study of vulvovaginitis in children. Unfortunately we have not had sufficient cases to form any decided opinions. The two cases which we have studied, however, seem highly significant.

Case 1.—A child of 8 years, suffering with acute vulvovaginitis, had come into the hospital about six months previously and had a gonococcic vaginitis at that time. This case was chronic and had not responded to treatment. At the time we first took over the case the condition had become acute with a marked discharge in which the gonococci were very numerous. All treatment was suspended for one week and then the vagina was flushed thoroughly with a culture of Lactobacillus acidophilus (strain D1) daily. This was the only treatment given. For two weeks the reaction of the vagina before flushing with the culture remained alkaline (PH 7.3) although smears showed the absence of the gonococci in 48 hours. At the end of 96 hours after the first flushing pus cells disappeared. Treatment was stopped after three weeks with a vaginal reaction PH 6.6. This case has been under observation for more than a year and weekly vaginal smears have not shown any gonococci. Once or twice pus cells have been noted but no laboratory or clinical signs of the vulvovaginitis have reappeared.

11. Recherches sur la flore intestinale normale et pathologique dus nourrisons, 1900, p. 85.

Case 2.—A child, three years of age, brought into the hospital, showed gonococci in vaginal smear. Vaginal flushings were made with a culture of Lactobacillus acidophilus (strain D1). Forty-eight hours later no gonococci were present in smears and only a few pus cells. The latter disappeared completely in five days. The child was taken home on the tenth day and no subsequent record was obtainable.

From the results of only two cases no definite statements as to the efficacy of this treatment are warranted. In the light of the fact that Lactobacillus acidophilus was not found in any case of gonorrhea in the female, and that the acid produced by this organism is decidedly detrimental to the growth of the gonococcus, the results are significant.

Laboratory cultures of the gonococcus on blood whey agar are killed within 18 hours when a whey broth culture of Lactobacillus acidophilus is spread thinly over them.

CONCLUSIONS

Döderlein's vaginal bacillus is Lactobacillus acidophilus. This organism is present in less than 10% of normal vaginas of children. It gets into the vagina by exterior passage from the intestinal tract, and can be introduced into the vagina by feeding a culture by mouth. It lives and develops acid either from a secretion of the vagina or in conveyed fermentable intestinal material or both. The organism is not present in the vagina in cases of gonococcal vaginitis. The organism has an inhibiting effect on the growth of the gonococcus in vitro, and Lactobacillus acidophilus vaginal implantation may present a rational cure for gonococcal vulvovaginitis and other gonococcal infections.

METHOD OF STAINING FLAGELLA

EMIL WEISS

From the Department of Bacteriology, Pathology and Preventive Medicine, Loyola University School of Medicine, Chicago

The need of a simple and reliable technic for staining flagella has prompted the following studies for obtaining smears with uninjured flagella, and for finding effective and stable mordants and contrasting stains.

Preparation of Slide.—A drop of bacterial suspension allowed to dry without spreading on the slide was found preferable to smears made in the usual way with the loop or by spreading with a slide as in making blood smears. Both of these methods tend to injure the flagella or leave them stretched along the bacterial bodies which have been dragged in the direction of the smearing. The use of chemicals to fix flagella in their natural positions as advised by some bacteriologists is also of use only with this undisturbed drop method. Too heavy a growth should not be used: heavy broth cultures should be diluted with distilled water, and to growth on agar slants 5 to 10 cc. of distilled water should be added and the tube shaken until suspension is sufficiently opalescent. The addition of acetic acid to the cultures (q. s. ad 50%) and a subsequent incubation at 37 C. in water bath for fifteen minutes is very satisfactory. Fluid cultures in medium containing serum or ascitic fluid should not be used for the demonstration of flagella, due to the fact that these proteins in the fixed slide take the stain as heavily as the flagella. The slides were cleaned by keeping them for a week in a 6% solution of commercial sulphuric acid mixed with equal parts of a 6% solution of potassium or sodium bichromate.

Mordants.—Tannic acid is used in almost every mordant described. It is soluble in water as high at 20%, but does not keep very well in a watery solution except in the presence of a disinfectant. Tannic acid in formalin (40% formaldehyde) affords a simple mordant which is stable, does not form a precipitate on standing, and is both a fixative and a disinfectant. The mordant consists of two solutions: solution A containing 100 grams of tannic acid in 100 cc. of 95% alcohol, and solution B containing 7.5 cc. of glacial acetic acid in 100 cc. of undiluted commercial formalin (40% formaldehyde). Both solutions keep

Received for publication, March 20, 1928.

indefinitely. Before use one part of solution A is mixed with two parts of solution B. This mixture also remains unchanged for several months.

Stains.—The use of a basic dye followed by a washing in water and a contrast staining with an acid dye was found effective.

The basic dyes used were: saturated solution of gentian violet in formalin, saturated solution of crystal violet in formalin, 5% alcoholic solution of brilliant green, 1% aqueous solution of malachite green, 1% aqueous solution of thionin blue, Loeffler's methylene blue, carbolfuchsin, 1% aqueous solution of safranin and pyronin. The demonstration of flagella with basic dyes is based on overstaining. The best basic dyes for that purpose are gentian violet and crystal violet. A saturated solution of gentian or crystal violet in formalin keeps very well and shows up the flagella better than any other basic dye. This stain is prepared as follows: 5 grams of gentian or crystal violet are added to 100 cc. of formalin, shaken, heated slightly over the flame, allowed to stand for a week at room temperature and then filtered.

This stain can also be used for other purposes, such as the Gram stain, and a capsule stain. The slides are either covered for 5 to 10 minutes with this stain or steamed for 2 to 5 minutes. In both instances the bacilli appear dark violet, almost black, the flagella slightly paler, bluish violet. In combination with the above stable mordant silver salts can be successfully used for the demonstration of flagella. By using only basic dyes the flagella appear less heavily stained than the bacterial bodies. This disadvantage was corrected by additional staining with a contrastive acid dye.

Several acid stains were used: eosin, acid fuchsin, acid blue-black, acid blue, azo-blue, acid violet and acid green. Eosin in 1% alcoholic or watery solution was absolutely useless. The other acid stains were dissolved in a concentration of 10% in diluted alcohol (two parts of distilled water and one part of 95% alcohol). A higher concentration of alcohol was not used, to avoid decolorization of basic stains, which were first applied in the staining procedure. These solutions of acid dyes kept very well. Watery solutions of the above acid dyes were less effective.

The results of the use of basic and acid dyes for the contrastive staining of bacterial bodies and flagella are as follows: gentian and crystal violet gave a very pronounced contrast-staining in combination with acid green; the contrast was less marked if acid fuchsin was used instead of acid green. Methylene and thionin blue gave good results in combination with acid fuchsin. Malachite and brilliant green were very successfully contrasted with acid fuchsin and acid violet; malachite green was less useful than brilliant green. Safranin, pyronin and carbol fuchsin gave satisfactory results with acid green or acid blue; carbolfuchsin was more effective than safranin and pyronin. The slides were more easily overstained with the acid dyes than with the basic dyes. If the slides were overstained with the basic dye, the acid stain would show up only slightly; if the slides were overstained with the acid stain, the basic dye would disappear entirely. The best results among the basic dyes were obtained with gentian and crystal violet, methylene and thionin blue, brilliant green and basic fuchsin. Among the acid dyes acid fuchsin, acid green and acid violet gave the most satisfactory results; acid blue, azo blue and aniline blue black were less useful. The results were less satisfactory if the acid stain was applied before the basic stain. Attempts were also made to prepare solutions containing both the basic and the acid dyes and in this manner stain simultaneously with both dyes; the results were not very encouraging.

In using contrastive stains for the demonstration of flagella, it was observed, that some individual bacteria are not stained with the basic stain, as expected, but take the acid stain. These irregularities in staining are not caused by errors in staining. These bacteria differ morphologically from the rest of the bacteria from the same culture. The possibility of contamination was eliminated by appropriate culture controls. These same bacteria if stained only with the basic dyes, appeared very pale. The morphological irregularities of these bacteria show a great resemblance to the degeneration and involution forms characteristic for the respective bacterial stain.

DISCUSSION

A new method is described for staining of flagella with the following procedure:

To an 18-hour broth culture glacial acetic acid is added (q. s. ad 5%). The culture tube is then kept in water-bath at 37 C. for 15 minutes. A drop is transferred with a loop from the culture to the slide and allowed to dry. The slide is then covered with the recommended mordant and steamed for 2-5 minutes. The slide is then washed with warm water for 1 to 2 minutes and covered with the basic stain. If the concentration of the basic stain is not higher than 1%, the slides are covered with it for 4 to 6 minutes or steamed for 2 to 3 minutes; if the concentration of the basic stain is higher than 1%, the slides are covered with it for 1 to 2 minutes. The slides are washed with water and covered with the solution of the acid dye for 10 minutes. The slides are then washed and dried.

The analysis of various mordants [1] shows, that tannic acid is the most effective constituent of all the chemicals used for that purpose. Gallic

1. Kolle, W., and Wassermann, A. (Friedberger u. Reiter): Handb. d. Path. Mikroorg., 1912, 1, p. 293; Ford, W. W.: Textbook of Bacteriology, 1927, p. 62.

acid is equally useful but keeps well only in an alcoholic solution. The other chemicals used in the various mordants are only slightly effective and their omission from the mordants does not decrease essentially the value of the mordant. The usefulness of glacial acetic acid for the preparatory treatment of bacterial cultures and as a constituent of the above mordant is demonstrated. The combination of a basic and an acid dye for the contrast staining of bacterial bodies and flagella has two distinct advantages over the simple use of a basic dye: the flagella appear plainer being stained with a different dye than the bacterial bodies; and normal and degenerated bacteria can easily be differentiated. The bacterial bodies take the basic dye, the flagella the acid dye. Some bacteriologists claim that the bacteria possess in their cytoplasm diffusely spread nuclei with the same affinity for basic dyes as the nuclei in tissue cells. The nuclei of degenerated tissue cells take the basic dye only slightly and the nuclei of necrotic cells cannot be differentiated from the cytoplasm by means of basic dyes. Similarly the affinity of irregularly shaped bacteria for the acid dyes is most likely based on degenerative changes of the nucleinic substances. These irregular forms are probably identical with the "so-called" degeneration and involution forms of bacteria. The above contrastive stains give very satisfactory results, when used for the demonstration of phagocytosed bacteria.

SUMMARY

A new method of staining flagella includes the treatment of young cultures with acetic acid (q. s. ad 5%) ; a drop of this suspension on slide allowed to dry untouched; and staining first with a basic dye and then with an acid dye. Useful contrastive stains were saturated gentian or crystal violet and acid green; Loeffler's methylene blue or aqueous thionin blue and acid fuchsin; brilliant green and acid fuchsin or acid violet; and carbol fuchsin and acid green. This method is also useful for the demonstration of degenerated or phagocytosed bacteria.

STUDIES ON THE METABOLISM OF THE ABORTUS-MELITENSIS GROUP

4. EFFECT OF VARIOUS CONCENTRATIONS OF CARBON DIOXIDE

James G. McAlpine and Charles A. Slanetz

From the Department of Animal Diseases, Storrs Agricultural Experiment Station, Storrs, Connecticut

The relation of Bact. abortus (bovine) to carbon dioxide has been the subject of several scientific investigations. During a study of the nitrogen metabolism of the abortus-melitensis group we[1] found that the members of this group do not all react in the same manner to various carbon dioxide concentrations. This paper is a continuation of those observations.

There are numerous references in the literature to the peculiar gaseous requirements of Bact. abortus (bovine). Bang[2] was able to isolate Bact. abortus from the uterus of a cow showing impending abortion, by supplying a modified gaseous environment for the culture. No multiplication of the organism took place under ordinary atmospheric conditions. By using deep tubes of serum-agar-gelatin they obtained growth in a zone 1.5 cm. below the surface of the medium, while the surface layer and the depth of the medium remained unchanged. Preisz[3] found that he could grow Bact. abortus on ordinary agar slants if oxygen was passed into the tubes and they were then sealed with wax. Nowak[4] proved that Bact. abortus can be grown on Petri dishes if they are enclosed in jars along with cultures of Bact. subtilis. In this way, he claimed, the oxygen tension was reduced. By the gradual reduction of the amount of Bact. subtilis growth on subsequent transfers, he showed that Bact. abortus can be acclimated to ordinary aerobic conditions. MacFadyean and Stockman[5] stated that different strains of Bact. abortus vary widely in their cultural characteristics and that the zone formation of Bang is not specific for Bact. abortus; they had obtained the same result with a strain of Mycobacterium tuberculosis isolated from the uterus. In their opinion the Bang bacillus was a strict aerobe. Zwick[6] also reported these variations in cultural characteristics, and cited one case in which growth was obtained under aerobic conditions directly from the animal body. Holth[7] used high oxygen tension over sugar-free agar for initial isolations. He also obtained excellent growths of

Received for publication, March 1, 1928.

1. J. Infect. Dis., 1928, 42, p. 66.
2. Ztschr. f. Thier. Med. 1897, 1, p. 241.
3. Centralbl. f. Bakt., 1. O., 1903, 33, p. 190.
4. Ann. de l'Inst. Pasteur, 1908, 22, p. 541.
5. Epizoötic abortion in cattle. Rpt. of Comm. appointed by Board of Agric. and Fisheries to inquire into epizoötic abortion, Appendix 1, 1909.
6. Centralbl. f. Bakt., 1 ref., 1910, 47, p. 219.
7. Ztschr. f. Infektionskr., parisit., Krank. u. Hyg. der Haustiere, 1911, 10, pp. 206 and 342.

the organism on slanted serum agar by merely sealing the cotton plugs with paraffin.

Smith and Fabyan[8] used Nowak's method of cultivation, with slight modifications. They stressed the importance of the correct amount of inoculated Bact. subtilis surface, since too much was found to inhibit the growth of Bact. abortus. Equally good results were obtained by using Bact. coli, Bact. megatherium, a staphylococcus, and a bacillus of guinea-pig pneumonia, for reducing oxygen tension. Various strains of Bact. abortus were found to have different growth requirements, but plain meat infusion agar and the simple sealing of tubes with wax gave good results.

Zwick and Wedemann[9] showed that the organism refused to proliferate under anaerobic conditions, and in an atmosphere of pure oxygen or nitrogen, but that it was not killed under either of these conditions. They compared the behavior of a strain which had been trained to grow aerobically with that of a typical newly isolated strain. Under five atmospheres pressure the aerobe remained unchanged, but the "microaerophile" grew deeper in the medium; under five atmospheres of oxygen the aerobic strain formed its colonies beneath the surface and the typical growths appeared still deeper in the agar. From these experiments they concluded that typical Bact. abortus strains have undergone "habitat" variations induced by the high oxygen tension in the uterus.

Huddleson[10] improved the method for the isolation of Bact. abortus from milk, The inoculated medium was placed in closed jars in which 10% of the air was displaced by carbon dioxide. In a later paper[11] he showed that it is not the reduced oxygen tension which facilitates the growth of Bact. abortus, but the increased amount of carbon dioxide. By inoculating tubes of sterile buffer solution connected by means of rubber tubing with freshly planted agar slants of Bact. subtilis, the original P_H of 7.0 was reduced to 6.5 in 48 hours. An increase in the amount of carbon dioxide was also demonstrated. Excellent results were obtained by growing newly isolated strains of Bact. abortus in an atmosphere containing 10% carbon dioxide. Meyer and Shaw[12] stated that the peculiar carbon dioxide requirements of Bact. abortus can be observed only in the strains which are isolated from the uterus. Smith[13] reported that freshly isolated strains of Bact. abortus yielded better growth under carbon dioxide than under ordinary aerobic conditions. It was impossible to initiate growth in certain strains in the open culture tube. When the carbon dioxide was removed by sodium hydroxide, growth was completely inhibited in freshly isolated strains and retarded in old cultures. He showed that the organism would tolerate 100% carbon dioxide, though there was some retardation of growth. With certain strains growth appeared in 11 days in tubes under carbon dioxide, but there was no indication of development in the tubes which were held under ordinary atmospheric conditions. He suggested that Bact. abortus (Bang) is perhaps the only pathogenic organism which possesses such a carbon dioxide relationship. In a later paper Smith[14] stated that by this

8. Centralbl. f. Bakt. 1, O., 1912, 61, p. 549.
9. Arb. a. d. kaiserl. Gesundheitsamte, 1913, 43, p. 130.
10. Michigan Agric. College Exper. Sta. Tech. Bull. 49, 1920.
11. Cornell Veterinarian, 1921, 11, p. 210.
12. J. Infect. Dis., 1920, 27, p. 173.
13. J. Exper. Med., 1924, 40, p. 219.
14. Ibid., 1926, 43, p. 317.

peculiar relationship to carbon dioxide it may be possible to differentiate the Bact. abortus strains into the bovine type on the one hand, and the so-called vaccinal or persistent udder strains on the other. Valley and Rettger [15] demonstrated that the growth of Bact. abortus (bovine) can be completely inhibited by the removal of all the carbon dioxide in the surrounding air.

In the literature on Bact. melitensis no mention is made of these peculiar gas requirements. Bruce [16] was able to isolate Bact. melitensis by inoculating spleen tissue from a fatal case on nutrient agar; he made no statement regarding alteration under ordinary aerobic conditions. Horrocks, Zammitt and Kennedy [17] and Shaw [18] isolated the organism from infected milk by plating the milk sediment on litmus-nutrose-agar plates.

TABLE 1.—HISTORY OF BACT. ABORTUS-MELITENSIS STRAINS

Strain	Source	Date	Place	From Whom Obtained
			BOVINE STRAINS	
66	Aborted fetus	Jan., 1925	Storrs, Conn.	Isolated by present authors
57	Milk	?	California ?	Univ. Calif., Davis, Calif.
68	?	?	California ?	Univ. Calif., Davis, Calif.
69	?	?	New York	C. M. Carpenter, Cornell Univ., Ithaca, N. Y.
			PORCINE STRAINS	
70	?	?	Iowa ?	P. R. Edwards, Agric. Exper. Sta., Lexington, Ky. Original from Ames, Iowa
71	Aborted fetus	?	New York	C. M. Carpenter, Cornell Univ., Ithaca, N. Y.
			HUMAN STRAINS	
72	Blood	June, 1926	Michigan	M. Crooks, Mich. Dept. of Health, Lansing, Mich.
73	Blood	June, 1927	Michigan	M. Crooks, Mich. Dept. of Health, Lansing, Mich.
74	Blood	?	New York	C. M. Carpenter, Cornell Univ., N. Y.
75	Blood	?	New York	C. M. Carpenter, Cornell Univ., N. Y.
76	Blood	?	New York	C. M. Carpenter, Cornell Univ., N. Y.
77	Blood	?	New York	C. M. Carpenter, Cornell Univ., N. Y.
78	Tonsil	?	New York	C. M. Carpenter, Cornell Univ., N. Y.
79	Blood	?	New York	C. M. Carpenter, Cornell Univ., N. Y.
80	Tonsil	?	New York	C. M. Carpenter, Cornell Univ., N. Y.
81	Blood	?	New York	C. M. Carpenter, Cornell Univ., N. Y.
82	Human fetus	?	New York	C. M. Carpenter, Cornell Univ., N. Y.
83	Blood	?	New York	C. M. Carpenter, Cornell Univ., N. Y.
84	Blood	?	New York	C. M. Carpenter, Cornell Univ., N. Y.
85	Blood	?	New York	C. M. Carpenter, Cornell Univ., N. Y.
86	Blood	?	New York	C. M. Carpenter, Cornell Univ., N. Y.
87	Blood	?	New York	C. M. Carpenter, Cornell Univ., N. Y.
88	Blood	?	Virginia	F. W. Shaw, Medical College of Virginia, Richmond, Va.
			MELITENSIS STRAINS	
89	Milk	May, 1923	Malta	Alice C. Evans, Hyg. Lab. Washington, D. C. Original from Pub. Health Dept., Malta

The strains of Bact. abortus obtained from porcine sources act more like those of Bact. melitensis. Good and Smith [19] isolated a strain from a case of swine abortion, using Nowak's method. Subcultures, however, developed immediately under atmospheric conditions. Doyle and Spray [20] obtained growth from guinea-pigs inoculated with placental material from an aborting sow. It may be assumed

15. J. Bact., 1927, 14, p. 101.
16. Practitioner, 1887, 39, p. 161.
17. Rpts. Comm. appointed by Admirality, War Off. and Civil Gov't of Malta for Investigation of Mediterranean Fever, 1905, pt. 3, p. 84-94.
18. Rpts. Comm. appointed by Admirality, War Office and Civil Gov't of Malta for Investigation of Mediterranean Fever, 1906, pt. 4, p. 16-26.
19. J. Bact., 1916, 1, p. 415.
20. J. Infect. Dis., 1920, 27, p. 165.

that normal atmospheric conditions were employed since no mention is made to the contrary.

Buck[21] made a comparative study of Bact. melitensis and Bact. abortus. He concluded that primary isolations of Bact. melitensis "develop with equal if not greater rapidity in a normal atmosphere than in one partially displaced by carbon dioxide gas. This characteristic permits the differentiation of Bacterium melitensis and Bact. abortus (bovine) in primary isolations." He found that artificially cultivated strains were not so exacting in their gas requirements when passed again through animals.

Source of Strains.—All the strains which were used in the nitrogen and glucose studies were used in this investigation, and others were added. There were 21 strains of Bact. abortus of bovine, 19 of porcine, and 28 of human origin, and 21 of Bact. melitensis. In table 1 are given the histories and sources of the organisms which have not been used and described previously.

Methods.—All strains were grown on Fairchild peptone agar slants for 24 hours. A small amount of the growth was suspended in sterile salt solution and 0.1 cc. of this added to 12 cc. of Fairchild peptone agar in large potato tubes. After thorough mixing these were poured into Petri dishes. A little experience was necessary before the proper suspension could be made. Eighteen plates were poured with each strain.

After hardening, three plates of each strain were placed under the various gaseous environments. One set was incubated under ordinary air conditions and four sets were placed in sealed bell jars provided with inlet and outlet tubes which could be hermetically sealed. The capacity of the bell jars averaged 2,000 cc. In one set the gaseous environment was left unchanged, and the jar tightly sealed; in the second, 10% by volume of the air was displaced by carbon dioxide; in the third 20% was displaced; in the fourth 30%, and in the fifth, 40%. Certain strains were found to be totally inhibited by 10% carbon dioxide; a second plating was made in which one set of plates was enclosed in a jar from which 5% of the air by volume was displaced with carbon dioxide. The carbon dioxide was allowed to flow in at the bottom of the bell jar and the displaced air to flow out at the top. When sufficient carbon dioxide had entered the jars, the outlet and inlet tubes were tightly sealed, and the jars incubated at 37°C. for three days. Results were recorded on the 1 +, 2 +, etc., scale, both the number of colonies and their size being considered.

In one set of experiments the effect of total exclusion of carbon dioxide was tried. Here the method of Valley and Rettger[15] was used. Broth tubes were substituted for the agar plates. After sterilization the broth was placed in bell jars which contained $Ca(OH)_2$ (moistened). When cool, they were incubated and returned to tightly sealed jars in the presence of $Ca(OH)_2$. These bell jars were then evacuated and refilled with carbon dioxide free air. Incubation was for five days at 37°C.

Effect of Different Concentrations of CO_2 with Plate Cultures.—In table 2 are given the results of different concentrations of CO_2 on all

21. J. Agric. Res., 1924, 29, p. 585.

of the strains employed in this study. The strains are arranged according to source, as was done in our previous reports. It will be noticed that, on the whole, the strains in each of the two main groups acted similarly toward the gas. The bovine cultures, with the exception of

Table 2.—Effect of Various Concentrations of Carbon Dioxide

Strains	Concentrations of CO_2					
Bovine	Air	Jar	10	20	30	40%
1	4*	5	5	2	2	0
2	6	8	9	8	2	0
3	5	6	6	3	2	0
4	8	9	0	0	0	0
5	5	6	7	5	1	contaminated
6	4	5	6	2	1	0
7	7	8	9	4	1	0
8	6	7	8	8	0	0
9	6	8	9	9	1	0
10	1	3	6	2	4	0
42	6	6	6	4	0	0
43	5	6	7	5	1	0
44	1	2	1	1	0	0
45	5	6	6	5	1	1
46	4	5	1	0	0	0
47	2	3	1	1	0	0
48	4	1	0	0	0	0
66	6	7	8	4	1	0
67	9	9	0	0	0	0
68	6	6	1	1	1	0
69	8	8	0	0	0	0
Porcine						
11	6	0	0	0	0	0
12	9	6	0	0	0	0
13	8	6	0	0	0	0
14	6	6	1	0	0	0
15	8	8	6	0	0	0
16	6	5	2	0	0	0
17	8	4	0	0	0	0
18	2	1	0	0	0	0
19	9	9	4	0	0	0
20	9	8	0	0	0	0
49	6	6	1	0	0	0
50	6	5	1	0	0	0
51	8	8	0	0	0	0
52	9	8	0	0	0	0
53	10	6	0	0	0	0
54	2	1	0	0	0	0
55	9	7	0	0	0	0
70	8	8	0	0	0	0
71	9	8	0	0	0	0

Strains	Concentrations of CO_2					
Human	Air	Jar	10	20	30	40%
21	9*	9	2	0	0	0
22	9	8	0	0	0	0
23	9	8	4	0	0	0
24	8	8	0	0	0	0
25	8	0	0	0	0	0
26	8	7	1	0	0	0
27	6	6	0	0	0	0
28	6	4	0	0	0	0
29	3	3	0	0	0	0
30	9	9	1	0	0	0
56	9	9	1	0	0	0
72	8	7	0	0	0	0
73	8	8	0	0	0	0
74	9	7	0	0	0	0
75	9	9	4	0	0	0
76	8	4	0	0	0	0
77	9	8	0	0	0	0
78	9	9	0	0	0	0
79	2	2	1	0	0	0
80	10	10	0	0	0	0
81	9	8	3	1	0	0
82	2	2	0	0	0	0
83	9	9	0	0	0	0
84	9	9	0	0	0	0
85	4	4	0	0	0	0
86	8	7	3	1	1	0
87	8	8	3	2	0	0
88	8	7	2	2	3	0
Melitensis						
31	8	4	0	0	0	0
32	6	6	0	0	0	0
33	3	3	0	0	0	0
34	8	8	0	0	0	0
35	2	2	1	0	0	0
36	5	4	0	0	0	0
37	6	6	5	0	0	0
38	9	8	2	0	0	0
39	10	8	0	0	0	0
40	6	6	1	0	0	0
41	4	3	1	0	0	0
57	9	8	0	0	0	0
58	8	6	0	0	0	0
59	9	8	0	0	0	0
60	2	1	0	0	0	0
61	1	1	0	0	0	0
62	2	2	0	0	0	0
63	6	5	0	0	0	0
64	3	3	0	0	0	0
65	1	1	0	0	0	0
89	5	4	0	0	0	0

* Figures indicate relative number and size of colonies.

strains 48, 67 and 69, were stimulated by the addition of 10% carbon dioxide, and in most instances tolerated 20%, and at times even 30% of the gas. More luxuriant growths took place within the sealed jars than under ordinary aerobic conditions. On the other hand, the porcine and human abortus, and the Bact. melitensis strains were markedly inhibited by the addition of 10% carbon dioxide. Frequently, the plates in the jars showed fewer and smaller colonies than those incubated in the air.

In chart 1 two typical strains from each of the four sources are given. The stimulatory effect of low concentrations of carbon dioxide on the bovine strains is well marked in these graphs. The sealed jars aid the growth of Bact. abortus (bovine), because there is a gradual accumulation of carbon dioxide resulting from the metabolism of the organism. Gas analyses of these jars after incubation have given results averaging 5% carbon dioxide. This chart also shows the close relationship between Bact. abortus of porcine and of human origin, and Bact.

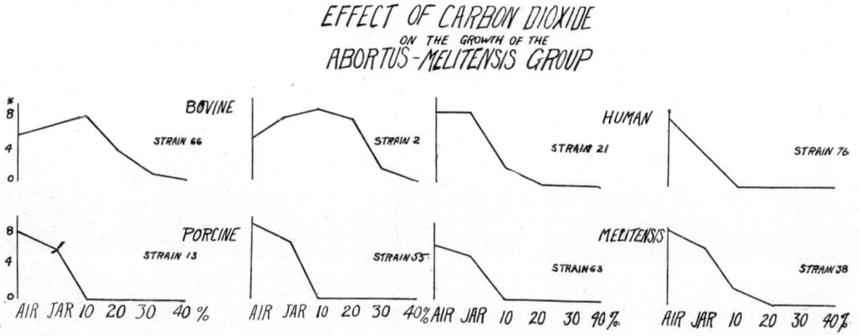

Effect of different concentrations of carbon dioxide on growth of two typical strains from each of the four groups (bovine, porcine, human, melitensis) of abortus-melitensis organisms.

melitensis. Any change from ordinary air conditions acted deleteriously on practically all cultures from these sources. There are a few strains of Bact. abortus of human origin which are typified by the graph for strain 21. In these cases the plates which were placed in the sealed jars without the addition of carbon dioxide grew as luxuriantly as those in the air.

Since a concentration of less than 10% carbon dioxide appeared to have a marked effect on most of the strains employed, a second series of experiments were conducted in which plates were placed under ordinary aerobic conditions in sealed jars and in concentrations of 5 and 10% CO_2. The results are given in table 3. It will be noticed that, although each individual strain has its own gas requirement, the bovine cultures are markedly different from all of the others. Three bovine strains proved to be exceptions, namely strains 48, 67 and 69. It has been shown in a previous paper [22] that strain 67 resembled more closely the porcine and human strains in that it utilized glucose in its metabolic activities. Glucose determinations have been made on strains 48 and 69 and both of these have been found to use this carbohydrate. Hence, although these three strains were isolated from bovine sources, they have certain of the physiologic characteristics of the porcine and human strains.

It was thought that the effect of carbon dioxide might be due to a lowering of the P_H of the agar in the higher concentrations of the gas. Therefore, hydrogen-ion concentration determinations of the plates in

TABLE 3.—EFFECT OF LOW CONCENTRATIONS OF CARBON DIOXIDE

Strains	Concentrations of CO_2			
	Air	Jar	5%	10%
Bovine				
1	4	5	6	6
2	4	5	6	6
4	8	9	9	0
6	3	4	6	6
43	4	6	7	5
46	4	5	8	1
Porcine				
12	9	6	0	0
13	8	4	0	0
53	6	2	2	0
70	5	3	0	0
71	6	5	0	0
Human				
72	8	8	6	0
73	8	0	0	0
76	6	6	5	0
83	8	8	7	6
Melitensis				
58	2	1	0	0
59	8	6	0	0
60	2	0	0	0
62	1	0	0	0

the various CO_2 atmospheres were made by the colorimetric method. It was found that 10% carbon dioxide depressed nutrient agar, the original P_H of which was 7.0, to P_H 6.8; 20 and 30% to around 6.4, and 40% to 6.2. A number of strains from each source were inoculated into agars having a P_H of from 6.6 to 5.8. Many of the strains grew throughout this P_H range, and none were inhibited at 6.2. The bovine strains did not differ in this respect from the Bact. abortus cultures of human and porcine origin and from those of Bact. melitensis.

Effect of Total Eclusion of CO_2 from Broth Cultures.—Three strains from each of the four sources of abortus-melitensis organisms

22. J. Infect. Dis., 1928, 42, p. 73.

were inoculated into broth tubes from which the carbon dioxide had been removed. They were incubated for five days in bell jars from which CO_2 had been completely excluded. All cultures used in this study failed to grow under these conditions.

DISCUSSION

In two previous papers [1,22] we showed that the abortus-melitensis group can be divided into two well marked subgroups. The strains of bovine origin, because of their inability to utilize glucose, are sharply separated from Bact. abortus porcine and human, and from Bact. melitensis, which use this carbohydrate in their metabolic activities. The results given here further support this grouping. The bovine strains, with very few exceptions, require the addition of 5 to 10% CO_2 for the promotion of their most luxuriant growth, while the porcine and human, and the Bact. melitensis strains, are more or less inhibited or rendered totally inert by like amounts of the gas.

Although all of the bovine strains employed in this study had been acclimated to aerobic conditions, they had retained their peculiar gas requirements, though somewhat modified by artificial conditions. The need for low concentrations of CO_2 became apparent only when different atmospheres were tried. On the other hand, Bact. melitensis and the porcine and human strains of Bact. abortus not only did not require the extra amounts of CO_2, but were actually inhibited by low concentrations of the gas beyond certain minimal amounts.

It has been shown that the effect of the various amounts of CO_2 is not due to an increase in the H-ions of the medium. Carbon dioxide at 40% did not depress the P_H of practically neutral nutrient agar plates in closed jars below 6.2, and it was observed that strains from all sources grew in mediums with as low P_H as this. Therefore, some other explanation for this inhibition must still be sought

The claim of Valley and Rettger [15] that Bact. abortus cannot multiply in the absence of CO_2 is substantiated by these results. The simple removal of carbon dioxide from the medium and surrounding atmosphere had a complete bacteriostatic action on all members of this group.

SUMMARY

By the addition of from 5 to 10% of CO_2 to bell jars containing inoculated plates, the growth of the bovine strains of Bact. abortus which had been acclimated to aerobic conditions was markedly accelerated.

On the other hand, this amount of the gas had a more or less inhibitory action on Bact. abortus strains of porcine and human origin, and on Bact. melitensis. This acceleration of growth for the bovine strains and inhibition for the porcine and human strains of Bact. abortus and of Bact. melitensis was apparently not due to changes in the H-ion concentration of the mediums. Total exclusion of CO_2 rendered the members of the abortus-melitensis group inert and unable to proliferate.

EXPERIMENTS RELATING TO THE PATHOLOGY AND THE ETIOLOGY OF MEXICAN TYPHUS (TABARDILLO)

1. CLINICAL COURSE AND PATHOLOGIC ANATOMY OF TABARDILLO IN GUINEA-PIGS

H. Mooser

From the Laboratory of the American Hospital, Mexico City, Mexico

The behavior of guinea-pigs inoculated with the virus of typhus has been extensively studied with respect to clinical course and pathologic changes since the time of Nicolle's first publications. With the exception of minor differences concerning the gross anatomic findings, there is complete agreement between all investigators: the only clinical sign accepted unanimously as pathognomic of typhus in guinea-pigs is a febrile reaction discoverable only with the thermometer and the necropsy findings are practically always negative except for a moderate enlargement of the spleen and lymphnodes, hyperemia of the brain and testicles with occasional petechial hemorrhages in the polar fat of the latter and beneath the skin. This rule is quite emphatically stated in the exhaustive study of Wolbach, Todd and Palfrey.[1] In 1917 M. H. Neill [2] published a short report on findings in male guinea-pigs inoculated with blood of patients with typhus during an outbreak among Mexicans in El Paso and Laredo, Texas. In 26 out of 37 males he noticed a more or less pronounced swelling and inflammation of the scrotum, and hemorrhages into the cremasteric fascia and beneath the parietal and visceral lamina of the tunica vaginalis. The histological examination of these parts revealed lesions consistent with typhus. Neill summarized his report as follows: definite gross, and minute pathologic changes in the genitals of male guinea-pigs reacting to Mexican typhus-fever have been described. The gross lesions occurred in about 70% of such animals examined. These depend on lesions of the blood vessels. These lesions are similar in process to those occurring in guinea-pigs infected with Rocky Mountain spotted fever, but are milder.

During several years the writer was engaged in experiments with guinea-pigs inoculated with blood from typhus patients. Out of 32 male

Received for publication, April 2, 1928.

1. The Etiology and Pathology of Typhus, 1922.
2. U. S. Pub. Health Rep., 1917, 32, p. 1105.

guinea-pigs inoculated with blood from ten typhus patients, 23 showed a transient rise of temperature to 104 or 104.5 F. lasting only from one to two days after an incubation period of twelve to eighteen days. Eighteen of these guinea-pigs developed a more or less marked swelling and reddening of the scrotum lasting only for a day or two. At necropsy the tunica vaginalis parietalis was found to be edematous, hyperemic and sometimes hemorrhagic. The tunica cremasterica beneath was also edematous and hemorrhagic. The same condition, although less pronounced, was found in the visceral part of the tunica vaginalis especially along the line which separates the fatty body from the testicle proper, where often pronounced edema and hemorrhage was met with. I was not able to start a strain from these animals as the virus invariably was lost in the first or second passage. These experiments were taken up again in November 1927 when a case of typhus fever was admitted to the hospital. The present paper presents the clinical and pathological findings in a larger series of guinea-pigs in which the strain isolated from this patient has been carried on. As these findings differ remarkably from the gross pathology described by all workers on the subject—except from those published by Neill—I find it necessary to give a short description of the clinical course of typhus in the patient from which the strain was started. The diagnosis of typhus was made by a clinician well acquainted with the disease. The patient presented the typical rash when I withdrew blood for guinea-pig inoculation on the seventh day of his illness. The Weil-Felix reaction was positive 1 : 3200 on the eleventh day of fever. There were no complications and the patient made an uneventful recovery which began on the 15th day after the fever had started. Blood cultures were negative.

CLINICAL COURSE OF TABARDILLO IN GUINEA-PIGS

Two male guinea-pigs, 1 and 2, were injected intraperitoneally with 3 cc. of blood from this patient diluted with an equal part of normal sterile salt solution. After a period of 11 days during which the animals had an average daily temperature of 102 one of them, guinea-pig 1, presented a sharp rise of temperature ranging between 104 and 105 F. accompanied by a moderate but distinct swelling and reddening of the scrotum. It was killed on the fifth day of fever and six other males inoculated intraperitoneally: two with 4 cc. of blood each diluted with salt solution, two with an emulsion of brain and two with an emulsion of spleen. On the second day of fever already two animals had been inoculated with 4 cc. of blood each, taken by heart puncture, so that eight animals were inoculated from guinea-pig one. This caution was taken to avoid most possibly the loss of the strain. The weight of these animals was from 250 to 300 grams as was the weight of nearly all animals used for these experiments. The necropsy of guinea-pig 1 did not reveal anything abnormal except for the lesions of the fascia cremasterica and tunica vaginalis to be described below. Guinea-pig 2 remained normal during an observation period of 30 days when it was inoculated with passage virus to which it reacted in a manner typical of Mexican typhus as described in this paper. Up to date 54 males and 4 females have been inoculated mostly with blood diluted with salt solution, occasionally with brain or with an emulsion made from the tunica vaginalis parietalis. The animals which served to maintain the strain invariably have been inoculated with blood whose sterility has always been controlled by a blood culture in glucose broth. Also from nearly all animals which have been killed for histological examinations, aerobic blood cultures were taken and frequently also cultures from the spleen. These numerous cultures did not show any growth with one single exception in which a bacillus of the enteritis group was isolated from the spleen. The animals of the first three passages presented a course of continuous fever, 104 to 106 F., lasting from three to nine days after an incubation period from 7 to 12 days. Later the incubation period was nearly always six to seven days and the period of constant fever (104 to 106 F.) became fixed to nearly exactly eight days. Animals inoculated with tunica presented a shorter incubation period. Whereas the females did not show any clinical signs of disease besides the febrile reaction, 50 out of the 54 males equalling 92.5% presented a more or less pronounced swelling of the scrotum which frequently appeared at the same time when the thermometer disclosed the beginning of the fever. Occasionally the beginning of the swelling was noticed several hours before the fever set in and in many animals the swelling became noticeable after the fever had lasted for already one or two days, very rarely later. The first sign of the scrotum lesion to be seen in adult males was generally complete descent of the testicles into the scrotal sac accompanied by a slight inflammatory edema of the proximal part of the scrotum. The swelling increased now rapidly under one's eyes i. e., in a few hours, spreading over the whole scrotum and in less than 24 hours the height of the swelling was generally reached, when it began to subside. Frequently the swelling increased and decreased during several successive days. At the height of the swelling the scrotum was decidedly edematous so that it could not be taken up in a fold. In animals with no or little pigment on that part of the body a distinct reddening appeared. The scrotum felt hot and clammy and was distinctly shiny. In one animal a distinct macular rash appeared over the scrotum and in two other animals with white scrotal skin a few irregular petechial spots were noticed (fig. 5). Frequently the edema spread to the prepuce. Swelling and reddening was only pronounced occasionally on one side or it appeared first on one side to spread shortly afterwards to the other side. A very characteristic symptom in nearly all animals with pronounced swelling was the fixation of the testicles within the scrotal sac. Whereas they are pushed back easily in normal animals, this became more and more difficult with increasing swelling and in well pronounced scrotal lesions they were absolutely fixed within the scrotal sac. As the animals showed signs of pain on handling the swollen part, naturally forced replacement was never tried. The scrotal swelling lasted only for a day or two, never more than four to five days but the testicles remained fixed within the scrotum for more than a week after the swelling had subsided in many animals. Not unfrequently the swelling appeared and nearly disappeared again within a day, although a very pronounced swelling always lasted for more than a day, generally two to three days at least. In six animals fever and swelling lasted only one day, but after an interval of only one single day of normal or nearly normal temperature the typical continuous fever of typhus started, accompanied by the renewed appearance of the scrotal swelling. With the exception of only three animals this swelling was pronounced and easily noticeable. In the latter three animals edema and reddening was only moderate and would probably not have been noticed if our attention had not been directed especially toward it. The height of the scrotal swelling was nearly invariably accompanied by the height of the febrile reaction but the duration of the fever was in no way related to the magnitude of the scrotal involvement. In animals in which the swelling fluctuated on successive days this fluctuation was generally accompanied by a corresponding slight rise and fall of the fever. In small males under 250 grams of weight in which the testicles had not yet completely descended into the depth of the scrotum reddening and swelling invariably appeared only over the proximal part of the scrotum. The swelling of the skin in these animals closely corresponded to the region in which the testicles were situated. The examination of our protocols revealed that of the four males which had not shown any swelling of the scrotum, three were very young males in which the testicles were still completely within the abdominal cavity.

GROSS PATHOLOGIC ANATOMY

Twenty-two animals were killed during the febrile reaction, either when the scrotal swelling was at its height or shortly afterwards to study its pathology or after the fourth or fifth day of fever to search for the specific lesions of typhus in the brains. This was sometimes done alternately, i. e. of an animal of the second passage for instance the scrotum and the testicles were examined and from an animal of the next passage the brain was examined. Or, as several animals always received injections at the same time with blood for passages, two animals were killed of the same series, one at the height of the scrotal swelling and the other after the fourth to fifth day of fever for study of the brain. With the exception of the scrotal and testicular lesions to be described, the necropsy findings were practically always negative. The spleen was frequently moderately enlarged and occasionally a fine coat of fibrin was found adherent to its edge. Frequently the fine adherent film described by Wolbach, Todd and Palfrey was found over the surface of the spleen. Cultures from these spleens and their fibrin coating proved sterile with one exception.

In an animal of the third passage a bacillus of the enteritis group was isolated from the spleen. We prepared a vaccine from the cultures and from then on vaccinated all our animals five to six times subcutaneously before using them for our experiments. Beginning with the fifth passage no fibrin was found any more around the spleen which was from then on found to be only moderately enlarged if at all. The fine adherent film however was still occasionally found over the spleens.

In one animal a few petechial spots were found beneath the visceral pleura and once a small hemorrhage over the psoas major muscle around the femoral artery. Smaller hemorrhages were occasionally met with beneath the skin. Animals with extensive scrotal and testicular involvement frequently presented decidedly congested inguinal lymph glands.

At necropsy swelling and inflammation of the scrotum was invariably less than during life—a few minutes before. The animals were deeply anesthetized with ether and as much blood as possible aspirated from the heart for transfer of the strain and blood cultures. The circumstance that this nearly complete exsanguination was followed by a noticeable decrease of the scrotal swelling indicates that it was partly due to congestion. Sometimes testicles which seemed to be firmly fixed within the scrotal sac in the living animal could be pushed back into the abdomen after it had been killed by bleeding. On incision the skin of the scrotum did not show alterations except for a more or less pronounced edema. The subcutaneous connective tissue however regularly presented pronounced edema especially in the cranial part of the scrotum where it loses itself in the abdominal wall. Even the lower part of the abdominal wall exceptionally showed a marked edema of its subcutaneous tissue. The edema of the subcutaneous tissue was sometimes so pronounced that a large drop of clear fluid could be collected with a capillary pipet from the depth of an incision. The most pronounced changes were invariably found in the fascia cremasterica and in the parietal part of the tunica vaginalis. These were characterized by edematous swelling, pronounced hyperemia of the fascia cremasterica accompanied by numerous petechial or diffuse hemorrhages beneath the tunica vaginalis parietalis. The fascia could easily be separated in toto with the testicles in place. As fascia cremasterica and tunica vaginalis are inseparable in these animals I shall refer to them simply as tunica. Occasionally the hemorrhage in the tunica involved the whole organ. Viewed from the inside the tunica presented itself as an intensely red membrane due to hyperemia and hemorrhages. Although it looked fairly moist it was found to be more or less opaque and milky as if it were covered with a grayish white membrane. This membrane was not always uniformly developed over the whole tunica vaginalis but looked thicker in some places. It was found to be especially thick where the testicles were adherent to the tunica. These changes of the tunica extended into the inguinal canal where they lost gradually into the normal peritoneum of the abdominal cavity. Only once thickening and hemorrhage extended beyond the inguinal canal into the peritoneum where it ceased abruptly. The same thickening was exhibited by the tunica of the testicles especially over the epididymis and along the shallow grooves between testicle and epididymis and testicle and polar fat. Frequently a film of fibrin was found covering the tunica which could be easily removed whereas the described thickening was firmly adherent but could be scraped off with a knife. The thickening of the tunica testiculi could best be noted when the organ was put for about ten minutes in Zenker's solution. Whereas the normal part of the tunica testiculi was still fairly shiny after this time, the thickened place looked now decidedly opaque. In two cases in which the testicles were found firmly fixed within the sac a large hemorrhage filled the sac. The obliteration of the processus vaginalis however was not due to hemorrhage as a rule, but the two leaves were generally found to be glued together without noticeable hemorrhage between them. On removing the testicles from within the sac, frequently pieces of the tunica vaginalis parietalis remained attached to the surface of the testicles. Generally hemorrhages were found to be less pronounced over the latter and its appendages than over the tunica parietalis. They were found especially along the proximal and distal part of the testicles along the mentioned shallow grooves, but occasionally a large part of their surface was covered by hemorrhage, and petechial spots were frequent and numerous over the polar fat and the epididymis. Testicles and adnexa were always decidedly swollen and hyperemic and their surfaces when cut revealed marked edema. Hemorrhages into the substance of the testicle proper were only occasionally found as small petechiae. They were more frequent in the polar fat along the border line between the latter and the testicle.

HISTOLOGIC EXAMINATION

A complete histologic examination of all internal organs was performed on two animals only. It was however done most carefully in the aim to look for the specific lesions of typhus and to exclude with the greatest degree of possibility signs of a secondary or concomitant infection. Because the lesions of scrotum and testicles described above are in such contrast to the findings of all the investigators on typhus, it necessarily constituted an important task of our investigation to separate etiologically—so far as this could be done with histological methods—the lesions universally accepted as pathognomonic of typhus in guinea-pigs, from the lesions of scrotum and testicles first described by Neill. For this reason we chose for the study of the internal organs two animals which had shown very pronounced scrotal swelling. Liver, spleen, lungs, kidneys, adrenals, heart and brain were examined. No lesions were found which could not unhesitatingly be taken as consistent with an uncomplicated typhus infection. These lesions, very few in number, consisted of swelling and proliferation of the endothelial cells of the intima of capillaries and small arteries with or without accompanying moderate perivascular infiltration with lymphocytes and plasma cells. Distinct peri and paravascular nodules formed chiefly by proliferated endothelial cells were only found in the myocardium of one of these animals. The typical nodular lesion of the gray matter of the brain were found in both. In the lung of one animal I found an occluding thrombus of a small artery which had caused a small hemorrhagic infarct. The parenchyma of kidneys, liver and adrenals was found to be normal.

The histology of the spleen which was examined in many animals was characterized by a diffuse overgrowth of endothelial cells especially pronounced within a broad line occupying the peripheral parts of the sections but also invading extensively the central parts. Large follicles with conspicuous central vessel were present, other follicles were replaced nearly completely by these large endothelial cells surrounding the central vessel which showed the typical endothelial lesion of typhus. This diffuse overgrowth of endothelial cells obliterated the land-marks of the organ more or less completely causing an intense red staining of the sections stained with hematoxylin-eosin or Giemsa's stain, whereas in a normal spleen the coloration of the sections is dominated by the dark staining of the nuclei of lymphocytes. Polymorphonuclear leukocytes and eosinophilic cells were present in some parts of the sections in fair numbers mixing diffusely with the endothelial cells. The latter were phagocytic, containing red cells, hemosiderin and nuclear debris. Mitoses of endothelial cells and probably of fibroblasts were found frequently outside and inside of follicles. Megakaryocytes and a similar large cell with a dark centrally situated multilobed nucleus were also met with in small numbers, and where these latter cells were found among endothelial cells, lymphocytes and polynuclears this part of the section had quite a striking resemblance with a spleen in Hodgkin's disease. Many red cells were always found outside of the vessels. The cells of the endothelial covering of the spleen frequently showed a more or less pronounced swelling and occasionally a layer of proliferated cells included in a mesh work of fibrinous material coated the surface.

Brain.—The brains of numerous animals were examined carefully in order to find the nodular lesion considered pathognomonic of a typhus infection (fig. 1). In animals killed before the fourth day of fever only the early vascular lesions accompanied by meningeal and perivascular infiltration with lymphocytes were found. After the fourth day the typical nodular lesion was present in all animals but as a rule their number was so small that a whole brain had to be cut in serial sections in order to find them. As a rule they were extremely scarce in animals inoculated with blood but quite numerous in animals inoculated with an emulsion of tunica vaginalis.

Scrotum, Tunica and Testicles.—As could be expected from the post mortem examinations the most numerous and most extensive lesions invariably were found in the scrotum, tunica cremasterica, tunica vaginalis, testicles and their adnexa. They were met with in these parts in such large numbers that they offered wonderful pieces for the study of the pathogenesis of typhus lesions. All stages of their development could often be found in one single section: beginning with swelling and vacuolization of individual groups of endothelial cells in small vessels, concentric proliferation of these cells toward the lumen to almost com-

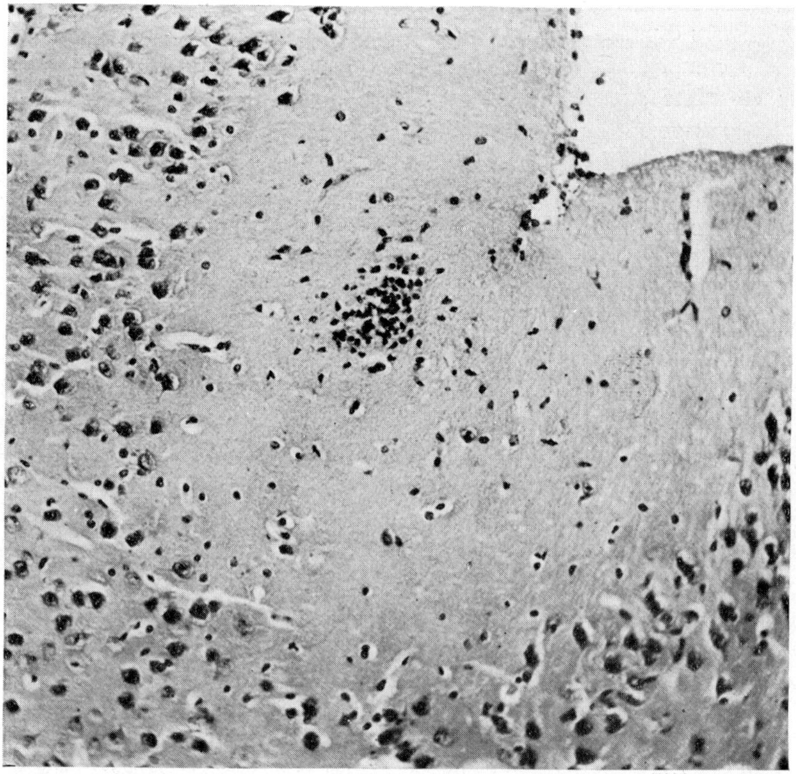

Fig. 1.—Small nodular lesion in the brain.

plete, and complete, obliteration of the vessel, accompanied often by extensive perivascular infiltration with lymphocytes, plasma cells and large mononuclear leukocytes. Nodular agroupation by these latter cells within the wall of arteries and veins and perivascular nodule formation was a constant finding. Occluding fibrin thrombi within necrosed blood vessels were found and large hemorrhages around very extended blood vessels showing more or less complete necrosis of all their coats.

Whereas in the upper layers of the skin of the scrotum only the early vascular lesions were present they increased in number and magnitude steadily towards the tunica vaginalis parietalis under which the most extensive changes invariably were found in all animals. The bundles of the cremasteric muscle were separated by abundant interstitial infiltration with lymphocytes, plasma cells, endothelial leukocytes, eosinophilic cells, polynuclears and often proliferated fibroblasts. Where this infiltration was especially pronounced the muscle cells showed signs of more or less complete degeneration from hyalin transformation to more or less complete granular disintegration. The endothelial lining of the tunica was generally destroyed and replaced by an exuberant proliferation of endothelial cells and infiltration with lymphocytes, polynuclears and endothelial leukocytes, which embedded in a mesh work of fibrin formed a coat of considerable thickness. Large and small hemorrhages were a constant finding within the tunica cremasterica and within the proliferated tunica vaginalis accompanied by pronounced edema of the connective tissue of the scrotum. Pronounced edema was also frequently found in the fatty body of the testicle which was second in respect to number and magnitude of the lesions to the tunica.

The most interesting results were gained by the careful study of the tunica vaginalis-parietalis and visceralis. I shall describe the findings with more detail because their histological analysis furnished new information on the pathogenesis of lesions produced in tissue by the presence of the virus of typhus. These lesions deserve a detailed description all the more as their correct interpretation led to the easy and constant demonstration of a minute intracellular microorganism in such large numbers as has been found so far only within the epithelial cells of the stomach of lice carrying the virus of typhus.

We have examined the tunica of animals killed between the first to the fourth day of the appearance of scrotal swelling. As the changes within the tunica parietalis were at this early date already so pronounced that it was not easy to gain an exact idea of their development, the description given in this paper on the successive changes of the tunica is mostly based on the observation of the tunica visceralis. The first sign of pathological changes in the endothelial lining of the tunica was a heaping up of the cells which were much larger and became cubical to cylindrical. The nuclei were also increased exhibiting a deep staining and increased chromatin substance. Frequently the protoplasma was vacuolated. Rare mitotic cell divisions were present. The next step was a pronounced proliferation of the swollen endothelial cell which formed frequently a layer of three, four and more cells. This proliferation generally took place at once over a large part of the tunica, but often circumscribed areas of proliferation were observed forming wart like protuberances (fig. 2). At the beginning of the endothelial swelling, but oftener when the proliferation was already in full progress an accumulation of large mononuclear cells, lymphocytes and plasma cells collected in the tissue beneath the tunica forming frequently a broad band of densely packed cells beneath the membrana limitans which was still intact. Frequently these cells were found penetrating through this membrane invading the coat of proliferated endothelial cells. The basal membrane disappeared frequently and it became then impossible to find out the limit between the proliferated tunica and the infiltrated underlying tissus. The cavity of the processus vaginalis was frequently completely obliterated and it was often not possible to find out which part of the proliferated and immigrated cells came from the tunica parietalis and which from the tunica visceralis. Hemorrhages took place, the infiltration increased and finally the proliferated tunica was replaced by a fibrinous material in whose meshes enormous numbers of endothelial cells, endothelial leukocytes, plasma cells, lymphocytes, polynuclears, red cells and nuclear debris collected. On the second day already newly formed capillaries entered these cell masses and mitotic fibroblasts were a frequent finding. These newly formed vessels were frequently the site of fresh typhus lesions and nodule formation by proliferated endothelial cells in their connection was often seen. These pronounced lesions took place regularly over the tunica parietalis, over the fat body and to a milder degree over the epididymis and the testicles proper. All stages were always present in a single section of these organs and as clinically the lesions retroceeded rapidly it is supposed that all these changes may stop rapidly at any phase of their development. When the proliferated cell masses however have been invaded from beneath by capillaries and fibroblasts a scar was formed which obliterated the peritoneal process to a greater or a lesser degree. Extensive fibrous adhesions have been found in animals several weeks after the experimental infection had subsided. At some places the changes did not occur in the manner described, the proliferation of the endothelium was here only slight but exudation of fibrin and endothelial leukocytes occurred early, coating the tunica as a broad line or the primary endothelial cells showed necrosis without proliferation and the underlying tissue was densely infiltrated with mononuclear cells, large number of polynuclears and lymphocytes covering or replacing the disappearing endothelial cells.

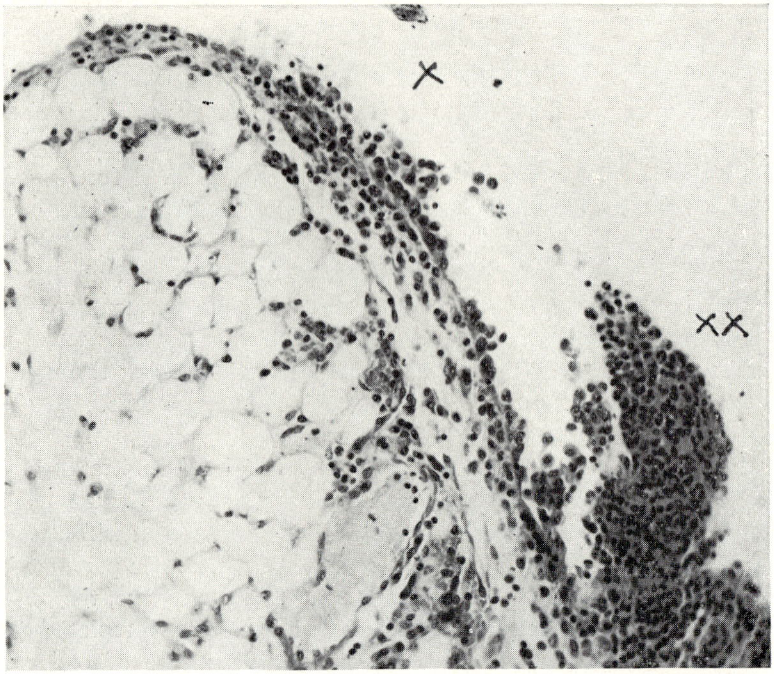

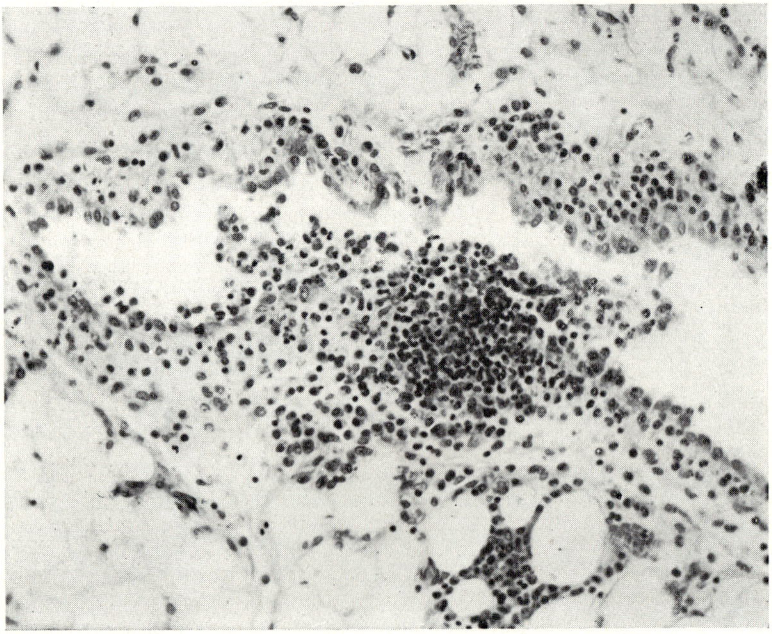

Fig. 2.—Proliferative lesions of tunica visceralis covering the polar fat of the testicle. X. Beginning proliferation; XX, wartlike protuberance formed nearly exclusively by proliferated endothelial cells of the tunica.

Fig. 3.—Nodular lesions beneath the tunica visceralis. Note proliferation of endothelial cells over the nodule and swelling and heaping up of the endothelial cells lining the fold of the tunica.

It seemed that the degree of proliferation was dependent on the degree of injury suffered by the endothelial cells. The place where the lesions occurred modified its character to some extent. Over the testicles for instance the proliferated coat was often quite extensive, yet the underlying tunica albuginea never showed such injury and cell infiltration as the cremasteric membrane and the superficial layers of the fat body. In the testicle proper the lesions were decidedly scarcer and distinct nodules were not found frequently but perivascular infiltration with lymphocytes and plasma cells were more frequent. Frequently typical nodules formed of densely packed endothelial cells were found immediately beneath the endothelial lining of the tunica, the tunica cells themselves taking part in the nodule formation (fig. 3). It looked decidedly as if these nodules were derived from the endothelial cells of the tunica and not from blood vessels. Moreover, distinct nodules composed of the typical pale endothelial cells so characteristic of the typhus nodule were seen projecting over the endothelial lining of the tunica into the cavity of the processus vaginalis. In the fatty body endothelial leukocytes or proliferated endothelial cells were found surrounding large fat cells, proliferating concentrically, forming a broad ring about the space left by the fat cells (fig. 3), exactly as was frequently seen within blood vessels and I got the impression that the numerous compact nodules often found in the fat body were at least in part due to such proliferation around fat cells. The most unexpected findings however were compact nodules of proliferated endothelial cells outside of the tissue, sit venia verbo. They were repeatedly found within the fibrinous material covering the tunica whose cell row though swollen and somewhat proliferated was still intact showing no signs of disintegration or perforation by blood vessels. The presence of the latter could be excluded with absolute security because the fibrinous material in which these nodules were embedded contained only relatively few leukocytes and mononuclear cells widely separted one from the other so that in our thin sections even the finest capillary could not have escaped detection (fig. 4). Moreover these nodules were often found to be far above the level of the swollen endothelial cells of the tunica. They only could have originated from desquamated endothelial cells. This was clearly evidenced from the finding of a mitotic cell division within such a nodule. The pathogenetic entity of the proliferative lesions of blood vessels and that of the endothelial lining of the tunica could nicely be demonstrated within narrow deep folds of the tunica covering the fat body. Proliferated tunica cells filled these narrow folds more or less completely and the surrounding tissue showed dense infiltration with endothelial leukocytes and lymphocytes as seen around blood vessels whose endothelial lining was proliferated. Indeed viewed under high power magnification it would have been absolutely impossible to distinguish an affected small blood vessel from these proliferated and infiltrated folds of the tunica without looking for the connection of them with the processus vaginalis.

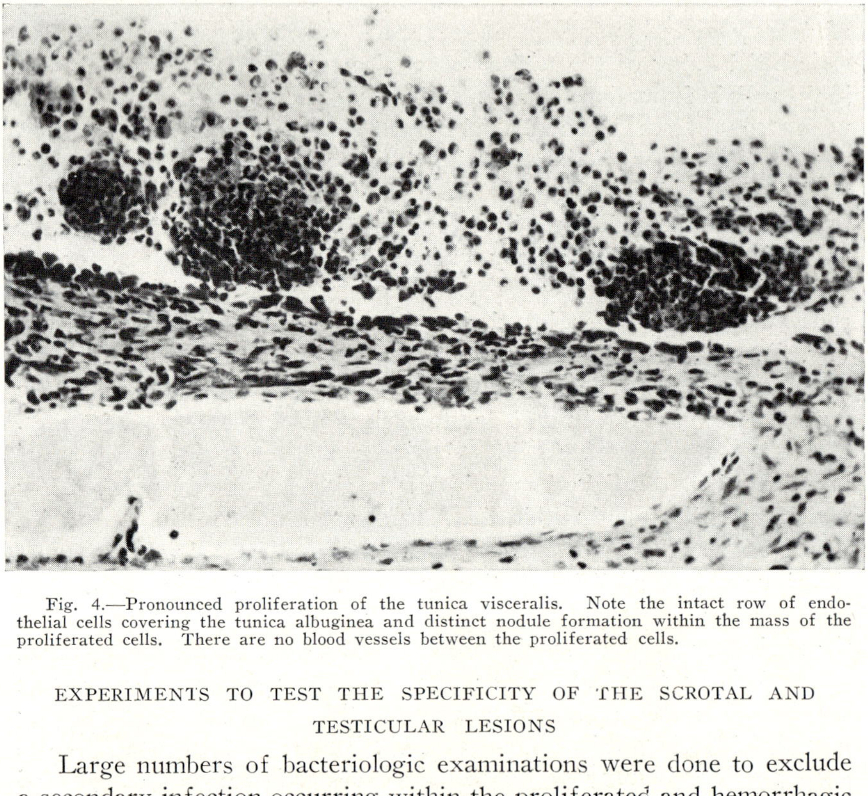

Fig. 4.—Pronounced proliferation of the tunica visceralis. Note the intact row of endothelial cells covering the tunica albuginea and distinct nodule formation within the mass of the proliferated cells. There are no blood vessels between the proliferated cells.

EXPERIMENTS TO TEST THE SPECIFICITY OF THE SCROTAL AND TESTICULAR LESIONS

Large numbers of bacteriologic examinations were done to exclude a secondary infection occurring within the proliferated and hemorrhagic tunica vaginalis, testicles and tunica cremasterica. Besides from the ordinary culture medium, ascites, blood serum agar and Noguchi's leptospira medium were inoculated with small pieces of these tissues. On no occasion did any bacterial growth develop and smears made from all animals did not show any microorganisms after staining with Loeffler's methylene blue and Gram's method.

As the large number of specific vascular lesions and nodules present in tunica and fat body indicated a possible accumulation of the virus of typhus in these parts, emulsions made from the tunica parietalis were injected into guinea-pigs. These inoculated animals invariably showed fever and swelling of the scrotum after an incubation period of only four days. The necropsy did not show any difference from animals given injections of blood, and the lesions of the brain were typical. A female injected with tunica showed the most numerous nodules in the brain of our series of animals. Two animals were given injections of the edema fluid which collected in the scrotal sac after removing the testicles and tunica cremasterica as a whole. Each received about 0.05 cc. diluted to 2 cc. with saline. One of them (33) received subcutaneously the fluid from an animal of the third blood passage, and the other (68) intraperitoneally the fluid from an animal of the ninth passage. The temperature chart of these two animals is as follows:

Guinea-pig 33		Guinea-pig 68
Dec. 21....102.4 F., inoculated	Jan. 1....104.4 F., enormous swelling and inflammation of scrotum	Feb. 10....101.8 F., inoculated
22....102	2....104.6	11....102.2
23....102	3....104.2	12....102.2
24....102.2	4....104	13....102
25....102.4	5....103.4	14....104.6, swelling of scrotum
26....102.6	6....102.8	15....104.4, swelling less
27....102	7....102.2	16....105.2, swelling very pronounced. Killed
28....104.4	8....101.6	
29....104.8	9....102.2	
30....105.2		
31....104.6, moderate swelling of scrotum		

Guinea-pig 33 remained refractory to a subsequent inoculation with passage blood. Guinea-pig 68 was negative at necropsy except for the scrotal swelling and testicular lesions. The typical nodular lesions, though very few, were found in its brain. Three cc. of blood taken from guinea-pig 68 and injected in guinea-pig 71 induced in the latter animal fever and scrotal swelling after an incubation period of five days only. Guinea-pig 71 did not show any signs of a secondary infection as revealed by autopsy, cultures and histological examinations and the lesions in brain and testicles were typical of typhus.

Guinea-pig 33 was given an injection on December 21, 1927, with edema fluid from animal 25 of the third passage. The fluid was collected with capillary glass pipets. During this manipulation a pipet broke and produced a superficial scratch on the back of my left hand. There was no bleeding and no attention was paid to this accident as we considered it harmless. On December 30th I went to bed because of a chilliness, fever, and severe headache. Fever and headache increased steadily for four days and on January 5 a scant macular rash appeared over the back, shoulders, arms and chest. The disease was then diagnosed as typhus and the laboratory reported Weil-Felix positive 1 : 200 on January 7, 1 : 400 on January 8. Blood cultures proved sterile. There were no complications except for a mild bronchitis and quite a marked deafness during the height of the fever, which dropped on the twelfth day. I am convinced that my disease was the result of this accident. I had not seen personally a case of typhus since the beginning of November when I started the strain which is the object of this

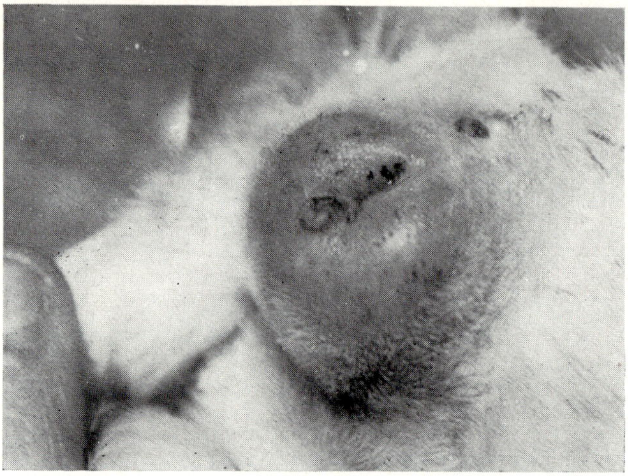

Fig. 5.—Swollen edematous and shiny scrotum covered by an irregular petechial rash.

paper. The possibility that I had acquired typhus by the bite of an infected louse is very small as all the cases reported in Mexico City during December were only four, all from other parts of the city than where I lived.

DISCUSSION

The observation of pronounced microscopic lesions of the genital organs in more than 90% of our male animals in which a supposed strain of Mexican typhus was carried on by blood passages required careful bacteriological, histological and experimental examinations to rule out a possible coexisting virus carried along with the virus of typhus. Although Neill had already observed the same lesions ten years before us in guinea-pigs inoculated with blood from Mexican typhus cases, his findings have not been confirmed by any other investigator. Wolbach, Todd and Palfrey [1] state: "Neil's brief description of the testicular lesions in guinea-pigs in our opinion overstates the degree of involvement" and: "the scrotal tissues and tunica remain normal and the reaction in our experience has been in no way comparable to that of Rocky Mountain spotted fever in guinea-pigs or as described with Mexican typhus by M. H. Neill (1917)." Considering that a large amount of research on typhus has been done with Mexican virus by Ricketts and Wilder,[3] Anderson and Goldberger,[4] Gavino and Girard,[5] Wolbach and Todd,[6] it seems almost impossible that such conspicuous lesions could have been overlooked. The observations of Neill and our previous observations on male guinea-pigs inoculated with blood from ten different cases of Mexican typhus indicate clearly that the lesions described in this paper are not a peculiarity of the strain described in this paper. The constantly negative bacteriological findings in our animals together with the absence of histological evidence in their tissues of another infection than that of typhus leads at least to strong suspicion that the testicular lesions, described by Neill and ourselves, are pathognomonic of a tabardillo infection in male guinea-pigs. This suspicion was strengthened by the histological findings in the tunica vaginalis.

Typhus has its specific histology by which it can be diagnosed by the pathologist. The lesions observed in the endothelial lining of the tunica vaginalis of our animals corresponded exactly to the lesions as described to occur in the vascular endothelium—in their histological appearance and pathogenesis: swelling, necrosis, proliferation and nodule formation. The endothelial lining of the processus vaginalis behaves in this respect exactly like the endothelium of a blood vessel and the surrounding tissues react equally in both. If swelling and proliferation of the endothelial cells of the blood vessel are the result of the presence of an intracellular parasite within these cells, the same must be true for the changes in the tunica of our animals. The experiments with emulsion made from the tunica and with the edema fluid collected from beneath the tunica cremasterica prove clearly that the virus is present there is considerable quantity. I suppose that the tunica is responsible for the often enormous numbers of typical typhus lesions just beneath it, because of the constant absence of a scrotal swelling in very young ani-

3. Ricketts, H. T., and Wilder, R. M.: J. Am. M. A., 1910, 54, pp. 1304 and 1373.
4. Collected Studies on Typhus, Hyg. Lab. Bull. no. 86, October, 1912.
5. Publicaciones del Instit. Bact. Nacional, 1910, no. 2.
6. Ann. de l'Inst. Pasteur, 1920, 34, p. 153.

mals in which the testicles are still within the abdominal cavity; and it is observed that the scrotal swelling in young animals, with only partly descended testicles, always closely corresponds to the place under which the testicles are situated. Moreover, we have never observed the slightest swelling of the external genital organs of females. But how did the tunica cells become infected with the virus of typhus, which circulates in the blood, and could so far only be demonstrated within endothelial cells of blood vessels and which was supposed to cause specific lesions only within and around these vessels? There are two possibilities. The first is that the peritoneal lining of the tunica became infected from nodular lesions situated immediately beneath it. Frequently typical nodules were found there involving the endothelium of the tunica and the possibility that these nodules were primarily derived from a capillary naturally could not always be excluded (fig. 3). The other possibility is that the cells of the tunica became primarily infected on account of the intraperitoneal inoculation of the virus. The processus vaginalis, with its testicles in place separated fairly well from the general peritoneal cavity, may constitute a good breeding place for the virus of typhus, a far better one perhaps than collodian sacs buried in the abdominal cavity. The observation of an animal with scrotal involvement after subcutaneous inoculation speaks against this possibility. The animal was however inoculated beneath the skin of the abdomen and the possibility that some of the material was injected into the abdominal cavity cannot be excluded. The limited number of animals at our disposal prevented the solution of this interesting problem. The presence of typical nodular agroupations of endothelial cells within the exudate which had collected in the processus vaginalis indicates at least that the virus of typhus was present here outside of any blood vessel. The observation of the narrow folds of the tunica over the fat body which exhibited a striking similarity to affected blood vessels hardly permits another explanation than that the tunica cells became infected with virus contained within the processus vaginalis. Besides the constant finding of the lesions of the tunica our strain differs also in respect to the incubation period from the strains of other sources. Wolbach, Todd and Palfrey [1] are of the opinion that a shorter period of incubation than seven days is due to a secondary infection. We observed only one case of proved secondary infection. After we had vaccinated all our animals against the germ isolated from this case before using them in our experiments, the incubation period was not lengthened in spite of the fact that from then on our animals presented without exception an absolutely clean peritoneum and their spleens were only moderately enlarged, if at all. The fact that fever and scrotal swelling usually occurred simultaneously also militates against the possibility that the short incubation period was due to something else than typhus. Our strain is now in the thirteenth passage showing still the lesions described, and we consider them as the most precious and valuable sign of tabardillo in guinea-pigs. The appearance of the scrotal swelling as an initial sign of the specific infection and the presence of pronounced histologic lesions on the first day of fever make me suspect that the virus had accumulated here considerably during the incubation period. I believe that the virus had multiplied here within endothelial cells until they ruptured spreading then into the surrounding tissue and blood causing the local reaction and the fever. The observation of a scrotal swelling shortly before the appearance of the fever fits very well into this conception. Moreover the fact that compact typical nodular lesions were found on the first and second day of fever in tunica cremasterica and in the fatty body beneath the tunica visceralis, and that such nodules could not be found in the brain before the fourth day hardly permits another assumption than that the virus had been present within the tunica before it reached the circulation and the brain.

The finding of these lesions will probably revive in Mexico the old dispute on the nosological entity of European typhus and tabardillo. This question was extensively discussed during the last Mexican Congress on Typhus in 1922, when Escalona [7] tried to prove again that tabardillo and typhus are different diseases. He did not, however, bring forth any single valuable argument for his point of view and curious enough the specific histology was not mentioned by him. There is no question that typhus and tabardillo are etiologically identical. Both are transmitted by the body louse, both give a positive Weil-Felix reaction in nearly 100% of the cases and the pathologic histology in both is indistinguishable. Finally both diseases have been proved to be identical by cross immunity tests. The peculiar localization of Mexican typhus in the tunica of guinea-pigs indicates that the virus from different countries may exhibit some biological differences by which they can be distinguished experimentally. Our animals show in the tunica cremasterica and in the fatty body besides the typical vascular lesions pronounced and often very diffuse perivascular infiltrations. Wolbach, Todd and Palfrey state that "diffuse perivascular infiltrations are not a conspicuous feature

7. Memorias del segundo congreso nacional del tabardillo, Mexico City, 1923.

of typhus in guinea-pigs." These considerable perivascular infiltrations in our animals may explain why the rash in man suffering from tabardillo is not infrequently decidedly papular.[8]

SUMMARY

Over 90% of the male guinea-pigs inoculated with the virus of Mexican typhus (tabardillo) presented more or less pronounced swelling and reddening of the scrotum which is due to extensive specific lesions in the tunica cremasterica, tunica vaginalis and testicles. The endothelial lining of the tunica vaginalis reacts exactly in the same manner to the presence of the virus of typhus as does the vascular endothelium. Evidence is forwarded that a considerable amount of virus was present in the swollen tunica and that it had accumulated there within the endothelial cells during the incubation period.

8. Escalona, Genaro: Ibid.

EXPERIMENTS RELATING TO THE PATHOLOGY AND THE ETIOLOGY OF MEXICAN TYPHUS (TABARDILLO)

2. DIPLOBACILLUS FROM THE PROLIFERATED TUNICA VAGINALIS OF GUINEA-PIGS REACTING TO MEXICAN TYPHUS

H. Mooser

From the Laboratory of the American Hospital, Mexico City, Mexico

Observation of the lesions of the endothelial lining of the tunica vaginalis in male guinea-pigs which showed scrotal swelling during the course of experimental typhus infection,[1] suggested that the etiologic agent of the disease could be demonstrated within the proliferated tunica. The lesions exhibited all the characteristics described by other investigators for the lesions in the endothelial lining of blood vessels consequent to the presence of Rickettsia prowazeki within the endothelial cells. The proliferation of the endothelial cells of the processus vaginalis was without exception so pronounced in our animals that it was reasonable to assume that the microscopical examination of these proliferated cells would disclose with adequate staining methods the presence of the intracellular parasite described in typhus literature. Moreover, if the assumption is correct that the minute intracellular bodies found in sections of tissues of typhus-infected man and animals are the cause of the disease and that the peculiar proliferation of the endothelial cells is really the immediate result of the presence of these bodies within the proliferated cells, it was also reasonable to expect that they were present in large numbers within the proliferated tunica. In no other tissue has such an abundant proliferation of endothelial cells been seen before in typhus-infected man and animal, in no tissue such a large number of supposedly specifically infected endothelial cells. The experimental demonstration that emulsions from the proliferated tunica and the fluid collecting within the tissues harbors a considerable amount of the virus, was also promising in this respect.

SECTIONS OF THE TUNICA

After a few trials on tissues fixed in Zenker's fluid and stained with Giemsa solution as devised by Wolbach, Todd and Palfrey,[2] we aban-

Received for publication, April 2, 1928.

1. Mooser, H.: J. Infect. Dis., 1928, 43, p. 240.
2. The etiology and pathology of typhus, 1922.

doned this method and fixed the tissues in Regaud's fluid before applying Giemsa's solution as a staining fluid. Although Zenker's fixation gives the most perfect histological pictures with Giemsa's stain, we were not able to find cell inclusions in such sections, which we could unreservedly have accepted as being microorganisms. In sections of tissue fixed in Regaud's fluid, however, a large number of cells were found within the proliferated tunica, containing an enormous number of minute bacilliform inclusions singly and in pairs. Within correctly differentiated parts of the sections their color was a light purple. When differentiation was not sufficient they stained a dark purple and when differentiation was carried on too far their color was a pale blue. As a rule these bacilliform inclusions were present in such large numbers within the cells that a dark coloration of the whole plasma of the cells resulted, by which they could be easily traced under low power. It was not exceptional to find three to six of such heavily filled cells within the field of the oil immersion lens. In well differentiated sections the outlines of these rods were always sharp and no surrounding halo was found as a rule. In cells, however, containing relatively few of these inclusions occasionally an indistinct clearer zone of the protoplasma was seen surrounding a single or paired rod. These inclusions were always found to be minute short rods, but as they were arranged in all directions within the cells, movement of the micrometer screw was frequently necessary to prove their rod form. Of course when they were directed perpendicularly to the lens they looked like granules. I do not pretend that my description of these bacilliform bodies found in sections is a definite one, because I have examined the tunica of two animals only for that purpose. As my acquaintance with mitochondria and other finer cell constituents is only rudimentary, the examination of these stained sections served only as a preliminary orientation for the search of microorganisms in the tunica with methods familiar to us.

SMEARS FROM THE TUNICA

The observation of cells within the proliferated tunica containing a considerable number of bacilliform inclusions suggested that these inclusions were microorganisms. As cell inclusions in sections of tissue, especially when there is inflammation, offer considerable difficulties for their correct interpretation, I took recourse to smears made from the proliferated tunica. Carefully made smears leave the cells intact and since they spread out flatly on the slide their intracellular constituents can be studied more accurately than within shrunken and rounded up cells within fixed tissue. Moreover, in smears stained with Giemsa's solution the granulations of cells cannot be confused so easily with intracellular parasites as in stained sections, because in smears the intracellular granulations show far greater specific affinities for the different staining bodies contained in Giemsa's solution than they do in sections of tissue and the form of intracellular parasites is far better preserved. Last but not least, mitochondria do not disturb the observer in smear preparations fixed with alcohol and less even in smears stained without previous fixation.

We made numerous smears from 20 animals. These were deeply anesthetized with ether, bled to death by heart puncture and after careful shaving, painting with iodine and thorough cleansing with alcohol of the abdominal wall and scrotum, the abdomen was opened and the incision prolonged on both sides over the scrotum. The testicles were carefully freed from the soft adhesions due to the proliferated tunica, and removed for histological examination. The soft layer of the tunica parietalis was then carefully scraped off with the sharp edge of a knife and spread gently over several slides. Each scraping of one tunica gave sufficient material for three to six smears. The entire scraping obtained from one tunica was spread with the edge of the knife on the first slide, the gross particles taken off carefully with the same knife and smeared on the next slide and so on. After thorough drying from 1 to 24 hours in closed dishes the smears were fixed in absolutely methyl-alcohol and stained with Giemsa's solution for one to three hours in staining jars.

The examination of the first smear revealed often an enormous number of reddish staining irregular granules, derived from destroyed endothelial leukocytes which contained such granules in great numbers collecting as large round masses within the plasma of these cells. Occasionally these granules had collected in form of a crescent along the margin of the nucleus. The granules exhibiting the typical staining properties of chromatin in Giemsa-stained smears are undoubtedly derivatives of destroyed nuclei within the phagocytic cells, as such nuclei have been found in all stages of granular disintegration within these cells. Leukocytes, lymphocytes, plasma cells and red cells were very numerous in these smears. In the first smear typical endothelial cells were relatively rare as compared with the second to sixth smears and they increased in number progressively in the subsequent smear, whereas the disturbing granulation outside of the cells became progressively less. The endothelial cells were easily recognized by their pale bluish protoplasm and their nucleus characterized by compact chromatin and several distinct blue staining nucleoli. Whereas these nucleoli are absent in the mature endothelial leukocytes and the chromatin of its nucleus forms a fine network, frequent transitional forms between the two were met with. Red cells and reddish granulations were found in both but the large majority of the endothelial cells showed only little reddish granulation or none at all, but not infrequently they contained dark blue and often greenish refractile granules. Whereas in single, well isolated and flatly spread out endothelial cells, the protoplasm was nearly homogenous showing only indistinct protoplasmic structure, in masses of not isolated cells a network of coarse dark blue staining structure was often seen, simulating occasionally large masses of accumulated bacilliform microorganisms.

In the smears of the first animal we found already typical endothelial cells containing an enormous number of a minute diplobacillus. This intracellular diplobacillus has been found quite easily in the smears of all twenty animals examined. In some smears these infected cells were so numerous that an examination of one to two minutes was sufficient to find them, in other smears ten to twenty minutes had to be spent before detecting them. They generally were so numerous within these cells as to completely fill their protoplasm and individual organism could only be recognized well at the margin of the cell where they frequently were found outside of the plasma, liberated because of the rupture of the latter. On account of the enormous number of this intracellular organism such heavily infected cells did not spread out on the slides as did normal or scantily infected cells, they rather ruptured. Other endothelial cells contained relatively few bacilli, distributed more or less evenly over the protoplasm or seldom collecting in small round or unequal shaped masses simulating colonies. Frequently they were arranged side by side not unlike diphtheroids. The individual diplobacilli exhibited as a rule a striking uniformity in respect to size, form and coloration within the same smear. They could best be studied when found outside of a ruptured cell. They were composed of two short rods separated by an often barely visible unstained space. The ends of the rods were rounded or less frequently bluntly pointed at both ends. Frequently there was no separation into the two segments visible and all transitions could be seen occasionally between a slender single bacillus and the diploform composed of the fragments. Generally the two fragments were joined end to end in a straight line, but pairs joined at an obtuse angle were not unfrequent.

Other endothelial cells were found containing a slightly larger bacillus. This bacillus frequently exhibited a decided polar staining and slightly lanceolated ends. The ends were stained blue or purplish whereas the intermediate line took a pale blue or was barely stained if at all. Such forms were found frequently with the diplobacillary form outside of ruptured endothelial cells. The diplobacillary forms usually stained reddish or purplish, the larger forms staining a deeper blue. The staining, however, was largely influenced by extrinsic conditions, as coloration of the protoplasm of the cells they were included in, length of staining and length of fixation. For instance, the diplobacilli, when massed compactly within a cell, almost without exception stained a light purple, whereas when lying isolated in or outside of the plasma they frequently stained blue. Cells containing very large numbers of bacilli could easily be traced under low magnification because the light purple stain dominated the whole protoplasm and frequently the outlines of the nucleus could not be made out under low power. Prolonged fixation of the smears with methyl alcohol resulted in a decided blue staining of the bacilli and their size was decidedly smaller. Twice a large filamentous form, staining a pale blue, was found alone in an endothelial cell, and occasionally pale, slender bacilli containing round blue or purplish staining granules were found outside of cells. Interesting information was gained by the examination of unfixed smears stained with Giemsa's solution. In such smears the diplo-arrangement of the bacilli was sometimes abolished, as was not infrequently the bipolar staining of the larger single forms; or the diplo-form was preserved but separation by a small unstained space was not complete because the pair was joined by a barely perceptible paler staining intermediate zone. Also the size of the bacilli was affected by not fixing the smears because they were found decidedly thicker and larger when not treated with alcohol. When lying isolated within the cells they also stained blue like the diplo-form in fixed preparations and like the latter had a tendency to stain a light purple when crowded in dense masses. Only exceptionally these bacilli were found within endothelial leukocytes and polynuclear leukocytes. The granulation of these cells did not disturb their recognition as these intracellular parasites never were granular and did not resemble cocci. Their outlines were always quite distinct and clear cut along the sides and an indistinct contour was only noticed at the place where the two segments of the pair joined. Their form and staining were so typical that they could always be easily recognized when found outside of cells.

Extracellular bodies have always been found evenly distributed in the smears, generally in scarce numbers, occasionally so numerous that they could be found in every field of the oil immersion. At the beginning I thought that they were derived from cells destroyed during the preparations of the smears. This assumption was abandoned because smears containing very numerous extracellular forms frequently contained only a few parasitical endothelial cells; whereas smears containing large numbers of these cells showed only scarce extracellular bacilli. This finding of larger numbers of extracellular bacilli in smears containing fewer intracellular ones as compared with smears containing numerous parasitized cells, indicates that these bacilli were liberated within the tissues by spontaneous rupture of the cells—as in the stomach of the louse—and that the intracellular masses of these parasites could probably best be found during the beginning of scrotal involvement.

The study of our protocols revealed that the most numerous intracellular parasites have been found in animals killed at a time when the scrotal swelling was in its beginning and that the most numerous extracellular forms associated with rare intracellular ones were found in animals killed after the first day of swelling. There was an exception to this apparent rule.

Animal 64 was killed on the fourth day of fever. The moderate scrotal swelling in this animal had fluctuated since the fever had started and this fluctuation was accompanied by slight increase or decrease of the fever. On the fourth day the fever rose suddenly to 106 F. and a pronounced edema began to appear over the scrotum when it was killed. Smears from the tunica revealed numerous endothelial cells crowded with parasites, and many extracellular parasites, lying in some places of the smear evenly distributed and in some places collected in large clusters.

A close study of a large number of these parasitical cells revealed that cells which were filled to rupture with these bacilli nearly invariably contained the minute diplobacillary form; whereas in scantily infected cells the larger rods frequently exhibiting bipolar staining was met with. But occasionally cells containing both were seen. One cell, for instance, contained a large number of densely packed minute red staining diplobacillary forms, among which the large blue staining rods were evenly distributed in small numbers. Giemsa's stain seems to be the only reliable stain for these microorganisms. They are gram-negative. This conclusion was drawn because we only were able to find them occasionally in smears stained by this method, and then as very pale, slender, single rods. Prolonged staining with hematoxylin stained them a pale grayish blue but they were found only after diligent search with this method. Other staining fluids generally used in bacteriological work stained them unsatisfactorily. These bacilli are not dissolved in the dried smears by distilled water because in smears stained with Giemsa's

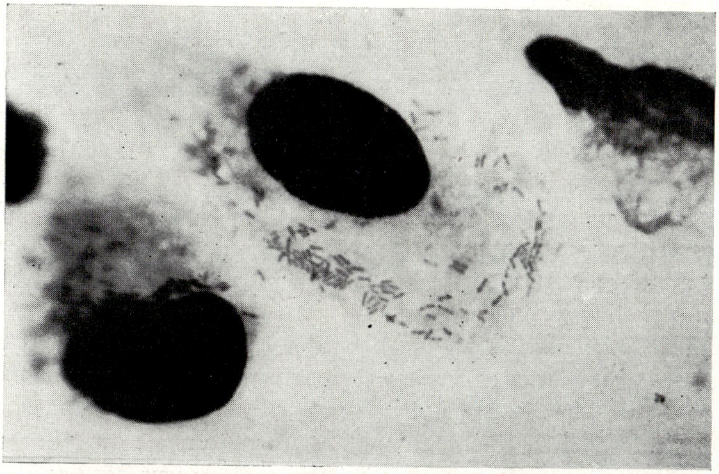

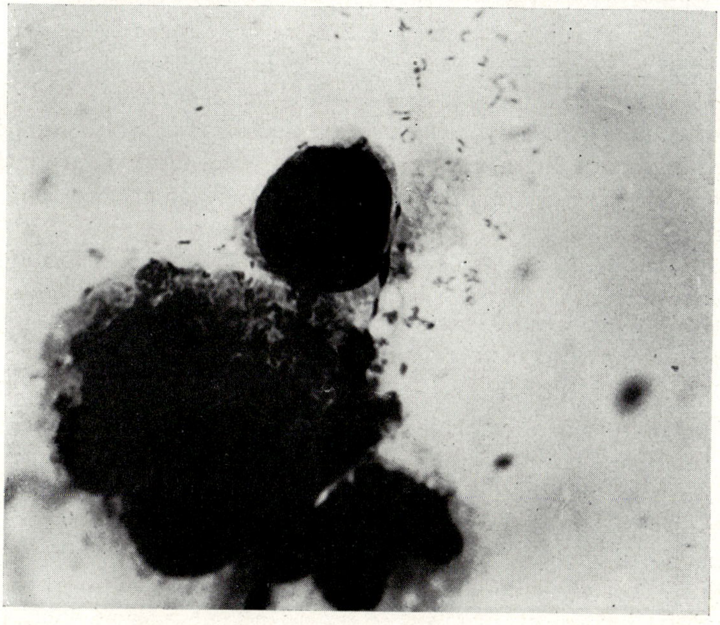

Fig. 1.—Scantily infected cells containing the relatively large bipolar-staining bacilli.

Fig. 2.—Heavily infected cell containing the smaller diplobacillus. Some bacilli were liberated by a scratch of the cell suffered when the smear was made.

solution, without previous alcohol fixation, they always were demonstrated easily as mentioned above. Unfixed smears have some advantage over fixed smears. They gave generally a clear background without granulations and many albuminous intracellular granulations were dissolved by the distilled water or stained only poorly. It was necessary, however, to apply this method only after thoroughly drying the smears because the protoplasm of endothlial cells, if not thoroughly dried, took such a dark blue coloration that the small diplobacilli frequently could not be seen satisfactorily. Of course, in fixed preparations, the cells looked prettier and their changes due to the infection with these parasites was only studied in fixed smears. Nucleus and protoplasm of scarcely infected endothelial cells looked normal. In heavily infected cells the protoplasm of the latter as a rule was found to be completely homogenous staining a pale blue. Frequently, however, their protoplasm seemed to be completely dissolved because nothing could be made out of it within the cell membrane. Where only a part of the cell was heavily infected, fading of the staining properties and more or less complete vacuolization of the whole cell protoplasm was noticed. Nuclear changes as a rule were also found only in heavily infected cells. They consisted in more or less complete indistinctness of the nucleoli and collecting of the chromatin around the nucleoli, and around small intranuclear vacuoles and towards the nuclear membrane. These cellular changes of protoplasm and nucleus was a common finding in our smears and was not found to be directly dependent on parasites as large numbers of such cells were found to be free of bacilli.

THE SPECIFICITY OF THE DIPLOBACILLI

From our former experiments we knew that the tissues of the proliferated tunica of animals inoculated with the supposed virus of typhus harbored a considerable quantity of it: 0.05 cc. of clear fluid collected from that part of the body conveyed the typical disease to guinea-pigs, and the involuntary autoinoculation of the writer with such material furnished clear evidence of its most infectious nature.* We thought that if we were able to demonstrate the diplobacilli within the highly infectious edematous fluid collecting in the tissues of the scrotum, especially beneath the tunica cremasterica, this would furnish considerable evidence that they are the causative agent of typhus.

* Recently one of my assistants who was making transfers of the virus and examining the tunica microscopically, came down with typhus. This occurred in May when typhus is not epidemic in Mexico City.

A little more than 0.1 cc. which could be collected from an animal with pronounced scrotal swelling was diluted with 2 cc. of salt solution. The mixture was then centrifugated at 1,000 revolutions per minute for one minute. The fluid became completely clear and after carefully removing three quarters of it without touching the wall of the tube with the pipet, no cells could be found in a drop deposited in the counting chamber. Smears made from the deposit in the tube used for centrifugation revealed mostly red cells, a few polynuclears and endothelial leukocytes and very few typical pale blue staining diplobacilli. The clear fluid was then injected intraperitoneally into a young male guinea-pig (57). The course of the disease in this animal is as follows:

January 28	29	30	31	February 1	2	3	4	5	6
102.6 F.*	102.4	102.4	102.2	102	102.4	102.6	102.8	104.8†	105.4‡

* Inoculated. † Scrotum swollen. ‡ Scrotum more swollen; guinea-pig killed.

Necropsy of this animal, guinea-pig 57, was completely negative with the exception of the pronounced hemorrhagic condition of the tunica and testicles and a large subcutaneous hemorrhage extending from the scrotum over the abdomen. Cultures from spleen, heart blood and tunica proved to be sterile. The histological examination of testicles, tunica and brain revealed the typical lesions of typhus. Smears from the tunica revealed large numbers of heavily infected endothelial cells. An emulsion of tunica from this animal was injected into male guinea-pig 61, heart blood into male guinea-pig 62 and an emulsion of brain into male guinea-pig 63. The following chart demonstrates the course of the disease in these three animals:

	Guinea-pig 61	Guinea-pig 62	Guinea-pig 63
Feb. 6	102.4, inoculated with emulsion of tunica	101.6, inoculated with blood	102.8, inoculated with brain
7	102.2	102.2	102.6
8	102.4	102	102.4
9	102.6	102.6	102.8
10	104.8, scrotum swollen	102.2	102
11	105.2, scrotum very swollen	102.6	102.2
12	106	102.8	102.2
13	105.2, killed	104, scrotum swollen	105, scrotum swollen
14		104.6, scrotum swollen	103.8, swelling disappeared
15		105, scrotum very swollen	105.2, scrotum very swollen
16		105, killed	105.4, killed

At necropsy these animals were completely negative with the exception of the typical scrotal and testicular lesions. Cultures from spleens, blood and tunicas were sterile. Diplobacilli were found in the tunica of these three animals and the typical nodular lesions, though scarce in number, were found in the brains of all three.

Controls.—Smears made with scrapings from both tunicas of two healthy male guinea-pigs, of two guinea-pigs several weeks after infection, and from the parietal peritoneum of three animals killed during the height of the experimental infection were stained with Giemsa's solution and carefully searched for intracellular bacilliform bodies. Nothing could be found that would have only remotely looked like the described diplobacilli inside and outside of cells. In the smears made from the tunica of the animals six weeks and two months, respectively, after infection, lymphocytes, plasma cells and endothelial cells containing freshly phagocytized red cells could still be found. Endothelial leukocytes containing large round masses of densely packed reddish granules were still present in quite large numbers in these cells. The injection of an emulsion of the tunica did not produce fever, scrotal swelling or immunity in the inoculated animals. Blue staining granules resembling sometimes closely coccoid bodies were also found within endothelial cells.

Cultures from the Tunica.—Large numbers of inoculations were made in different mediums, fluid, semifluid and solid, containing blood, serum and plasma from man, rabbit, guinea-pig and horse, and egg albumen with and without addition of yolk. Most of them were kept under aerobic conditions, but frequently we kept them under partial oxygen tension and under anaerobic conditions. With the exception of two instances in which a diphtheroid bacillus developed, in only one tube of a series of twelve inoculated ones, these cultures proved to be sterile.

DISCUSSION

The constant finding of an intracellular minute diplobacillus in the smears of our animals reacting to the virus of Mexican typhus and its absence in smears from the tunica of normal animals and animals recovered from the experimental infection is highly suggestive that these bacilliform bodies are the cause of tabardillo. The demonstration that edematous fluid freed of cells was highly infectious causing the typical experimental disease in guinea-pigs and that these small diplobacilli could be found, and only these, in the sediment of such fluid in our opinion furnishes considerable evidence of the correctness of our point of view. The enormous multiplication of these microorganisms within the endothelial cells of the tunica causing considerable extension and finally rupture of the cells gave pictures highly simulating the infected epithelial cells of the stomach of lice containing the virus of typhus. I am not in the position to discuss on the entity of these bacilli and Rickettsia prowazeki as I never had the opportunity to study infected lice.

The different forms found, however, in the tunica of our animals resemble so closely the form found by Rocha Lima and other investigators of infected lice that their identity is highly suggestive. Wolbach, Todd and Palfrey [2] are of the opinion that the different forms found by them in sections of lice represent different stages of the development of the same microorganism. They found that in scarcely infected epithelial cells of the louse they were always bacilliform, whereas in heavily infected cells they found the minute coccoid form. We found a similar behavior of these parasites within the tunica of our animals. In scarcely infected cells the larger bacilliform rods were the rule, whereas in heavily infected cells the minute diplobacillus was present. In addition to these two forms we found forms first described by Ricketts and Wilder [3] and since then considered to be the type form of Rickettsia—small bacilliform bodies exhibiting bipolar, slightly metachromatic staining, and even larger forms of pale staining bacilli including darker staining around granules. These forms have heretofore only been described in lice and their presence within mammalian tissue in our opinion supports the Rickettsia theory of typhus. In addition we found the filamentous form heretofore found only in the epithelial cells of the gut of the infected lice.

The possibility that the described diplobacilli are not the causitive agent but a mere secondary invader was carefully considered at the beginning of our work. The failure of cultivating them with the help of all possible devised and not yet devised mediums, although very suggestive, of course does not exclude such a possibility. Olitsky [4] found that the typhus infection readily opens the door to secondary infections in guinea-pigs. My own observations do not concur with the findings of this investigator. Our strain is at present in the 18th passage carried along in more than one hundred animals and although we always have practiced a blood culture and frequent cultures from the spleens, we have only once been able to demonstrate a secondary invader. During the past seven years we have worked with a large number of blood cultures from cases of typhus and in no instance did we get any growth from such cultures when they had been taken by us personally, and we are convinced that secondary infections are not more frequent in typhus than they are in other acute febrile systemic infections. Indeed a negative blood culture in the first days of a serious looking disease, with high fever, in our experience in Mexico City, is suspicious of typhus. There is no doubt in our minds that these described rods are really microorganisms. Only exceptionally have they been seen as filaments like mitochondria and never as granules like normal and pathological cell constituents. Moreover, their form and shape have never been found to be affected by serious damage suffered by the

3. J. Am. M. A., 1910, 54, p. 1373.
4. Memorias del segundo congreso nacional del tabardillo, Mexico City, 1922.

including cells. They looked exactly alike in scarcely infected cells showing no signs of degeneration, and in heavily infected cells whose protoplasm and nucleus exhibited the marks of almost complete disintegration. The evidences forwarded in this paper for the specificity of this diplobacillus are numerous and serious ones: constant presence in animals reacting to the virus of typhus; absence in normal animals, and in recovered animals; presence within endothelial cells of tissues exhibiting the specific lesions of typhus; absence in endothelial cells of the same animals not exhibiting these specific lesions; high specific infectiousness of the pathological tissues in which they invariably could be found, and their failure to grow on artificial mediums.

The observation of large numbers of extracellular diplobacilli in our smears indicates that they are able to live at least temporarily outside of the cells. Multiplication, however, seems to take place in living cells only. In our previous publication on tabardillo in guinea-pigs we forwarded evidence that the virus of typhus multiplies abundantly within the endothelial cells of the tunica vaginalis during the incubation period. The presence of large numbers of heavily infected endothelial cells on the first day of fever, at a time when no conspicuous lesions can be found in other organs, hardly permits another explanation. So long as these microorganisms are intracellular they only cause swelling and proliferation of the infected cells, but once liberated by rupture of the heavily infected cells, they are spread into the connective tissue and into the blood immediately, in large numbers, causing sudden extensive local reaction and sudden appearance of fever. They are distributed as extracellular forms through the blood stream and invade secondarily the endothelial cells of all organs to repeat there the same play.

SUMMARY

A minute intracellular diplobacillus has been demonstrated in sections and smears of the proliferated tunica vaginalis of guinea-pigs reacting to the virus of Mexican typhus (tabardillo). Considerable evidence is forwarded that this diplobacillus is the causative agent of typhus.

RECENT CASES OF UNDULANT FEVER IN NEW YORK STATE

RUTH GILBERT AND MARION B. COLEMAN

From the Division of Laboratories and Research, New York State Department of Health, Albany

In recent years there have been reports from a number of districts in the United States, of the occurrence of undulant fever where it was known that the patients had neither had contact with goats, nor used goats' milk or its products. Of 213 blood specimens, received during the past two years from cases with continued fever, which gave no reaction with Bacillus typhosus, 16 agglutinated organisms of the abortus-melitensis group in a dilution of 1:40 or higher. So little information was obtained concerning 5 of the patients that, although the symptoms reported suggested undulant fever, their histories have not been included in this study. At the branch laboratory in New York City Miss Langworthy and Miss Owen have studied 17 specimens, two of which agglutinated organisms of the abortus-melitensis group in a dilution of 1:40 or higher. An investigation of the cases from which these were obtained has indicated a diagnosis of undulant fever. Nineteen blood specimens also were received to be examined for evidence of undulant fever. Of these, 6 gave a definite reaction. In addition 2 cases of infection were incurred in the course of laboratory work, one with a strain of B. melitensis and the other with a strain of B. abortus.

Thus, there was an opportunity to make a limited study of 26 cases in which the clinical manifestations and laboratory findings indicated diagnoses of undulant fever. A summary of the clinical histories follows.*

Case 1.—That of a man, 33 years of age, resident in Lewis County. Serum was collected three months after the onset of illness. It agglutinated B. abortus in a dilution of 1:640 and B. melitensis in a dilution of 1:160. This case was mild but of 4 or 5 months' duration. The patient was able to attend to business, but complained of being tired and showed a loss of 20 pounds in weight. He was seen only occasionally by his physician. Other symptoms reported were a high pulse rate, a temperature at times of 101 F., night sweats, and, on one occasion, the left knee was sensitive and painful for 2 days. Cows' milk, raw, was used by the patient's household. The occurrence of abortion in the herd from which this was obtained was not determined. A few months later a specimen of citrated blood was submitted from the patient's brother, who was reported by his attending physician to have developed a similar illness. No organisms other than those obviously due to contamination were found. No other specimens were sent.

Case 2.—That of a woman, 20 years of age, resident in Saratoga County. A specimen of serum was submitted by the director of a local laboratory to be examined for evidence of

Received for publication, May 2, 1928.

* Since this report was prepared, 9 other cases have come to our attention in each of which the clinical manifestations and the agglutination with blood specimens have indicated a diagnosis of undulant fever.

undulant fever. Definite agglutination of B. melitensis was obtained in a dilution of 1: 80 and of B. abortus in a dilution of 1: 160. The leukocyte count, which was made in the sanatorium in which she was employed, was reported to be between 3,000 and 4,000 per cubic millimeter. The duration of the illness was about 2 weeks, 5 days being spent in the infirmary. The symptoms at onset were vomiting, pain in the abdomen, and weakness, following which the patient fainted. Constipation was noted throughout the illness. The highest temperature recorded was 101 F. She had apparently had no contact with animals and had drunk no raw milk except that used in her coffee. It was learned, however, that 5 of the cows in the herd from which the milk was obtained, had aborted within a few months previously. Specimens of milk and blood were obtained from the two cows which had aborted most recently, and B. abortus was isolated from the milk of one. The serums of both agglutinated a stock strain of B. abortus in a dilution of 1: 250 and the strain of B. abortus isolated from the milk, in a dilution of 1: 1,000. The patient's serum also agglutinated this strain of B. abortus in a dilution of 1: 500.

Case 3.—That of a man, 26 years of age, resident in Erie County. The disease continued 4 months. The patient had been ill 1 month at the time the first specimen of blood was examined and found to agglutinate B. melitensis in a dilution of 1: 160. The symptoms were headache, gurgling, chills, constipation, enlarged and tender spleen, profuse night sweats, temperature from 98.4 F. in the morning to 102 F. in the evening. The physician reported a leukocyte count of 5,200 per cubic millimeter. The patient had had no contact with goats nor had he ever knowingly drunk goats' milk. Raw cows' milk had been taken in small quantities, but none of the herds from which the milk was obtained for use in his household showed contagious abortion. The patient had traveled about the state, however, and had taken the usual small quantities of milk as occasion required.

Case 4.—That of a woman, 34 years of age, resident in Columbia County. Serum collected 6 weeks after the onset of illness agglutinated B. melitensis in a dilution of 1: 640. The leukocyte count was 6,600 per cubic millimeter, with 63% lymphocytes. The patient first had a mild attack of what was diagnosed as grip, having a temperature of from 100 to 101 F. for 6 days. She then seemed well, but 2 days later her temperature rose to 103 F. and she complained of headache, malaise, slight cough, pains in the back and extremities, and some constipation. At no time were there any sweats and there had been no arthritis. Occasional chilly sensations occurred. For 5 weeks the temperature varied from 99 to 100 F., usually down in the morning and up in the afternoon. The impression was that she was only moderately ill. The physical examination showed normal conditions. The x-ray revealed a slight cloudiness in the apex of the right lung, but it was not considered evidence of tuberculosis. This study was made about 6 weeks after the onset of the illness. The outcome of the case was not learned. The patient had never knowingly drunk goats' milk. She used cows' milk in average quantities. The milk was said to have been purchased at various stores.

Case 5.—That of a woman, 20 years of age, resident in Albany County. The duration of the illness was 10 weeks. This was a case of infection contracted in a laboratory, the organism having undoubtedly been ingested while the patient was pipetting. B. melitensis was agglutinated by the serum in a dilution of 1: 160 on the 12th day of illness and in a dilution of 1: 1,280 4 weeks later. Definite agglutination of B. typhosus was also obtained in a dilution of 1: 320. The patient had been inoculated with typhoid-paratyphoid vaccine 2 years previously. Four months later her serum had been tested and no agglutination had been obtained with B. typhosus. Repeated cultural examinations of feces and urine failed to show any typhoid bacilli. B. melitensis was isolated from a specimen of blood collected during the 2d pyrexial period. It is interesting to note that only 2 colonies of this organism developed. This examination was made by pipetting 0.5 cc. of citrated blood onto each of 8 plates, 4 containing blood agar and 4 dextrose serum agar. Half of the plates were incubated in an atmosphere of about 10% carbon dioxide, and the other half under the usual aerobic conditions. Several liver infusion agar slants were also inoculated and incubated with the plates. Seven days after inoculation, no growth was observed on any of the media. Four days later, one colony was found on a dextrose serum agar plate incubated aerobically, and 1 colony on a blood agar plate incubated under partial carbon dioxide tension. Transfers of these colonies showed definite growth in 24 hours, and the cultural and serologic characteristics corresponded with those of the strain of B. melitensis with which the patient had been working. No growth other than that obviously due to contamination was found in any of the other cultures. From a specimen of urine collected 10 days after the onset of illness and from guinea-pigs inoculated with a specimen of urine collected 6 months later, an organism was isolated which had the morphologic and cultural characteristics of B. melitensis, but which was not agglutinated in serums immune to this organism. The guinea-pigs from which the 2d culture was obtained were autopsied 11 weeks after inoculation, and were found to have enlarged nodular spleens and enlarged retroperitoneal glands. Blood counts made on the 12th and 17th days of the patient's illness showed 6,800 and 4,800 leukocytes per cubic millimeter, with 42% and 30.2% lymphocytes, respectively. The onset of the disease was sudden, with severe frontal headache and fever. A physician, called on the 2d day, made a diagnosis of influenza. After 5 days, the temperature had returned to normal and the patient felt able to be about the house, although she was weak and had no appetite. On the 10th day, there was a rise in temperature and she returned to bed. The temperature varied from 100 to 104 F. for 8 days, after which it gradually returned to normal. There were no more relapses. The symptoms noted were headache, profuse sweating, constipation, prostration and depression. Ten weeks after onset the patient was able to return to her duties at the laboratory. At the end of 10 months, her weight had returned to normal and she felt well, but tired much more easily than formerly.

Case 6.—That of a man, 47 years of age, resident in Albany County. The duration of the illness was 2 months. A specimen of blood collected about 1 month after the onset agglutinated B. melitensis in a dilution of 1: 1,280, and B. abortus in a dilution of 1: 2,500. The onset was sudden, with urticaria and fever. The temperature varied from 100 to 103 F., with 1 remission about 10 days after the onset. The other complaints were marked constipation and distention, as well as profuse night sweats. The urticaria cleared up in a few days, but the other symptoms persisted. The patient was able to return to his business about 10 weeks after the date of onset. About 1 year previous to this illness, the patient had had a nervous breakdown and at that time was advised by his physician to build up his general health by a liberal diet, 1 of the chief items of which was milk. After that, he drank from 3 to 6 glasses of milk a day. At times, the milk was purchased from a dealer, but for the most part was obtained from a cow which he had purchased about 16 months previously. The cow's serum agglutinated B. abortus in a dilution of 1: 40 only. In the cultural examination of 6 samples of milk, no B. abortus was found. Fifteen guinea-pigs were inoculated with these specimens and only 1 showed any evidence of infection. In the latter the spleen was enlarged and nodular. A culture was obtained from the spleen which was found to have the morphologic and cultural characteristics of B. abortus, but which was not agglutinated in serum immune to this organism. Moreover, other guinea-pigs inoculated with emulsions of the spleen and liver did not show any abnormalities when autopsied 8 weeks later.

Case 7.—That of a man, 30 years of age, resident in Steuben County. The duration of the illness was 3 months. Serum collected about 2 weeks after the date of the onset agglutinated B. melitensis in a dilution of 1: 1,280 and 6 weeks later definitely agglutinated the bacillus in a dilution of 1: 160 only. The symptoms reported were fever, tenderness in the right iliac region, gurgling, palpable spleen, bronchitis, chills and sweating. No information as to the probable sources of the infection could be obtained.

Case 8.—That of a man, 23 years of age, resident in Cattaraugus County. A specimen of serum was submitted by the bacteriologist in charge of the county laboratory, 3 weeks after the onset of the illness. B. melitensis was agglutinated in a dilution of 1: 320. A report of this case has already been made.[1] Raw milk had been used from a herd in which abortions

1. Fisher, M. E., and J. P. Garen: N. Y. State J. M., 1927, 27, p. 706.

had occurred.

Case 9.—That of a man, 27 years of age, resident in Orange County. Serum from the patient was submitted for the agglutination test with typhoid bacilli by the bacteriologist in charge of the St. Luke's Hospital Pathological Laboratory, Newburgh, New York. Agglutination of B. melitensis was obtained in a dilution of 1: 320. Since this man was connected with the quartermaster's department at the West Point Military Reservation, he was transferred to the government hospital as soon as the result of this examination was known. From a memorandum by Dr. F. W. Laidlaw, district state health officer, it was learned that the results of our tests were confirmed at the Hygienic Laboratory in Washington. The clinical course was stated to be indefinite, with a nightly rise of temperature, a low leukocyte count, and the chest, in x-ray examination, normal.

Case 10.—That of a man, 30 years of age, resident in Albany County. The illness lasted 3 or 4 weeks. This was a case of infection incurred in a laboratory. While autopsying a guinea-pig 6 days previous to the observation of the first symptoms, the patient cut his finger with a broken glass push pin which had been used to fasten the animal to the board. This guinea-pig was infected with a virulent strain of B. abortus of bovine origin. Serum collected 1 week after the first symptoms were noted, gave agglutination of B. melitensis and B. abortus in a dilution of 1: 80. The patient's serum had been previously tested with these organisms and no reaction had been obtained. No growth was obtained on cultural examination of the blood. The leukocyte count was 4,000, with 51% lymphocytes. The symptoms complained of were general muscular pains, stiff neck, pain in the eyes, nausea and headache. The patient remained at home only 1 week. The temperature was not taken regularly, but when determined it was found to be within normal limits.

Case 12.—That of a man, 28 years of age, resident in Oneida County. A specimen of collected 4 weeks after the onset of the illness, agglutinated B. melitensis and B. abortus in a dilution of 1: 1,280. Profuse sweating, chills, fever and a moderately high pulse rate were the symptoms reported. The patient was still in the hospital 6 weeks after the onset. The outcome of the case was not reported. The physician stated that there was a history of at least 3 abortions among this farmer's cows during the year previous to his illness.

Case 12.—That of a man, 28 years of age, resident in Oneida County. A specimen of blood was submitted by the director of the Faxton Hospital Laboratory in Utica. Agglutination of B. melitensis was obtained in a dilution of 1: 640, and of B. abortus in a dilution of 1: 1,280. A leukocyte count of 4,000 was reported. On August 16, 17 and 18 the patient was ill in bed, with a temperature of about 100 F. The illness was diagnosed as grip. He returned to work on the 19th of August and felt well until September 6. He was then kept in bed for 5 weeks, with a temperature ranging from 99.1 F. in the morning to 102 or 103 F. in the evening. The only other symptom noted was constipation. No recurrence of fever has been reported. The milk used in this man's household was from the same dairy as that used by the patient in case 18. Occurrence of abortions in the herd was not determined.

Case 13.—That of a man, 47 years of age, resident in Wayne County. Serum collected 2 weeks after the onset of the illness agglutinated both B. melitensis and B. abortus in a dilution of 1: 1,280. The symptoms reported were headache, chills, sweating, severe backache and some constipation. The temperature ranged from 99 to 104.6 F. The patient drank raw cows' milk from a herd in which cows were found (by Carpenter[2]) to be heavily infected with B. abortus.

Case 14.—That of a man, 46 years of age, resident in Wayne County. Serum collected 2 weeks after the onset of the illness agglutinated B. melitensis in a dilution of 1: 1,280 and

2. Personal communication, Jan. 4, 1928.

B. abortus in a dilution of 1: 320. The symptoms reported were headache, chills, sweating and severe backache. The temperature ranged from 100 to 103 F. The patient drank raw cows' milk from the same source as the patient in case 13.

Case 15.—That of a boy, 5 years of age, resident in Wayne County. Serum collected about 3 weeks after the onset of the illness agglutinated B. melitensis in a dilution of 1: 160, and B. abortus in a dilution of 1: 320. The symptoms reported were headache, chills, sweating and constipation. The temperature ranged from 99 to 104.6 F. The patient drank raw cows' milk from the same source as the patient in case 13.

Case 16.—That of a woman, 55 years of age, resident in Chautauqua County. Serum collected about 3 weeks after the onset of the illness agglutinated B. abortus and B. melitensis in a dilution of 1: 320. The symptoms reported were headache, chills, sweating, fever, rose spots (?), diarrhea, gurgling and weakness. The patient, who lives on a farm, used raw milk from her own cows. Agglutination tests made with serums from the cows, indicated that one of them was heavily infected with B. abortus. Unfortunately, samples of milk could not be secured for bacteriologic examination.

Case 17.—That of a woman, 28 years of age, resident in Oneida County. Serum collected about 6 weeks after the onset of the illness agglutinated B. melitensis in a dilution of 1: 320, and B. abortus in a dilution of 1: 640. The symptoms reported were chills, sweating, arthritis, enlarged spleen, somewhat enlarged lymph glands, rash, constipation, and slight bronchitis and râles at the base of the right lung, heard posteriorly. The temperature ranged from 99 to 104 F. The patient drank raw cows' milk, but so far as her physician could learn, there had been no abortion in the herd from which this was obtained.

Case 18.—That of a man, 43 years of age, resident in Oneida County. Serum collected about 3 months after the onset of illness agglutinated B. abortus and B. melitensis in a dilution of 1: 320. The symptoms reported were headache, chills, sweating, enlarged spleen, constipation, lung involvement and depression. The temperature ranged from 98.6 to 103 F. The patient drank raw cows' milk. No information concerning abortion in the herd from which this was obtained could be secured.

Case 19.—That of a man, 60 years of age, resident in Chautauqua County. In a specimen of serum collected 5 weeks after the onset of illness, agglutination of B. abortus and of B. melitensis was obtained in a dilution of 1: 1,280. The symptoms reported were headache, febrile reaction, nosebleed, diarrhea, delirium, gurgling, palpable spleen and sweating. The patient drank raw cows' milk. Abortions were reported to have occurred in the herd from which this was obtained.

Case 20.—That of a man, 56 years of age, resident in Suffolk County. The illness continued for 3½ months. In a specimen of serum collected 6 weeks after the onset of the illness, agglutination was obtained with B. melitensis in a dilution of 1: 320 and with B. abortus in a dilution of 1: 640. B. typhosus was also agglutinated in a dilution of 1: 80. A blood count made 10 days later showed 6,100 leukocytes, with 56% lymphocytes. The onset was sudden, with severe frontal headache, general malaise, chilly sweats, anorexia and constipation. The temperature ranged from 99.5 F. at 9: 00 a. m. to 101-102 F. at 9: 00 p. m. The symptoms persisted for 2 months and then gradually disappeared except that the patient still complained of weakness 3½ months after the onset. It was learned that the patient had drunk raw cows' milk and that abortions had occurred in the herd from which this was obtained. B. abortus was isolated from guinea-pigs inoculated with milk from 2 of the cows, and definite agglutination of this organism was obtained in the serum of 1 of them in a dilution of 1: 320, and in that of the other in a dilution of 1: 80. These data were collected at the branch laboratory in New York City.

Case 21.—That of a man, 48 years of age, resident in Orange County. Serum collected about 4 weeks after the onset of the illness agglutinated B. melitensis in a dilution of 1: 160, and B. abortus in a dilution of 1: 320. The symptoms reported were: variable temperature, sweating, neuralgia and weakness. The outcome of this case was not determined, but the duration was at least 7 weeks. These data were collected at the branch laboratory in New York City.

It will be noted that cases have occurred in 13 counties in various sections of the state. In all except one case, agglutination of B. abortus or B. melitensis was obtained in a dilution of serum 1 : 160 or higher. In serum of case 12 a marked proagglutinoid zone was observed. No agglutination of B. abortus was noted in the dilutions ranging from 1 : 10 through 1 : 160; a partial reaction occurred in the dilution of 1 : 320, and definite agglutination in that of 1 : 640 and in that of 1 : 1280. B. melitensis was only partially agglutinated in the dilution of 1 : 40 and was definitely agglutinated in dilutions ranging from 1 : 80 through 1 : 640. This phenomenon was observed frequently, but in no other instance to such a marked degree. In 3 cases (5, 10, and 20) definite agglutination was obtained with typhoid bacilli in dilutions of 1 : 320, 1 : 40, and 1 : 80, respectively. Two of these cases (5 and 10) were infections incurred in the course of laboratory work. Both patients had received typhoid vaccine within the previous 2 years. The other (see case 20) may have had a double infection or a previous undiagnosed case of typhoid fever. In this case, laboratory examinations were not made until about 6 weeks after the onset of the illness when repeated examinations failed to show typhoid bacilli in feces or urine. The fact that this patient's serum agglutinated B. melitensis in a dilution of 1 : 320 and B. abortus in a dilution of 1 : 640, and that B. abortus was isolated from the cow's milk which was used in a raw state by the patient, indicates strongly a diagnosis of undulant fever, possibly as a secondary infection.

Fecal and urinary specimens from 10 patients were examined for organisms of the enteric group but none was found.

B. melitensis was isolated form 1 of 2 blood specimens collected in citrate solution from the patient in case 5. Evidently few of the organisms were present, since only 2 colonies developed on the plates. In the examination of similar specimens from 10 other cases, neither B. abortus nor B. melitensis was isolated. These results indicate that the organisms can seldom be isolated from the blood of a patient unless a series of specimens is examined.

A leukopenia with lymphocytosis was noted in the 5 instances in which blood counts were made.

The symptom complex corresponded with that reported by other workers,—sudden onset with severe headache, malaise, muscular pains, chills, profuse sweating, and constipation. The characteristic undulating fever was noted from 2 weeks to 5 months except in one case (10) in which no rise in temperature was observed at any time. In but 3 instances was a rash reported and this persisted for only a short period. There was enlargement of the spleen in 6 cases and involvement of the lungs or of the bronchi in four cases.

No history of contact with goats or swine was reported in any instance. The source of the milk supply of 14 of the patients was determined, and in every case raw milk had been used. In 9 of these instances, the milk used had been obtained from herds in which abortions had occurred, and B. abortus was isolated from the milk of cows belonging to 2 of the herds. Also, the serums from these cows agglutinated B. abortus; one in a dilution of 1:160, and the other in a dilution of 1:250.

In 3 cases (13, 14, and 15) which occurred in October and November, 1927, in a small city in the central part of the state, the patients had used raw milk from the same dairy. Blood specimens from 3 other patients in the same city, having similar symptoms, gave no agglutination with B. abortus and B. melitensis.* It seems probable that these illnesses also were undulant fever, since, as Carpenter [3] has pointed out, agglutination is not essential to such a diagnosis.

An interesting contrast in clinical manifestations is afforded by the two infections contracted in the laboratory. The mode of infection is not definitely known in case 5, but was probably by mouth. As may be seen from the case history, the illness, although of shorter duration than in some of the other cases reported, was severe. Cultural characteristics of the organism isolated from the blood stream and absorption tests made with the patient's serum indicated that the infection was due to a strain of B. melitensis with which she had been working. This strain had been isolated from a guinea-pig infected with human blood in 1922 at the Bureau of Animal Industry in Washington.[4] At present, it is pathogenic for guinea-pigs only when given in doses sufficiently large to produce a septicemia.

Case 10, the other infection incurred in the laboratory, was probably traumatic in origin. This was an unusually mild infection, which would not have been recognized but for the accident which was known to have occurred. The strain of B. abortus responsible for this infection induces typical tubercle-like lesions in guinea-pigs.

For purposes of comparison, 500 serums submitted for the complement-fixation test for syphilis were tested for agglutination with B. melitensis. Six of these or 1.2% gave a definite reaction in a dilution of 1:80 or higher. There were 3 which reacted in a dilution of 1:320. All efforts to obtain further information and specimens for confirmatory examination from these cases were unsuccessful. Ten of the serums tested reacted in a dilution of 1:40 only. No investigation of these cases was attempted. The proportion of definite reactions is somewhat higher than that reported by Evans [5] and by McAlpine and Mickle.[6]

* Specimens of blood which failed to agglutinate cultures of B. abortus or B. melitensis have been received from several other patients with clinical symptoms of undulant fever.

3. J. Infect. Dis., 1926 (Sept.), 39, p. 220.
4. J. Agric. Research, 1924, 29, p. 585.
5. Hygienic Laboratory Bulletin, 1925, 143.
6. Connecticut Health Bull., 1927, 41, p. 255.

The relative infrequency of agglutination of organisms of the abortus-melitensis group by serums of normal persons is of questionable significance, since it has been shown [3] that agglutinative properties may be entirely lacking in serums from patients with undulant fever.

CONCLUSIONS

This investigation demonstrates that cases of undulant fever are not uncommon and that they are distributed rather generally throughout New York State. In none of the cases studied, was there a history of contact of patient with goats or hogs, but 14 patients were known to have used raw cows' milk. In 9 instances, abortions were found to have occurred in the herds from which the milk was obtained. A consideration of the data available indicates 3 possible reasons why cases of undulant fever are not reported more frequently in districts where unpasteurized milk is used from herds in which contagious abortion is prevalent: Many of the severe infections have probably been diagnosed as atypical cases of typhoid fever, influenza, or even tuberculosis or malaria; mild forms may have presented so few symptoms that physicians have not been consulted; and the blood from some cases of undulant fever may not have agglutinated cultures of B. melitensis or B. abortus.

RHEUMATIC FEVER

2. ALLERGIC REACTIONS WITH A TOXIN-PRODUCING STRAIN OF THE NONMETHEMOGLOBIN-FORMING STREPTOCOCCUS ISOLATED FROM RHEUMATIC FEVER

KONRAD E. BIRKHAUG

From the Department of Bacteriology, the University of Rochester School of Medicine and Dentistry, Rochester, N. Y.

Recently, Birkhaug[1] described 68 strains of a streptococcus which failed to form methemoglobin, but which fermented inulin and remained insoluble in bile. These organisms were isolated from the blood, tonsils, feces, and apical dental abscesses of patients with rheumatic fever. When grown in tryptic digest broth, they produced a soluble toxic principle similar to the Dick toxin or the erysipelas toxin described by Birkhaug,[2] in that it produced typical lesions of the skin when injected intradermally into susceptible individuals. About 70 per cent of persons with a definite history of rheumatic fever reacted positively with this toxic principle when 0.1 cc. of a dilution of 1 : 100 was injected intradermally. Approximately 20 per cent of normal persons without a history of rheumatic fever gave positive reactions with the same dose. It was further demonstrated that when large doses of this toxin were injected intra-articularly and intramuscularly into an hypersensitive person, typical polyarthritis developed rapidly, which responded favorably to administration of salicylates. From these observations, I concluded that these reactions constituted "possibly a form of allergy in relation to the group of non-methemoglobin-forming streptococci associated with rheumatic fever."

These studies were further elaborated by Kaiser,[3] who performed intradermal tests with the toxic filtrate of the non-methemoglobin-forming streptococcus on 801 children. In this group, 72.2 per cent of the children with a definite history of rheumatic fever reacted strongly with 0.1 cc. of the toxin in a dilution of 1 : 100. On the other hand, only 20 per cent of the normal children, without any history of rheumatic fever or of repeated attacks of sore throat, reacted positively with a similar dose. In order to ascertain the degree of specificity of this test, Kaiser made parallel Schick and Dick tests on

Received for publication, May 24, 1928.

1. Proc. Soc. Exper. Biol. & Med., 1927, 24, p. 541; J. Infect. Dis., 1927, 40, p. 549.
2. Proc. Soc. Exper. Biol & Med., 1925, 23, p. 201.
3. J. Infect. Dis., 1928, 42, p. 25.

the same series of children. The results demonstrated that no correlation existed between these respective tests.

Swift, Derick, and Hitchcock,[4] also, confirmed the results obtained by Birkhaug[1] with the filtrates of the non-methemoglobin-forming streptococcus. In addition, these investigators found that most patients in the acute stages of rheumatic fever, and many who have apparently recovered, show a similar hypersensitiveness of the skin to filtrates of certain strains of Streptococcus viridans. This apparent overlapping may possibly be explained by the study of Clawson,[5] who found that his nonhemolytic streptococcic strains often produced green on transfers. As early as 1914, Holman[6] reported a similar observation and many workers have agreed or disagreed with the notion that certain mutations from one definite type of streptococcus to another type do occur. During two years' careful observation of about 200 strains of the non-methemoglobin-forming streptococcus isolated from rheumatic fever, I have not been able to find any indication that this form undergoes mutation to a typical Streptococcus viridans. A simpler explanation of the overlapping observed by Swift, Derick, and Hitchcock between the toxic filtrates of the non-methemoglobin-forming streptococcus and Streptococcus viridans might be that these organisms contain common allergenic properties. A better approach to this assumption might be made by the production of allergic reactions in man or animals with fractions of the respective bacterial cells.

A careful study of the ill-defined clinical picture of rheumatic fever makes it increasingly difficult to attribute the many variable manifestations of this disease to the action of a single microorganism. In a most comprehensive and elaborate critical review of rheumatism, Holman[7] has carefully outlined this uncertainty. Even the most generous critic must admit that the recent assertion by Small[8] that his Streptococcus cardioarthritidis is the specific cause of rheumatic fever, is based on meager experimental evidence.[9]

I sought to ascertain experimentally in animals the existence of a specific or nonspecific hyperallergic state responding to sensitization with the non-methemoglobin-forming streptococcus, an organism which is isolated quite readily from the throats of persons with rheumatic

4. J. Am. M. A., 1928, 90, p. 906.
5. J. Infect. Dis., 1925, 36, p. 444.
6. Ibid., 1914, 15, p. 293.
7. Arch. Path., 1928, 5, p. 68.
8. Am. J. M. Sc., 1927, 173, p. 101.
9. J. Am. M. A., 1927, 88, p. 326; ibid., p. 405 (editorials).

fever, and occasionally from the blood, dental abscesses, and feces of such persons. The possibility of sensitization of guinea-pigs and rabbits with streptococcic cultures and filtrates had been demonstrated by Davis,[10] who in 1913 attempted a biologic classification of streptococci by anaphylactic reactions. Zinsser[11] also had demonstrated the possibility of sensitizing animals with bacterial substances, and he observed subsequently that materials from the site of a bacterial infection played an important part in this. Zinsser and Mallory[12] further studied bacterial anaphylaxis with the pneumococcus and Zinsser and Grinnell[13] with the streptococcus. They found that streptococci could live in foci for long periods after the animals had become insensitive. Mackenzie and Hanger[14] were also able to elicit allergic reactions in a number of patients with filtrates of nonhemolytic as well as hemolytic streptococci. They failed, however, to discover any definite relationship between these reactions and wellknown types of disease.

Derick and Andrewes[15] obtained responses in the skin of rabbits with living and killed sedimented cultures in about 50 per cent of normal animals. Bristol,[16] Paraf,[17] Dochez and Sherman,[18] Mackie and McLachlan,[19] and Dochez and Stevens[20] demonstrated allergic reactions in guinea-pigs and rabbits with strains from scarlet fever and erysipelas. Birkhaug[21] accidentally produced typical erysipelatous eruptions by injections of large doses of a toxin-vaccine of Streptococcus erysipelatis into persons hypersensitive with the toxic filtrate of this streptococcus. I explained the recurrence of erysipelas in certain individuals on the basis of anaphylaxis. Bearing in mind the many studies of previous workers on bacterial anaphylaxis, I undertook a study of allergic reactions in guinea-pigs and rabbits, using as the allergenic agent, the non-methemoglobin-forming streptococcus from rheumatic fever.

Methods and Materials.—Thirty-four normal guinea-pigs and 24 normal rabbits, after depilation of the abdominal skin, received intradermal injections of toxic filtrates of the following organisms respectively: nonmethemoglobin-forming

10. J. Infect. Dis., 1913, 12, p. 386.
11. Proc. Soc. Exper. Biol. & Med., 1924, 22, p. 35.
12. J. Immunol., 1924, 9, p. 75.
13. Ibid., 1925, 10, p. 725.
14. Proc. Soc. Exper. Biol. & Med., 1924, 21, p. 442.
15. Ibid., 1925, 23, p. 116.
16. Am. J. M. Sc., 1923, 166, p. 853.
17. Bull. et Mém. Soc. méd. d. Hôp. de Paris, 1925, 49, p. 395.
18. Proc. Soc. Exper. Biol. & Med., 1925, 22, p. 282.
19. Brit. J. Exper. Path., 1927, 8, p. 129.
20. J. Exper. Med., 1927, 46, p. 487.
21. J. Am. M. A., 1928, 90, p. 1997.

streptococcus, RF.24, isolated by Birkhaug from rheumatic fever, Streptococcus cardioarthritidis, 4159, isolated by Small from rheumatic fever, Streptococcus viridans, A-179, isolated by Dr. H. F. Swift and Dr. R. A. Kinsella, from rheumatic fever, Streptococcus erysipelatis, E-1 (Birkhaug), Streptococcus scarlatinae, N.Y.5 (Dochez), and Pneumococcus 1. The skin test dose consisted of 0.1 cc. of the filtrate in a dilution of 1 : 5, obtained by passing a 5-day broth culture through a Seitz filter. Observations were made in the course of 20 hours following inoculation. Six guinea-pigs, or 17.6%, and 3 rabbits, or 12.5%, were found hypersensitive to several of the filtrates, presenting lesions at the site of the inoculations, which measured from 1 cm. to 3 cm. in diameter. These animals were subsequently discarded. The rest of the animals remained insensitive to all the filtrates.

The filtrates used were prepared by inoculating respective portions of Douglas'[22] tryptic medium digest with the six organisms mentioned. The cultures were incubated for 5 days at 37 C. At the end of the period of incubation, a 0.5% solution of phenol was added and the cultures were passed through Seitz filters. The filtrates were purified by the Mackie and McLachlan method[23] of precipitating the active toxic principle with 6 volumes of absolute alcohol. The resultant white and flaky precipitate was readily redissolved in carbolized saline solution and in this manner made up in the desired dilutions.

The sensitizing bacterial agent was the non-methemoglobin-forming streptococcus, RF.24, isolated from rheumatic fever. This organism was grown in Douglas' tryptic medium digest broth at 37 C. for 24 hours. The culture was then centrifugated at high speed for 30 minutes. The supernatant fluid was discarded and the bacterial residue washed twice with normal saline solution. The final residue was adjusted to desired amounts of bacteria per cc. both by the opacity and by methods of direct counting. Fresh cultures were employed for every injection and the calculated dose of living organisms was injected intraperitoneally.

Sensitization.—Twenty guinea-pigs received injections of the following doses of streptococcus RF.24, 3 days being allowed to elapse between inoculations: 10^9, 2×10^9, 2.5×10^9, 3×10^9, 4×10^9 and 5×10^9 (6th dose). Eight guinea-pigs were used as controls.

Sixteen rabbits received injections of the following doses: 10^9, 2.5×10^9, 5×10^9, 5×10^9, 5×10^9, 6×10^9 7×10^9, and 8×10^9. Six rabbits were used as controls. None of the animals died during this period of sensitization.

Allergic Reactions.—As soon as the second day after the injection of the last sensitizing dose of streptococcus RF. 24, most of the guinea-pigs and rabbits showed typical cutaneous allergic reactions with 0.1 cc. of the purified toxic filtrate of the streptococcus RF. 24 in the lower dilutions of 1 : 5 and 1 : 10 (table 1). With the higher dilutions of 1 : 100 and 1 : 500, the lesions of the skin were almost nil during the early days of cutaneous allergy and irregular during the height of cutaneous allergy. The most typical lesions were elicited with the dilution of 1 : 5 and this strength was chosen as the standard in all subsequent cutaneous tests. The lesions of the skin produced by the

22. Lancet, 1914, 2, p. 891, modified by Hartley, P.: J. Path. & Bact., 1922, 25, p. 479; and by Watson, A. F., and Wallace, U.: ibid., 1923, 26, p. 447.

23. Brit. J. Exper. Path., 1926, 7, p. 41.

dilution of 1 : 5 resembled in many respects a moderately positive Schick test in the human skin in which the local redness and edema are sharply limited and circular in distribution. In many instances, the local swelling became papular in form. In all instances, the lesion developed in the course of from 8 to 10 hours after inoculation and reached its maximal size in from 18 to 20 hours. In about 30 hours, the lesion had completely disappeared, leaving the skin unpigmented. Desquamation usually followed at the site of the lesion in the course of from 4 to 6 days. The diameter of the lesions varied between 0.5 cm. and 2.3 cm. The height of cutaneous allergy was reached about the 30th day after the last sensitizing injection and most animals became

TABLE 1.—ALLERGIC REACTIONS PRODUCED WITH VARIOUS DILUTIONS OF HOMOLOGOUS FILTRATE INJECTED INTRADERMALLY INTO GUINEA-PIGS SENSITIZED WITH NONMETHEMOGLOBIN-FORMING STREPTOCOCCUS RF. 24

Day After Last Sensitizing Dose	Dilutions of Filtrate 0.1 Cc.	Guinea-Pigs												
		50	51	52	53	54	55	56	57	58	59	60	61	Controls
2	1:5	0.5	0.5	1.2	0	0.8	0.5	0.8	0	0.4	0.7	0.8	0.4	0
	1:10	0.4	0.3	0.6	0	0.4	0	0.4	0	0	0.3	0.3	0	0
	1:100	0	0	0	0	0	0	0	0	0	0	0	0	0
15	1:5	1.4	1.5	1.2	0	1.5	1.1	0.9	0	1.7	0.8	1.6	1.8	0
	1:10	1.1	1.0	0.6	0	0.8	0.5	0.4	0	1.2	0.4	1.0	1.3	0
	1:100	0.4	0	0	0	0	0	0	0	0.4	0	0.3	0.2	0
25	1:5	1.6	1.9	1.7	0	1.8	1.6	0	0	1.5	0	1.9	2.3	0
	1:10	0.8	1.4	1.1	0	1.2	1.1	0	0	1.5	0	1.4	1.6	0
	1:100	0.4	0.9	0.5	0	0.6	0.4	0	0	1.0	0	0.7	0.7	0
45	1:5	0.2	0.4	0.6	0	2.1	1.3	0	0	0	0	1.4	1.1	0
	1:10	0	0	0	0	1.5	0.8	0	0	0	0	0.6	0	0
	1:100	0	0	0	0	0	0	0	0	0	0	0	0	0

Observations of allergic reactions were made 20 hours after the intradermal injection. The measurements represent maximal diameters of the lesions in centimeters.

insensitive about the 50th day after the injection of the last sensitizing dose.

Tables 2 and 3 show that guinea-pigs and rabbits sensitized with streptococcus RF. 24 displayed cutaneous allergy with toxic filtrate RF. 24 during the first week after the injection of the last sensitizing dose. During the first days of cutaneous allergy, the reactions were nullified in some animals and in others were greatly reduced in intensity when 0.1 cc. of the dilution of 1 : 5 had been heated at 98 C. for 4 hours. However, a few days afterward the allergic reactions elicited with the heated filtrate were similar to those obtained with the unheated filtrate. When filtrate RF. 24 was mixed with equal parts of either the guinea-pig or the rabbit antiserum RF. 24 and the mixtures allowed to remain in the icebox for 12 hours, it failed to elicit any cutaneous lesions when these mixtures were subsequently injected into hypersensitive

Day After Last Sensitizing Dose	Substances Injected, 0.1 Cc.	Guinea-Pigs 1	2	3	4	5	6	7	8	9	10	11	12	13	14	Controls
2	Streptococcus RF. 24															
	Unheated toxin	++	+++	+	+	++	+	+	++	+++	++	++	0	+	++	0
	Heated toxin	0	0	+	0	0	+	+	0	+	0	0	0	0	0	0
	Toxin-antitoxin	0	0	0	0	0	0	0	0	0	0	0	0	0	0	0
	Str. cardioarthritidis															
	Unheated toxin	++	+++	+	+	+	+	+	++	+++	++	++	0	+	++	0
	Heated toxin	0	0	0	0	0	+	+	+	+	0	0	0	0	0	0
	Toxin-antitoxin	0	0	0	0	0	0	0	0	0	0	0	0	0	0	0
5	Str. viridans															
	Unheated toxin	0	0	0	0	0	0	0	0	0	0	0	0	0	0	0
	Str. erysipelatis															
	Unheated toxin	0	0	0	0	0	0	0	0	0	0	0	0	0	0	0
	Str. scarlatinae															
	Unheated toxin	0	±	0	0	0	0	0	0	±	0	0	0	0	0	0
	Pneumococcus 1															
	Unheated toxin	0	0	0	0	0	0	0	0	0	0	0	0	0	0	0
33	Streptococcus RF. 24															
	Unheated toxin	+++	+++	++	++	+++	+++	++	+	++	±	+	0	+++	++	0
	Heated toxin	+++	+++	++	+	+++	+++	+++	+	++	±	+	0	++	++	0
	Toxin-antitoxin	0	0	0	0	0	0	0	0	0	0	0	0	0	0	0
	Str. cardioarthritidis															
	Unheated toxin	+++	+++	++	+	++	+++	++	+	+	+	+	0	+++	++	0
	Heated toxin	+++	++	++	+	++	++	+	+	+	+	+	0	+++	+	0
	Toxin-antitoxin	0	0	0	0	0	0	0	0	0	0	0	0	0	0	0
35	Str. viridans															
	Unheated toxin	+	0	0	0	+++	+	0	0	+	0	0	0	+	0	0
	Heated toxin	+	0	0	0	++	+	0	0	+	0	0	0	+	0	0
	Toxin-antitoxin	0	0	0	0	0	0	0	0	0	0	0	0	0	0	0
	Str. erysipelatis															
	Unheated toxin	++	0	0	+	+++	0	0	0	0	0	0	0	++	0	0
	Heated toxin	++	0	0	+	++	0	0	0	0	0	0	0	++	0	0
	Toxin-antitoxin	+	0	0	0	++	0	0	0	0	0	0	0	+	0	0
72	Streptococcus RF. 24															
	Unheated toxin	0	0	0	0	0	0	0	0	0	0	0	0	0	0	0

Intraperitoneal injections of living RF. 24 streptococci in following doses, 10 days interval between doses: 2.5×10^9, 3.5×10^9, 4×10^9, 5×10^9, 5×10^9, 5×10^9, and 8×10^9.

Day After Last Sensitizing Dose	Substances Injected, 0.1 Cc.	Guinea-Pigs 1	2	3	4	5	6	7	8	9	10	11	12	13	14	Controls
140	Streptococcus RF. 24															
	Unheated toxin	+++	+++		+++	+++	+++	0	+++	+++	0	+++	+++	+++	++	0
	Heated toxin	+++	+++	0	+++	+++	++	0	+++	+++	0	+++	+++	+++	++	0
	Toxin-antitoxin	+++	++	0	+++	+++	+++	0	+++	+++	0	+++	+++	+++	+++	0
	Str. cardioarthritidis															
	Unheated toxin	+++	+++	0	+++	+++	++	0	+++	+++	0	+++	+++	+++	+++	0
	Heated toxin	+++	++	0	++	++	++	0	+++	+++	0	+++	++	+++	+++	0
	Toxin-antitoxin	+++	+++	0	+++	+++	++	0	+++	+++	0	+++	+++	+++	+++	0
145	Str. viridans															
	Unheated toxin	+++	+++	0	++	++	+	0	++	++	0	+++	++	++	++	0
	Str. erysipelatis															
	Unheated toxin	+++	+++	0	+++	+++	+++	0	+++	+++	0	+++	++	++	+++	0
	Str. scarlatinae															
	Unheated toxin	+++	+++	0	++	+++	++	0	+++	++	0	+++	++	++	+++	0
	Pneumococcus 1															
	Unheated toxin	++	++	0	++	+++	++	0	+++	++	0	+++	++	++	++	0
	Staphylococcus aureus															
	Unheated toxin	+++	+++	+++	+++	+++	+++	++	+++	+++	++	+++	+++	+++	0	+++
210	Streptococcus RF. 24															
	Unheated toxin	+++	++	0	+	+++	++	0	+++	+	0	+++	++	++	+	0
	Heated toxin	+++	++	0	0	+++	++	0	+++	0	0	+++	++	++	0	0
	Toxin-antitoxin	+++	++	0	0	+++	+++	0	+++	0	0	+++	++	+	0	0

Observations of allergic reactions were made 20 hours after the intradermal injection. Each + equals to 0.5 cm. of maximal diameter of lesion; +++ indicates any reaction in excess of 1.5 cm. in diameter. Heated toxin represents toxic filtrate heated at 98 C. for 4 hours. Toxin-antitoxin stands for equal parts of 1:5 dilution of toxin and undiluted specific guinea-pig or rabbit serum.

Table 3.—Allergic Reactions Produced by Intradermal Injections of Specific and Nonspecific Culture Filtrates into Rabbits Sensitized with Non-Methemoglobin-Forming Streptococcus RF. 24

Rabbits previously had received intraperitnoeal injections of living RF. 24 streptococci in the following doses, 3 days interval between doses: 10^9, 2.5×10^9, 5×10^9, 5×10^9, 5×10^9, 6×10^9, 7.5×10^9, 7.5×10^9, and 8×10^9

Day After Last Sensitizing Dose	Substances Injected, 0.1 Cc.	Rabbits 1	2	3	4	5	6	7	8	9	10	11	12	13	Controls
4	Streptococcus RF. 24														
	Unheated toxin	++	+++	++	++	0	+++	+++	++	++	0	+++	+++	+	0
	Heated toxin	0	+	+	0	0	+	+	0	0	0	+	+	0	0
	Toxin-antitoxin	0	0	0	0	0	±	0	0	0	0	0	0	0	0
	Str. cardioarthritidis														
	Unheated toxin	++	+++	+++	++	0	+++	+++	+	++	0	+++	+++	+	0
	Heated toxin	0	+	±	0	0	±	+	0	0	0	0	++	+	0
	Toxin-antitoxin	0	0	0	0	0	0	0	0	0	0	0	0	0	0
8	Str. viridans														
	Unheated toxin	0	0	+	0	0	0	0	0	+	0	0	0	0	0
	Str. erysipelatis														
	Unheated toxin	0	++	+	0	0	0	±	0	±	0	0	0	0	0
	Str. scarlatinae														
	Unheated toxin	0	+	0	0	0	0	0	0	±	0	0	0	0	0
	Pneumococcus 1														
	Unheated toxin	0	0	0	0	0	0	0	0	+	0	0	0	0	0
24	Streptococcus RF. 24														
	Unheated toxin	+++	+++	+++	++	0	+++	+++	+++	++	0	+++	+++	+++	0
	Heated toxin	+++	+++	++	++	0	+++	++	++	++	0	++	++	++	0
	Toxin-antitoxin	0	±	0	0	0	±	0	0	0	0	0	0	0	0
	Str. cardioarthritidis														
	Unheated toxin	+++	+++	+++	++	0	+++	+++	+++	+++	0	+++	+++	+++	0
	Heated toxin	+++	++	++	++	0	+++	++	++	+++	0	++	++	+++	0
	Toxin-antitoxin	0	+	0	0	0	+	0	0	0	0	0	0	0	0
27	Str. viridans														
	Unheated toxin	0	0	++	0	0	0	+	0	+	0	0	0	0	0
	Heated toxin	0	0	++	0	0	0	+	0	+	0	0	0	0	0
	Toxin-antitoxin	0	0	0	0	0	0	0	0	0	0	0	0	0	0
	Str. erysipelatis														
	Unheated toxin	0	++	++	0	0	++	0	0	+	0	0	0	0	0
	Heated toxin	0	++	++	0	0	++	0	0	±	0	0	0	0	0
	Toxin-antitoxin	0	0	0	0	0	0	0	0	0	0	0	0	0	0
68	Streptococcus RF. 24														
	Unheated toxin	0	0	0	0	0	0	0	0	0	0	0	0	0	0

Intraperitoneal injections of living RF. 24 streptococci in following doses, 10 days interval between doses: 5×10^9, 7.5×10^9, 8×10^9, 8×10^9, 8×10^9, 8×10^9, and 9×10^9

Day After Last Sensitizing Dose	Substances Injected, 0.1 Cc.	Rabbits 1	2	3	4	5	6	7	8	9	10	11	12	13	Controls
158	Streptococcus RF. 24														
	Unheated toxin	+++	+++	+++	+++	0	0	+++	+++	0	0	+++	0	+++	0
	Heated toxin	+++	+++	+++	+++	0	0	+++	+++	0	0	+++	0	+++	0
	Toxin-antitoxin	+++	+++	+++	+++	0	0	++	+++	0	0	++	0	+++	0
	Str. cardioarthritidis														
	Unheated toxin	+++	+++	+++	+++	0	0	+++	+++	0	0	+++	0	+++	0
	Heated toxin	+++	+++	+++	+++	0	0	+++	+++	0	0	+++	0	+++	0
	Toxin-antitoxin	+++	+++	+++	+++	0	0	+++	+++	0	0	++	0	+++	0
163	Str. viridans														
	Unheated toxin	+++	+++	+++	+++	0	++	0	++	0	0	+++	0	++	0
	Heated toxin	+++	+++	+++	+++	0	+	0	+	0	0	+++	0	+	0
	Toxin-antitoxin	++	++	+++	++	0	±	0	+	0	0	++	0	++	0
	Str. erysipelatis														
	Unheated toxin	+++	++	+++	++	0	0	++	0	0	0	±	0	0	0
	Heated toxin	+++	++	+++	++	0	0	++	0	0	0	0	0	0	0
	Toxin-antitoxin	+++	++	+++	+++	0	0	++	0	0	0	++	0	0	0
166	Pneumococcus 1														
	Unheated toxin	++	+	++	0	0	+	++	0	0	0	0	0	++	0
	Heated toxin	+++	++	++	+	0	++	++	0	0	0	0	0	+++	0
	Toxin-antitoxin	+++	++	+++	+	0	++	++	0	0	0	0	0	+++	0
	Staphylococcus aureus														

animals. Similar results were obtained in these animals with the filtrate produced by Small's Streptococcus cardioarthritidis, which might indicate a close biologic relationship between this organism and the non-methemoglobin-forming streptococcus RF. 24, likewise isolated from rheumatic fever.

In cutaneous tests with heterologous filtrates produced by S. viridans, S. erysipelatis, S. scarlatinae and pneumococcus 1 these guinea-pigs and rabbits remained insensitive to standard doses during the first week of cutaneous allergy produced with the homologous allergen RF. 24. But coincident with the maximal cutaneous allergy with filtrates RF. 24, about 30% of all the animals displayed cutaneous allergy with the heterologous filtrates. These reactions, however, remained much less pronounced than those elicited with the homologous allergen. Heating the respective heterologous filtrates at 98 C. for 4 hours failed to inactivate the allergenic constituents in the filtrates. By mixing the filtrates with their respective antiserums and allowing the mixtures to remain in direct contact in the icebox for a period of 12 hours, complete neutralization of the allergen principle was obtained so that lesions did not develop at the site of injections in sensitive animals.

Simultaneously with the loss of the cutaneous allergy produced with filtrate RF. 24 in both guinea-pigs and rabbits, loss of cutaneous sensitiveness was observed with the heterologous filtrates. The guinea-pigs became insensitive approximately 40 days after the last sensitizing dose of streptococcus RF. 24 and the rabbits became insensitive about 60 days after the last sensitizing dose. Two guinea-pigs and 3 rabbits treated in similar manner with the reacting animals, remained completely insensitive to all the filtrates mentioned. In none of the control animals were cutaneous reactions obtained during this period.

Dochez and Stevens,[20] in their recent study of allergic reactions in rabbits with strains from erysipelas, observed a period of cutaneous insensitivity to the toxic filtrates of the erysipelatous strains taking place about the 50th day after the injection of the first sensitizing dose. They continued to immunize these rabbits for 3 months intracutaneously and 3 months intravenously, until on the 187th day after the first intracutaneous inoculation cutaneous reactions reappeared. Stimulated by these studies, I continued sensitization of these colonies of previously hypersensitive guinea-pigs and rabbits.

Second Period of Sensitization.—Into 20 guinea-pigs were injected intraperitoneally for a period of 8 weeks the following gradually increasing doses of living and broth-free streptococcus RF. 24, about 10 days being allowed to elapse between injections: 2.5×10^9, 3.5×10^9, 4×10^9, 5×10^9, 5×10^9, and 8×10^9. On the 140th day after the injection of the last sensitizing dose previous to the appearance of the first phase of cutaneous allergy, the guinea-pigs displayed an extraordinary hypersensitivity not only to the homologous but also to the heterologous filtrates. No difference was observed between the lesions produced by the unheated and the heated filtrates, and the specific antiserums failed to nullify the property that called forth the cutaneous reactions to the filtrates. The cutaneous sensitivity during this second phase persisted until approximately 230 days after the onset of the first phase of allergy, or about 80 days after the last injection of the living culture RF. 24. One immunized guinea-pig that remained insensitive to cutaneous injections of toxic filtrates during the first phase of allergy of the other sensitive guinea-pigs, became strongly sensitive during their second phase. The necrosing reactions of the skin which followed the injections of the toxic filtrate produced by Staphylococcus aureus must be dissociated from the typical allergic reactions elicited by the remaining filtrates, since control animals reacted equally well with the staphylococcic toxin.

Desensitization of cutaneously allergic guinea-pigs was attempted approximately 210 days after the last sensitizing dose of streptococci RF. 24, which produced the first phase of cutaneous allergy. This was accomplished by injecting intracardially 10 cc. of undiluted filtrate RF. 24 to which no preservative had been added. Ten guinea-pigs which reacted hyperallergically with a dilution of 1 : 5 received the intracardial injections. The etherized animals did not display any typical anaphylactic shock following the injection. All the animals, however, reacted immediately with tremors which rapidly passed off in the course of 20 minutes. For control purposes, 4 guinea-pigs which likewise reacted hyperallergically with filtrate RF. 24 in the dilution of 1 : 5 received intracardial injections of 10 cc. of Douglas' tryptic broth from the identical lot of broth in which toxic filtrate RF. 24 was produced. Only transitory tremors were observed following the injection of the broth.

The first indication of desensitization was observed on the fourth day following the intracardial injection of the undiluted toxin, when 6 guinea-pigs failed to react cutaneously with 0.1 cc. of filtrate RF. 24 in the dilution of 1 : 5. On the 6th day 8 guinea-pigs and on the 10th day 10 guinea-pigs failed to react with filtrate RF. 24. The 4 guinea-pigs receiving intracardial injections of 10 cc. of Douglas' broth remained hyperallergic for approximately 30 days following the injections. At this time no cutaneous reactions were elicited with the unheated or heated filtrates of RF. 24 and Streptococcus erysipelatis. Failure of the hyperallergic guinea-pigs to respond violently to the large intracardial injection of filtrate RF. 24 may possibly be explained on the basis that the animals at this stage were beginning to become spontaneously insusceptible.

During the second phase of cutaneous allergy, 3 guinea-pigs died from peritonitis and respiratory disease. Eight control guinea-pigs remained consistently insensitive with all the filtrates used.

Fourteen rabbits likewise received intraperitoneal injections for a period of 10 weeks, of the following doses of living and broth-free streptococci RF. 24, about 10 days being allowed to elapse between injections: 5×10^9, 7.5×10^9, 8×10^9, 8×10^9, 8×10^9, 9×10^9, 9×10^9. The first reappearance of cutaneous allergy with filtrate RF. 24 occurred about 158 days after the last sensitizing dose was injected previous to the onset of the first phase of cutaneous allergy. No semblance of specificity of allergic reactions was observed in the rabbits during the second phase. Both heated and unheated heterologous filtrates produced lesions of the skin identical with those elicited with filtrate RF. 24. Neutralization of the property calling forth cutaneous reactions was not accomplished by the respective specific antiserums. Allergic reactions were produced in the rabbits until approximately the 240th day after the last sensitizing dose previous to the appearance of the first phase, or the 90th day after the last sensitizing dose previous to the appearance of the second phase of cutaneous sensitivity. Two rabbits which displayed cutaneous allergy during the first phase of sensitization did not develop a second phase of sensitivity. Here again necrosing reactions of the skin to Staphylococcus aureus in both sensitized and normal control rabbits nullified any notion of a relationship between the results obtained with this and with the other filtrates.

Attempts were made to desensitize cutaneously allergic rabbits by the intravenous injection of toxic filtrate RF. 24. Among 13 surviving sensitized rabbits, 11 reacted hyperallergically with the filtrate on the 216th day after the last sensitizing dose before the appearance of the first phase of cutaneous allergy. Four of these rabbits received intravenous injections of 20 cc. of unheated and undiluted filtrate RF. 24, to which no preservative had been added, and four others received intravenous injections of 20 cc. of heated undiluted filtrate RF. 24, free from any preservative. For control purposes, the remaining 3 susceptible rabbits received intravenous injections of 20 cc. of

Douglas' tryptic broth of the same lot as that employed for the production of the filtrate. No violent general reactions were observed in any one of these 11 rabbits following the injections, except a series of tremors which passed off in the course of half an hour. Daily intradermal injections of 0.1 cc. of the filtrate in a dilution of 1 : 5 revealed that complete desensitization had taken place in 3 rabbits on the 3rd day after the injection. Two of these rabbits received intravenous injections of the unheated and one of the heated filtrate. On the 5th day, 7 rabbits became insusceptible, 4 of these having received intravenous injection of the unheated and 3 of the heated filtrate. The 8th rabbit remained cutaneously allergic with the diluted filtrate until the 12th day after the intravenous injection of the desensitizing dose. The 3 susceptible control rabbits remained cutaneously allergic following the intravenous injection of 20 cc. of Douglas' broth, respectively for 22, 28, and 36 days.

These studies confirm the observations made by Mackie and McLachlan [19] that it is possible under certain conditions to produce cutaneous sensitiveness in guinea-pigs to filtrates of cultures of scarlatinal streptococci by injection of living organisms and that generally the active principle in the filtrates is not inactivated at 100 C. even after 3½ hours exposure. These writers failed, however, to observe an early phase of specificity in the sensitive state.

The observations presented in this paper are almost identical with those made by Dochez and Stevens,[20] who were able to produce cutaneous allergy in rabbits with filtrates of cultures of erysipelatous streptococci. They were the first observers to report the existence of two types or phases of allergic reactions, the property of the filtrate eliciting reactions in the first phase being completely nullified with erysipelas immune serum.

The two periods of allergy observed by Dochez and Stevens with Streptococcus erysipelatis do not appear, from the experiments presented in this paper, to be an attribute of the erysipelas organism particularly. The non-methemoglobin-forming streptococcus isolated in blood cultures from a patient during an acute attack of articular rheumatism is also found to possess certain allergenizing properties in the guinea-pig and the rabbit, which strongly resemble those observed of S. erysipelatis by Dochez and Stevens. Whether any significance should be attached to the observation that a brief period of apparently specific hypersensitiveness existed in these animals treated experimentally with the homologous allergenic substance, is a question which necessitates further investigation, since specific antiserums seemed to nullify the property eliciting the cutaneous allergic reactions during the early phase. The subsequent loss of the specific cutaneous allergic response and the introduction of a phase of susceptibility to a variety of bacterial filtrates of cultures of heterogeneous bacteria are observations which might be linked up with the clinical findings of Swift, Derick, and Hitchcock[4] that patients with rheumatic fever show hypersensitiveness to filtrates of both the non-methemoglobin-forming and the viridans types of streptococci. With the aid of the Committee of Scientific Research of the American Medical Association, these studies will be extended to include a series of determinations of cutaneous bacterial allergy in patients with rheumatic fever with a variety of substances obtained from nonhemolytic and hemolytic streptococci.

CONCLUSIONS

Guinea-pigs and rabbits sensitized to the non-methemoglobin-forming streptococcus isolated from rheumatic fever may be rendered cutaneously hypersensitive to filtrates of cultures of this organism. A brief period of specificity in the sensitive state is recorded. This period is shortly followed by a sensitive state that is nonspecific. During this phase of the cutaneous reactions, the allergenic property of the filtrate can be nullified completely with specific antiserums. After the end of the cutaneous allergy of this first phase, continued sensitization of the animals with living non-methemoglobin-forming streptococci produces the reappearance of cutaneous allergy. During the second phase, the reactions of allergy are nonspecific and the allergic principle of the filtrate is nonneutralizable with specific antiserums. For this phase, filtrates heated at 98 C. for 4 hours are not inactivated as allergic substances. Heterogeneity in the cutaneous responses of patients with rheumatic fever to filtrates of the non-methemoglobin-forming streptococcus and to certain strains of Streptococcus viridans might be explained on the basis of prolonged sensitization to any one dominant strain of the nonhemolytic streptococci. Desensitization of bacterially hyperallergic guinea-pigs and rabbits was accomplished during the second phase of cutaneous allergy by intracardial or intravenous injections of bacterial filtrates.

DETOXIFYING, DIFFUSING, GERMICIDAL, AND SURFACE TENSION DEPRESSING PROPERTIES OF SOAPS

Forrest R. Davison

From the Department of Physiology, Rutgers University, New Brunswick, N. J.

Considerable work has been done on soaps during the last few years. Various outstanding properties of soaps have been studied. Larson and Nelson [1] showed that sodium ricinoleate (castor oil soap) possessed the property of detoxifying soluble toxins and endotoxins. Larson, Evans and Nelson [2] found that oleic, stearic and palmitic acid soaps had no detoxifying properties against diphtheria and tetanus toxins, while the soaps of lauric, myristic, ennenoic and hendeconoic possess some, and castor oil soap possesses high detoxifying ability. Larson and Nelson [3] showed that rabbits could be immunized against fatal doses of pneumococcus. Netter, Andre, Cesari and Catoni [4] showed that sodium ricinoleate (castor oil soap) immunized rabbits against pneumococcus and streptococcus. Larson, Evans and Nelson [2] found that soaps which detoxify bacterial toxins readily, form clear solutions and dialyze readily through collodium sacs.

While there is considerable difference of opinion, the general view is that soaps are not highly germicidal. Rosenau [5] states "ordinary soaps have but limited disinfecting power." Reichenbach [6] found potassium stearate, palmitate and myristate germicidal to B. coli, but soaps made from oleic, erucic, linolic were inactive. Reasoner [7] found soaps active against Spirochaeta pallida, Tilley and Schaeffer [8] found coconut oil soap effective against B. typhosus, B. pyocyaneous and Staphylococcus aureus. Walker [9] found chemically pure soaps very different in germicidal ability, while commercial soaps showed considerable germicidal activity against streptococcus, pneumococcus, diphtheria bacillus, and to a lesser extent against typhoid bacillus. He found coconut oil soap active against typhoid bacillus. Larson [10] found that pneumococcus and streptococcus will not grow in the presence of even small quantities of castor oil soap.

Bacteriologists are becoming more interested in the importance of surface tension on bacterial growth and activity. Larson, Cantwell and Hartzell [11] pioneers in this field, found lowering of the surface tension of broth caused pellicle formers to grow down in the medium, and spores formed more slowly. Larson [12] found pneumococcus and streptococcus grew poorly at a low surface tension. Ayers,

Received for publication, April 2, 1928.

1. Proc. Soc. Exper. Biol. & Med., 1924, 21, p. 278.
2. Ibid., 1924-5, 22, p. 194.
3. Ibid., 1925, 22, 357.
4. Compt. rend. Soc. de Biol., 1927, 96, p. 184.
5. Prev. Med. & Hyg., 1927, p. 1367.
6. Ztschr. T. Hyg. in Infektionskr., 1908, 59, p. 296.
7. J. Am. M. A., 1917, 68, p. 73.
8. J. Infect. Dis., 1925, 37, p. 358.
9. J. Infect. Dis., 1924, 35, p. 557; 1925, 37, p. 151.
10. Proc. Soc. Exper. Biol. & Med., 1921, 19, p. 62-3.
11. J. Infect. Dis., 1919, 25, p. 41.
12. Absts. Bact., 1921, 5, p. 2.

Rupp and Johnson[13] found lowered surface tension depressed the growth of streptococci. Hastings and Anastasia[14] showed surface tension effected the agglutinizing power of bacteria. Gibbs, Batchelor and Sickel,[15] Pizarro[16] showed the importance of the nature of the surface tension depressant used.

This brief résumé will serve as a background for the following account of studies of the detoxifying, diffusion, germicidal and surface tension depressing properties of several common soaps.

EXPERIMENTAL WORK

Preparation of Soaps.—Twelve soaps were prepared from their respective oils by the usual methods employed in saponification: the saponification number of each oil was found and from this number the theoretical amount of alcoholic solution of sodium hydroxide was added and heated on a steam bath until complete saponification took place. Sodium soaps of castor, linseed, olive, coconut, lard, peanut, maize, sesame, corn, cotton-seed, palm and apricot oils were made according to the above method. Approximately 5% soap solutions were made and adjusted to approximately a P_H of 7.0 with their respective fatty acids and sodium hydroxide. The soap solutions were made to exactly 5% strength and stored in pyrex flasks stoppered with rubber stoppers. These were considered the stock solutions for future work.

Detoxifying Action.—The twelve soaps prepared were studied to determine their ability to protect guinea-pigs from fatal doses of tetanus toxin. Tetanus toxin was chosen in preference to any other toxin because it was available and is one of the most deadly toxins. In determining the detoxifying or protective ability of the various soaps, a measured quantity of soap to be tested was mixed with a definite amount of standardized toxin and injected subcutaneously in a guinea-pig.

Standardization of Tetanus Toxin: Tetanus toxin may be secured in the powdered form or in solution. A solution will lose its activity slowly and keeps best in a refrigerator. The dry powder keeps very well. It was necessary to standardize the toxin and the following method was used: The standardization of tetanus toxin is based on the fact that when sufficient tetanus toxin is injected subcutaneously in a guinea-pig it will show symptoms of paralysis, convulsions, and death will soon follow. An arbitrary unit was chosen for a standard, as that amount of tetanus toxin necessary to kill a 300 gm. guinea-pig in 24 hours. This was designated as one fatal dose or one minimum lethal dose (MLD). It is

13. J. Infect. Dis., 1923, 33, p. 202.
14. J. Immunol., 1924, 9, p. 365.
15. J. Bact., 1926, 11, p. 393.
16. J. Bact., 1927, 13, p. 387.

necessary to have at least 8 guinea-pigs of about 300 grams weight, to carry out a standardization of this toxin.

Determination of Detoxifying Power.—Guinea-pigs weighing 300 to 350 grams were used for the experiment. They were placed in separate cages and numbered. From the standardized tetanus toxin a solution was made so 1 cc. of solution contained exactly ten fatal doses of toxin for a guinea-pig weighing 300 gms. The exact amount of toxin was calculated for each guinea-pig: a guinea-pig weighing 350 grams received 1.17 cc. measured by a Folin buret. To each quantity of toxin solution (10 MLD, the volume depending on the weight of the guinea-pig) was added 1 cc. of 1% soap solution. This soap-toxin mixture was left for fifteen minutes, then injected subcutaneously in a guinea-pig. Care was exercised in this injection not to pierce the peritoneal membrane or lose any of the soap-toxin mixture by its coming out near the site of the injection. Table 1 shows the relative detoxifying or protective ability of these soaps. One MLD of tetanus toxin kills in 24 hours; 10 MLD, in 16 hours. This relation is due to the fact that there is a period of incubation necessary for tetanus toxin.

TABLE 1.—RELATIVE PROTECTIVE ACTION OF SOAPS AGAINST TETANUS TOXIN

Figures indicate hours of survival of guinea-pig after injection of soap-toxin mixture.

Soap (oil)	Exper. 1 Hours Survival	Exper. 2 Hours Survival	Average
Castor	124	128	126
Coconut	89	67	78
Linseed	80	72	76
Cottonseed	80	70	75
Palm	68	68	68
Olive	64	70	67
Lard	64	70	67
Peanut	60	63	62
Corn	53	48	51
Sesame	52	48	50
Maize	54	46	50
Apricot	44	44	44
Toxin control (no soap)	17	16	17

The results of the study of the detoxifying abilities of several soaps with respect to tetanus toxin are found in table 1. In the control experiments 1 cc. of physiologic salt solution was used in place of the soap solution.

Diffusion.—In this work a study of the ability to dialyze or diffuse through a semipermeable membrane was made for the twelve commercial soaps. Dialyzing bags prepared from collodium proved unsatisfactory so parchment sacs were used, calibrated by a method suggested by Eggerth,[17] by measuring the dialysate.

Method: Soaps which had been adjusted to a P_H 7.0 and stored in pyrex flasks were diluted to 1% solutions with neutral distilled water. Equivalent quantities of soap in solutions (15 cc.) were placed in 25 cc. diffusion shells, and dialyzed against six liters of distilled water for 24 hours at 20 C. The necks of the shells were wrapped carefully around long glass tubing to prevent a development of pressure in the liquid inside the shell. This size of shell, amount of soap and

17. J. Biol. Chem., 1921, 47, p. 203.

water surrounding the shell worked well for this particular series. The rate of diffusion or dialyzing of the soaps was determined by getting the dry weight of the dialysate. The parchment dialyzing shells were previously standardized against 1% soap solution and those shells chosen that gave the same rate of dialysis.

Table 2 shows the relative rate of diffusion of various soaps, under identical conditions of temperature, amount of water used in dialysis and time.

Germicidal Action.—The method used for the testing of the germicidal ability of soaps is very similar to the method that Larson of Minnesota used and not unlike the method of Rideal and Walker [18] in determining the phenol coefficient of a disinfectant.

TABLE 2.—RELATIVE RATES OF DIFFUSION OF PURE SOAPS

Percentage of soap dialyzed (dry weight of dialysate) in 24 hours at 20 C.

Soap	1st Shell, %	2nd Shell, %	3rd Shell, %	Average Diffusion, %
Sodium ricinoleate	75.6	73.8	75	74.8
Apricot	49.2	51.3	47.5	49.3
Coconut	41.6	49.4	48.8	46.6
Sesame	34.3	33.3	34	33.8
Corn	25.2	35.3	23.4	27.9
Linseed	20.3	33.3	26.8	26.8
Cotton	24	24.2	24.3	24.1
Peanut	16.4	24.1	24.5	21.6
Maize	17.8	17.3	18.9	18
Olive	15	16.6	15	15.5
Palm	13	12.3	12.4	12.5
Lard	3.5	3.6	....	3.55

TABLE 3.—ACTION OF CASTOR OIL SOAP ON STREPTOCOCCUS HEMOLYTICUS

Growth = +, no growth = 0.

Soap Concentration, %	Time in Minutes						
	0	3	5	7	10	15	20
.25	+	+	+	+	+	+	0
.5	+	+	0	0	0	0	0
.75	+	+	0	0	0	0	0
1.0	+	0	0	0	0	0	0
2.0	+	0	0	0	0	0	0

Method: A young 24 hour culture of the organism of a known concentration was placed in the desired strength of soap solution, then reinoculated at intervals of time into suitable sterile broth mediums, and allowed to incubate for 48 hours. The clearness and cloudiness was taken as the indication of the killing, and lack of killing action of the soap. The organisms used were Streptococcus viridans, Streptococcus hemolyticus and Staphylococcus.

It is impossible to present all the tables of the killing time and dilution for all the bacteria, by the twelve soaps, so the results with castor oil soap are given in table 3 as an illustration, and the results for the other soaps.

18. J. Sanitary Inst., 1903, 24, p. 424.

The results show that .25% castor oil soap kills Streptococcus hemolyticus in twenty minutes, 0.5% concentration in five minutes and 1.0% in three minutes, etc. The concentration of soap and time necessary to destroy bacteria may vary considerably for different strains depending on the source and previous history of the organism. It was found in some cases that Streptococcus hemolyticus, which had been cultivated in our laboratory for six months on artificial medium, was much more difficult to kill in this manner than was a fresh virulent strain. For this reason the tests were carried out on bacteria that had just been received from a patient at the Cincinnati Hospital. This would represent the virulency of bacteria under their natural conditions.

The soaps are listed as follows in the order of their bactericidal action.

Streptococcus Hemolyticus	Streptococcus Viridans	Staphylococcus
Castor	Castor	Castor
Coconut	Coconut	Cottonseed
Linseed	Linseed	Coconut
Cottonseed	Apricot	Olive
Olive	Cottonseed	Corn

The soaps not mentioned (peanut, maize, sesame, palm and lard oil soap) were very poor in their germicidal power and in some cases it required two hours time for them to kill so they are left out of the table.

Surface Tension Depression.—The drop weight or drop number method has almost invariably been employed in the study of the surface tension of soap solutions. Harkins, Davies and Clark [19] used the drop weight method, later Hillyer [20] used the same method.

Method: The value of surface tension can be obtained by determining the weight of the drop of liquid which freely falls from the end of a tube. The weight of fifty drops of the soap solution falling from a carefully ground tip of a capillary buret, was taken by running the drops in a tared weighing flask and re-weighing. The temperature of the liquid was kept at 20 C. by holding the buret in a constant temperature water bath which did not vary 0.1 C. A regular interval of 20 seconds was allowed for each drop to form and fall. The liquid in the capillary was kept at the same initial height at the beginning of the 50 drop count. Consistent results could be obtained from day to day with the same solution by holding the temperature constant, and regulating the time of each falling drop to twenty seconds.

$$\frac{\text{wt. of 50 drops of soap solution}}{\text{wt. of 50 drops of water}} \times 72.8 = \text{surface tension in dynes}$$

Surface tension of water at 20 C. equals 72.8 dynes per cm.

19. J. Am. Chem. Soc., 1917, 39, p. 586.
20. Ibid., 1903, 25, p. 515.

Table 4 gives the surface tension of the soaps at 5%, 2%, 1%, 0.1% and 0.05% concentrations. The density factor has not been taken into consideration in the above equation because the density of all soap solutions have approximately the same density as water even in extreme concentration. For example a normal solution of sodium palmitate has a density equal to 0.997 of that of water at the same temperature.

TABLE 4.—SURFACE TENSION OF SOAP SOLUTION

At 20 C. surface tension of water equals 72.8 dynes per cm.

Soap (Oil)	Dynes per Cm.				
	5%	2%	1%	.1%	.05%
Castor (1)	34.8 34.5	35.2 35.1	33.8 34.6	39.8 40.0	55.6 55.9 55.7
Castor (2)	34.9 34.8	35.6 35.2	35.2 35.0 34.9	46.1 45.8	52.1 52.0 52.1
Coconut	27.8 28.0	27.1 27.1	31.0 21.1	35.9 36.7	48.1 48.0 48.1
Cottonseed	Solid	Solid	26.4 26.5	25.5 25.4	29.1 29.1 29.3
Linseed	28.0 28.1	26.9 27.1	26.9 26.8	29.2 29.3	33.0 33.1 33.0
Palm	Solid	Solid	38.9 38.1 38.4	28.4 27.6 27.0	34.8 34.7 34.8
Olive	27.8 28.8 27.8	25.5 25.3 25.1	25.5 25.6	26.1 25.7	27.4 24.5 27.5
Lard	36.9 36.5 35.5	31.2 31.2 30.3	29.7 29.3	27.5 27.3 27.2	30.1 20.0
Peanut	38.1 37.4	34.1 33.4 33.7	29.7 29.3	27.5 27.3 28.2	30.1 30.0
Corn	27.6 27.6 27.5	27.2 27.0 26.9	25.4 25.1 24.8	23.6 26.2 27.4	29.2 29.4 29.1
Sesame	26.8 27.4 27.2	26.1 26.3	23.4 24.3	26.9 27.2	30.1 30.0 30.1 29.4
Maize	28.3 28.6 28.8	28.6 28.7	27.7 27.5	27.5 27.3 27.2	30.1 30.0 29.4
Apricot	25.7 26.0 26.6	26.2 26.1	25.1 25.6	26.6 26.7	31.7 31.6 31.7

DISCUSSION

The question of the manner in which soaps detoxify toxins is not known. Larson, Halvorson and Evans [21] consider it an adsorption phenomena. That is, the soap forms a film about the toxin and thus

21. Colloid symposium monograph 3, 1925 (Chemical Catalogue Company).

puts it out of the sphere of action. Gradually the film may be removed by dissolving or a similar action thus freeing the toxin. The germicidal action also seems an adsorption phenomena. That is, a film seems to form around the bacteria, killing them in some cases and in other cases not, because after 48 hours the culture tubes have become cloudy showing that the bacteria are alive. In such cases it might appear that the film is gradually removed and the bacteria set free. Another possibility of the action of soaps on toxins might be a simple neutralization, as the neutralization of an acid by an alkali.

One outstanding feature of this study is the fact that castor oil, coconut oil, linseed oil and cottonseed oil soaps have the highest detoxifying ability, also the highest germicidal ability, and an outstanding dialyzing ability. The soaps which have a high detoxifying ability, and which diffuse most readily and also are more germicidal have the lesser ability to reduce the surface tension. The germicidal action of the soaps tested was proportional to their ability to diffuse or dialyze through the dialyzing thimbles, and it might also be considered as proportional to their ability to diffuse through membranes of bacteria, thus destroying them.

The relation between detoxification and surface tension is somewhat obscure. The possible significance of surface tension in this connection was first pointed out by Berczeller [22] who claims that detoxification of foreign solutions give rise to solutions of higher surface tension approximating water. This is shown to be quite true for the synthesis in the body of hippuric acid from benzoic acid and glycocoll. The soaps studied which gave the higher surface tensions in solution (approaching water) were the best detoxifyers of tetanus toxin. It is possible that the soaps of higher surface tensions form soap-toxin mixtures of higher surface tensions which are less toxic because of their greater ability to diffuse through membranes due to their higher surface tension. Substances with higher surface tension are conceded to be better able to pass semipermeable membranes.

Soaps with greatest diffusing or dialyzing abilities also had the greatest detoxifying power. This might be due to the fact that the soaps of high diffusing ability formed soap toxins, solutions of high diffusing abilities and were more easily removed from the body or distributed so widely as to be less harmful.

22. Biochem. Ztschr., 1917, 84, p. 75.

CONCLUSIONS

Twelve common soaps were prepared and their detoxifying, diffusing, germicidal and surface tension depressing properties studied. Soaps possessing high detoxifying ability, diffuse readily, are highly germicidal, but are correspondingly ineffective surface tension depressants.

INFECTION OF LABORATORY WORKER WITH BACILLUS INFLUENZAE

JOHN E. WALKER

From the Department of Immunology, School of Hygiene and Public Health, The Johns Hopkins University, Baltimore, Maryland

The importance of Pfeiffer's bacillus as a pathogenic organism often associated with respiratory infections is generally recognized. It is a very difficult matter, however, to determine whether the organism is the primary cause of an infection. In measles and whooping cough the organism is unquestionably to be regarded only as a frequent secondary invader. There is a large group of infections diagnosed as colds, sporadic influenza, or epidemic influenza in which it is by no means certain that the organism, when found, is merely a secondary invader as in measles and whooping cough. It is the purpose of this paper to report an accidental infection in which it seems reasonably certain that Pfeiffer's bacillus was the primary etiological agent.

Previous accidental or experimental inoculations of Pfeiffer's bacillus in human beings have been reported by several authors. Davis[1] inoculated a volunteer intranasally with a culture of Peiffer's bacillus isolated from whooping cough. Headache, cough, and a temperature of 100.2 F. developed. The symptoms lasted three days. Cultures from the nose, throat, and sputum showed many organisms similar to those inoculated. The volunteer remained a carrier for four weeks. Tedesko[2] in 1907 stated that the pathologist Kretz contaminated his hands by breaking a culture of Pfeiffer's bacillus over them. A condition resulted which was described as a typical attack of influenza. The sputum remained positive for Pfeiffer's bacillus for a period of two months. An extensive series of experiments was performed in 1919 under the direction of Rosenau and McCoy.[3] Volunteers were inoculated intranasally with strains of Pfeiffer's bacillus recently isolated from cases of influenza. The results were entirely negative. Other volunteers were inoculated with unfiltered nasopharyngeal secretions from influenza patients, likewise with negative results as far as the production of any syndrome resembling influenza. Sellards and Strum[4] inoculated volunteers with strains of Pfeiffer's bacillus isolated from measles. No symptoms developed, nor did any of the volunteers become carriers. Wahl, White, and Lyall[5] inoculated five volunteers intranasally with old strains of Pfeiffer's bacillus. There was no clinical response, although the organisms persisted in the nares for two days and in the nasopharynx for one to three weeks. In another experiment by the same authors, two

Received for publication, March 19, 1928.

1. J. Infect. Dis., 1906, 3, p. 1.
2. Centralbl. f. Bakteriol., 1, O., 1907, 43, p. 322.
3. Public Health Reports, 1919, 34, p. 33.
4. Bull. Johns Hopkins Hosp., 1919, 30, p. 331.
5. J. Infect. Dis., 1919, 25, p. 419.

volunteers were inoculated intranasally with a strain recently isolated from the lung of a fatal case of influenza. The results were likewise practically negative clinically, though one of the two subjects had an elevation in temperature of 0.5 F. Bloomfield[6] inoculated 14 volunteers with three strains of Pfeiffer's bacillus obtained from healthy carriers. No symptoms were produced, and in every instance where Pfeiffer's bacilli were recovered later than 24 hours after inoculation, the strains were shown to be serologically different from the strains inoculated. Park and Cooper[7] report an infection following the accidental inoculation of the throat of a laboratory worker with a culture of Pfeiffer's bacillus. Two weeks later a temperature of 101 F. developed, and the patient was confined in bed. Throat culture showed many colonies of Pfeiffer's bacillus, serologically identical with the strain accidentally inoculated. In another instance, inoculation occurred through sucking a culture into the mouth. This was followed by pharyngitis on the fourth day, accompanied by moderate prostration and a slight rise in temperature. Here, again, cultures of the pharynx yielded organisms serologically identical with those accidentally inoculated. Cecil and Steffen[8] inoculated six volunteers with two strains of Pfeiffer's bacillus obtained from clinical cases of influenza. In five of the individuals symptoms followed which could be classified either as a severe cold or as afebrile influenza. Organisms serologically identical with the organisms inoculated were isolated from the volunteers for periods of from two weeks to two months. The authors stress the fact that certain strains of Pfeiffer's bacillus have a marked power of attacking healthy mucous membranes. Cecil and Steffen controlled their results by inoculating other volunteers with sterile broth filtrates of the organisms. None of these volunteers developed any symptoms. The most recent work relating to the inoculation of humans with Pfeiffer's bacillus is that of Fenyvessy and Kopp.[9] These authors worked with an organism isolated during an epidemic of influenza which occurred in 1925. Three of five individuals inoculated developed syndromes that were described as mild influenza. One of them had a temperature of 38 C. The symptoms lasted from 3 to 4 days. Organisms similar to those inoculated were recovered from the nasopharynx. Nasopharyngeal cultures before inoculation were negative.

Summarizing this previous work, five reports (Davis, Tedesko, Park and Cooper, Cecil and Steffen, and Fenyvessy and Kopp) describe the development of definite infections after the inoculation of humans with cultures of Pfeiffer's bacillus. Tedesko, and Fenyvessy and Kopp unqualifiedly believe the disease produced in this manner to be influenza. Cecil and Steffen consider the disease produced by them probably to be influenza, while Park and Cooper consider the cases reported by them definitely not to be influenza.

Source of Culture.—The strain of Pfeiffer's bacillus with which the present report is concerned was obtained through the courtesy of Dr. Irmgard Dresel, who isolated it at necropsy from the lungs of a five months old infant. This strain has been labeled "10068," the Johns Hopkins Hospital necropsy number. The clinical diagnosis was lobular pneumonia following pertussis. During the life of the infant, Dr.

6. Bull. Johns Hopkins Hosp., 1920, 31, p. 85.
7. J. Immunol., 1921, 6, p. 81.
8. J. Infect. Dis., 1921, 28, p. 201.
9. Centralbl. f. Bakteriol., 1, O., 1926, 98, p. 477.

J. Howard Brown isolated B. pertussis from the sputum on the potato-glycerol-blood agar of Bordet and Gengou. Necropsy showed lobular pneumonia, pulmonary abscesses, and bronchiectatic cavities. Cultures of the lungs on ordinary blood agar showed Pfeiffer's bacillus, and pneumococcus, group 4. The almost universal occurrence of Pfeiffer's bacillus in pertussis is well known. This fact has been recently emphasized by Povitsky [10] who found Pfeiffer's bacillus present in almost every case of pertussis examined. It was invariably present in great numbers at the beginning of the second week of the whoop.

Morphologically, the 10068 strain is the classical coccobacillus described by Pfeiffer in his original communication. This morphology has been constantly preserved when grown in chocolate broth and transferred at intervals of 3 to 6 days. Elongated rods and filamentous forms, however, develop in chocolate broth cultures kept at room temperature for several weeks. The elongated forms reproduce true for at least several generations. The organism grows much more profusely on chocolate mediums than on red blood. There has been no tendency for it to grow on ordinary mediums. Nitrates are reduced. Indol is not formed. The organism is not hemolytic.

An antiserum was prepared by rabbit injection. This serum agglutinated the homologous strain in the dilution of 1:1280, and failed to agglutinate another strain of Pfeiffer's bacillus even in the dilution of 1:10. A third strain of Pfeiffer's bacillus (from meningitis) was agglutinated by the serum in the dilution of 1:80.

Medical History. Mode of Inoculation.—The infection occurred in a laboratory worker (E), male, 35 years of age. In the past he has been very susceptible to colds, averaging 3 or 4 severe colds a year. There has been 3 attacks of influenza, in 1918, in 1920, and in 1923. In each instance influenza was present in epidemic form in the locality. All three attacks were febrile (at least 103 F.). Conjunctivitis and bronchitis were present. Prostation during convalescence was marked. No bacteriological examinations were made.

On October 27, 1927, E. inoculated a rabbit intranasally with a chocolate broth culture of the 10068 strain. The animal sneezed as each drop was allowed to fall from the pipet, and the fluid was expelled as droplets and fine spray. E. felt many of the droplets strike his face.

It is believed, beyond any reasonable doubt, that the above incident represents the moment of inoculation. The culture had been in the

10. J. Infect. Dis., 1923, 32, p. 8.

laboratory only 12 days, and there was no other known opportunity for E. to acquire the infection. The strain had been isolated at autopsy 16 days previously.

Course of Infection.—The symptoms and bacteriological examinations are listed chronologically, October 27th being considered as the first day.

Day

1 Accidental inoculation.

2 At 7 p. m. (28 hours after inoculating the rabbit) a severe frontal headache developed. Two hours later E. began sneezing. This was accompanied by a profuse watery nasal discharge. The mucous membranes of the nose were swollen, and breathing through the nose was difficult. Nasal culture: many colonies of Staphylococcus albus and of a delicately growing diphtheroid.

4 The watery nasal discharge and sneezing have continued. Nasal culture: very heavy growth of Pfeiffer's bacillus. A few colonies of Staphylococcus albus.

6 The nasal discharge has become mucopurulent, and somewhat yellowish in color. Herpes has developed on the skin above the upper lip in two places, one just below the midline, and the other just lateral to the left nostril. Nasal culture: very heavy growth of Pfeiffer's bacillus. No other organisms.

10 There is a bilateral conjunctivitis, with a small amount of mucoid exudate. Culture of conjunctivae: Pfeiffer's bacillus in almost pure culture. There are a few colonies of Staphylococcus albus and of gram-negative cocci.

12 The mucopurulent nasal discharge continues though it is not so profuse. A cough has developed, especially marked in the morning. The expectoration is purulent, and of a uniform yellowish green color. Culture of sputum: very heavy growth of Pfeiffer's bacillus.

15 This date may be roughly taken as marking the end of definite symptoms. The conjunctivitis, rhinitis, and cough have markedly improved. The temperature was taken at irregular intervals throughout the infection, usually in the evening. At no time was the temperature above 99.2 F. During the infection, E. went to the laboratory daily as usual. There was constantly present a marked feeling of oppression, and nothing much was accomplished in the way of work.

17 Nasal Culture: very heavy growth of Pfeiffer's bacillus with a few colonies of Staphylococcus albus.

30 Nasal cultures, sputum cultures, and throat cultures during the past 13 days have been negative for Pfeiffer's bacillus.

35 There has been present today a definite sense of nasal obstruction. The obstruction was transient, passing away in the evening. Nasal culture: a few colonies of Pfeiffer's bacillus and of Gram negative cocci.

39 Nasal Culture: Pfeiffer's bacillus, Staphylococcus albus, and diphtheroids in about equal numbers.

75 Repeated nasal cultures and throat cultures since the 39th day have been negative for Pfeiffer's bacillus. There have been no further respiratory symptoms.

In every instance where Pfeiffer's bacillus was isolated the organisms were morphologically and culturally similar to the 10068 strain. The strains isolated from the nose on the fourth day, from the conjunctivae on the 10th day, from the sputum on the 12th day, and from the nose on the 39th day were agglutinated by an antiserum for 10068 to its full titer, 1280. In no instance was any evidence of serological change observed in the organisms isolated.

E's blood serum was examined on six occasions during and after the infection for the presence of agglutinins for the 10068 strain. The results were entirely negative.

DISCUSSION

It is of considerable interest that the first nasal culture, made at the time of the initial symptoms, was entirely negative for Pfeiffer's bacillus. This might lead one into considering the possibility of the Pfeiffer bacillus having been grafted upon some pre-existing infection. While the possibility cannot be ruled out entirely, it must be recognized as a pure speculation. The production by Cecil and Steffen of definite symptoms in 5 out of 6 experimental subjects, renders such an assumption entirely unnecessary. I believe that Pfeiffer's bacillus was the primary cause of the infection just described for the following reasons: the symptoms began about 28 hours after an opportunity of acquiring by spray inhalation a large dose of the organisms; cultural examinations showed the organism to be present in predominating numbers in all inflammatory exudates examined during the height of the symptoms; the symptoms agree fairly closely with the symptoms of some of the experimental inoculations described by other authors. The fact that the first culture was negative for Pfeiffer's bacillus I interpret as showing that bacteriological examination may miss entirely the causative organism in infections of this kind, and may show other organisms of a very doubtful significance.

On account of the absence of definite fever, the infection would ordinarily be classified as a severe cold. The absence of fever, however, does not necessarily rule out the diagnosis of influenza. Bloomfield and Harrop [11] state that 11% of the patients studied by them during the 1918 epidemic were entirely afebrile. The case described here, though, can be strictly interpreted as demonstrating only that Pfeiffer's bacillus is able to attack the normal respiratory mucous membrane as a primary incitant of disease, rather than throwing any definite light on the possible relation of Pfeiffer's bacillus to influenza.

This avidity of some strains of the organism for attacking normal mucous membrane is, in general, favorable to the hypo-

11. Bull. Johns Hopkins Hosp., 1919, 30, p. 1.

thesis that Pfeiffer's bacillus is the cause of influenza. The evidence which still led him to consider the organism as the cause of influenza was reviewed by Pfeiffer[12] in 1921. A more recent review is by Zinsser.[13] The latter, while admitting the incompleteness of the evidence, is also inclined to consider Pfeiffer's bacillus as the etiological agent.

SUMMARY

The course of a laboratory infection with Pfeiffer's bacillus is described. The symptoms consisted of rhinitis, conjunctivitis, and bronchitis. There was no fever. Organisms serologically identical with the laboratory strain were isolated from the nose, conjunctivae, and sputum. The disease would ordinarily be classified as a severe cold, though the diagnosis of sporadic influenza cannot be entirely eliminated. The infection demonstrates anew that some strains of the organism have an extraordinary avidity for attacking respiratory mucous membrane as the primary cause of disease.

12. Centralbl. f. Bakteriol., 1, O., 1921, 85, p. 43.
13. Textbock of Bacteriology, 1927.

STAPHYLOCOCCUS AUREUS CONJUNCTIVITIS OF THE NEWBORN

ARTHUR B. THOMAS

From the Pathology Laboratory, Elizabeth Steel Magee Hospital and Department of Pathology, University of Pittsburgh, Pa.

Twenty years ago Sydney Stephenson reviewed the subject of ophthalmia neonatorum with special reference to etiology. After a thorough study of the literature he concluded that two-thirds of the cases of acute purulent conjunctivitis of the newborn were due to the gonococcus,[1] while in the remaining one-third the conjunctivitis was caused by other organisms or by mechanical or chemical injury. Stephenson [2] further asserted that all cases were directly or indirectly the result of an infective vaginitis in the mother. May [3] stated that two-thirds of all cases of ophthalmia neonatorum were produced by infection from a gonorrheal vaginitis; in one-third the infection resulted from a simple catarrhal vaginitis. The prevailing conception regarding the nature and the origin of the causative agents in purulent conjunctivitis in the newborn is in keeping with the opinion of these authors.

The list of microorganisms associated with ophthalmia in the newborn is moderately long. In 1914,[4] a general survey of the causative microorganisms revealed the following: of every 100 cases of ophthalmia neonatorum 65% were due to the gonococcus, 10% to the pneumococcus, 5% to B. coli, 5% to other organisms, the most important of which were Streptococcus pyogenes and the Koch-Weeks bacillus, and in the remaining 15% no organisms were found in the exudate. In the readily available literature on the subject [5] from 1790 to the present time it was impossible to find more than passing mention of the staphylococci as causative agents in the production of a purulent conjunctivitis of the newborn. Collins and Mayou [6] dismissed the subject with the

Received for publication, April 19, 1928.

1. Ophthalmia Neonatorum, 1907, p. 62.
2. Practitioner, 1914, 93, p. 382.
3. Diseases of the Eye, 1924, p. 108.
4. Ref. 2, p. 380.
5. De Schweinetz: Diseases of the Eye, 1924. Am. Encyclopedia of Ophthalmology, —?—, p. 3163. Duane, Alexander and Hastings: New York M. J., 1906, 83, p. 1058. Groenouw: Arch. Ophthalmol., 1898, 27, p. 557. Love, L. F.: New York M. J., 1920, 112, p. 242. Lehrfeld, Louis: Am. J. Ophthalmol., 1923 (series 3), 6, p. 380. Waldeck, G. M.: J. Mich. M. Soc., 1922, 21, p. 591. Nehl, W.: M. Record, N. Y., 1922, 101, p. 623. Thompson, J. H.: J. Missouri M. A., 1917, 14, p. 7. Luedde, W. A.: Am. J. Ophthalmol., 1907, 24, p. 195. Wilder, William H. and Davis, David J.: Trans. Am. Ophthal. Soc., 1913, p. 377.
6. The Pathology and Bacteriology of the Eye, 1925, p. 495.

statement that Staphylococcus aureus is associated with one of the more virulent forms of ophthalmia neonatorum. Because of the prevailing impression that the staphylococcus plays a minor role in the etiology of this disease it is thought pertinent to report a series of 100 cases in which the causative agent was an atypical staphylococcus aureus.

In 1926-27 a small epidemic of acute purulent conjunctivitis occurred among the infants in the hospital. It was characterized by a sudden onset, a thick greenish-yellow creamy discharge, redness and swelling of the eyelids. The first signs were usually apparent six to 12 days after birth. One or both eyes became involved and after three to four days of treatment with argyrol the inflammation subsided, with no permanent damage. From the clinical picture the casual observer would have had difficulty in distinguishing the disease from gonorrhoeal ophthalmia. Indeed, at the outset there was also some difficulty in the bacteriological diagnosis due to the fact that smears of the exudate showed, in addition to pus and fibrin, a gram-negative intracellular diplococcus. It was the study of this organism which proved to be of interest and eventually led to the isolation of a virulent atypical staphylococcus. The following characteristics of the organism were studied: the morphology and staining, in direct smears of the exudate, and in smears of the organism from various culture mediums; the reaction on mediums and gross appearance of the colonies; carbohydrate metabolism; thermal death points; agglutination reactions, and the pathogenicity for animals.

In direct smears of the exudate stained by Gram's method, the organisms appeared as small cocci arranged usually in pairs but sometimes in small agglomerations. There was apparently a moderate degree of pleomorphism. It was difficult to determine, however, that this apparent difference in size may not have been due to the staining since the smaller cocci invariably gave up the dye when stained by Gram's method. The larger cocci were gram-positive. These characteristics of pleomorphism and metachromasia were exhibited by all of the cultures studied. In many instances a diplococcus was both pleomorphic and metachromatic in which case the smaller half was gram-negative. Phagocytosis was demonstrated in many of the smears and the picture often closely resembled that seen in gonorrheal exudate. The cultures, however, were all negative for gonocci. The microscopic pictures of the staphylococci taken from the various culture mediums were similar to those seen in smears of the exudate, both in pleomorphism and polychromasia.

The organism grew readily on all ordinary mediums, including broth, plain agar, blood agar, gelatin and Loeffler's medium. In broth the organism produced a general turbidity in 24 hours with a granular sediment in 48 hours. On plain agar the colonies were moist, raised, slightly irregular in outline and showed within four to five days a rich orange pigment. On blood agar hemolysis occurred in 18 hours. Proteolysis of Loeffler's mediums occurred in three days. Stab cultures in gelatin medium showed saccate liquefaction of the medium in 24 hours becoming stratiform in three to six days. Staphylococci used as controls showed a saccate liquefaction which did not become stratiform. The reaction of the organism to various carbohydrates differed from control staphylocci principally in the fermentation of mannitol with the production of acid. Dextrose, galactose, sucrose, maltose, lactose, mannitol and dextrin were fermented with the production of acid but no gas. Raffinose, dulcitol, xylose, inulin, salicin and inositol were not fermented. Lead acetate was not reduced. Indol was not formed.

The thermal death point was ascertained by heating freshly inoculated broth medium in a water bath at 56 C., incubating the tubes at 37 C. for 24 to 48 hours and then transferring to solid medium. Two hours were required to kill the most resistant culture.

With these characteristics of the staphylococcus definitely established an attempt was made to classify it further according to agglutination reactions. For this purpose five rabbits were given 3 intravenous injections with salt solution suspensions of killed organisms at intervals of three days, and were bled five days after the last injection. The serum obtained was used to study the agglutination reactions of cultures of the the organism and of five controls. The results of the agglutination test while not conclusive are at least suggestive that the organisms belonged to one group.

Pathogenicity for animals was tested as follows: Salt solution suspension of the organism from a 12-hour agar culture was used. Five cc. of the suspension were injected into the stomach of a rabbit in an effort to produce an enteritis. The result of this test was negative. A drop of the suspension was introduced into each eye of a white mouse. There was a transient congestion of the conjunctivae lasting about 12 hours but no exudate developed. The experiment was repeated on two more mice with the same results. An attempt was then made to produce lesions in the eyes of rabbits. The right cornea in each of three rabbits was scarified with a sharp scalpel and a few drops of the material were introduced. Two of the animals developed a mild conjunctivitis lasting three to four days. Two other rabbits treated in a like manner with control organisms did not develop lesions. One cc. of the material was injected subcutaneously into the abdominal wall of a guinea-pig. Two days later a definite abscess had developed. A purulent exudate drained from this lesion for six weeks, the animal became extremely emaciated and finally died. On two different occasions a staphylococcus was isolated from the lesion which was in all respects identical with the organism being studied. Similar injections with control staphylococcus aureus gave negative results. Three rabbits were given subcutaneous injections of the material into the abdominal wall. Two developed abscesses, two similarly treated with control organisms did not.

Further evidence of the virulence of the organism was furnished by its ability to produce lesions in other parts of the body. It was obtained in pure culture from six cases of breast abscess, the wounds of two abdominal incisions, one axillary abscess, two of dermatitis, one of rhinitis, one from a carbuncle of the nose which was probably the result of an accidental inoculation, and from the stools of ten cases of enteritis in infants.

With this evidence it seemed reasonable to conclude that the epidemic of conjunctivitis was due to a single virulent strain of an atypical staphylococcus. An attempt was then made to ascertain its origin and to determine the mode of transmission. The organism was obtained for the first time from the stool of a premature infant dying of enteritis. Further than this is was impossible to trace it. As to the mode of transmission there were several possibilities. Due to the variety of lesions produced, it seemed that the infection was not derived from a vaginitis in the mothers. Attention was, therefore, directed to an examination of materials with which the infant came in contact soon after birth. Various materials were cultured but found to be sterile or containing only nonpathogenic organisms with two exceptions.

From these two sources an organism was obtained which was identical with that cultured from the conjunctival exudate. The first was a large bottle of supposedly sterile olive oil used by the nurses to cleanse the skin of the infants. The second was a dish of saturated boric acid solution used to bathe the breasts and nipples of the mothers immediately before the infants were fed. In 1927 Garretson and Cosgrove [7] showed that boracic acid could harbor pathogenic organisms and reported a series of cases of ulceration of cornea and panophthalmitis due to B. pyocyaneus and Staphylococcus aureus, the organisms possibly having been transferred from the boracic acid to the eyes. More careful use of the boric acid solution and sterilization of the olive oil in our wards were followed by a disappearance of the epidemic. It, therefore, seemed probable that the epidemic was produced by the use of contaminated olive oil or boric acid or by both.

7. J. Am. M. A., 1927, 88, p. 700.

CONCLUSIONS

An acute purulent conjunctivitis may occur in infants without evidence of a preexisting vaginitis in the mother. In 100 consecutive cases of purulent conjunctivitis of the newborn none appeared to be caused by the gonococcus. Cultures of Staphylococcus aureus, isolated from the conjunctivitis and some other lesions that were present, seemed to belong to a single strain and were atypical in staining qualities, metabolic reactions with carbohydrates, and in pathogenicity for animals. This organism was considered to be the causative agent in all the cases and was probably transmitted through contaminated olive oil or boric acid or both.

CHEMICAL AND BACTERIAL INHIBITION OF GAS FORMATION IN BACTERIAL CULTURES

Mitsuteru Ishikawa

From the Department of Research Bacteriology, Northwestern University Medical School, Chicago

Inhibitory influences, chemical and bacterial, on the production of gas by bacteria have been noticed by few investigators. Pakes and Jollyman [1] found that sodium nitrate has a suppressing effect on the generation of gas from sodium formate by B. coli-communis, B. enteritidis Gärtner and the pneumobacillus of Friedlander. Herter [2] noticed that sodium benzoate added to nutrient broth inhibits the evolution of gas from a carbohydrate by bacteriums, such as B. coli and B. aerogenes, and that calcium carbonate prevents the inhibition by the benzoate. Theobald Smith and D. E. Smith [3] described that certain strains of paratyphoid bacilli exert a definite inhibitory influence on the liberation of gas from lactose by the colon bacillus.

In this article are reported studies of the inhibitory effect of various chemical substances on the production of gas by both single and associative cultures, and of the mechanism involved in the symbiotic phenomenon reported by Smith and his associate.

CHEMICAL INFLUENCE

Bismuth subnitrate, potassium bichromate, potassium chlorate, sodium fluoride, sodium iodate and sodium salicylate were used in the experiments, sodium benzoate and potassium nitrate also being employed in the hope of obtaining further informations of their influences. Stock solutions of these substances were prepared with distilled water, except that of bismuth salt which was dissolved in a dilute hydrochloric acid solution, to make following concentrations:

Bismuth subnitrate, 0.1 mol.	Sodium iodate, 0.1 mol.
Potassium bichromate, 0.01 mol.	Sodium salicylate, 0.15 mol.
Potassium chlorate, 0.01 mol.	Sodium benzoate, mol.
Sodium fluoride, mol.	Potassium nitrate, mol.

Single Cultures.—With pure cultures of various organisms five following experiments were conducted.

Received for publication, May 11, 1928.

1. J. Chem. Soc., 1901, 79, p. 457.
2. J. Biol. Chem., 1909, 7, p. 59.
3. J. Gen. Physiol., 1920-1921, 3, p. 21.

Method: Three kinds of medium were used: broth, synthetic, and broth agar. The broth was composed of peptone 10 gm., meat extract 2 gm., sodium chloride 5 gm., monobasic acid potassium phosphate 1 gm. and 1000 cc. of water. The synthetic medium consisted of sodium chloride 5 gm., magnesium sulphate 0.2 gm., ammonium chloride 10 gm., monobasic acid potassium phosphate 1 gm., a trace of calcium chloride and a liter of water. The broth agar was prepared by melting 10 gm. of washed agar in a liter of broth. The reaction was adjusted to approximately neutral, and Andrade indicator or brom-cresol-purple solution was added for the detection of changes of reaction. The fluid mediums were used in Smith fermentation tubes and the agar medium in ordinary test tubes; 13 cc. of the fluid into a fermentation tube and 7 cc. of the agar into a test tube were poured. Then, varying amounts, from 0.1 cc. to 0.5 cc. to a tube, of chemical solutions mentioned above were added to tubes, which was followed by giving proper amounts of distilled water to make the total volume of the solution and water thus added to tubes equal. The reaction of tubes was adjusted carefully with a dilute solution of NaOH when the acid solution of bismuth salt was added. These tubes having been sterilized by autoclaving, sterile 20% solutions of carbohydrates were added to them, by giving 1 cc. of the solution to a Smith tube and 0.5 cc. to an agar tube. Bacteria were planted by taking 0.1 cc. of broth cultures to a fermentation tube and one loopful of the same to an agar tube. Inoculated tubes were kept in the incubator at 37 C. usually for two days.

Exper 1: It was intended to detect influences of the chemicals on the acid and gas production of various types of bacteria. B. alkaligenes, B. foetidus, B. enteritidis, B. morgani, B. proteus, B. paratyphosus B, B. mucosus, B. coli and B. aerogenes were cultivated in glucose agar tubes containing varied amounts of the chemical substances. Effects exerted by bismuth subnitrate and potassium iodate are as follows:

	Bismuth Subnitrate					Sodium Iodate				
Cc.	0.1	0.2	0.3	0.4	0.5	0.1	0.2	0.3	0.4	0.5
B. alkaligenes	0	0	0	0	0	0	0	0	0	—
B. foetidus	a	a	a	a	a	a	a	a	a	a
B. enteritidis	ag	a	a	a	a	ag	a	a	a	—
B. morgani	ag	a	a	a	a	ag	a	a	a	a
B. proteus	ag	a	a	a	a	ag	ag	a	a	a
B. paratyphosus	ag	a	a	a	a	ag	a	a	a	—
B. mucosus	ag	ag	a	a	a	ag	a	a	a	a
B. coli	ag	ag	a	a	a	ag	ag	a	a	a
B. aerogenes	ag	ag	ag	a	a	ag	ag	a	a	a

ag = acid and gas, a = acid, 0 = no acid and no gas, — = no growth.

Essentially similar results were shown by the other substances, save the nitrate which neither exhibited any deleterious effect on bacterial growth nor allowed marked acid production in tubes without gas. The experiments brought out, therefore, that B. alkaligenes which does not ferment glucose, and B. foetidus which produces acid, were not affected noticeably in their fermentative ability by the presence of the chemicals, that the presence of certain amounts of these substances permitted aerogenous bacilli to yield only acid, while smaller amounts allowed the production of both acid and gas and greater amounts even inhibited their growth, and that different kinds of aerogenous bacilli were influenced by the substances in practically the same manner.

Exper. 2: Comparisons were made of the inhibitory effects of the subcarbonate, subgallate, nitrate and subnitrate of bismuth, of ammonium and sodium benzoates, and of ammonium, potassium and sodium nitrates. Bismuth salts were used—subgallate was dissolved with NaOH solution and the others with

HCl solution—at the concentration of 0.1 mol., and benzoates and nitrates at 1.0 mol. Glucose agar tubes to which varying amounts of these salt solutions had been added were employed. B. coli, B. morgani and B. proteus were seeded in the tubes. It was found that subcarbonate, subgallate, subnitrate and nitrate of bismuth were analogous in their suppressing effect on gas formation; so with benzoates and nitrates. In addition, bismuth subcarbonate was compared to calcium and sodium carbonates in like manner. The results revealed that calcium and sodium carbonates did not, contrary to bismuth subcarbonate, inhibit the generation of gas to a noticeable degree. This seems to indicate that bismuth itself is responsible for the inhibition exerted by bismuth compounds.

Exper. 3: The object of these experiments was to determine the influence of the salts of bismuth (bichromate, chlorate, fluoride, iodate, salicylate, benzoate, and nitrate) on the liberation of gas from various carbohydrates by B. coli, B. morgani, B. aerogenes. Glucose, lactose, sucrose, maltose and mannitol were used. To agar tubes containing these carbohydrates varied amounts of chemical solutions were added, as in the first experiments. In tubes which contained proper amounts of chemicals, definite acid reaction was brought forth from glucose by B. morgani, from glucose, lactose, maltose and mannitol by B. coli and from glucose, lactose, sucrose, maltose and mannitol by B. aerogenes. This finding intimates that evolution of gas from lactose and others was suppressed by the presence of these substances as well as from glucose. Moreover, the results showed that an aerogenous bacillus which is unable to attack certain carbohydrates under ordinary conditions produced neither acid nor gas under the influence of such chemical substances.

Exper. 4: This study was to ascertain any differences between the broth and the synthetic mediums with regard to the influence of the chemicals. The medium, broth and synthetic, contained glucose as the source of gas production. These were held in Smith tubes to which various amounts, from 0.1 cc. to 0.5 cc. as in other cases, of the chemical solutions were added. B. coli and B. proteus were used. In brief, this resulted in showing a slight difference between the two kinds of mediums: generally speaking, less amounts of the solutions were required for inhibiting gas formation in the synthetic medium than in the broth. If the fact that the growth of bacteria was more luxuriant in the broth than in the synthetic medium is considered, this outcome would seem rather natural.

It has been reported by Hoppe-Seyler,[4] Pakes and Jollyman[5] and Harden[6] that several microorganisms are able to generate gas from salts of formic acid. And, in the light of investigations by Frankland and associates,[7] Franzen and Braun[8] and Franzen and Steppuhn,[9] the formation of gas from carbohydrates appears to originate mainly in the decomposition of formic acid, an intermediate product of fermentation. It is of significance, therefore, in interpreting the nature of the inhibitory effect studied herein to know how the chemical substances affect gas formation from formic acid.

Exper. 5: These were carried out to determine if the chemicals affected formation of gas from formic acid. The experiments were practically the duplicates of the first experiments with glucose, except that 20% solution of

4. Ztschr. f. physiol. Chem., 1887, 11, p. 556.
5. J. Chem. Soc., 1901, 79, p. 386.
6. Ibid., 1901, 79, p. 610.
7. Ibid., 1892, 61, p. 270.
8. Ztschr. f. physiol. Chem., 1908, 68, p. 29.
9. Ibid., 1912, 77, p. 129.

sodium formate, which had been filtered through Berkefeld filter, was used instead of the sugar solution.

Neither gas nor acid was produced by B. alkaligenes and B. foetidus in any of the tubes, while B. enteritidis, B. morgani, B. proteus, B. paratyphosus B, B. mucosus capsulatus, B. coli and B. aerogenes evolved gas in tubes containing 0.1 cc. of the chemical solutions but not in tubes of 0.5 cc.: it should be remembered that B. alkaligenes and B. foetidus are not able but all of the aerogenes bacilli experimented with are able to liberate gas from sodium formate in ordinary mediums. The results illustrate, it appears, that organisms which possess the ability to decompose sodium formate into gases under ordinary conditions do not produce gas from the substance in the presence of proper amounts of bismuth and other chemicals.

Now, it is evident that the production of gas from carbohydrates and from sodium formate are equally vulnerable to the inhibitory influence of the chemical substances which have been studied.

Associative Cultures.—I [10] have already studied the production of gas by associative cultures of bacteria: a gas-forming organism with one that is acid-producing; a gas-producing bacillus with a proteolytic organism, and a gas-forming and acid-producing organism with a proteolytic bacterium. How these three types of bacterial associations are influenced, in their gas-producing activity, by bismuth subgallate, potassium bichromate, potassium chlorate, sodium fluoride, sodium iodate, sodium salicylate, sodium benzoate and sodium nitrate, is the subject of the following experiments. Solutions of these substances were used at the same concentrations as in the preceding experiments.

For different types of synergic cultures, broth, milk and gelatin mediums were employed. Fresh pasteurized milk was used as the milk medium. And the gelatin medium was prepared by using 5 gm. of pure gelatin, instead of ammonium chloride, as the sole source of nitrogen in a liter of the synthetic base described before. They were poured into Smith tubes, 13 cc. being given to a tube, to each of which 0.5 cc. of the above mentioned chemical solution was added. Otherwise, adjustment of reaction, sterilization, incubation were accomplished in the same manner as in the experiments with single cultures.

Gas-Forming and Acid-Producing Organisms: B. morgani was selected for the gas-forming and B. foetidus for the acid-producing organism. It must be recalled that B. morgani yields acid and gas from glucose but not from lactose and other carbohydrates, while B. foetidus produces acids but not gas from glucose, lactose and the like, and that when these two organisms are cultured symbiotically they produce not only acid but also gas from lactose and other carbohydrates which can not be attacked by B. morgani alone. Into lactose broth containing the chemicals, these microbes were inoculated simultaneously. In the tube which contained any of the chemical substances, they produced acid but failed to form gas, in contrast to a noticeable generation of gas by them in the control tube. The growth of bacteria in tubes of chemicals was not so luxurious as in the control, yet it was not so scanty as to justify the assumption that the

10. J. Infect. Dis., 1927, 41, p. 238.

failure of generating gas was due to insufficient growth. The experiment with sucrose broth gave rise to identical results.

Gas-Producing Bacillus with Proteolytic Organism: B. coli, as a producer of gas, and B. subtilis, as a proteoclastic organism, were inoculated at the same time into milk, to which the chemical substances had been added. It has been shown [10] that the colon bacillus alone does not yield an appreciable amount of gas in milk, unless it is cultured in association with a proteolytic bacterium or one of certain nitrogenous substances, such as digested products of proteins, peptone, amino acids and ammonium salts, is added intentionally to the medium. This experiment showed that the two organisms failed to generate gas to any extent in the tubes containing the substances, bismuth and others.

In addition to the foregoing experiment, the colon bacillus was grown in milk tubes, each of which contained 1 cc. of 5% peptone or glutamic acid solution and 0.5 cc. of one of the chemical solutions. Here again the colon bacillus failed to generate gas. Of course control tubes for both experiments—symbiosis of B. coli with B. subtilis in plain milk, and B. coli alone in milk containing peptone or the amino acid—produced gas.

It may be stated, therefore, that in the presence of the chemicals B. coli does not yield gas in milk, either in association with a proteolytic organism or under the accelerating influence of nitrogenous substances.

Gas-Forming and Acid-Producing Organisms with a Proteolytic Organism: In the gelatin medium held in Smith tubes, to which lactose and one of the chemical substances had been added, three strains of bacteria, B. morgani, B. foetidus, B. mesentericus, were cultivated. B. mesentericus, which decomposes gelatin vigorously but does not attack lactose, had been grown for 24 hours before the other two organisms were inoculated. It should be noted here that B. morgani and B. foetidus can not produce gas symbiotically from lactose in this gelatin medium, in contrast to their gas-forming activity in lactose broth, but they do produce acid and gas in the lactose gelatin medium, in the presence of proper nitrogenous substances or through the association with a proteolytic bacterium. Yet, gas could not be noticed in the mixed culture tubes containing the chemical substances. It was also found, as in the preceding experiment, that peptone and glutamic acid did not exhibit their accelerating effect, in the presence of the chemicals, on the formation of gas by the symbiosis of B. morgani and B. foetidus in the lactose gelatin medium.

These findings are indicative, it may be interpreted, of the inhibitory effect of bismuth and other substances on the evolution of gas in mediums containing only complex proteins, by the associative cultures of three kinds of bacteria, or by the symbiosis of an acid-producing and a gas-forming organism under the accelerating influence of proper nitrogenous substances.

Throughout these experiments with associative cultures, it was noticed that potassium nitrate was not quite identical to the other inhibitory substances in its effect, that is, as pointed out in the experiments of single cultures, nitrate showed no detrimental influence on bacterial growth, yet, did not allow bacteria to produce definite acid reactions, whereas all of the others exhibited a tendency of hindering bacterial growth, though decisive acid reactions took place in the presence of them.

BACTERIAL INFLUENCE

In the light of previous work,[10] it appears that the intensive production of gas by aerogenous bacilli requires the presence of certain simple types of nitrogenous substances in culture mediums. This leads to the assumption that the inhibitory action involved in the phenomenon described by Smith and Smith,[3] of the paratyphoid bacillus may be caused, partly at least, by the insufficiency of proper nitrogenous substances necessary for the gas-producing activity of the colon bacillus. To determine the validity of such an assumption, the following experiments have been carried out.

Effect of B. Paratyphosus B on B. Coli.—Method: Broth and synthetic mediums like those used in the preceding experiments were prepared, with the difference in some instances of including varying amounts of peptone (the sole source of nitrogen in the synthetic medium). To 13 cc. of fluid in each Smith tube, after sterilizing, 1 cc. of sterile lactose solution was added. Bacteria were inoculated by carrying 0.1 cc. of broth cultures to the tube, which subsequently was kept at 37 C. One of our stock cultures of paratyphoid bacilli, which is B. paratyphoid B serologically, was selected to be used, on account of its definite inhibitory effect on gas production of B. coli.

Varying Amounts of Peptone: It was desired in this experiment to detect the relation between varied amounts of peptone and grades of inhibition. To Smith tubes containing the synthetic base varying amounts of peptone and water, 0.1, 0.2, 0.3, 0.4 and 0.5 cc. of 20% peptone solution and 0.5, 0.4, 0.3, 0.2 and 0.1 cc. of water to correspond, were added before autoclaving. The paratyphoid bacillus had been grown for three days in those tubes when the colon bacillus was inoculated. At the end of 24 hours incubation, unequal amounts of gas were formed by this synergic culture. In five control tubes of the colon bacillus, which contained different amounts of peptone but no paratyphoid bacillus, approximately equal amounts of gas were generated. In contrast to this, volumes of gas evolved in the tubes of associative culture were roughly proportional to the amounts of peptone added to tubes. The tube of 0.1 cc. peptone yielded less than the tube of 0.2 cc., and the 0.3 cc. tube produced more than the 0.2 cc. tube. Thus, the 0.1 cc. tube contained the least and the 0.5 cc. tube the greatest amounts of gas. Yet, even the tube of 0.5 cc. did not liberate so much gas as the control tubes.

These observations would indicate that the paratyphoid bacillus lessened the amount of simple nitrogenous substances which apparently are indispensable for gas formation by the colon bacillus, and that the amounts of such substances remaining in tubes were nearly in proportion to the amounts of peptone originally added, consequently, gas being generated to varied extents corresponding to amounts of suitable nitrogenous substances.

Additional Nitrogenous Substances: The aim of this experiment was to reveal the effect on the inhibitory phenomenon produced by adding peptone, glutamic acid and ammonium chloride to the culture medium. Lactose broth was heavily seeded with the paratyphoid bacillus, and incubated for 4 days; then, 1 cc. of sterile 5% solution of peptone, glutamic acid or of ammonium chloride was added to tubes, the colon bacillus was planted, and the culture results were examined after incubation for 1 day. The tube without additional substances showed just a trace of gas, while those with peptone, glutamic acid or ammonium chloride contained greater amounts of gas. In the control tube without any additional substance, the single culture of the colon bacillus generated gas most vigorously.

It would seem that these substances, peptone, glutamic acid, and ammonium chloride accelerated the formation of gas by providing nitrogenous substances.

Associative Culture.—In association with the paratyphoid and the colon bacilli, B. mesentericus was cultivated to find out what effect, if any, the latter has on the synergic phenomenon of the former two organisms. Lactose broth was used. The paratyphoid bacillus had been grown for three days before B. coli and B. mesentericus were inoculated simultaneously. The results obtained by 24-hour incubation after the final inoculation were; the associative culture of the colon bacillus with B. mesentericus yielded a larger amount of gas than the single culture of the colon bacillus, the mixed culture of the three organisms produced as much gas as the colon bacillus alone, and the tube which contained the symbiotic culture of the colon and the paratyphoid bacilli had a decidedly smaller volume of gas than any of the other tubes.

Thus, B. paratyphosus and B. mesentericus seem to have exerted antagonistic influences, inhibitory and accelerating, on the production of gas by B. coli. Probably the antagonism originated in their opposing actions toward simple nitrogenous substances; the paratyphoid bacillus has a tendency not to increase markedly amino and ammonia nitrogens at an early period of cultivation, as will be discussed in the following chapter, whereas B. mesentericus shows a definite increase of such nitrogens under similar conditions.

Production of Ammonia.—According to the extensive investigation of Kendall, Day and Walker [11] on changes of milk induced by diverse microorganisms, B. paratyphosus B first decreased and later increased the amount of ammonia in milk, while many other bacteria increased it from the beginning of cultivation. One of the tables given by them shows that the increase of ammonia nitrogen due to this organism was — 0.70, 0.00, + 1.40 (expressed as mg. per 100 cc. of milk) in 1, 3 and 7 days respectively. And the work by Kendall and Haner [12] brought out clearly the nature of nitrogen metabolism of this bacillus and others, through the determination of total, protein, nonprotein, polypeptid, amino and ammonia nitrogens. They found that the paratyphoid bacillus produced in the plain gelatin medium 35, 23, 31 of amino nitrogen and 60, 60, 69 of ammonia nitrogen (both expressed as mg. per 100 cc. of the medium) on the first, third, sixth days respectively, while the control free from bacteria contained, without change during the period, 32 of amino and 57 of ammonia nitrogens. They also found that

11. J. Am. Chem. Soc., 1914, 36, p. 1937.
12. J. Infect. Dis., 1922, 30, p. 236.

the bacillus increased to a marked degree, progressively from the first to the sixth days, the amount of protein nitrogen at the expense of polypeptid nitrogen.

These results suggest that the paratyphoid bacillus is, particularly in early days of cultivation, more active in converting simple nitrogenous substances into complex ones than in decomposing complex substances into simpler forms.

An attempt was made to compare B. paratyphosus B (1), which has been used in the preceding experiments, with more or less similar organisms as to the formation of ammonia. Two strains of B. paratyphosus B, and one strain each of B. morgani and B. paratyphosus A were inoculated in plain broth. After the incubation of 4 days, the cultures were tested for ammonia, the determination being conducted as described by Kendall.[13] The results expressing mg. of ammonia nitrogen per 100 cc. of culture medium are as follows:

B. paratyphosus B (1).........	36.4	B. paratyphosus A..............	56.0
B. paratyphosus B (2).........	47.6	B. morgani	57.4

It should be noted that the bacteria other than B. paratyphosus B (1) showed no definite inhibitory effect on the gas-producing activity of B. coli. This result indicates that the strain of B. paratyphosus responsible for the inhibitory phenomenon generated the least amount of ammonia.

DISCUSSION

The finding that the generation of gas by single cultures of aerogenic bacilli, from carbohydrates and from sodium formate is influenced by bismuth and other chemical substances, and the assumption that gas formation from carbohydrates is due to the decomposition of formic acid, lead to the interpretation that the inhibitory effect of such substances, except ammonium, potassium and sodium nitrates, is the result of their detrimental influence on the formation or the activity of formiase, which is regarded as responsible for the disintegration of formic acid. It is probable that nitrates, differing from other chemical substances used, suppress the generation of gas through a chemical reaction with formic acid as described by Pakes and Jollyman.[1]

As to the nature of the inhibitory effect on the formation of gas by the synergism of a gas-forming and an acid-producing organism, nothing can be deduced, inasmuch as the mechanism underlying this phenomenon still remains obscure.

13. J. Infect. Dis., 1922, 30, p. 211.

The previous study [10] on the mechanism involved in the generation of gas through the symbiosis of an aerogenous bacillus and a proteolytic organism revealed that the rôle played by the proteolytic bacterium is to pave the way, by decomposing complex proteins, for the fermentative activity of the other. Accordingly two suppositions may arise concerning the inhibitory effect considered herein; the one is to suppose that it is a result of deleterious influence of the chemical substances on protein-decomposing activity of the proteolytic organism, and the other is to assume that it originates in their effect on fermentative activity as is the case with single cultures. An experiment in regard to the effect of bismuth subgallate, potassium bichromate, potassium chlorate, sodium benzoate, sodium fluoride, potassium iodate, sodium benzoate and potassium nitrate upon the proteolytic action of bacteria was conducted. This was carried out in the same manner as described in the experiment with casein of a previous paper,[10] save that gelatin was used instead of casein and that varying amounts of the chemicals were added to tubes, wherein B. mesentericus, B. proteus and Staphylococcus were cultivated. The result showed that these substances did not arrest, when used at the concentrations similar to those of foregoing experiments, the proteoclastic activity of bacteria on gelatin. Probably the chemicals exerted some influence on the proteolysis, although this can not be stated definitely, since the method was not a quantitative one. Yet, it was revealed, beyond doubt, that the chemicals did not inhibit proteolysis so definitely as they did the formation of gas. It may reasonably be assumed therefore, that the inhibition of gas formation is due to the detrimental effect on fermentative process rather than to the deleterious influence on proteolysis.

Direct influence of these chemicals on the gas-producing activity of a gas-forming and an acid-producing organism in symbiosis would seem to account for the inhibition of gas formation caused by the associative culture of these two kinds of bacteria with a proteolytic organism, because in this association the proteolytic organism apparently accelerates the generation of gas which takes place initially through the symbiosis of the other two, and because the experiment mentioned above has shown that the presence of the chemical substances does not arrest completely the protein-splitting activity.

It was found that peptone or glutamic acid added to milk and gelatin mediums did not prevent the inhibitory action of bismuth and other chemicals. This finding provides an evidence in support of the assumption that the inhibitory effect of the chemical substances is dependent on their detrimental influence on fermentative process rather than on protein hydrolysis, since it is probable that if the insufficiency of proper nirogenous substances, resulting from the arrest of proteolysis, is responsible for the suppression of gas production, the addition of simple nitrogenous substances ought to accelerate gas production.

Series of experiments concerning the symbiotic phenomenon described by Smith and Smith seem to have shown that the inhibitory effect of the paratyphoid bacillus on the generation of gas from lactose by the colon bacillus is likely due, partly at least, to the insufficiency of simple nitrogenous substances, which appears to be caused by a somewhat characteristic metabolical activity of the paratyphoid bacillus.

SUMMARY

Subcarbonate, subgallate, nitrate, subnitrate of bismuth, ammonium and sodium benzoates, potassium bichromate, potassium chlorate, sodium fluoride, sodium iodate, ammonium and sodium nitrates, and sodium salicylate definitely suppress the evolution of gas, not only from carbohydrates by single cultures of gas-producing bacilli and by three types of associative cultures (a gas-forming with an acid-producing organism, an aerogenous bacillus with a proteolytic organism, and gas-forming and acid-producing organisms with a proteolytic bacterium), but also from sodium formate by pure cultures of aerogenous bacteria. The inhibitory effect of the paratyphoid bacillus on gas production of the colon bacillus appears to depend, partly at least, on a deficiency of proper nitrogenous substances apparently resulting from the metabolic activity of the paratyphoid bacillus.

INFLUENCE OF IODIDE ON BACTERIAL DECOMPOSITION OF NITROGENOUS SUBSTANCES

Mitsuteru Ishikawa

From the Department of Research Bacteriology, Northwestern University Medical School, Chicago, and the Department of Bacteriology and Public Health, Washington University School of Medicine, St. Louis

The effect of iodides on the nitrogen metabolism of human and animal bodies has been studied by several investigators. Grabfield, Alpers and Prentiss[1] reported that there was an increase in the nitrogen excretion from the human body following the ingestion of iodides. Hesse[2] found that the influence of potassium iodide was practically the same, either administered parenterally or given by mouth. Boothby and Rowntree[3] stated that iodides did not cause any noticeable change in the basal metabolic rate of normal persons. Grabfield and Prentiss[4] showed that iodides of sodium, lithium, calcium, potassium, strontium and magnesium had an increasing effect on the nitrogen excretion in the human urine. They[5] concluded, in their study of the effect of iodides on the nitrogen partition, that the increase did not change the partition of total nitrogen, ammonia nitrogen, uric acid and creatinine in both urine and blood. According to Grabfield, Gray, Flower and Knapp,[6] sodium iodide injected subcutaneously increased the nitrogen excretion of a normal dog but not of a dog from which the thyroid gland had been removed.

In the light of such studies, particularly of the last mentioned work by Grabfield and associates, it appears of interest to determine the influence of iodides on the activity of microorganisms (comparatively simple, unicellular structures) toward nitrogenous substances. The present work has been carried out to determine how potassium iodide influences the disintegration of gelatin and the decomposition of urea by diverse bacteria.

DISINTEGRATION OF GELATIN

Generation of Ammonia.—Urea in the urine and ammonia in cultures of bacteria have approximately analogous significance as the manifestation of nitrogen metabolism of human beings and microorganisms. In the following experiments, therefore, through the determination of ammonia produced in mediums, the effect of iodine compounds on the disintegration of gelatin by cultures of proteolytic bacteria was detected.

Received for publication, April 4, 1928.

1. J. Pharm. & Exper. Therap., 1924, 22, p. 393.
2. Arch. f. exp. Path. u. Pharm., 1924, 102, p. 63.
3. J. Pharm. & Exper. Therap., 1924, 22, p. 99.
4. Ibid., 1925, 25, p. 411.
5. Ibid., 1926, 27, p. 231.
6. J. Clinic. Invest., 1927, 4, p. 323.

Method.—Nutrient broth used as the base of mediums was prepared by dissolving peptone, 10 gm.; meat extract, 1 gm.; sodium chloride, 5 gm., in 1 liter of water. Eighty cc. of the broth were poured into 200 cc. flasks, and 10 cc. of 10% gelatin solution were added to every flask. Then, different amounts of 1% solution of potassium iodide or potassium iodate were added to the flasks, and the content of a flask was made up to 100 cc. with proper amounts of distilled water, e. g., when 1 cc. of the iodine solution was used 9 cc. of water were added. The reaction was adjusted to approximately neutral. The flasks were covered with small beakers, instead of being plugged with cotton, and sterilized in the autoclave. Inoculation of bacteria was accomplished by adding 0.1 cc. of plain broth culture of an organism to a flask. Inoculated flasks were kept in the incubator at 37 C. Ammonia was determined by the air current method modified by Kendall[7] to be suitable for bacteriological experimentation.

In the first experiment, effects of potassium iodide and potassium iodate on the ammonia production of B. proteus vulgaris were compared. Ammonia was measured on the second, fourth and sixth days of cultivation, and the results recorded as follows:

Ammonia Nitrogen (Mg. per 100 Cc.) Produced by B. proteus in Mediums Containing Iodide or Iodate in Different Percentages

		0	0.005%	0.01%	0.05%	0.1%
Potassium iodide	2 days	24.5	23.8	23.8	23.1	22.4
	4 days	42.7	39.2	39.2	38.5	37.1
	6 days	63.0	58.1	57.4	54.6	47.6
Potassium iodate	2 days		23.8	23.1	22.4	22.4
	4 days		37.8	37.1	37.1	35.0
	6 days		56.7	55.3	54.6	49.0

The results indicate that both substances exerted, progressively from 0.005% to 0.1%, a definite inhibitory effect, that the effects of the two compounds were nearly of the same intensity, and that the influence did not vary to a noticeable degree at different periods of incubation.

In the second experiment, three kinds of proteolytic bacteria: B. mesentericus, B. proteus-vulgaris and B. pyocaneus, were compared in their ability of generating ammonia under the influence of potassium iodide. After 5 days' incubation, the ammonia nitrogen (mg. per cc.) was determined as previously described and recorded as follows:

KI	0	0.002%	0.01%	0.02%	0.04%	0.06%
B. mesentericus..................	91.0	81.2	77.0	72.8	70.0	67.2
B. proteus.........................	35.0	33.6	33.6	32.9	30.8	30.1
B. pyocyaneus....................	56.0	51.8	53.9	52.5	51.1	49.0

B. mesentericus produced decisively greater amounts of ammonia than B. proteus and B. pyocyaneus not only in the absence but also in the presence of the iodide, and B. pyocyaneus, compared with B. proteus, generated more ammonia in both the iodide mediums and the plain medium. This intimates that potassium iodide did not have a noticeable

7. J. Infect. Dis., 1922, 30, p. 211.

selective action, so far as its influence upon the bacterial decomposition of gelatin was concerned. In addition, these results seem to corroborate the findings of the preceding experiment.

Production of Amino Acids.—The two experiments provided sufficient evidence that potassium iodide exerts an inhibitory effect on the generation of ammonia by proteolytic organisms. Since the iodide was added to culture mediums, however, the possibility that the influence might be due to its impedimental effect on the growth of bacteria still remains.

Kendall and Walker [8] found that the liquefaction of gelatin by a sterile solution containing the soluble proteolytic enzyme of B. proteus is not associated with an increase of ammonia; this is interpreted by them as indicating that hydrolytic cleavage of the protein, shown by the liquefaction of gelatin, is independent of deaminization.

Therefore, by means of the soluble proteolytic enzyme of the proteus bacillus it was intended, in the experiment to be described, to elucidate mainly two points: what is the effect of the iodide on the activity of bacteria-free enzyme, and, how the iodide affects decomposing action other than deaminization of proteolytic bacteria.

Method.—B. proteus-vulgaris was inoculated from an agar slant into some 300 cc. of plain broth contained in a 500 cc. flask, and cultivated for 7 days at 37 C. Then, the culture was filtered through a Berkefeld filter. Ten cc. of the filtrate were added to each of 200 cc. flasks containing sterile mixed solution of gelatin and potassium iodide; one flask had 50 cc. of distilled water containing the iodide, at concentrations from 0.001% to 1.0%, and 10 cc. of 10% gelatin solution. The flasks had been kept for 5 days at 37 C. before they were tested for amino nitrogen.

Amino nitrogen was determined by formol titration, as described by Kendall.[7] At the time of titration, sterility of the flasks was examined by inoculating small portions of the contents, 1 cc. from each flask, into plain broth tubes, none of which indicated bacterial growth. The results were as follows:

KI, %....................	0	0.001	0.01	0.05	0.1	0.2	0.4	0.6	0.8	1.0
Amino N (mg. per 100 cc.).	39.2	39.2	37.8	36.4	36.4	33.6	32.2	31.5	30.1	28.0

The iodide, the results appear to illustrate, had a detrimental effect upon the activity of the proteolytic enzyme, not associated with bacterial growth, and that its presence decreased the amounts of amino acids produced from gelatin by the enzyme.

DISINTEGRATION OF UREA

It is an established fact that urea is split into ammonia and carbon dioxide by the urease activity of diverse microorganisms. I have made a

8. J. Infect. Dis., 1915, 17, p. 442.

study [9] of the bacterial decomposition of urea, with special reference to the influence of carbohydrates. It has brought out, among other things, that utilizable carbohydrates actually accelerate the liberation of ammonia from urea by several bacteriums, cultured and washed, and that thymol has an inhibitory effect on the urease activity.

For the purpose of detecting how potassium iodide affects the decomposition of urea by cultured or washed bacteria, the following experiments were made. Disintegration of urea was measured by the determination of ammonia, which was accomplished in the same way as described before.

Bacteria in Culture.—The methods used were like those for studying ammonia production from gelatin, save that 10% urea solution instead of gelatin solution was used. The urea solution was filtered through a Berkefeld filter, and was added to sterilized contents of flasks to made its final concentration 1%. B. proteus-vulgaris and B. ammoniagenes were studied. B. ammoniagenes has been described by Cooke and Keith [10] as a vigorous urea-splitting organism, and two strains used in this experiment were obtained through the courtesy of Dr. Cooke. Ammonia was determined on the first and third days of incubation at 37 C., with following results:

		KI%	0	0.002	0.01	0.02	0.04	0.06
Ammonia N (mg. per 100 cc.)	B. ammoniagenes	1 day	145.6	140.0	140.0	135.8	114.8	106.4
		3 days	380.8	343.0	343.0	334.6	308.0	299.6
	B. proteus	1 day	308.0	305.2	305.2	299.6	294.0	285.6
		3 days	343.0	333.2	330.6	330.6	324.8	322.0

The outcome reveals that the liberation of ammonia by both organisms was impaired by the presence of potassium iodide, that the decrease in ammonia production was roughly proportional to the amounts of iodide in the medium, and that both bacteria did not exhibit a distinctly different susceptibility to the deleterious influence.

Washed Bacteria.—There is the possibility, as pointed out before, that the foregoing effect on urea decomposition might have originated in the harmful effect of the iodide on bacterial growth, inasmuch as it was added to culture medium. But the following experiments with washed bacteria made it certain, it would seem, that the decreasing effect is intrinsically associated with the urea-splitting activity of bacteria.

The organisms used were B. ammoniagenes, B. lactis-aerogenes, B. proteus and Staphylococcus aureus, all of which actively disintegrated urea in culture mediums. The method for the preparation of washed bacteria has been described

9. J. Infect. Dis., 1928, 43, p. 67.
10. J. Bact., 1927, 13, p. 315.

in a previous publication[9] In this experiment, all bacteria were grown on 1% glucose agar plates.

The mixture of physiological salt solution containing potassium iodide, bacterial suspension and urea solution was held in ordinary test tubes: the tube contained 8 cc. of physiologic salt solution with varying percentage of iodide, 1 cc. of bacterial suspension and 1 cc. of 10% urea solution, but when glucose was added, 7 cc. instead of 8 cc. of physiologic salt solution and 1 cc. of 10% glucose solution. Ammonia was determined after keeping the tubes at 37 C. for 10 to 20 hours—tubes of an organism were, of course, tested simultaneously. B. ammoniagenes and B. proteus were examined in the absence of glucose, while B. lactis aerogenes and Staphylococcus were tested in the presence of the sugar. But, the results of B. ammoniagenes and B. lactis-aerogenes are omitted from the tabulation, because these organisms gave rise to a similar outcome to that of the other two bacteria.

In the light of the author's previous work the question of bacterial growth can be excluded from the interpretation of these results with washed, suspended bacteria. Accordingly, the table may be regarded as indicating that the iodide had a deleterious effect on the urease activity of bacteria, and that the effect was definite in the presence, as well as in the absence, of glucose: glucose has been proved to have a marked accelerating effect on the decomposition of urea by the suspensions of B. lactis-aerogenes, Staphylococcus and others.[9]

	KI %	0	0.01	0.05	0.1	0.2	0.4	0.6	0.8
Ammonia N (mg. per 100 cc.)	B. proteus	178.6	169.8	155.8	154.4	151.6	148.4	148.4	137.6
	Staphylococcus	142.8	140.0	134.4	128.8	127.4	128.8	123.2	121.8

DISCUSSION

The experiments reveal that potassium iodide exerts an inhibitory influence on bacterial decomposition of nitrogenous substances, gelatin and urea. Thus, it would seem that the effect of potassium iodide on such activities of microorganisms and on nitrogen metabolism of higher organisms are not in accord, since, as referred to at the begining of this paper, the administration of iodides increases the nitrogen excretion of animal bodies.

The deleterious influence of the iodide on the disintegration of nitrogenous substances by bacteria is due, it would seem, to its detrimental effect on the activity of enzymes, according to observations of the experiments with the filtrate containing the soluble enzyme of B. proteus and with the washed bacteria of several kinds.

The experiment with the bacteria-free filtrate has shown clearly that the iodide has an inhibitory effect on the activity of the enzyme responsible for the production of amino acids from gelatin. This leads to the assumption that this decreased production of ammonia from gelatin by bacteria in culture mediums is very likely concerned with two factors: the decreased production of simple forms of nitrogenous substance, as mentioned, and the impaired activity of deaminase, owing to the iodide. The results which brought out that the iodide exerts an analogous influence to both cultured and washed bacteria upon the liberation of ammonia from urea appears to offer an evidence in support of the foregoing statement.

Urease and protease are quite different enzymes: this is obvious in the light of various evidences, e. g., urea-splitting organisms are not always proteolytic bacteria; the proteolytic enzyme may be obtained in the filtrate free from bacteria, but it has failed so far to secure urease in such a way; and the presence of an utilizable carbohydrate accelerates urea decomposition but inhibits proteolysis. Therefore, from the ground that the iodide undoubtedly affects the activity of the proteolytic enzyme, it is not warranted to draw a definite conclusion, but it may be assumed that the iodide has an inhibitory effect on the activity rather than on the formation of urease.

On the whole, the experiments described seem to show that the disintegration of nitrogenous substances by bacteria is more or less impaired by the presence of potassium iodide, and that the inhibitory influence of the substance is chiefly, if not entirely, due to its deleterious effect on the activity of enzymes. It is of interest to note, in this connection, that Grabfield and his associates [6] stated, "It seems likely that this increase (by iodides) in nitrogen excretion without a corresponding increase in sulphur excretion represents mobilization and excretion of deposit nitrogen."

CONCLUSIONS

Potassium iodide and potassium iodate exert an inhibitory effect on the formation of ammonia by cultures of proteolytic organisms and on the production of amino acids by the proteolytic bacteria-free enzyme. In this effect, potassium iodide has practically no demonstrable selective action; different bacteria are affected almost equally by the presence of the iodide. The liberation of ammonia from urea by urea-splitting bacteria, cultured or washed, is decreased under the influence of the iodide, apparently through an inhibitory effect on the activity of the enzymes.

THE THERMAL DEATH POINT OF BRUCELLA ABORTUS IN MILK

Ruth Boak and C. M. Carpenter

From the Diagnostic Laboratory, New York State Veterinary College, Cornell University, Ithaca

Inasmuch as it has been demonstrated that certain strains of Brucella abortus are pathogenic for man and that these may occur in milk and other dairy products,[1] more information concerning the thermal death point of the organism is desirable. There is only meager information in the literature concerning its resistance to heat, the prevailing opinion being that Brucella abortus is very sensitive to heat and easily destroyed at a comparatively low temperature. This opinion probably is based on the fact that it does not grow readily and abundantly on the ordinary culture mediums under normal atmospheric conditions.

MacFadyean and Stockman [2] observed that Brucella abortus was destroyed in two hours when exposed to a temperature of 55 C. Zwick and Wedeman [3] state that it is killed in from ten to fifteen minutes at 60 C., and in five to ten minutes at 65 C. At a recent meeting of the American Public Health Association, Park [4] reported results upon data he obtained by mixing several strains of Brucella abortus isolated from cattle and swine with cultures of Brucella melitensis. He observed that all cultures were killed when exposed for ten minutes at 140 F., for seven minutes at 142 F., and for five minutes at 145 F. The suspension used by Park contained 5,000 million bacteria per cc.

Observations have been made on the thermal death point of eight strains of Brucella abortus. Four of these, 1, 2, 3 and 4 were isolated from milk by guinea-pig injection. Cultures 1 and 4 were recovered from certified milk and culture 3 from milk which was being drunk by a patient who had undulant fever. Culture 2 was isolated from the Ithaca City milk supply. The three human cultures, 5, 6 and 7, were recovered in culture from the blood of patients suffering from undulant fever. The porcine strain, 8, was isolated from a fetus.

Received for publication, April 16, 1928.

1. Carpenter and Baker: Cornell Veterinarian, 1927, 17, p. 236. Carpenter and Boak: Am. J. Pub. Health, 1928, to be published.
2. Report of Dept. Com. to inquire into epizootic abortion, London, 1909, part 1, p. 10.
3. Arb. a. d. k. Gsndhtsamte, 1912, 63, part 1.
4. Unpublished paper read at 56th annual meeting of Am. Pub Health Assoc., October, 1927.

Test tubes containing 10 cc. of sterilized whole milk were inoculated with the growth from agar slants of the above cultures and incubated 48 hours at 37 C. Sternberg bulbs [5] of an approximate 2 cc. capacity were filled with this inoculated milk and sealed. The filled bulbs were immersed completely in an electrically controlled water bath for successive intervals of 5, 10, 15 and 20 minutes, at a temperature of 140 F. With the exception of the 20 minute intervals, the same exposures were used at 142 F. and 145 F. At the end of the desired exposure the bulbs were removed and placed immediately in an ice water bath. After breaking the seal by filing off the end of the bulb stem, the bulb was warmed and several drops of the treated milk were forced out into a tube containing 10 cc. of liquefied agar to which 1 cc. of sterile defibrinated blood had been added. This inoculated medium was then plated. Guinea-pigs received intraperitoneally the amount remaining in the bulb which varied from 1 to 1.5 cc. The plate cultures were allowed to incubate at 37 C. for one week before they were considered negative.

TABLE 1.—VIABILITY (+) OF ORGANISMS EXPOSED TO DIFFERENT TEMPERATURES FOR 5 TO 20 MINUTES AND THEN TESTED IN CULTURES (C) AND BY GUINEA-PIG INOCULATION

Temperature of exposure			140 C.				142 C.			145 C.		
Minutes exposed.......			5	10	15	20	5	10	15	5	10	15
Organism from milk	1	c	+	+	0	0	+	0	0	0	0	0
		gp	+	+	0	0	+	0	0	0	0	0
	2	c	+	+	0	0	+	0	0	+	0	0
		gp	+	+	0	0	+	+	0	+	0	0
	3	c	+	+	0	0	+	0	0	0	0	0
		gp	+	+	0	0	+	0	0	0	0	0
	4	c	+	+	0	0	+	0	0	0	0	0
		gp	+	+	0	0	+	0	0	0	0	0
Human	5	c	+	+	0	0	+	0	0	0	0	0
		gp	+	+	0	0	+	0	0	0	0	0
	6	c	+	+	0	0	+	+	0	+	0	0
		gp	+	+	0	0	+	+	0	+	0	0
	7	c	+	0	0	0	+	0	0	0	0	0
		gp	+	+	0	0	+	0	0	0	0	0
Porcine	8	c	+	+	+	0	+	+	0	+	0	0
		gp	+	+	+	0	+	+	0	+	0	0

The guinea-pigs were necropsied from three to five weeks following their inoculation with the milk. They were examined for macroscopic lesions of the abortion disease, their serum was tested for abortus agglutinins, and the spleens were removed and cultured for Br. abortus.

Cultures were made and guinea-pigs given injections with milk from control bulbs that were filled as were the bulbs that were exposed to the various temperatures. The cultures from the control bulbs showed luxuriant growths of Brucella abortus. The guinea-pigs injected with the untreated milk showed typical lesions of abortus infection. The exact number of organisms per cc. was not determined but it greatly exceeded the number occurring in naturally infected milk. The results of these studies are shown in the table.

It will be noted that the temperature and time of exposure required to destroy the several strains of Brucella abortus used in this work

5. Am. J. Med. Sci., 1887, 94, p. 146.

varied. The porcine culture was the most resistant, withstanding temperatures of 140 F. for 15 minutes, 142 F. for 10 minutes, and 145 F. for 5 minutes. It failed to grow in cultures or to infect guinea-pigs when exposed for 20 minutes at 140 F., for 15 minutes at 142 F., and for 10 minutes at 145 F.

One bovine culture (2) and one human culture (6) were somewhat less resistant than the porcine strain (8). They were killed after 15 minutes exposure at 140 F., although they were viable for 10 minutes at 142 F., but dead at 15 minutes, while neither was viable after 10 minutes at 145 F. The other three bovine cultures, 1, 3, 4, and the two remaining human strains, 5 and 7, showed similar resistance, being killed after 15 minutes exposure at 140 F., 10 minutes exposure at 142 F. and 5 minutes exposure at 145 F. In two instances guinea-pigs became infected with the treated milk while the cultures remained negative. No growth was obtained from strain 2 after exposure for 10 minutes at 142 F. but the guinea-pig showed typical lesions of abortus infection. Culture 7 infected a guinea-pig after 10 minutes exposure at 140 F. but the culture remained negative.

In the two cases where it was observed that guinea-pigs became infected when the cultures were negative, the result may have been due to the fact that more of the treated milk was injected into the guinea-pig than was used for making cultures. We believe, however, that in general guinea-pig injection is more satisfactory and more dependable than the use of culture mediums. Hagan [6] has demonstrated that only a very few of the organisms are required to infect a guinea-pig.

Four of the cultures 1, 2, 3 and 4, grown in whole milk, were exposed at 160 F. for ½, 1, 1½ and 2 minutes successively. The organisms were viable at the one-half minute exposure but failed to grow in cultures or to infect guinea-pigs after a one minute exposure.

CONCLUSIONS

The thermal death point of eight strains of Brucella abortus of porcine, human and bovine origin grown in milk was variable. The porcine strain was most resistant. An exposure of 15 minutes at 140 F. (60 C.) destroyed the human and bovine cultures that were examined. The porcine strain, however, was still viable at this temperature.

Injection into guinea-pigs was more reliable than cultures for determining the viability of Brucella abortus in milk.

6. J. Exper. Med., 1922, 36, p. 697.

CLASSIFICATION OF BACTERIUM ALCALIGENES, PYOCYANEUM, AND FLUORESCENS

Bruno Leo Monias

From Uihlein Memorial Laboratory, Grant Hospital, Chicago, and the Pathological Laboratory of Rush Medical College, University of Chicago

The following article is a continuation of a previous study on classification of bacteria of the human intestines [1] It deals with the classification of different strains of E. Pribram's microbiological collection isolated by different investigators at various times.

Original Names and Sources of 30 Cultures Used in Study

1. Bacterium faecale alcaligenes nr. 198, 1887..............Petruschky, Danzig
2. Bacterium faecale alcaligenes, 1916......................Petruschky, Danzig
3. Bacterium faecale alcaligenes, 1911.........................Basel, Wurzburg
4. Bacterium vitulinum.......................Lehmann Neumann, Weissenberg
5. Bacterium pyogenes foetidum................................Jaiser, Stuttgart
6. Bacterium faecale alcaligenes.....................................Frankfurt
7. Bacterium faecale alcaligenes, 1925...................... Path. Dept., Vienna
8. Bacterium faecale alcaligenes nr. 58...........................Jaffé, Vienna
9. Bacterium faecale alcaligenes nr. 68...........................Jaffé, Vienna
10. Bacterium faecale alcaligenes nr. 1053.........................Jaffé, Vienna
11. Bacterium faecale alcaligenes nr. 1097a.......................Jaffé, Vienna
12. Bacterium faecale alcaligenes nr. 1097b.......................Jaffé, Vienna
13. Bacterium denitrificans ....Jensen
14. Bacterium faecale aromaticum 1.......................................Stutzer
15. Bacterium faecale aromaticum 2.......................................Stutzer
16. Bacterium pyocyaneum alpha, 1893...................................Gessard
17. Bacterium pyocyaneum beta, 1893..Ernst
18. Bacterium pyocyaneum, 1917..............................Herbert, Vienna
19. Bacterium pyocyaneum...................................University, Vienna
20. Bacterium pyocyaneum Carnforthvigss.........Jaffé, Grant Hospital, Chicago
21. Bacterium pyocyaneum....................................Schnürer, Vienna
22. Bacterium viride Lodzense, 1916..................................Wolf, Lodz
23. Bacterium pyocyaneum, 1921............................University, Vienna
24. Bacterium syncyaneum beta...........................Lehmann, Wuerzburg
25. Bacterium fluorescens liquefaciens...................Lehmann, Wuerzburg
26. Bacterium fluorescens aureus......................................Zikes, Vienna
27. Bacterium putidum (Spirillum)........................Lehmann, Wuerzburg
28. Bacterium fluorescens liquefaciens...................Grassberger, Vienna
29. Bacterium fluorescens...Jaiser, Stuttgart
30. Bacterium fluorescens, 1913..............................Piorkowski, Berlin

The methods used in this work are described in the first paper: [1] the Gram stain, Zettnow's method for demonstrating flagella, tests for milk

Received for publication, April 4, 1928.

1. J. Infect. Dis., 1927, 40, p. 570.

coagulation, Ehrlich's indol test. Pribram and Halle's test for acid and gas production from carbohydrates and for liquefaction of gelatin.

Organisms 1 to 5 of the tabulation are gram-negative, almost as long as wide, motile by means of peritrichous flagella, form smooth colonies on agar, do not liquefy gelatin, and grow in broth forming a sediment. They produce indol in broth, alkali in litmus milk, acid and gas on different carbohydrates. There are some morphological and biological differences among these strains regarding the length and width of the rods, the formation of colonies on agar plates and sugar fermentation: organisms 1 and 2 ferment almost all carbohydrates, 3 and 4 ferment only a few, 5 ferments dextrose and galactose only. Organisms 6 to 15 differ from the first 5 strains. They are also gram-negative rods, some straight, some curved with polar flagella. The growth on agar is smooth with entire colonies, gelatin is not liquefied, indol is not formed, nor is acid in any carbohydrate, but milk is made alkaline. All organisms except 6 and 9 grow brown on potatoes and all except 9 form sediments in broth. Some of them liquefy gelatin, 6, 7 and 13 do not.

Organisms 16 to 24 are gram-negative rods with monotrichous flagella, form alkali, produce a green color, liquefy gelatin and have no ferments for carbohydrates. Organisms 16 and 18 are slender, 17, 19 and 22 are short and thick, 17 and 19 grow smooth and all others grow luxuriantly. Number 24 differs somewhat from all others by producing indol in broth and showing a slight tendency to ferment dextrose and maltose.

Organisms 25 to 30 are straight or curved rods and carry polar flagella. They coagulate milk. Organisms 25, 26 and 27 have no ferments for carbohydrates, 28 ferments many carbohydrates, 29 ferments all except sucrose and raffinose, and 30 ferments all carbohydrates. Only one of this group, 28, produced indol.

DISCUSSION

Among the cultures isolated by different authors under the name of Bacterium faecale alcaligenes (1-15), two morphologically as well as biologically different groups could be distinguished. The organisms of the first group which includes Petruschky's [2] original culture isolated from decomposed beer, are motile with peritrichous flagella. Cultures of this group ferment all monosaccharides and especially the hexoses.

2. Centralbl. f. Bakteriol., 1. O., 1889, 19, p. 187.

Some of these strains form acid only, others develop gas from carbohydrates. Some of these cultures ferment monoses only, others act on the bioses (disaccharides). The organisms of the second group are also motile, have polar flagella and do not ferment any carbohydrates.

The first of these two groups is related to the group of Bacterium coli. Their fermentative power is much less than that of the coli group and to a great extent no acid can be produced from lactose. Alcaligenes * faecalis Petruschky named according to the nomenclature of the Society of American Bacteriologists typifies this species, and is described by Bergey [3] as being "motile by means of peritrichous flagella." The further remark that it does not form acid or gas in carbohydrate mediums, does not agree with my findings on cultures examined. It might be that if solid mediums under purely aerobic conditions (agar stroke) were used, different results would be obtained. The method used in this examination was that of an anaerobic culture in a liquid medium (Congo red broth).

The second group with polar flagella corresponds to the group of Pseudomonas Migula. According to the classification of the Society of American Bacteriologists this group belongs to the genus Pseudomonas. The species should be called "Pseudomonas alcaligenes." Lehmann and Neumann [4] change the former name of "Bacterium alcaligenes" into "Vibrio alcaligenes," referring to Strecker's article. Strecker evidently worked on cultures having polar flagella only. Petruschky's strain on the contrary has peritrichous flagella.

A few other cultures have been examined and classified with regard to their relationship to the two groups. Two organisms, Bacterium vitulinum Weissenberg and Bacterium pyogenes foetidum Jaiser, had peritrichous flagella and fermented carbohydrates to variable degrees. Another culture, Bacterium denitrificans, isolated by Jensen from horse feces, is closely related to the species Pseudomonas alcaligenes. It has peritrichous flagella and no ferments for carbohydrates. A similar culture, Bacterium denitrificans Christensen, is described in Bergey's manual as possessing "peritrichous (?) flagella." A question mark after the word peritrichous signifies that the morphology of this microorganism is still questionable. The photograph of Jensen's organism shows how difficult it is to decide whether the flagella are peritrichous or polar in this case. But there is no doubt that the insertion of the flagella is extra polar. In

* "Alcaligines" in Bergey's Manual.[3]

3. Manual of Determinative Bacteriology, 1923.
4. Bacteriological Diagnosis, 1927.

this case the culture cannot be classified as Pseudomonas and the correct classification according to the American nomenclature should be: Alcaligenes denitrificans.

There is further a close relationship between the Bacterium alcaligenes and pyocyaneum. The second group, Pseudomonas alcaligenes, resembles in all its characteristics Bacterium pyocyaneum except in the color production. All cultures of Pribram's collection belonging to this group are unable to ferment carbohydrates and do not produce indol. The species Pseudomonas aeruginosa of the American nomenclature is characterized in Bergey's manual as indol-producing. It would

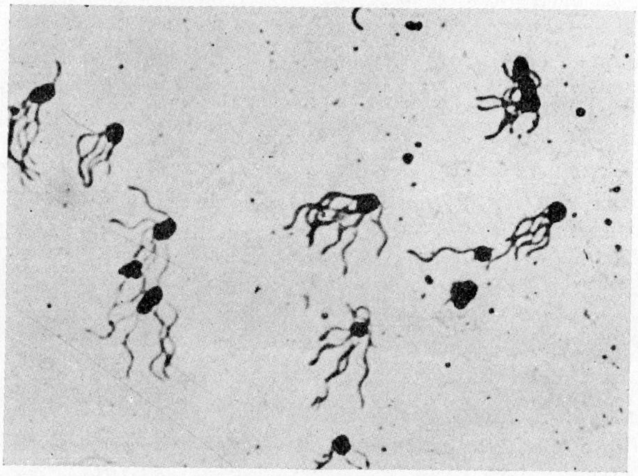

Microphotograph of Bacterium denitrificans Jensen, showing extra-polar insertion of flagella.

be correct therefore to distinguish this group from the Pseudomonas pyocyanea which does not form indol.

The cultures of Pseudomonas fluorescens which we examined coincide in all their characteristics with the qualities of this species mentioned in Bergey's Manual. There are no statements regarding the fermentation of carbohydrates by this species. The biological examination revealed that only one of the examined cultures lacked ferments for carbohydrates. Another culture fermented all carbohydrates, even mannitol, dulcitol, sorbitol and dextrin. Between these two classes we found transitional forms, some of which fermented carbohydrates, and others which affected only a few of them. Among many of them were also a few strains which produced acid but no gas. Pribram and Pulay demonstrated the relationship of this group to other groups, which extends primarily to the genus Vibrio. They further proved the relationship of these organisms to the group Pseudomonas alcaligenes. Strecker and recently Lehmann and Neumann demonstrated that the group Pseudomonas ("Vibrio") alcaligenes belongs to the species Vibrio.

The following tabulation will assist in the understanding of the results of the systematic classification of the microorganisms, which have been examined in this paper. For the classification of the fluorescens group 1 Pribram and Pulay's [5] paper and their outline may be consulted.

Alcaligenes faecalis: gram-negative, straight rods; motile by means of peritrichous flagella; indol production; alkali formation in milk; fermentation of dextrose; some strains likewise ferment other carbohydrates.

Pseudomonas alcaligenes: gram-negative, straight and curved rods; motile by means of polar flagella; no indol production; milk alkaline; no fermentation of any carbohydrates.

Pseudomonas pyocyaneum: same characteristics as Pseudomonas alcaligenes, plus production of pyocyanin.

Pseudomonas fluorescens: same characteristics as Pseudomonas alcaligenes, plus production of a small amount of pyocyanin; some strains have active ferments for carbohydrates.

Vibrio fluorescens (Vibrio putidus): same characteristics as Pseudomonas fluorescens; greater tendency to form curved rods; transitional form to the genus Vibrio, as Vibrio saprophiles and others.

SUMMARY

A microbiological collection of 30 cultures has been classified systematically on the basis of morphology and of biochemical reactions with special reference to their relationship to two main groups of bacteria, the one group related to Bacterium coli, and the other to Pseudomonas Migula.

5. Centralbl. f. Bakteriol., 1. O., 1915, 76, p. 321.

ANTIGENIC ANALYSIS OF STRAINS OF BACILLUS TYPHOSUS

LEON C. HAVENS

From the Laboratories of the Alabama State Board of Health, Montgomery

The antigenic composition of B.typhosus has been studied by a number of investigators. Observations range from close similarity between strains, on the one hand, to evidence that distinct differences exist. Hooker,[1] for example, concluded from results of agglutinin absorption and particularly complement fixation that his strains could be separated into three groups.

Aside from purely bacteriological and immunological considerations, the question of the uniformity of strains of B.typhosus presents certain practical aspects. A laboratory which does any considerable amount of diagnostic work needs for Widal tests a strain of typhoid which is readily and consistently agglutinable. The search for such a strain sometimes presents difficulties. The same problem occurs in the selection of a suitable culture for the manufacture of typhoid vaccine, local strains sometimes being employed for this purpose, on the assumption that they will be antigenically similar to most other strains of the locality. Antigenic similarity or dissimilarity also affects the identification of unknown cultures.

Attempts to obtain information bearing on these problems led to the examination of the serologic relationships of a number of cultures of B.typhosus. Evidence has been sought from the results of agglutination, agglutinin absorption, complement fixation and bactericidal tests. Eight strains have been studied intensively. Thirty additional cultures have been included in agglutinin absorption experiments.

The eight cultures on which this study was largely based are the following: 1. Rawlings: obtained from Army Medical School in 1922. 2. Mississippi: obtained from Dr. Wm. Krauss, Memphis, Tenn., in 1921; originally isolated from blood culture, 1918. 3. Pfeiffer: Rockefeller Institute, 1925. 4. Talladega: obtained from blood culture, 1923. 5. 391: obtained from blood culture, 1923. 6. Feces: carrier, 1924. 7. Blood: culture, 1924. 8. Blood: culture, 1924.

Received for publication, May 7, 1928.

1. J. Immunol., 1926, 2, p. 1.

Immune serums were prepared by the injection of rabbits with each of the eight cultures just described and these eight serums were used throughout the experiments. The injections were made with live unheated bacteria from agar cultures, suspended in physiologic salt solution. The rabbits received three injections on successive days, followed by a rest of three days, until nine injections had been given. Initial doses of about 100,000,000 bacilli were increased gradually to 2 billion for the final doses. The rabbits were bled 7 to 9 days after the last dose, the serum was removed from the clot and stored without the addition of a preservative.

TABLE 1.—AGGLUTINATION REACTIONS OF 8 STRAINS OF B. TYPHOSUS

	Strains							
Serum	1	2	3	4	5	6	7	8
1	1600	40	1600	400	1600	800	200	800
2	3200	6400	6400	800	3200	3200	1600	3200
3	320	200	3200	40	800	1600	40	200
4	6400	400	400	3200	1600	800	3200	3200
5	400	200	3200	400	3200	1600	400	400
6	800	200	3200	800	3200	3200	800	400
7	3200	1600	800	6400	1600	1600	3200	100
8	800	400	1600	800	1600	1600	800	3200

TABLE 2.—COMPARISON OF AGGLUTINABILITY OF TWO STRAINS OF B. TYPHOSUS IN WIDAL TESTS

Number Serums Tested	Total Positive	Positive with Strain 2	Positive with Strain 7
270	25	24	11

AGGLUTINATION TESTS

In table 1 are given the results of cross agglutination tests with the eight cultures and their corresponding serums. The figures refer to the highest dilution of serum in which definite clumping occurred. Marked differences in the ability of the serums to agglutinate the different strains are evident. Serum 1 varies in titer from 1 : 1600 for its homologous strain to 1 : 40 for strain 4. Serums 3, 5, 6 and 7 show similar variations in their titers for the eight strains tested. When the agglutinability of strains is compared in a large number of different serums, as in the Widal test, differences again appear. Table 2 gives the results with strains 2 and 7 in agglutination tests of 270 serums received from patients.

Positive results were obtained in 25 cases. The superiority of strain 2 over strain 7 for Widal tests is obvious. Positive results were obtained in 24 cases with the former as compared with only 11 for the latter. In only two serums did strain 7 agglutinate in a higher dilution than strain 2.

AGGLUTININ ABSORPTION

Technic: Cultures were grown for 24 hours on beef infusion agar (P_H 7.6) in Kolle flasks. The growth was washed off with salt solution, centrifugated for 20 minutes at 2,000 r.p.m. and the supernatant fluid removed. The organisms packed at this constant speed were diluted 1:20 with salt solution and the minimum absorbing dose was determined for a definite amount of the homologous serum. Absorption was carried on at 37 C. for two hours. The absorbed serum was centrifugated to remove the absorbing bacteria and serial dilutions of the absorbed serum from 1:100 to the titer of the unabsorbed serum were then tested for agglutinins. Absorption by a given strain was considered complete if the titer of the serum was diminished to 15% or less, i. e., if no agglutination occurred in a dilution of 1:100.

TABLE 3.—AGGLUTININ ABSORPTION OF 7 SERUMS BY 38 STRAINS OF B. TYPHOSUS

Strain	Years Isolated	Serum 2	4	5	6	7	8	9
1	20	+	—	—	—	—	—	+
3	15	+	+	+	—	+	+	—
2	10	—	+	—	—	—	—	—
4	4	+	+	+	+	+	+	+
5	4	+	—	+	+	+	+	+
6	4	+	—	+	+	+	+	+
7	4	+	—	—	+	—	—	+
8	4	+	+	+	+	+	+	+
9	3	+	+	—	—	—	—	—
10	3	+	+	+	+	+	+	—
11	3	+	+	+	+	+	+	+
12	3	+	—	—	+	—	+	—
13	3	+	—	+	+	+	+	—
14	3	+	—	+	+	+	+	+
15	3	+	—	+	+	—	+	—
16	3	+	+	+	+	+	+	—
17	3	+	—	+	+	+	+	+
18	2	+	+	+	+	+	+	—
19	1	+	+	+	—	—	+	—

Strain	Time Isolated	Serum 2	4	5	6	7	8	9
20	1 year	+	—	+	—	—	+	—
21	1 year	+	+	+	—	—	—	—
22	1 year	+	+	—	—	—	—	—
23	1 year	+	+	+	—	+	—	—
24	1 year	+	—	—	+	+	+	—
25	1 year	+	+	+	—	—	+	—
26	14 days	+	—	—	+	—	—	+
27	14 days	+	+	+	+	+	+	+
28	14 days	+	+	+	+	+	+	+
29	12 days	+	+	+	+	+	+	+
30	12 days	+	—	+	+	—	—	+
31	10 days	+	—	+	+	—	—	+
32	10 days	+	+	+	+	+	+	+
33	9 days	+	—	—	—	+	+	+
34	8 days	+	+	—	+	—	+	—
35	7 days	+	—	+	+	+	+	—
36	7 days	+	+	—	—	—	—	—
37	6 days	+	—	+	+	+	+	+
38	4 days	+	+	+	—	+	+	—

+ = absorption; — = no change in titer of absorbed serum.

Results: In table 3 are given the agglutinin absorption reactions of 38 strains with 7 serums. A (+) sign indicates complete absorption, a (—) sign, failure to absorb. The absorbing dose in each test was 1.5 the minimum dose found for the homologous strain. Eleven of the 38 strains absorbed all of the seven serums. Eight strains absorbed six serums and one (strain 2) failed to absorb the agglutinins from any serum but its own. Between the eleven strains which gave positive results with each serum and the one which was negative with all but its homologous serum are gradations, strains absorbing five serums, strains absorbing four, and strains absorbing only two or three serums. Rarely, however, does there occur the same combination of serums with any two of these intermediate strains.

The results of these tests indicate that antigenic differences exist between strains of B.typhosus, as determined by agglutinin absorption. About one-third of the strains examined appear to be similar in their agglutinogenic character, absorbing completely all the serums tested. Five others (5, 6, 14, 17 and 37), are similar in that they absorb the agglutinins from all but serum 2. But the tests reveal among the other strains differences of varying degree, scarcely any two showing the same absorbing capacities.

Cross absorption tests between strains illustrates these differences more sharply. Each one of eight serums was tested with each of the

TABLE 4.—CROSS ABSORPTION TESTS

Serums 1, 2, 3, 4, 5, 6, 7, 8 absorbed with strains 1, 2, 3 and tested for agglutinins with the homologous strains.

	Absorption with																
	Strain 1								Strain 2								Strain 4
Serum	1	2	3	4	5	6	7	8	1	2	3	4	5	6	7	8	1-8
1	0 1600	0 80	0 1600	0 400	0 1600	0 800	0 400	0 800	1600	0	1600	400	1600	800	400	800	0
2	100 3200	6400 6400	6400 6400	100 800	3200 3200	0 3200	0 1600	400 3200	0	0	0	0	0	0	0	0	0
3	0 3200	0 200	1600 1600	0 40	1600 1600	0 1600	0 40	0 200	0	0	1600	0	800	0	0	0	0
4	100 3200	800 800	3200 3200	1600 3200	1600 1600	1600 3200	400 3200	3200 3200	3200	0	3200	3200	1600	1600	3200	3200	0
5	0 400	0 200	3200 3200	0 400	3200 3200	1600 1600	0 400	0 400	100	0	3200	200	3200	0	100	400	0
6	0 800	0 200	3200 3200	0 800	3200 3200	1600 3200	0 800	0 800	800	0	3200	800	3200	3200	800	800	0
7	200 3200	0 1600	0 400	200 3200	100 400	100 1600	0 3200	0 160	3200	0	200	1600	0	0	1600	0	0
8	0 800	0 800	0 1600	100 800	3200 3200	200 1600	100 800	3200 3200	100	0	0	400	3200	1600	400	3200	0

strains used in producing the serums and the absorbed serum was then tested for agglutinins with each of the eight cultures. The absorbing dose here was again 1.5 the absorbing dose of the homologous strain. No two of the eight strains so examined were identical in their absorption capacities. One culture (4) absorbed all the agglutinins for all of the eight cultures from every serum. Strain 1, on the other hand, completely absorbed the agglutinins for every culture only from its own serum, and less completely from serum 7. The other strains varied between these limits.

Table 4 gives the results with strains 1, 2 and 3 and is illustrative of the irregularity of the results obtained. The figures indicate the highest dilution of the absorbed serum which agglutinated the test organism. Under the results for strain 1 the lower figure in each section is the result obtained with the unabsorbed serum. The figure at the head of each column is the strain with which the absorbed serum was tested for agglutinins.

Although these tests with full absorbing doses indicate the agglutinogenic variability of the typhoid bacillus, further experiments, summarized in table 5, furnish additional evidence of this complexity. Each of three serums (1, 3 & 7) was absorbed with four strains in fractional doses, from 1.5 to 0.05 dose. The serums thus absorbed with graduated doses of the several strains were then tested for agglutinin content with the strains whose numbers are given at the heads of the columns. The figures are the highest dilutions of the absorbed serums with which agglutination occurred.

Table 5.—Fractional Agglutinin Absorption

Absorbing Dose	Serum 1: 1	3	4	5	7	8
	Absorbed with Strain 1					
1.5	0	0	0	0	0	0
1.0	0	0	0	0	0	100
0.75	100	0	0	100	0	100
0.5	200	200	0	100	0	200
0.3	200	200	0	100	0	200
0.2	400	200	100	100	100	400
0.1	800	800	200	400	200	800
0.05	800	800	400	400	200	800
0	1600	1600	400	1600	400	1600
	Absorbed with Strain 3					
1.5	200	0	200	100	400	0
1.0	400	0	400	100	400	0
0.75	800	0	400	100	200	0
0.5	1600	0	400	100	400	0
0.3	1600	0	400	200	400	0
0.2	1600	0	400	200	400	0
0.1	1600	0	400	400	400	100
0.05	1600	100	400	800	400	100
0	1600	800	400	1600	400	800
	Absorbed with Strain 4					
1.5	0	0	0	0	0	0
1.0	0	200	0	0	0	0
0.75	0	400	0	0	0	0
0.5	100	400	0	200	0	0
0.3	100	400	0	100	0	0
0.2	200	800	0	200	0	0
0.1	200	800	100	400	100	100
0.05	200	800	200	400	200	200
0	800	800	400	800	400	800
	Absorbed with Strain 5					
1.5	0	0	0	0	0	—
1.0	100	0	0	0	0	—
0.75	100	100	0	0	0	—
0.5	200	100	100	100	100	—
0.3	200	200	100	100	100	—
0.2	100	400	100	100	100	—
0.1	200	400	100	200	200	—
0.05	400	800	200	200	200	—
0	800	800	400	800	400	—

Absorbing Dose	Serum 3: 1	3	5	6
	Absorbed with Strain 1			
1.5	0	800	1600	0
1.0	0	800	800	100
0.75	0	800	1600	200
0.5	0	800	1600	800
0.3	0	800	1600	1600
0.2	0	1600	1600	1600
0.1	100	1600	1600	1600
0.05	200	800	1600	1600
0	800	800	1600	1600
	Absorbed with Strain 3			
1.5	0	0	0	0
1.0	0	0	0	0
0.75	0	0	100	0
0.5	0	100	100	100
0.3	0	200	200	200
0.2	100	400	400	400
0.1	200	800	800	800
0.05	100	800	1600	1600
0	800	800	1600	1600
	Absorbed with Strain 4			
1.5	0	0	0	0
1.0	0	800	800	800
0.75	100	1600	1600	800
0.5	100	1600	1600	1600
0.3	200	1600	1600	1600
0.2	200	1600	1600	1600
0.1	400	1600	1600	1600
0.05	800	1600	1600	1600
0	800	1600	1600	1600
	Absorbed with Strain 5			
1.5	0	0	0	0
1.0	0	0	0	0
0.75	0	100	0	0
0.5	0	100	0	0
0.3	100	100	100	100
0.2	100	200	200	200
0.1	100	800	400	800
0.05	400	1600	800	1600
0	800	1600	1600	1600

Absorbing Dose	Serum 7: 1	3	5	7
	Absorbed with Strain 1			
1.5	200	0	0	0
1.0	200	0	100	100
0.75	200	0	100	100
0.5	400	0	200	200
0.3	800	0	400	400
0.2	1600	0	400	800
0.1	3200	0	400	1600
0.05	3200	100	800	3200
0	3200	800	800	3200
	Absorbed with Strain 3			
1.5	3200	0	400	3200
1.0	3200	0	400	3200
0.75	3200	0	400	3200
0.5	3200	0	400	3200
0.3	3200	0	400	3200
0.2	3200	0	400	3200
0.1	3200	100	400	3200
0.05	3200	200	400	3200
0	3200	400	400	3200
	Absorbed with Strain 5			
1.5	0	0	0	0
1.0	0	0	0	100
0.75	100	0	0	400
0.5	200	0	0	400
0.3	400	0	0	400
0.2	400	0	0	400
0.1	800	0	100	1600
0.05	800	0	200	3200
0	1600	400	800	3200
	Absorbed with Strain 7			
1.5	0	0	0	0
1.0	0	0	0	0
0.75	100	100	0	100
0.5	100	100	100	200
0.3	400	100	100	400
0.2	800	200	200	800
0.1	1600	200	200	1600
0.05	1600	200	200	1600
0	3200	800	400	3200

Great variability in absorption and agglutination is evidenced between the different strains. When serum 1 is absorbed by strain 3, 0.1 of the absorbing dose is sufficient to completely remove the agglutinins for strain 3, while 1.5 doses does not affect the agglutinins for strain 7. Numerous other examples of extreme variability in agglutinin content are apparent.

BACTERICIDAL EXPERIMENTS

Technic.—Twenty-four hour broth cultures were diluted so that 1.0 cc. contained approximately 100,000 bacilli. To 0.5 cc. of such suspensions in sterile tubes were added 0.5 cc. of the dilution of serum used, and 0.5 cc. of fresh guinea-pig serum, diluted 1:20. The tubes were incubated at 37° C. for two hours and 0.1 cc. of the mixture was

TABLE 6.—BACTERICIDAL TESTS

Serums 1, 2, 3, 4, 6 and 8 and strains 1, 2, 3, 4, 5, 6, 7 and 8

		Culture							
Serum	Dilution	1	2	3	4	5	6	7	8
1	2000	0	0	5000*	1	0	0	100	0
1	5000	0	0	5000	50	500	0	100	0
2	500	0	0	60	4	0	30	500	0
2	1000	0	0	40	300	1000	80	2000	0
3	5000	0	0	0	0	0	0	100	0
3	10,000	0	0	0	0	0	0	50	0
4	500	0	0	0	0	0	0	10	0
4	1000	0	0	0	0	0	0	0	0
6	5000	0	0	0	0	0	0	0	0
6	10,000	0	0	0	100	100	0	100	0
8	5000	50	10	100	0	0	0	0	0
8	10,000	30	20	100	0	0	0	0	0
0.5 cc. complement		2000	500	5000	2000	5000	1000	2000	2000
0.5 cc. salt solution		2000	1000	5000	2000	5000	2000	2000	2000

* Figures refer to number of colonies on each plate.

then plated in agar. The plates were incubated overnight and the number of colonies counted the following morning.

Of the serums tested 5 and 7 were found to be very low or entirely lacking in bactericidal antibodies. These were necessarily omitted from the bactericidal tests. Table 6 presents the results of an experiment in which serums 1, 2, 3, 4, 6 and 8 were tested for bactericidal power against strains 1, 2, 3, 4, 5, 6, 7 and 8. In each test, two dilutions of serum were used, the smallest amount which showed marked bactericidal action against the homologous culture, and twice that amount. The figures refer to the number of colonies on the plate from each test. These experiments, which yielded consistent results on repetition, do not support the evidence of antigenic complexity obtained by agglutinin absorption. With the exceptions of the tests of culture 3 with serum 1, and culture 7 with serum 2, all serums exerted an approximately equal bactericidal action on all strains.

COMPLEMENT FIXATION

Antigens.—Cultures were grown on infusion agar for 24 hours. The growth was washed off with 0.85% salt solution, centrifugated, resuspended in fresh salt solution, and again centrifugated. This washing was repeated three times. The washed bacteria were suspended in 0.85% salt solution containing 0.5% phenol. The anticomplementary dose was determined in the presence of two units of complement and one-fourth this amount was used in the tests. Strains 1 and 3 were high in anticomplementary properties, requiring dilution to 1:300 and 1:200 respectively, compared with 1:10 or 1:20 for the other antigens.

Serums.—The same serums as in the preceding experiments were used in the complement fixation tests. The titers of the serums were determined by using one-fourth of the anticomplementary doses of the homologous antigen with 0.5 cc. of increasing dilutions of the serum in

Table 7.—Complement Fixation

Antigens 1, 2, 3, 4 and 7

Antigen	Anticomplementary Dose	Serum 1		Serum 2		Serum 3				Serum 4		Serum 7	
		1:50	1:100	1:50	1:100	1:50	1:100	1:250	1:500	1:500	1:1000	1:1000	1:2000
1	0.01 cc.	4+	3+	—	—	4+	4+	2+	—	3+	1+	4+	1+
2	0.03 cc.	4+	2+	4+	4+	4+	4+	4+	2+	4+	2+	4+	3+
3	0.01 cc.	4+	4+	4+	3+	4+	4+	4+	4+	4+	4+	4+	4+
4	0.05 cc.	4+	4+	4+	4+	4+	4+	4+	3+	4+	4+	4+	—
7	0.05 cc.	4+	—	4+	1+	4+	1+	—	—	4+	4+	4+	4+
Titer of serum		1:100		1:100		1:500				1:1000		1:2000	

an anti-sheep system. The primary incubation was for 1 hour at 37 C.; final incubation was for 30 minutes. Two units of complement and two units of amboceptor were used throughout the tests. The titers of the serums for their homologous antigens were found to be as follows: serum 1, 1:500; serum 2, 1:100; serum 3, 1:500; serum 4, 1:2000; serum 5, 1:500; serum 6, 1:1000; serum 7, 1:2000; serum 8, 1:2000.

Cross complement fixation tests were then made with amounts of each serum of one-half the titer and full titer, with results as given in table 7. Here, again, as in the bactericidal experiments, evidence of close identity contrasts with the wide variations revealed by agglutinin absorption.

DISCUSSION

In these experiments we have evidence gained from four methods of testing for antibodies. These experimental methods apparently vary in the exactness with which they reveal the true antigenic composition and in the delicacy with which they elicit differences between strains. The observed differences probably vary with the sensitiveness of the various methods used to detect them. Of the methods used—agglutination, agglutinin absorption, both with full absorbing dosage and fractional dosage, complement fixation and bactericidal antibody tests—the results of agglutinin absorption, particularly where fractional doses were used, demonstrated the greatest disparity.

The results of agglutinin absorption confirm the evidence of a lack of uniformity between strains which is shown by their agglutinating capacity in the several serums (tables 1 and 5). While agglutination reactions by themselves might be an indication only of a difference in agglutinability, rather than an inherent difference of antigenic composition, the results of fractional absorption show that the components of different strains vary in agglutinogenic content (table 5). When serum 7 is absorbed with strain 5, 0.1 of the absorbing dose is sufficient to remove all of the agglutinins for culture 5, while 15 times this amount does not affect its agglutinating capacity for cultures 1, 5 and 7. The absorption of serum 1 with strain 3 produces similar results. On the other hand, in the absorption of serum 1 with strain 5, the different doses affect equally the agglutinins for all of the 5 strains tested.

The results of agglutinin absorption of a larger number of cultures with full dosage (table 3) indicate that they can be roughly divided into those with the most representative antigenic composition, as shown by complete absorption of all or most of the serums tested; those with incomplete or imperfect antigenic representation, absorbing the agglutinins from only one or two serums; and those strains with an antigenic complex lying between these extremes. While no two strains in these groups may be identical, as indicated by fractional absorption, differences between the strains of a group are less marked than those between strains of different groups.

These results agree with those obtained by Hooker,[1] who suggests that strains which give incomplete absorption, such as our strains 1 and 2, are degraded, having lost, by long cultivation on artificial mediums, some of their original antigenic components. There is some evidence in our results that this may be true. Cultures 1, 2, 3 and 7 have been on artificial mediums for years, while all the freshly isolated strains which we have studied completely absorb the agglutinins from all of the test serums. That old strains do not necessarily lose their agglutinogenic properties, to any marked degree, is shown by strains 4, 5 and 6, which are from 4 to 6 years old.

The evidence furnished by these agglutinin absorption tests points to a complexity of antigenic composition best described, as Stevens and Doche [2] have pointed out for the hemolytic streptococcus group, by comparison with a mosaic. It is probable that this method of antigenic analysis is too delicate for the crude material with which it deals. If the antigens could be purified, closer and more consistent relationships might be established between strains of the same species.

Complement fixation does not show such a disparity of antigenic composition as we have found by agglutinin absorption. Here the results show uniformity (table 7), all of the antigens fixing complement in the presence of each serum to about the same degree, with the exception of antigen 1 with serum 2 and antigen 7 with serum 3.

The bactericidal tests (table 6) also show little variation between the strains examined. The serums were equally potent in their bactericidal action, the only exceptions here being serum 1 with culture 3 and serum 2 with culture 7.

If we attempt to answer the questions which prompted this study, we are confronted by this conflicting evidence. In the selection of a suitable culture to use in Widal tests, the method of trial, results of which are given in table 2, indicates the superiority of strain 2 over strain 7. Yet we find in table 1 that this culture does not agglutinate so well with the serums used as some of the other strains. Furthermore, agglutinin absorption indicated a great dissimilarity between strain 2 and other strains. The two lines of evidence may be reconciled on the basis of the theory that strain 2 contains common or group agglutinogens for many strains, but is poor in specific or strain components.

The question of the selection of a suitable culture for use in vaccine is not answered by the agglutinin absorption results. Our strain 1 is the Rawlings culture widely used for this purpose, and yet the results indicate that it is one of the incomplete or degraded strains. Probably the bactericidal and complement fixation tests give better evidence regarding this point. Certainly they correspond more closely with the vast experience with this culture in the field. A culture is not necessarily unfit for vaccine because of its lack of agglutinogens common to many other strains. When the crude antigen represented by the whole, unmodified bacterial cell is used, the antigenic nature of a strain of B.typhosus cannot be determined with certainty by testing a single antibody or by tests which are based on only one antigenic function.

2. J. Exper. Med., 1926, 44, p. 439.

Agglutinin absorption elicited the most marked differences, but a limited antigenic composition as shown by this method apparently bears no relation to the ability of such a strain to stimulate the production of a high degree of protection against many other strains.

SUMMARY

The antigenic identity of strains of B.typhosus has been studied by agglutinin absorption, complement fixation, and bactericidal activity. The greatest differences between strains were obtained by agglutinin absorption with fractional doses. Complement fixation and bactericidal tests indicated only minor differences between the strains tested.

Agglutinin absorption is probably the most sensitive method of bringing out differences in antigenic composition. The results indicate that the method is more delicate than practical uses demand. The suitability of a particular culture for the Widal test or for vaccine cannot be definitely determined by means of these experiments, but they indicate that complement fixation and bactericidal tests conform most closely to the empirical evidence gained from practical application in the field.

COMPARISON OF GLYCEROL AND BRILLIANT GREEN BILE FOR TREATMENT OF FECES FOR ISOLATION OF TYPHOID ORGANISMS

Leon C. Havens and Catherine Ridgway

From the Laboratories of the Alabama State Board of Health, Montgomery

Our first description [1] of the use of brilliant green bile in feces to be examined for typhoid organisms included a comparison with glycerol, using feces inoculated with a known small number of typhoid bacilli. The results indicated the superiority of the bile, the organisms being recovered in 90% of the specimens as compared with 35% with glycerol. Since that time field observations [2] have been made which also indicate the superiority of brilliant green bile. The purpose of this study is a further comparison of the two methods.

Technic.—The brilliant green used was a domestic commercial product, presenting no demonstrable superiority over any other brand. Prior to its use, the dye was digested with hydrochloric acid and carefully titrated, using known quantitities of feces and typhoid bacilli. This procedure has been described in detail heretofore.[2] The glycerol used was Merck's "Reagent" diluted to 30% with 0.85% NaCl. Both bile and glycerol were put up in 15 cc. amounts in 1 ounce bottles. Endo agar containing a suitable amount of brilliant green as determined by titration [2] was used for plating the specimens. A constant amount of feces (0.1 gm.) was used throughout the tests. The number of B. typhosus added to each specimen of feces was determined by colony counts of serial dilutions of broth cultures plated on agar at the time of inoculation of the feces.

The specimens in brilliant green bile were incubated at 22 to 25 C.; the same specimens in glycerol were kept at room temperature (15 to 20 C.). Comparative specimens in glycerol kept at 2 to 4 C. yielded similar results. The specimens were plated 24, 48 and 72 hours after preparation, using one loopful from each bottle, without agitation of the contents. Platings from the surface were found to give better results, both in numbers of typhoid colonies and prevention of overcrowding with fecal bacteria.

Results.—Six hundred and sixty-one specimens of feces inoculated with typhoid were examined in both 30% glycerol and brilliant green bile. Four different dosages of typhoid bacilli were used, 1,000,000; 100,000; 10,000 and 1,000. The results with each method are given in table 1. Specimens containing large numbers of typhoid bacilli (1,000,000) gave positive results with all but seven specimens (95%) in brilliant green bile, while 23 of these were missed in glycerol (84% positive).

Received for publication, May 7, 1928.

1. Havens, L. C., and Dehler, S. A.: J. Lab. & Clin. Med., 1924, 10, p. 238.
2. J. Prev. Med., 1927, 1, p. 359.

When fewer bacilli (100,000) are added to the feces specimens the recoveries from glycerol decreased to 46%, while 85% still were positive in brilliant green bile. With a further decrease in dosage (10,000) the glycerol recoveries fall to 20%, the bile recoveries to 58%. Eighteen specimens containing as few as 1,000 bacilli were all negative in glycerol, but yielded five positive results from bile.

In table 2 are given the results of the platings on each successive day. There was a progressive decrease in the recoveries from day to day, with the exception of the series containing 1,000 bacilli. Here, it is interesting to note, none was positive on the first day, 5 recoveries being obtained on the succeeding days, 1 on both the second and third days, 2 only on the second, and 2 only on the third. Thus, while 5 of these specimens, or

TABLE 1.—RECOVERY OF B. TYPHOSUS FROM FECES IN GLYCEROL AND BRILLIANT GREEN BILE

Dose of B. typhosus	Number of Specimens	B. Typhosus Obtained From: Glycerol		Brilliant Green Bile	
		Number	Per Cent	Number	Per Cent
1,000,000	144	121	84	137	95
100,000	261	119	46	221	85
10,000	238	47	20	139	58
1,000	18	0	0	5	28
Total	661	287	43	502	75

TABLE 2.—RESULTS OF SUCCESSIVE PLATINGS OF SPECIMENS

Number of Organisms Put in Specimen	Percentage of Specimens Yielding B. Typhosus: 24 Hours		48 Hours		72 Hours	
	Glycerol	B. G. Bile	Glycerol	B. G. Bile	Glycerol	B. G. Bile
1,000,000	84	95	70	88	57	79
100,000	40	69	24	63	11	32
10,000	17	39	7	36	2	15
1,000	0	0	0	17	0	17

28%, were positive, the percentage for the second and third days platings is, in each case, only 17. The specimens in bile frequently yielded typhoid colonies on the second or third day, when the results were negative on the first day. This was particularly true with dosages of 100,000 or less. When the glycerol specimens were negative on the first plating, positive results on the later days rarely occurred.

Table 2 further shows the necessity of rapid immediate examination of specimens in glycerol. Even with large dosage the percentage of recoveries decreased in 48 hours from 84 to 70, whereas the specimens in brilliant green bile yielded a larger number of positive results after 48 hours than were obtained from glycerol in 24 hours. With smaller dosages the time element is even more important. Decreases with glycerol as great as 65% occurred, as against less than 10% decrease in bile during the 48-hour interval.

With few exceptions, more typhoid colonies appeared on the plates streaked from bile, and there were usually fewer colonies of fecal bacteria. In other words, the plates were less crowded and examination was easier. Table 3 gives the ratios between typhoid and fecal colonies, obtained by approximating the total number of each on all the plates.

The glycerol specimens were positive and the bile specimens negative in a total of eleven specimens, three where the dosage of typhoid bacilli was 1,000,000, three with a dosage of 100,000 and in five with a dosage of 10,000. In each one of these specimens fewer than 10 typhoid colonies appeared on the plates.

DISCUSSION

Under the conditions of these observations, the advantages of brilliant green bile for the collection of feces are obvious. The superiority of this medium over glycerol increases rapidly as the numbers of typhoid bacilli in the specimen become fewer. With large doses of typhoid bacilli, recoveries can be expected in 95% of specimens in brilliant green bile and in 84% when preserved in glycerol, but if smaller numbers of typhoid bacilli are added, the percentage of recoveries falls rapidly with the glycerol method, reaching 20% with 10,000 dosage, while 58% of such specimens in bile were positive. Even with as few as 1,000 typhoid bacilli in the specimen, brilliant green bile frequently produced positive results, while all of these specimens in glycerol were negative.

TABLE 3.—RATIO OF TYPHOID TO FECAL COLONIES

	Total Typhoid	Total Fecal	Ratio	
			Typhoid	Fecal
Glycerol	13,700	324,000	1	24
Brilliant green bile	57,200	334,000	1	6

When the age of the specimen is considered, the advantage is with brilliant green bile. The platings on successive days of the specimens in this medium showed a much smaller decrease with lapse of time. As a matter of fact for 48 hours the number of recoveries is practically constant, while on the plates streaked with the same specimens in glycerin, the numbers of typhoid colonies rapidly diminish. This is particularly true for dosages below 1,000,000.

These experiments further permit an estimate of the minimum number of typhoid bacilli which can be detected in a specimen of feces. Positive results cannot be expected with the glycerol method if the number of bacilli is less than 10,000 and consistently positive results are not obtained when the number is below 1,000,000. In brilliant green bile positive results are obtained when as few as 1,000 bacilli are present in the specimens and the results are consistently positive with numbers above 10,000. Thus a tenfold sensitiveness for brilliant green bile is indicated.

So far as we are aware, no quantitative determinations of the efficiency of methods for the examination of feces for the presence of typhoid have hitherto been reported. These experiments indicate that even under the most favorable conditions, positive results cannot usually be expected even with feces containing fairly numerous typhoid bacilli. If we apply this information to field conditions, it is reasonable to expect that active cases of typhoid fever, who usually excrete the bacilli in enormous numbers, will yield consistently positive results. Healthy carriers, who may excrete variable numbers from time to time, constitute the most important problem for the laboratory. These experiments indicate that when the specimen is collected in glycerol there is a favorable chance of detection, only when a carrier is excreting 1,000,000 bacilli per 0.1 gram of feces. Collected in brilliant green bile the same likelihood of detection exists with the presence of only 100,000 organisms. On the other hand, fewer than 10,000 bacilli per 0.1 gram will only rarely be detected in 30% glycerol, while such specimens will yield from 25 to 50% positive results in brilliant green bile. The minimum detectable number for glycerol appears to be 10,000 while for brilliant green bile it is 1,000 or less. It is possible that, with further refinement of technic, the typhoid carrier may be found to excrete the bacilli with considerable constancy, his supposed intermittency being a matter of the minimum detectable number of organisms excreted.

SUMMARY

Six hundred sixty-one specimens of feces containing known numbers of typhoid bacilli were inoculated into both 30% glycerol and brilliant green bile. Positive results were obtained in 43% of the specimens in glycerol, in 75% in brilliant green bile. Dosages of at least 100,000 typhoid bacilli per 0.1 gram of feces are necessary to obtain consistently positive results in glycerol, while one-tenth of this number will yield the same percentage of recoveries from brilliant green bile. In glycerol the minimum detectable number of typhoid bacilli in feces appears to be 10,000; in brilliant green bile, 1,000. The effect of the age of the specimen has been studied. Specimens in brilliant green bile show a very slight decrease in positive results for 48 hours, while the typhoid bacilli in the same specimens in glycerol disappear rapidly.

SEPTIC INFECTION DUE TO BACTERIUM MORGANI 1

TH. THJÖTTA

From the Bacteriological Laboratory of the Norwegian Army, Oslo, Norway

A woman, aged 45, had for some time complained of oppression in the right hypochondrium. She gave a history of 3 or 4 typical attacks of cholelithiasis. On Dec. 17, 1928, the patient's biliary colic grew worse and a surgeon was called in consultation. The patient was jaundiced and febrile. In the absence of alarming symptoms, the patient was unwilling to undergo operation. On December 20, her general condition was aggravated and her temperature ranged between 38 and 39 C. The patient was transferred to a surgical clinic and cholecystostomy was performed. Pus was freely evacuated and sent to the bacteriologic laboratory for examination. No stone was found at the operation. Shortly before the operation the temperature had risen to 40.5 C., but a few hours after the operation the temperature fell to 37.6 C. and the patient remained comfortable for 3 days. On December 24, blood was taken from the patient for bacteriologic cultures and also to obtain serum for agglutination tests. The patient's condition became gradually worse, and she died on December 28, the 12th day after the onset of acute symptoms.

The examination of the fluid evacuated from the gall-bladder revealed gram-negative, motile bacilli of the colon-typhoid morphology. When these bacilli were cultured on lactose and blood agar plates two types of colonies were easily differentiable. The colony which failed to ferment lactose was rather small, while the colony that fermented lactose was large, thick, and mucoid and on further cultivation was found to consist of bacterium aerogenes.

The gram-negative bacilli that do not ferment lactose were found, on further examination, to ferment dextrose, levulose, and galactose, with formation of gas. The bacilli did not ferment mannitol or maltose. Indol was formed in peptone water and turned lead acetate agar brown. Gelatin was not liquefied. According to the English classification, this organism is Bacterium morgani 1. The Danish investigators call it B. metacoli, and Bergey [1] called it Salmonella morgani.

Received for publication, April 21, 1928.

1. Manual of determinative bacteriology, 1925.

The blood culture taken from the patient on December 24, showed an abundance of the nonlactose-fermenting, gram-negative bacilli, which were agglutinated by the patient's serum in a titer of 1:320. The patient's serum failed to agglutinate B. typhosus, B. paratyphosus A and B, or any of the dysentery bacilli, or the strain of B. aerogenes isolated from the fluid of the gallbladder. It is reasonable to conclude from these bacteriologic and serologic studies that B. morgani 1 was the etiologic agent causing the death of the patient.

B. morgani 1 was first described in 1905 and 1906 by Morgan, who made a large number of isolations of this organism from the stools of children with diarrheal diseases.[1a] These studies were shortly confirmed by Morgan and Ledingham,[2] Öhrum and Bahr,[3] and Bahr and Thomsen.[4] Other investigators were able to isolate the organism from the stools of children with summer diarrhea. Tribondeau and Fichet [5] and d'Herelle [6] found it in severe cases of dysentery and seriously considered the organism as the cause of this disorder. Fridtjof Bang,[7] in 1917, studied a number of strains of Morgan's bacillus not only in stools of children with diarrheal diseases, but also in feces of infants that were without any gastrointestinal disorders. Bang scouted the idea of a relationship existing between Morgan's bacillus and infant diarrhea. On the other hand, he seriously considered the bacillus as a rare type of B. coli. Thjötta,[8] in 1918, studied 9 patients with severe colitis. He was able to isolate Morgan's bacillus from the intestines and the feces of these patients. Two patients died and at necropsy large ulcers were observed in the intestinal mucosa. Morgan's bacillus was isolated from these lesions in large numbers. All the patients' serums, however, failed to agglutinate the organisms, even in the fatal cases. In tests for agglutination and for complement-fixation with serums produced by immunization of rabbits against B. morgani 1, the homologous strains called forth positive reactions in high dilutions, while, in all tests, the heterologous strains elicited no reactions. Thjötta concluded from these observations that this organism was nonpathogenic and that it most likely was an unusual type of B. coli supervening on the ordinary intestinal bacterial flora during diarrheal disorders.

1a. Brit. M. J., 1906, 1, 908; ibid., 1907, 2, 16.
2. Proc. Roy. Soc. Med., 1908-1909, 2, p. 133.
3. Meddelelser fra det Kgl. Veterinaer og Landbohöiskoles Serumlaboratorium, no. 5, 1910.
4. Ibid., no. 19, 1912.
5. Ann. de l'Inst. Pasteur, 1916, 30, p. 357.
6. Bull. Acad. de med., Paris, 1916, 76, p. 425.
7. Meddelelser fra Statens Seruminstitut, 1917, 19.
8. Medicinsk Revue, 1918, no. 4; J. Bact., 1920, 5, p. 67.

In 1920, Olaf Bang [9] isolated B. morgani 1 in the feces of a patient with purpura abdominalis, after a considerable intestinal hemorrhage. Zinsser,[10] in a recent review of the literature on Morgan's bacilli, points out the possibility of variants, in the form of unknown species of these organisms, regarded from the standpoint of fermentations of sugar, agglutinability, and other characteristics, and he cautions against accepting as new species, organisms which differ from the well-known types in only one or another of such characteristics.

In consideration of the case presented in this paper it is evident that B. morgani 1 was the cause of the fatal illness and that this organism can become highly pathogenic. The evidence for an etiologic relationship of B. morgani 1 to the acute septicemia of the patient was strengthened by the appearance of specific agglutinins for Morgan's bacillus in the patient's serum. In the absence of specific antibodies for the bacillus in the serums of persons from whose intestinal lesions this organism was isolated, it is reasonable to believe that the intestinal disorders were not caused by Morgan's bacillus, but that the latter was just an occasional saprophyte present in the intestinal tract. This view is favored when one considers this bacillus as a type of B. coli. B. coli occasionally becomes pathogenic and brings about generalized infection, starting from such foci as the kidney, the bile-ducts, or other parts of the body which serve as portals of entry. Under such circumstances, one always finds agglutinins and complement-fixing bodies in the patient's serum. The case presented in this paper is such a case in point, with B. morgani 1, as the infective agent. It is unlikely, on the other hand, that this organism should have been the etiologic agent in the severe and fatal colitis of patients earlier described by Thjötta [8] in whose serums no production of antibodies was detected.

In considering B. morgani 1 as a special and an unusual type of B. coli, it then becomes questionable whether or not the name Salmonella morgani applied to this organism by the commission appointed by the Society of American Bacteriologists in 1920, and later employed by Bergey,[1] is the correct appellation. In the opinion of trained bacteriologists this generic name embraces the large group of bacteria in which one finds B. enteritidis (Gaertner), B. aertrycke, B. typhi-murium, and others. The only similarity of Morgan's bacillus to these organisms is its inability to ferment lactose and saccharose. Morgan's bacillus is usually a strong producer of indol, while all

9. Tidskr. f. d. Norske Laegeforening, 1920, 13, p. 441.
10. Textbook of bacteriology, 1927, p. 609.

typical Salmonella lack this property. Further, Morgan's bacillus is only slightly motile, while all Salmonella are strongly so, and finally, Morgan's bacillus is different from Salmonella in point of pathogenicity. For these reasons, the more logical name for this organism is Bacillus metacoli, as it was called by the Danish investigators; it does, in fact, belong to the genus Escherichia, despite its fermentative reactions.

SUMMARY

A case of septic infection due to Bacterium morgani 1 is reported which originated in the gallbladder and terminated fatally on the 12th day after the onset of acute symptoms. Bact. morgani 1 was isolated from the gallbladder and the blood. The patient's serum agglutinated the organism in a dilution of 1 : 320.

B. morgani 1 is generally considered a nonpathogenic, rare type of B. coli, which under certain conditions may become highly virulent. The generic name Salmonella morgani is found to be inappropriate. This organism should property be called either B. morgani 1, B. metacoli, or Escherichia morgani.

BACTERIOLOGIC AND BACTERIOPHAGIC STUDY OF INFECTED URINES

JANET ANDERSON CALDWELL

From the Baylor Hospital Laboratory, Dallas, Texas

Few studies have been made of infected urines from a bacteriophagic point of view. Bacteriologic studies are more numerous but the author is unaware of any report including the dissociative phenomena of such cultures. The present report is based on 112 cases of urinary tract infections. The specimens were collected during cystoscopic examinations and were sent to the hospital laboratory for routine examination which included cultures on plain agar plates. The urines were then neutralized and filtered through Berkefeld N candles. In this way were made available for comparison, cultures, filtrates, microscopic and smear findings. The study was limited to cases yielding pure cultures of gram-negative bacilli.

BACTERIOLOGIC CLASSIFICATION

Technic.—The original plain agar plate culture was transplanted to 2 agar slants, one of which was stored in the icebox for any necessary future examination. Individual colonies were not used as the source of the cultures, as the idea of the author was to study the whole culture as soon after isolation as possible and in its mass condition, much as it is in the body. Data arrived at in this manner may be of use in indicating the expectancy from therapeutic use of the bacteriophage.

The usual differential mediums were used; Russell's double sugar agar, dextrose and lactose broth, litmus milk, gelatin, and citrate agar[1] which was useful in differentiating B. aerogenes from B. coli. Gram's stain and hanging drop examinations were also used. When the cultural characteristics suggested that the organism was B. typhosus, paratyphosus A or B, or B. dysenteriae, agglutination tests were made.

Spore-Forming Aerobes.—Twelve of the 112 cultures proved to be sporeformers. They all passed the routine urine sediment smear, and agar culture smear, as ordinary gram-negative bacilli. They grew fairly readily on plain agar forming a thin, bluish, slightly adherent film, like the R types of certain species and sometimes showed flecks or rims of more opaque culture. In smears, the bacilli were moderately long and slender, uniform in appearance, and without the variations in size and shape so common with gram-negative bacilli recently isolated from the body. In plain, and in dextrose broth, the growth of these bacilli was

Received for publication, April 14, 1928.

1. Simmons: J. Infect. Dis., 1926, 39, p. 209.

slow, meager, and often in the form of scum or agglutinated masses. Gram-positive bacillary forms were searched for diligently on many smears but in only two of the cultures were a few eventually found. In 11 of the 12 cases spores were found after repeated examinations from old slants or after several transfers. They were oval, refractive, non-staining, subterminal or terminal, formed late and in only small numbers. In the other case no spores have been found but a suspension gave growth after being heated in a water bath 1½ hours at 80 C. All 12 cultures gave the same cultural reactions i.e. no change on Russell's, gelatin, citrate agar, or in litmus milk, dextrose or lactose broth.

When this bacillus was present in the urines it was practically always in pure culture and was associated either with no pus or with only one or two pus cells in each high-power field. There were only a few colonies present on the agar plates inoculated directly from the urines. One would be inclined to consider the bacilli only as chance contaminations but in 6 cases repeated ureteral catheterizations were made and practically the same findings and identical cultures were obtained over periods of many weeks. Bacteriophage was demonstrated in 2 of the 12 urines containing this organism.

A number of gram-negative, spore-forming aerobic bacilli have been described and these are classified by Ford and Laubach.[2] These cultures are probably best classified as B. pseudotetanicus. Few references to such an organism in human disease are present in the literature. Batchelor [3] found B. pseudotetanicus present in the intestinal tract of 9 of 50 children examined for cultures of aerobic spore-forming bacilli. Dick and Dick [4] mention finding a gram-negative aerobic spore-forming bacillus in the urine of a patient free from nephritis but they do not describe it further. Such cultures have probably been overlooked frequently in routine smears and cultures of catheterized specimens and probably also in reported bacteriologic studies of urines.

Gram-Negative Aerobes Not Spore-Forming.—The remaining cultures are tabulated as follows:

Organisms	%
B. coli	47
B. lactis-aerogenes	12
Slow lactose-fermenters	9
Alkaligenes fecalis	5
Fluorescing bacilli	8
Atypical fluorescing bacilli	12
Proteus: irregular sugar and citrate fermentation, slow gelatin liquefaction. Colony covers plate in 24 hours (fig. 7)	6
Proteolytic: less spreading colony, negative sugar fermentation, rapid gelatin liquefaction	1

2. J. Bact., 1926, 1, pp. 273 and 518.
3. Ibid., 1919, 4, p. 23.
4. J. Am. M. A., 1915, 65, p. 6.

The first two groups are clear cut and need no further description. They were not subdivided. No typhoid, paratyphoid or dysentery cultures were obtained in the 100 urines. Urea-splitting cultures were not encountered, but as Proteus ammonii is found by Hager and MacGath [5] in only a fraction of 1% of urine cultures this is not surprising.

Much has been written about slow lactose-fermenting bacilli (group 3). Monias [6] in a recent classification considers them as transition forms between the true B. coli and the enteritidis groups and subdivides them into 4 groups. The literature on water and soil analysis [7] is rich in descriptions of slow fermenters of lactose. As to the clinical significance of the group, Castellani [8] has isolated cultures from human feces and named them B. metadysenteriae. His cultures formed no gas in any sugar, but acid in many, including lactose. Agglutination tests were negative. Several cultures in group 3 were similar. Dudgeon and Pulvetaft [9] described a type of culture found in severe acute pyelitis which has the peculiar reaction of hemolysis and delayed fermentation of lactose, but Herrold [10] denies that there is any constant relationship between hemolysis and fermentation or specific agglutination. Young [11] recognizes a group of paradysentery organisms in urine cultures and MacKenzie and Cochrane [12] report 2% of para- or pseudo-organisms in urine cultures related to B. dysenteriae and B. coli.

The bacilli of group 5 are like B. pyocyaneus except that they did not give a positive pyocyanin test. Probably at least some of these cultures were originally B. pyocyaneus but have undergone slight modification in the body, losing first their power to produce pyocyanin. That such modifications of bacilli producing diffusing pigment occur is brought out in the discussion of group 6.

The 12 bacilli grouped as atypical fluorescing bacilli (group 6) have the cultural reactions of that group (no sugar fermentation but growth on citrate agar). They do not all give diffusing pigment but several illustrations will make clear the reason for diagnosing them as I have. One culture was obtained from a patient from whom many later specimens were received. In one of these a very definite lavender pigment diffused through the agar. Another culture after 6 passages on agar

5. J. Am. M. A., 1925, 85, p. 1352.
6. J. Infect. Dis., 1927, 40, p. 570.
7. Kliger: J. Bact., 1919, 4, p. 35.
8. J. Trop. Med., 1923, 26, p. 123.
9. J. Hyg., 1927, 26, p. 285.
10. J. Urol., 1923, 7, p. 473.
11. Personal communication.
12. Canadian M. A. J., 1924, 14, p. 293.

developed a yellowish diffusing pigment. A third frequently showed a slight greenish diffusing pigment after incubation for 48 hours. One culture was obtained several months after the patient had received two series of bacteriophage treatments. The organism obtained previously in this case was a definite fluorescent bacillus. The colonies of the second culture are very different being small, round, opaque and without pigment but the cultural reactions of the two organisms are identical. As this change has been seen before in fluorescent bacilli during bacteriophage treatment and gradual reversion to type observed,[13] there is little doubt that 114 helps to identify other members of the group identical culturally but whose pedigrees are unknown. A fifth culture produced a dirty yellow diffusing pigment on slants 2 or 3 weeks old. In summarizing this group, diffusing pigment was observed in 4 of 12, a fifth was derived from a typical fluorescent bacillus and finally, all cultures were culturally identical in having the unique combination of reactions of no change in sugar mediums but growth on citrate agar, which is the same combination given by the definite fluorescent bacilli.

CLASSIFICATION BASED ON ARTIFICIAL COLONIES

Technic.—Freshly hardened plain agar plates 5 to 7 mm. thick were stabbed in the center with a platinum wire which had been carried across a 24-hour agar slant culture. The plates were examined at 24 hours, and at 4, 7, 10 and 14 days, often more frequently. Measurements were recorded with descriptions which took note chiefly of thickness, opacity by reflected and transmitted light, shape, color, and any variation in density in different portions of the colony. If varying density occurred, the colonies were watched to see if the change spread into new or old portions of the culture. After the first few months of this study Hadley's[14] monograph appeared and since that time the artificial colony observations have been worded in terms of dissociation change.

Review of Dissociative Changes.—The salient evidence of the cultural variations which are now considered to be stages in the cyclogeny of the species, and whose superficial picture is called microbic dissociation, are here reviewed. These changes in a broad sense are similar in many, probably all, bacterial species, and doubtless include many fine gradations from one type to another, but certain landmarks in the cycle which are striking in their characteristics have been carefully described, and they, at least, can be used as the basis for classification of colony types.

The S or "normal," smooth, homogeneous colony is the textbook colony for the bacterium under consideration. For bacilli of this series the artificial colony of an S type is round, with regular margin, of medium or marked opacity, usually

13. Caldwell: Arch. Int. Med., 1928, 41, p. 189.
14. J. Infect. Dis., 1927, 40, p. 1.

somewhat fluorescent and of perfectly uniform density (fig. 1). In the entire series of 100 cultures there was probably no single culture which is a pure, typical S type but there were a number which gave artificial colonies like that of figure 1 which qualifies as an S culture save for its finely serrated margin. These cultures are probably best considered to be SR meaning that the tendency to dissociation is initiated in the culture but is inconspicuous and is making little progress.

The R is the large, rough, i. e., irregular shaped colony, flat, thin, bluish by reflected light, quite transparent and never fluorescent (fig. 2). Unfortunately this type may approximate the regular round colony so that the best criteria are the rough surface, the bluishness and the thinness. Of the R type, there appears in the organisms under consideration, a certain extreme variety which will tentatively be put in a subdivision. This type begins as a small colony, not over 1 cm. in diameter, which is very thin and transparent. It spreads slowly and continually to cover most of the plate with a very filmy irregular growth, the center usually being thicker. The outer extension is practically invisible except in favorable light. No pits, bands or other areas of clearing or changed growth are present (fig. 3). A description which fits the three members of this group is given by Hadley (page 24[14]). As the R type of culture develops from the S it is to be expected that the two types may coexist in the same artificial colony and this finding is very common when dissociation is constantly occurring as in urinary bacilli. Several types will be recognized where the two types S and R coexist in a single artificial colony.

S-R 1: Those cultures in which the two densities are strikingly different giving a very remarkable appearance. Here the S usually forms the irregular shaped center with margin, wedges or scallops of R. The change may spread inward and always continues outward in the enlarging colony. This type of colony is described perfectly by Hadley as marginal dissociation and is well known to bacteriologists (fig. 4).

S-R 2: Those cultures in which there are two different densities in the colony but the variation is only slight in degree. It assumes the same arrangement and is probably of the same significance as S-R 1 (fig. 5).

S-R 3: Those cultures in which there are two different densities in the colony but where there is no sharp line of change from one to the other. These colonies are very pretty. They are large, irregular with the central portion distinctly thinner than the margins which are of a definite S like density. There are 8 cultures in this class (fig. 6).

On the basis of the above descriptions the 100 cultures are classified as follows:

S or SR type culture	23
R type culture	14
filmy, spreading variety	3
S and R mixed	
in striking contrast	24
less striking contrast	10
without sharp transition	8
Proteus colony type	6
Suicide cultures	3
Mucinous	1
Definite fluorescing bacilli	8

The table demonstrates that only about 23% of the cultures of bacilli isolated freshly from urine, give colonies approximating the "normal" in mass inoculation. Practically half are obviously in the process of dissociation and the others have already attained the R type.

Comparison of Dissociative and Cultural Classification.—The dissociation groups were compared with the groups classified by cultural methods to see if any significant relationship existed. It was noted that the B. lactic-aerogenes cultures were always splitting into S and R. The atypical fluorescing bacilli furnished most of the unusual colony forms of the spreading sort, being R and S and R. As any bacillus related to B. pyocyaneus is likely to have a spreading filmy growth the association probably means nothing but some confirmation for considering the cultures related to B. pyocyaneus.

BACTERIOPHAGE STUDY

The bacteriophagic study consisted of two parts, first, the testing of the cultures for susceptibility to lysis and, secondly, the testing of the urines for the presence of native bacteriophage.

Susceptibility to Lysis.—The gram-negative bacilli described were tested for susceptibility to bacteriophagic lysis with sewage filtrate which is rich in lytic principle.[15]

Technic: To 3 tubes of broth lightly inoculated with suspensions of the organisms were added respectively 2, 10 and 30 drops of sewage filtrate. Observations of clearing were made after 3, 6 and 24 hours of incubation and at the 6th hour subcultures on agar slants were made from the 10 or 30-drop tube. Lytic plaques on agar were considered essential in a result recorded as positive. When no evidence of lysis on agar or in broth occurred, 5 serial passages were made and tested in the same manner before a negative result was recorded. The negative cases were all tested with 2 or 3 samples of sewage collected at intervals of 2 months. There would have been 3 other negative cases if only one sample had been used. The object was to ascertain the proportion of cultures in urinary infection which could be lysed by bacteriophage and the proportion in which the action was sufficiently strong so that they might be hopefully treated with the bacteriophage.

The results of tests with sewage filtrate on 100 cultures follow:

Degree of Lysis	Number of Cultures	
A, maximum lysis	39	72%, good lysis
B, satisfactory lysis	33	
C, good lysis but with secondary cultures	10	21%, poor lysis
D, weak lysis always	11	
No lysis, negative	7	

15. Zdansky: Wien. klin. Wchnschr., 1924, 37, p. 501. Cowie: Ann. Clin. Med., 1926, 5, p. 57. Caldwell: J. Infect. Dis., 1927, 40, p. 575.

The table shows that 74% of cultures can be readily and quickly lysed by sewage filtrate. This is so readily accomplished that concentrated treatment filtrate can be available within 72 hours of obtaining the patient's urine.

Relation of Susceptibility to Lysis to Dissociative Pnenomena.—It was expected that the cultures which failed to lyse would be found to belong to some one stage of the dissociation cycle, for such is the intimation in the literature, incriminating especially the R type as resistant to lysis. In fact, this conviction is held so universally that it has come about that the letter R is used to mean a rough colony, a certain stage in the dissociation cycle and resistance to bacteriophage action. The tabulation condenses this comparison:

	Degree of Lysis		
Colony Type	A, %	B, %	Poor or No Lysis, %
SR "normal" colonies	59	16	25
R rough colonies	20	40	40
S and R dissociating colonies	42	36	18
Rare colonies	36	21	43

The percentages show that cultures in every phase of the dissociation cycle have been lysed with maximum and good reactions and, on the other hand, that even the S "normal" cultures exhibit poor lytic reactions in as high as 25%. This is convincing evidence that no colony type or stage of dissociation has inherent resistance to bacteriophage action. It is entirely a matter of having a source of bacteriophage sufficiently rich in strains. When one finds eventually a bacteriophage to an unusual type of organism the reaction is as good as with one of the every day colon bacilli, or as with the S stage of dissociation.

NATIVE BACTERIOPHAGE

Incidence.—Native bacteriophage was demonstrated in the filtrates of 26 urines by the following method.

The filtrate of each urine was added in 2-, 10-, and 30-drop quantities to 3 sets of broths. One set was inoculated with the patient's own bacillus; the second with a stock Shiga dysentery culture and the third with a stock B. coli. Observation for clearing and for evidence of lysis on agar slants was made during each of five serial passages unless the test was positive with one or more of the organisms, in which case, the test was discontinued as positive. A culture of the Shiga dysentery bacillus was used because it is lysed by a large number of bacteriophage strains and is as sensitive to bacteriophage action as any bacillus known at present. The culture of B. coli used had been proved by frequent use to have average susceptibility to anticolon bacteriophage. The technic used in these tests is practically identical with that used by Larkum [16] although it was selected some months before his article was published.

16. J. Bact., 1926, 12, p. 203.

The demonstration of bacteriophage was accomplished for 15 urines in the first passage, for 5 urines in the second passage, and for 2 more urines in the third, 2 in the fourth, and 2 in the fifth passage. Thirteen demonstrations occurred with B. dysenteriae (8 with B. dysenteriae only), 9 demonstrations with B. coli (4 with B. coli only), and 10 demonstrations were with the patient's own organism (8 with this organism only). Twenty of the 26 native bacteriophage reactions were thus shown by only two passages. This means either that the method picks out only strong, rather "polyvalent" bacteriophage or that many serial passages are of little advantage in enhancing urine strains. A striking fact in this connection is that Larkum [16] with similar technic obtained the same percentage of positive urine filtrates. Naturally his B. dysenteriae, B. coli, and urine organisms were different strains from those used by the author. But as he examined subsequent specimens of urine in a number of cases he raised his percentage of native bacteriophage to 36, so that one can almost believe that if specimens were obtained and tested repeatedly that bacteriophage would probably be found to be quite common in infected urines.

Significance of Native Bacteriophage.—The cultures obtained from the 26 urines containing native bacteriophage were compared with the cultures obtained from negative cases, the idea being to see if there was any relation between the presence of native bacteriophage and the ease with which the associated culture is lysed or, secondly, if such associated cultures have any constant growth characteristics or belong to any one stage of the dissociation cycle. If there is no constant relationship, there is here further proof that contact with bacteriophage does not produce a general resistance to bacteriophage lysis or any consistent cultural change. The following table condenses this comparison:

	26 Positive Filtrate Urines %	Remaining 74 Urines %
Organism Represented		
B. coli	40	47
Slow lactose-fermenting	4	9
B. lactis-aerogenes	15	12
B. pyocyaneus	11	8
Atypical B. pyocyaneus	15	11
B. proteus	4	6
B. alkaligenes	8	5
Susceptibility to Sewage Filtrate		
Maximum lysis A and B	37	39
Moderate, satisfactory	33	33
Weak or absent lysis	30	28
Type of Colony		
SR "normal"	15	25
R rough	15	15
S and R active dissociation	**52**	**32**
Odd colony types	11	20

The first division in the table shows that there is no special cultural group more often associated with native bacteriophage than not. Noting the class of atypical fluorescing bacilli which have been shown to have high percentage of odd colony types and of weak lysis, it will be seen that they are not more frequently associated with native bacteriophage than are other organisms.

The second division shows that contact with native bacteriophage cannot be the cause of the failure of lysis of a culture.

As for the R type, in the third division it is shown to be no oftener associated with native bacteriophage than not. One effect of native bacteriophage on cultures is seen in the much higher per cent of cultures showing a mixture of S and R which represent cultures in active dissociation. This is only confirmation of the already known fact that bacteriophage is one of many agents which can initiate dissociative change.

Type of Native Bacteriophage.—Since a lytic substance which produces plaques with unusual diffuse margins[17] on agar has been described (the α component of Hadley[18]), it is of interest to note the type of lytic principle found in the urine filtrates. Is it ever the α type, or do the native bacteriophage strains always produce sharp-margined plaques? In 19 of the 26 urines containing native bacteriophage, isolated plaques were seen on the early agar slants and their number and size recorded. These are all of the β type. In 5 other cases, the record shows that although only sterile agar slants were obtianed, the clearing in broth was still marked at 24 hours. This is fairly conclusive evidence that the principle acting was of the β type as the α commonly allows the early development of secondary cultures so that lysis in broth is transient. Another case showed marked and permanent clearing with no evidence on agars made at 3 hours which could only mean that the usual sharp-margin, β, plaque type of lytic principle was responsible. Only one case suggested the presence of an α component. In this case the clearing was much reduced at 24 hours and scattered colonies varying in size were present on the agar slants. Although the questionable cases should have been diluted to give isolated plaques on agar, the data is sufficiently conclusive to warrant the statement that lytic principle native in infected urines is usually of the β type. Whether the α principle may have existed in the case at some earlier stage in the infective process cannot be stated.

17. Goodwin and Caldwell: J. Lab. & Clin. Med., 1928, 13, p. 724.
18. Proc. Soc. Exper. Biol. & Med., 1928, 25, p. 359.

SUMMARY

In the classification of 112 bacilli from infections of the urinary tract, a group of 12 aerobic, gram-negative bacilli which produce spores was recognized and described. Seventeen cultures related to fluorescing bacilli were also described.

Sewage filtrate produced marked lysis of 74% of the 100 nonspore-forming cultures and failed to produce lysis of 7%. These 100 cultures were classified into colony types on the basis of dissociative changes. The susceptibility of the various dissociative types to lysis by sewage filtrate was tested. The results strongly suggest that there is no stage of dissociation of urinary bacilli which is resistant to bacteriophage action.

Native bacteriophage was demonstrated in the filtrates of 26 of the 100 urines: in 20 only two passages were required. It can be demonstrated with the organism found in the same urine about as often as by using stock cultures of colon and dysentery bacilli. Native bacteriophage was found associated with every cultural group; with cultures in every stage of dissociation and with cultures having all degrees of sensitiveness to lysis. Therefore, contact with bacteriophage in the body does not produce in a culture resistance to lysis or any constant change in its growth characteristics, nor does it force the culture into any one stage of the dissociation cycle.

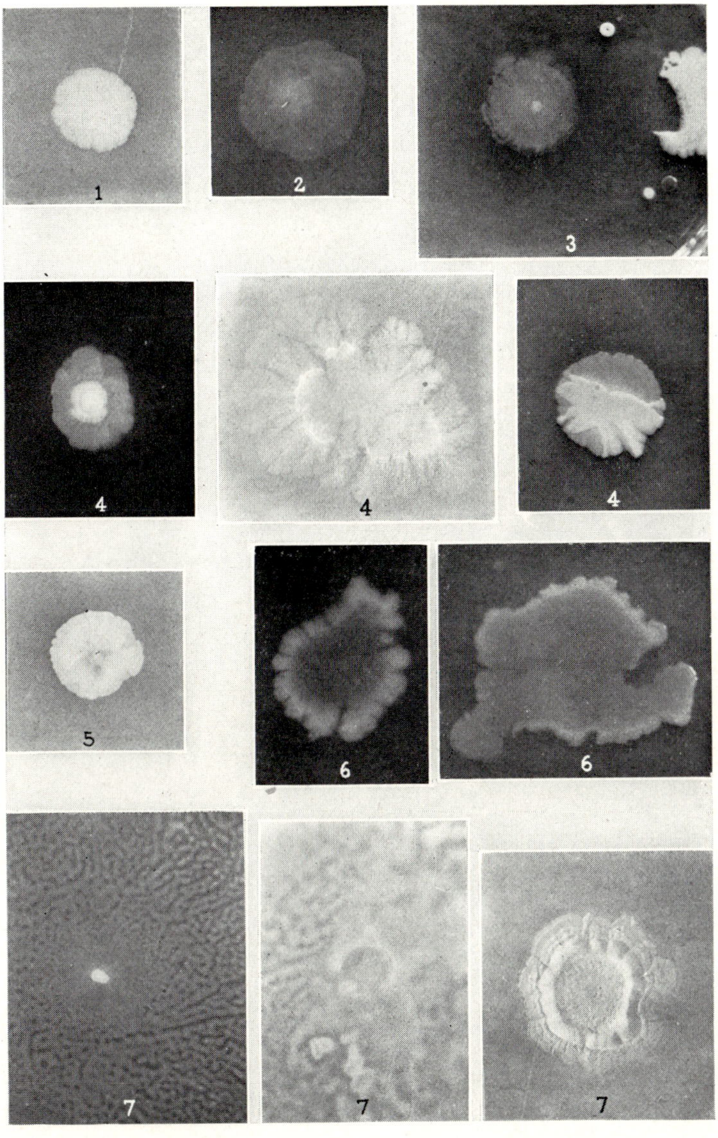

Fig. 1.—S type colony, "normal."

Fig. 2.—R type colony, "rough."

Fig. 3.—Special form of R type colony: entire plate covered with filmy almost invisible growth.

Fig. 4.—S and R dissociation obvious: several varieties.

Fig. 5.—S and R variation in density less obvious than in figure 4.

Fig. 6.—S and R transition gradual.

Fig. 7.—S and R rare colony types: B. proteus. (Right) Mucinous.

PRODUCTION OF HISTAMINE, TYRAMINE, BRONCHO-SPASTIC AND ARTERIOSPASTIC SUBSTANCES IN BLOOD BROTH BY PURE CULTURES OF MICROORGANISMS

KARL K. KOESSLER, MILTON THEO. HANKE
AND
MARY S. SHEPPARD

From the Otho S. A. Sprague Memorial Institute and the Department of Pathology, The University of Chicago

A study of the metabolism of histidine and tyrosine by bacteria was started, in this laboratory, ten years ago.[1] These two amino acids were selected because their decarboxylation products, histamine and tyramine, show pronounced pharmacological activity. We were, at first, chiefly interested in the nature of the products that would be formed from histidine and tyrosine by the action of bacteria, particularly in the kind of bacteria that produce histamine and tyramine, and the conditions under which these amines are produced. We soon found that the histamine and tyramine producers are few in number; but there was still the possibility that other products, possibly other amines of therapeutic significance, might be produced. The study was then expanded to include two pharmacological tests, namely: a test for bronchospastic, and one for arteriospastic substances.[2] The present report, which deals with the production of histamine, tyramine, and bronchospastic and arteriospastic substances by a selected group of microorganisms belonging to the American Type Culture Collection, has led to a few new observations; but it has more particularly strengthened the conclusions drawn, from time to time, in the course of these experiments. We wish, therefore, to summarize briefly the information that has been accumulated in the course of this work.

SUMMARY OF THE PREVIOUS RESULTS [1]

We have never observed the production of histamine and tyramine excepting in a medium that has become acid. Decarboxylation of the respective amino acids with the production of amines appears to be a protective mechanism that is resorted to when the H-ion concentration

Received for publication, May 31, 1928.

1. This summary has been derived from a series of articles published by Karl K. Koessler and Milton Theo. Hanke under "Studies on Proteinogenous Amines," J. Biol. Chem., 1919, 39, p. 497; 1922, 50, p. 131; 1924, 59, p. 835.

2. Koessler, Karl K.; Lewis, Julian H., and Walker, Jennie A.: Arch. Int. Med., 1927, 39, p. 163.

of the bacterial protoplasm, and of the medium, becomes sufficient to threaten the life of the organism. The faculty of decarboxylation is not common, and it can not be correlated with any of the common cultural characteristics. This faculty seems to be quite permanent in some instances, and transitory in others. It may be lost; and it may be acquired. One strain of colon bacillus, a histidine decarboxylator, has quantitatively retained its ability to produce histamine for ten years that we know of. We have on record one gram-positive histamine producer and five gram-positive tyramine producers that lost the faculty of decarboxylation after six months growth on laboratory mediums. The gram-positive organisms seem to lose the faculty of decarboxylation when grown on laboratory mediums. We have not as yet encountered a gram-negative organism that did not retain this faculty under similar conditions. One colon bacillus when freshly isolated produced no tyramine during a 14-day incubation period. Six months later, an 80% conversion of tyrosine to tyramine was regularly obtained. No microorganisms has yet been isolated that will decarboxylate both histidine and tyrosine. The chemical mechanism of the decarboxylation does not appear to be identical for these two amino acids. This conclusion is strengthened by the fact that, whereas tyrosine can be rather easily decarboxylated by heat, histidine does not lose carbon dioxide under these conditions. Decarboxylation is a fairly common property of the mixture of microorganisms found in feces. More than 50% of all whole-stool inoculations lead to a production of histamine, of tyramine, or both. It is rarely possible to isolate an amine-producing organism, and we are inclined to believe that the decarboxylation is due to the symbiotic activity of the mixture of bacteria. The mixture of bacteria contained in sputum does not, as a rule, produce either histamine or tyramine.[2]

The metabolism of histidine with the production of imidazole acetic, propionic, or lactic acids (our method does not differentiate between them) has been noted in a few cases. The amount produced is never large. The corresponding production of hydroxyphenyl-lactic acid from tyrosine has also been noted in a few cases. The amount produced is small.

Whereas tyramine is produced only in acid medium, phenol is produced only in alkaline medium. As much as 87% of the tyrosine may be converted into phenol. Paracresol was not produced by any of the bacteria that we studied.

The compounds that correspond chemically to phenol and to cresol in the imidazole series are imidazole and methyl imidazole. Bacteria do not appear to convert histidine into these imidazoles. This is probably due to the comparative instability of the imidazole ring. Chemists consider the imidazole ring to be very stable; and it is, excepting for one very well known reaction. Suitable acid chlorides, in alkaline solution, rupture the imidazole ring instantly with the production of substituted ethylene diamine derivatives. The imidazole ring is very rapidly ruptured by bacteria. The rupture of the ring is probably more easily accomplished than is the degradation of the carbon chain.

The mixtures of bacteria contained in sputum grow luxuriently on a blood-broth medium containing either histidine or tyrosine. They do not, as a rule, decarboxylate either histidine or tyrosine; but they do lead to the production of arteriospastic and bronchospastic substances in over 50% of the samples examined.[2] The chemical identity of this substance, or substances, has not yet been determined; but certain facts that will be presented later in this paper indicate that the active substance is an amine.

EXPERIMENTAL REPORT

This part of the paper deals with the production of histamine from histidine, tyramine from tyrosine, bronchospastic, and arteriospastic substances in a blood-broth medium by the action of a selected group of microorganisms belonging to the American Type Culture Collection. Most of them will probably be available for some time.

These organisms have all been grown on a liquid blood-broth medium that contains 1% Bacto-peptone, 2% glycerol, 0.4% beef extract, 5% of whole sheep blood, and 1% of either histidine or tyrosine.[3] Of this medium, 200 cc. portions are inoculated with approximately nine billion microorganisms and incubated at 37.5 C. for 14 days. A two cc. portion of the incubated mixture is transferred to a small collodion sack and dialyzed against distilled water for 24 hours. The colorimetric P_H determinations are conducted on the diffusate. The final mixtures are usually so highly colored that accurate P_H determinations can not be conducted directly on the medium.

The remaining liquid is heated on the water-bath. In most cases sufficient acid is present to give a cleancut coagulation. When this is not the case, acetic acid is added to the hot liquid until a good flocculation is obtained. The mixture is filtered, and the clear, pale-colored, filtrate is evaporated in a glass dish on the water-bath. The residue is dissolved in water, treated with 0.5 cc. of 95% sulfuric acid, and diluted to exactly 25 cc. This liquid can be kept indefinitely. It is referred to as the "total concentrated filtrate."

A ten cc. portion of the total concentrated filtrate is treated with three grams of solid, powdered, sodium hydroxide, and the cooled, alkaline mixture is extracted with

3. The liquid medium containing peptone, glycerol and beef extract is treated with Pfanstiehl's charcoal and filtered before adding the amino acid. This treatment is essential because certain peptones and beef extracts contain bronchospastic and arteriospastic substances.

amyl alcohol six times, using 20 cc. for each extraction. The combined amyl alcohol extractions are extracted with N sulfuric acid. The acid is neutralized with sodium hydroxide, the liquid evaporated and finally diluted to 25 cc.[4] This is the amine fraction, and contains all of the histamine or tyramine and other amines that may be present, and it could also contain neutral compounds. The broncho-spastic and arteriospastic substances, when they are produced, are always found in this fraction.

The alkaline aqueous residue left after the amyl alcohol extractions is treated with seven cc of 37% hydrochloric acid, and evaporated to dryness. The residue is dissolved in water and diluted to 25 cc. This is the amino acid fraction. It has never been found to contain pharmacologically active substances. It is not discussed further in this paper.

The amine fractions were, in every case, tested chemically for histamine and tyramine.[1, 5] Pharmacological tests were conducted on both the total concentrated filtrate and on the amine fractions. The results are always identical on these two fractions, i. e., the activity always appears in the amine fraction. The values given in the tables for bronchospasms and arteriospasms represent the response obtained, in every case, with one cc. of the total concentrated filtrate. The responses have been designated as 2 +, 3 +, and 4 +, and the accompanying figure illustrates our interpretation of these responses. The experimental results have been summarized in the table.

The first part of this table is a summary of the results obtained with bacteria that are commonly classified as belonging to the colon-typhoid group. Of the 94 bacteria studied, nine, approximately 10%, converted histidine into histamine. There were no tyramine producers in this group. Of the nine histamine producers, two belong to the Escherichia group, and seven to the Salmonella group.[6] The fact that five of the eight Salmonella morgani strains produce histamine may be of significance in certain types of diarrhea with which this microorganism has been found to be associated. The Salmonella group contains a high percentage of bacteria that produce bronchospastic and arteriospastic substances. Of the 49 strains of Salmonella studied, 38 produced bronchospastic substances, and 36 produced arteriospastic substances.

Of the 18 dysentery bacilli (Eberthella dysenteriae) studied, the first 12 listed in the table are B. paradysenteriae Flexner, Strong, Hiss, or

4. For a detailed description of the process see J. Biol. Chem., 1919, 39, p. 521.

5. It will be noted that tyramine is being extracted from a 30% sodium hydroxide solution instead of from a sodium carbonate solution as originally specified. We were rather surprised, but gratified, to find that tyramine either does not form a sodium phenate derivative, or, if such a derivative is formed, it is soluble in amyl alcohol. Tyramine can be quantitatively extracted from aqueous sodium hydroxide solution with amyl alcohol. This procedure also, of course, separates tyramine quantitatively from tyrosine.

6. The cultural characteristics of the histamine producers were rechecked in this laboratory. We are able to corroborate the classification, as given in the table in every case but one, namely, Salmonella Schottmüller 980. This strain ferments salicin, forms indol and does not agglutinate with a Schottmüller antiserum. The cultural characteristics of 980 indicate that it may be Salmonella Columbiensis.

Collins. The last six are B. dysenteriae Shiga. Five of the six Shiga strains produced arteriospastic and bronchospastic substances. Of the 12 paradysenteriae bacilli, five produced bronchospastic, and six, arteriospastic substances.

All nine bacilli belonging to Escherichia produced bronchospastic and arteriospastic substances. In seven of the nine cases, the active substance certainly was not histamine.

All the true typhoid bacilli, Eberthella typhi, produced both bronchospastic and arteriospastic substances.

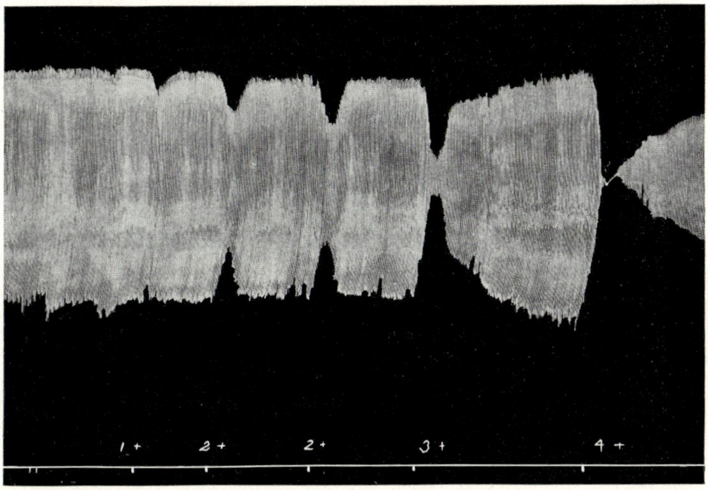

Fig. 1.—Illustration of the interpretation of the 1+, 2+, 3+ and 4+ bronchospasms of the pithed guinea-pig.

Bronchospastic and arteriospastic substances are rarely produced by microorganisms other than those belonging to the colon-typhoid group. Of the 44 pyogenic cocci studied, only nine produced bronchospastic substances, and 17 produced arteriospastic substances. In the diphtheria and diphtheroid group, one out of five produced spastic substances. Fifteen aerobic spore-forming bacteria were studied, and, of these, three produced bronchospastic and four arteriospastic substances. Of the 13 bacteria isolated from dairy products, none produced bronchospastic, and three produced arteriospastic substances. The remaining three groups, other bacteria, higher bacteria, yeast and molds, includes 32 microorganisms. Three produced bronchospastic and two produced arteriospastic substances.

Production of Histamine, Tyramine and Bronchospastic and Arteriospastic Substances in Pure Cultures of Microorganisms

COLON TYPHOID GROUP

Name of Microorganism	Amino Acid Added to Blood-Broth Medium	Broncho-spasm	Arterio-spasm	Histidine Converted Into Histamine	Tyrosine Converted Into Tyramine	Reaction After Incubation, P_H
1. Aerobacter aerogenes 211......	Histidine	None	None	None		5.8
	Tyrosine	None	None		None	5.6
2. Aerobacter aerogenes 541......	Histidine	None	None	None		5.0
	Tyrosine	2+	2+		None	5.0
3. Aerobacter aerogenes 129......	Histidine	None	None	None		6.4
	Tyrosine	None	None		None	5.6
4. Aerobacter cloacae 222........	Histidine	4+	4+	None		6.2
	Tyrosine	4+	4+		None	5.6
5. Aerobacter cloacae 529........	Histidine	None	None	None		5.8
	Tyrosine	None	None		None	6.4
6. Alcaligenes fecalis 57..........	Histidine	None	None	None		8.2
	Tyrosine	None	None		None	8.4
7. Alcaligenes fecalis 212.........	Histidine	2+	None	None		7.7
	Tyrosine	3+	2+		None	7.0
8. Alcaligenes fecalis 213.........	Histidine	None	None	None		7.8
	Tyrosine	None	None		None	8.2
9. Eberthella alkalescens 4.......	Histidine	4+	4+	None		5.8
	Tyrosine	4+	4+		None	5.2
10. Eberthella dispar 29...........	Histidine	4+	4+	None		5.8
	Tyrosine	4+	4+		None	5.2
11. Eberthella dysenteriae 32......	Histidine	None	None	None		5.2
	Tyrosine	None	None		None	6.2
12. Eberthella dysenteriae 33......	Histidine	4+	4+	None		5.0
	Tyrosine	None	None		None	5.2
13. Eberthella dysenteriae 34......	Histidine	3+	3+	None		5.8
	Tyrosine	None	None		None	5.0
14. Eberthella dysenteriae 35......	Histidine	None	None	None		5.2
	Tyrosine	None	None		None	5.8
15. Eberthella dysenteriae 36......	Histidine	4+	4+	None		5.4
	Tyrosine	4+	4+		None	5.4
16. Eberthella dysenteriae 38......	Histidine	None	None	None		5.7
	Tyrosine	None	None		None	6.8
17. Eberthella dysenteriae 40......	Histidine	None	None	None		5.8
	Tyrosine	None	None		None	7.0
18. Eberthella dysenteriae 41......	Histidine	None	3+	None		6.4
	Tyrosine	None	None		None	7.2
19. Eberthella dysenteriae 42......	Histidine	None	None	None		5.2
	Tyrosine	None	None		None	5.8
20. Eberthella dysenteriae 44......	Histidine	4+	4+	None		5.6
	Tyrosine	4+	4+		None	5.2
21. Eberthella dysenteriae 47......	Histidine	None	None	None		7.8
	Tyrosine	None	None		None	8.2
22. Eberthella dysenteriae 48......	Histidine	4+	3+	None		6.4
	Tyrosine	None	None		None	6.6
23. Eberthella dysenteriae 51......	Histidine	4+	4+	None		5.4
	Tyrosine	None	None		None	5.8
24. Eberthella dysenteriae 52......	Histidine	4+	4+	None		5.8
	Tyrosine	4+	None		None	7.0
25. Eberthella dysenteriae 204.....	Histidine	None	None	None		7.0
	Tyrosine	None	None		None	7.0
26. Eberthella dysenteriae 871.....	Histidine	4+	4+	None		6.4
	Tyrosine	4+	4+		None	6.4
27. Eberthella dysenteriae 873.....	Histidine	4+	4+	None		5.6
	Tyrosine	2+	2+		None	5.6
28. Eberthella dysenteriae 968.....	Histidine	4+	4+	None		5.2
	Tyrosine	4+	4+		None	5.2
29. Encapsulatus pneumonie 218..	Histidine	None	None	None		4.6
	Tyrosine	None	None		None	5.4
30. Encapsulatus rhinoscleromatis 219	Histidine	None	2+	None		5.2
	Tyrosine	None	None		None	5.8
31. Escherichia acidi-lactici 128....	Histidine	2+	2+	None		6.2
	Tyrosine	4+	4+		None	5.8
32. Escherichia coli 26.............	Histidine	4+	4+	None		6.2
	Tyrosine	4+	4+		None	6.0

PRODUCTION OF HISTAMINE, TYRAMINE AND BRONCHOSPASTIC AND ARTERIOSPASTIC SUBSTANCES IN PURE CULTURES OF MICROORGANISMS—*Continued*

COLON TYPHOID GROUP

Name of Microorganism	Amino Acid Added to Blood-Broth Medium	Broncho-spasm	Arterio-spasm	Histidine Converted Into Histamine	Tyrosine Converted Into Tyramine	Reaction After Incubation, P_H
33. Escherichia coli 205	Histidine	4+	4+	None		6.2
	Tyrosine	4+	4+		None	6.0
34. Escherichia coli 206	Histidine	4+	4+	99%		5.8
	Tyrosine	None	None		None	6.0
35. Escherichia communior 130	Histidine	4+	4+	None		5.8
	Tyrosine	4+	3+		None	6.2
36. Escherichia communior 207	Histidine	4+	4+	None		5.0
	Tyrosine	None	None		None	5.2
37. Escherichia communior 208	Histidine	4+	4+	None		5.0
	Tyrosine	4+	4+		None	5.6
38. Escherichia communior 209	Histidine	4+	4+	None		5.0
	Tyrosine	4+	4+		None	4.8
39. Escherichia neopolitana 133	Histidine	4+	4+	40.2%		4.8
	Tyrosine	4+	4+		None	6.2
40. Lactobacillus acidophilus 314	Histidine	None	None	None		5.0
	Tyrosine	None	None		None	5.4
41. Lactobacillus acidophilus 332	Histidine	None	None	None		4.8
	Tyrosine	None	None		None	4.8
42. Salmonella abortivo-equina 127	Histidine	None	None	None		6.2
	Tyrosine	None	None		None	6.6
43. Salmonella anatum 817	Histidine	None	None	None		5.4
	Tyrosine	None	None		None	6.0
44. Salmonella anatum 818	Histidine	None	None	None		5.2
	Tyrosine	None	None		None	6.2
45. Salmonella columbiensis 747	Histidine	4+	4+	None		6.0
	Tyrosine	4+	4+		None	6.2
46. Salmonella pestis-caviae 902	Histidine	4+	3+	None		5.6
	Tyrosine	4+	3+		None	5.4
47. Salmonella aertrycke 633	Histidine	4+	4+	None		5.4
	Tyrosine	4+	4+		None	5.2
48. Salmonella aertrycke 532	Histidine	4+	4+	None		5.2
	Tyrosine	2+	2+		None	6.4
49. Salmonella aertrycke 854	Histidine	4+	4+	None		5.8
	Tyrosine	4+	4+		None	5.2
50. Salmonella aertrycke 855	Histidine	4+	4+	None		5.4
	Tyrosine	4+	4+		None	5.6
51. Salmonella aertrycke 856	Histidine	4+	3+	None		5.0
	Tyrosine	2+	2+		None	5.8
52. Salmonella enteritidis 56	Histidine	4+	None	None		6.8
	Tyrosine	None	None		None	6.8
53. Salmonella enteritidis 210	Histidine	None	None	None		5.4
	Tyrosine	None	None		None	5.6
54. Salmonella enteritidis 525	Histidine	4+	4+	31%		5.8
	Tyrosine	None	None		None	5.8
55. Salmonella enteritidis 904	Histidine	4+	4+	None		6.2
	Tyrosine	4+	4+		None	6.8
56. Salmonella gallinarum 811	Histidine	4+	4+	None		5.0
	Tyrosine	4+	4+		None	5.8
57. Salmonella muriotitis 915	Histidine	3+	3+	None		6.0
	Tyrosine	3+	None		None	5.2
58. Salmonella morgani 79	Histidine	4+	4+	80%		5.6
	Tyrosine	4+	4+		None	5.8
59. Salmonella morgani 746	Histidine	4+	4+	62%		5.5
	Tyrosine	4+	4+		None	5.4
60. Salmonella morgani 973	Histidine	4+	4+	None		5.4
	Tyrosine	4+	4+		None	5.0
61. Salmonella morgani 974	Histidine	4+	4+	68%		5.6
	Tyrosine	4+	4+		None	6.0
62. Solmanella morgani 975	Histidine	4+	4+	None		5.8
	Tyrosine	4+	4+		None	5.0
63. Salmonella morgani 976	Histidine	4+	4+	None		5.6
	Tyrosine	4+	4+		None	5.8
64. Salmonella morgani 977	Histidine	4+	4+	68%		5.4
	Tyrosine	4+	4+		None	5.8

PRODUCTION OF HISTAMINE, TYRAMINE AND BRONCHOSPASTIC AND ARTERIOSPASTIC SUBSTANCES IN PURE CULTURES OF MICROORGANISMS—*Continued*

COLON TYPHOID GROUP

Name of Microorganism	Amino Acid Added to Blood-Broth Medium	Broncho-spasm	Arterio-spasm	Histidine Converted Into Histamine	Tyrosine Converted Into Tyramine	Reaction After Incubation, P_H
65. Salmonella morgani 978.......	Histidine	4+	4+	74%		5.4
	Tyrosine	4+	4+		None	6.0
66. Salmonella paratyphi 83......	Histidine	4+	4+	None		5.2
	Tyrosine	4+	4+		None	5.4
67. Salmonella paratyphi 84......	Histidine	4+	4+	None		5.2
	Tyrosine	4+	4+		None	5.8
68. Salmonella paratyphi 202.....	Histidine	4+	4+	None		5.4
	Tyrosine	4+	4+		None	5.6
69. Salmonella paratyphi 979.....	Histidine	4+	4+	None		5.5
	Tyrosine	None	None		None	5.0
70. Salmonella paratyphi 199.....	Histidine	4+	4+	None		5.0
	Tyrosine	4+	4+		None	5.4
71. Salmonella psittacosis 96......	Histidine	4+	4+	None		5.2
	Tyrosine	4+	4+		None	5.6
72. Salmonella pullorum 812......	Histidine	None	4+	None		6.2
	Tyrosine	None	2+		None	6.2
73. Salmonella pullorum 813......	Histidine	None	None	None		6.6
	Tyrosine	None	None		None	7.0
74. Salmonella pullorum 814......	Histidine	4+	4+	None		6.0
	Tyrosine	4+	4+		None	6.6
75. Salmonella pullorum 815......	Histidine	None	None	None		6.4
	Tyrosine	None	None		None	6.6
76. Salmonella pullorum 819......	Histidine	None	None	None		6.8
	Tyrosine	None	None		None	6.8
77. Salmonella pullorum 820......	Histidine	4+		None		5.8
	Tyrosine	4+			None	5.6
78. Salmonella schottmülleri 200..	Histidine	4+	4+	None		5.6
	Tyrosine	4+	4+		None	6.0
79. Salmonella schottmülleri 201..	Histidine	None	None	None		5.4
	Tyrosine	None	None		None	5.2
80. Salmonella schottmülleri 744..	Histidine	4+	4+	None		5.6
	Tyrosine	None	None		None	6.4
81. Salmonella schottmülleri 980..	Histidine	4+	4+	77%		5.8
	Tyrosine	2+	3+		None	5.8
82. Salmonella typhi-murium 198.	Histidine	4+	4+	None		5.2
	Tyrosine	4+	4+		None	5.2
83. Salmonella typhi-murium 905.	Histidine	4+	4+	None		5.4
	Tyrosine	4+	2+		None	5.4
84. Salmonella typhi-murium 903.	Histidine	4+	4+	None		5.8
	Tyrosine	4+	4+		None	6.0
85. Salmonella suipestifer 105.....	Histidine	4+	4+	None		5.6
	Tyrosine	None	None		None	5.6
86. Salmonella suipestifer 214.....	Histidine	4+	4+	None		5.4
	Tyrosine	None	None		None	5.2
87. Salmonella suipestifer 215.....	Histidine	None	None	None		7.1
	Tyrosine	None	None		None	6.0
88. Salmonella suipestifer 539.....	Histidine	4+	4+	None		5.4
	Tyrosine	4+	4+		None	5.6
89. Salmonella suipestifer 787.....	Histidine	None	None	None		8.4
	Tyrosine	None	None		None	8.0
90. Salmonella suipestifer 800.....	Histidine	None	None	None		7.0
	Tyrosine	None	None		None	7.0
91. Eberthella typhi 166...........	Histidine	3+	2+	None		5.2
	Tyrosine	3+	2+		None	5.2
92. Eberthella typhi 167...........	Histidine	4+	4+	None		6.2
	Tyrosine	2+	2+		None	7.0
93. Eberthella typhi 191...........	Histidine	3+	4+	None		6.4
	Tyrosine	None	None		None	5.6
94. Eberthella typhi 193...........	Histidine	4+	4+	None		5.6
	Tyrosine	None	None		None	6.0

PRODUCTION OF HISTAMINE, TYRAMINE AND BRONCHOSPASTIC AND ARTERIOSPASTIC SUBSTANCES IN PURE CULTURES OF MICROORGANISMS—*Continued*

PYOGENIC COCCI

Name of Microorganism	Amino Acid Added to Blood-Broth Medium	Broncho-spasm	Arterio-spasm	Histidine Converted Into Histamine	Tyrosine Converted Into Tyramine	Reaction After Incubation, P_H
1. Staphylococcus 149............	Histidine	3+	2+	None		5.2
	Tyrosine	None	None		None	5.0
2. Staphylococcus acne 150.......	Histidine	4+	4+	None		
	Tyrosine	4+	4+		None	
3. Staphylococcus acne 151.......	Histidine	None	None	None		8.0
	Tyrosine	None	None		None	8.0
4. Staphylococcus aureus 152....	Histidine	None	None	None		4.6
	Tyrosine	None	None		None	5.2
5. Staphylococcus aureus 153....	Histidine	None	None	None		4.8
	Tyrosine	None	None		None	5.2
6. Staphylococcus candicans 154	Histidine	None	None	None		4.8
	Hyrosine	None	None		None	6.2
7. Staphylococcus epidermidis	Histidine	None	None	None		4.8
155	Tyrosine	None	None		None	5.6
8. Staphylococcus aureus 156....	Histidine	None	None	None		5.0
	Tyrosine	None	None		None	5.2
9. Staphylococcus aureus 157....	Histidine	None	None	None		5.0
	Tyrosine	None	None		None	5.2
10. Staphylococcus aureus 158....	Histidine	None	2+	None		5.2
	Tyrosine	None	3+		None	5.2
11. Staphylococcus tetragenes 159	Histidine	None	None	None		5.2
	Tyrosine	None	None		None	5.2
12. Staphylococcus albus 251......	Histidine	3+	2+	None		8.0
	Tyrosine	None	None		None	8.6
13. Staphylococcus citreus 395....	Histidine	None	None	None		5.8
	Tyrosine	None	None		None	6.6
14. Staphylococcus aureus 426.....	Histidine	None	None	None		4.8
	Tyrosine	None	4+		None	4.8
15. Staphylococcus albus 427......	Histidine	None	None	None		7.6
	Tyrosine	None	None		None	7.6
16. Staphylococcus aureus 476.....	Histidine	None	None	None		4.4
	Tyrosine	None	None		None	5.0
17. Staphylococcus aureus 477.....	Histidine	None	None	None		4.8
	Tyrosine	None	None		None	5.0
18. Streptococcus 160..............	Histidine	None	None	None		6.8
	Tyrosine	None	None		None	7.0
19. Streptococcus 161..............	Histidine	None	None	None		5.2
	Tyrosine	None	None		None	5.7
20. Streptococcus viridans 162....	Histidine	None	None	None		5.8
	Tyrosine	None	None		None	6.4
21. Streptococcus mastitis 342....	Histidine	None	None	None		4.6
	Tyrosine	None	None		None	4.6
22. Streptococcus (stomach ulcer)	Histidine	None	None	None		5.2
344	Tyrosine	None	None		43%	5.4
23. Streptococcus ulcer colitis 345.	Histidine	None	None	None		4.6
	Tyrosine	None	None		45%	5.2
24. Streptococcus chorea 346......	Histidine	4+	3+	None		5.4
	Tyrosine	4+	None		None	5.7
25. Streptococcus chronic ar-	Histidine	4+	2+	None		5.8
thritis 348	Tyrosine	4+	4+		50%	5.8
26. Streptococcus 349..............	Histidine	None	None	None		5.2
	Tyrosine	None	None		None	6.2
27. Streptococcus sepsis 420.......	Histidine	None	None	None		5.8
	Tyrosine	None	None		None	6.6
28. Streptococcus measles 422.....	Histidine	4+	3+	None		5.6
	Tyrosine	None	None		None	6.2
29. Streptococcus measles 423.....	Histidine	None	None	None		5.8
	Tyrosine	None	4+		None	6.0
30. Streptococcus erysipelas 425...	Histidine	None	3+	None		6.4
	Tyrosine	None	None		None	7.0
31. Streptococcus german measles	Histidine	None	None	None		5.0
433	Tyrosine	None	None		None	6.4
32. Streptococcus scarlatina 543..	Histidine	None	None	None		6.4
	Tyrosine	None	4+		None	7.0

Production of Histamine, Tyramine and Bronchospastic and Arteriospastic Substances in Pure Cultures of Microorganisms—*Continued*

PYOGENIC COCCI

Name of Microorganism	Amino Acid Added to Blood-Broth Medium	Broncho-spasm	Arterio-spasm	Histidine Converted Into Histamine	Tyrosine Converted Into Tyramine	Reaction After Incubation, P_H
33. Pneumococcus type 1 134......	Histidine	None	2+	None		7.1
	Tyrosine	None	None		None	7.4
34. Pneumococcus type 1 306......	Histidine	None	None	None		5.2
	Tyrosine	None	None		None	6.2
35. Pneumococcus type 1 309......	Histidine	None	None	None		7.1
	Tyrosine	None	None		None	7.4
36. Pneumococcus type 1 350......	Histidine	None	None	None		6.4
	Tyrosine	None	None		None	7.0
37. Pneumococcus type 2 307......	Histidine	None	3+	None		5.8
	Tyrosine	None	None		None	6.2
38. Pneumococcus type 2 310......	Histidine	None	None	None		5.6
	Tyrosine	None	None		None	6.2
39. Pneumococcus type 3 308......	Histidine	None	3+	None		6.2
	Tyrosine	None	3+		None	7.0
40. Pneumococcus type 3 311......	Histidine	4+	4+	None		6.0
	Tyrosine	4+	4+		None	7.0
41. Pneumococcus type 3 351......	Histidine	4+	4+	None		6.0
	Tyrosine	4+	4+		None	6.4
42. Pneumococcus type 3 556......	Histidine	4+	4+	None		6.6
	Tyrosine	None	4+		None	7.3
43. Neisseria catarrhalis 835.......	Histidine	None	None	None		7.7
	Tyrosine	None	None		None	8.0
44. Neisseria intracellularis 837....	Histidine	None	None	None		7.7
	Tyrosine	None	None		None	8.0

DIPHTHERIA AND DIPHTHEROID GROUP

Name of Microorganism	Amino Acid Added to Blood-Broth Medium	Broncho-spasm	Arterio-spasm	Histidine Converted Into Histamine	Tyrosine Converted Into Tyramine	Reaction After Incubation, P_H
1. Corynebacterium diphtheriae 170	Histidine	None	None	None		5.8
	Tyrosine	None	None		None	5.0
2. Corynebacterium diphtheriae 291	Histidine	None	None	None		4.6
	Tyrosine	None	None		None	4.6
3. Corynebacterium diphtheriae 296	Histidine	None	None	None		5.2
	Tyrosine	None	None		None	7.2
4. Corynebacterium pseudodiphtherium 371	Histidine	None	None	None		6.2
	Tyrosine	None	None		None	6.2
5. Corynebacterium xerosis 373..	Histidine	4+	2+	None		7.8
	Tyrosine	4+	None		None	8.0

AEROBIC SPORE-FORMING BACTERIA

Name of Microorganism	Amino Acid Added to Blood-Broth Medium	Broncho-spasm	Arterio-spasm	Histidine Converted Into Histamine	Tyrosine Converted Into Tyramine	Reaction After Incubation, P_H
1. Bacillus anthracis 240.........	Histidine	2+	3+	None		6.8
	Tyrosine	3+	4+		None	7.0
2. Bacillus anthracis 241.........	Histidine	None	None	None		7.0
	Tyrosine	None	None		None	6.2
3. Bacillus anthracis 247.........	Histidine	None	None	None		8.0
	Tyrosine	None	None		None	8.0
4. Bacillus mesentericus 76.......	Histidine	None	None	None		6.6
	Tyrosine	None	None		None	6.3
5. Bacillus megatherium 72......	Histidine	None	None	None		6.4
	Tyrosine	None	None		None	7.1
6. Bacillus subtilis 102............	Histidine	None	None	None		5.0
	Tyrosine	3+	2+		None	5.0
7. Bacillus subtilis 243............	Histidine	None	None	None		6.2
	Tyrosine	None	None		None	6.4
8. Bacillus subtilis 465............	Histidine	None	None	None		7.6
	Tyrosine	4+	3+		None	7.6
9. Bacillus subtilis 466............	Histidine	None	None	None		7.6
	Tyrosine	None	None		None	6.8
10. Bacillus vugatis 123...........	Histidine	None	2+	None		7.4
	Tyrosine	None	2+		None	7.4
11. Bacillus panis 82..............	Histidine	None	None	None		7.7
	Tyrosine	None	None		None	7.8
12. Bacillus lactimorbi 246........	Histidine	None	None	None		7.7
	Tyrosine	None	None		None	7.8

PRODUCTION OF HISTAMINE, TYRAMINE AND BRONCHOSPASTIC AND ARTERIOSPASTIC SUBSTANCES IN PURE CULTURES OF MICROORGANISMS—*Continued*

AEROBIC SPORE-FORMING BACTERIA

Name of Microorganism	Amino Acid Added to Blood-Broth Medium	Broncho-spasm	Arterio-spasm	Histidine Converted Into Histamine	Tyrosine Converted Into Tyramine	Reaction After Incubation, P_H
13. Bacillus cereus 21..............	Histidine	None	None	None		6.8
	Tyrosine	None	None		None	6.6
14. Bacillus petasites 89...........	Histidine	None	None	None		7.0
	Tyrosine	None	None		None	6.8
15. Bacillus subtilis viscosis 103...	Histidine	None	None	None		7.5
	Tyrosine	None	None		None	7.5

ANAEROBIC SPORE-FORMING BACTERIA

Name of Microorganism	Amino Acid Added to Blood-Broth Medium	Broncho-spasm	Arterio-spasm	Histidine Converted Into Histamine	Tyrosine Converted Into Tyramine	Reaction After Incubation, P_H
1. Clostridium botulinum 458....	Histidine	None	None	None		
	Tyrosine	None	None		None	
2. Clostridium botulinum 320a...	Histidine	None	None	None		6.4
	Tyrosine	None	None		None	7.0
3. Clostridium chauvei 11a.......	Histidine	None	None	None		6.0
	Tyrosine	None	None		None	7.2
4. Clostridium chauvei 12b.......	Histidine	None	None	None		6.0
	Tyrosine	None	None		None	6.8
5. Clostridium histolyticum 611..	Histidine	None	None	None		7.0
	Tyrosine	None	None		None	6.8
6. Clostridium oedematis-maligni 53a	Histidine	None	None	None		7.2
	Tyrosine	None	None		None	7.2
7. Clostridium oedematis-maligni 54a	Histidine	None	None	None		7.0
	Tyrosine	None	None		None	7.0
8. Slostridium oedematis-maligni 55	Histidine	None	None	None		6.2
	Tyrosine	None	None		None	6.4
9. Clostridium sporogenes 459...	Histidine	None	None	None		7.0
	Tyrosine	None	None		None	7.0

ACIDFAST BACTERIA

Name of Microorganism	Amino Acid Added to Blood-Broth Medium	Broncho-spasm	Arterio-spasm	Histidine Converted Into Histamine	Tyrosine Converted Into Tyramine	Reaction After Incubation, P_H
1. Mycobacterium butyricum.. 362	Histidine	None	None	None		7.2
	Tyrosine	None	None		None	7.2
2. Mycobacterium avium 118.....	Histidine	None	None	None		7.2
	Tyrosine	None	None		None	7.0
3. Mycobacterium phlei 354......	Histidine	None	None	None		7.2
	Tyrosine	None	None		None	7.6
4. Mycobacterium leprae 68......	Histidine	None	None	None		7.3
	Tyrosine	None	None		None	7.5
5. Mycobacterium leprae 283.....	Histidine	None	None	None		7.0
	Tyrosine	None	None		None	7.6
6. Mycobacterium ranae 110.....	Histidine	None	None	None		6.2
	Tyrosine	None	None		None	7.0
7. Mycobacterium smegma 101...	Histidine	None	None	None		7.0
	Tyrosine	None	None		None	7.0
8. Mycobacterium smegma 361...	Histidine	None	None	None		7.5
	Tyrosine	None	None		None	7.4
9. Mycobacterium tuberculosis bovis 112	Histidine	None	None	None		7.8
	Tyrosine	None	None		None	7.7
10. Mycobacterium tuberculosis hominis 115	Histidine	None	None	None		7.3
	Tyrosine	None	None		None	7.5
11. Mycobacterium tuberculosis hominis 119	Histidine	None	None	None		7.2
	Tyrosine	None	None		None	7.3

BACTERIA ISOLATED FROM DAIRY PRODUCTS

Name of Microorganism	Amino Acid Added to Blood-Broth Medium	Broncho-spasm	Arterio-spasm	Histidine Converted Into Histamine	Tyrosine Converted Into Tyramine	Reaction After Incubation, P_H
1. Lactobacillus bulgaricus 521..	Histidine	None	None	None		4.6
	Tyrosine	None	None		None	4.4
2. Lactobacillus bulgaricus 522..	Histidine	None	None	None		5.0
	Tyrosine	None	None		None	6.2
3. Lactobacillus bulgaricus 523..	Histidine	None	None	None		5.2
	Tyrosine	None	None		None	5.2
4. Lactobacillus casei 336........	Histidine	None	None	None		5.2
	Tyrosine	None	None		None	5.8
5. Streptococcus kefir 341........	Histidine	None	None	None		5.4
	Tyrosine	None	None		None	5.0

Production of Histamine, Tyramine and Bronchospastic and Arteriospastic Substances in Pure Cultures of Microorganisms—*Continued*

BACTERIA ISOLATED FROM DAIRY PRODUCTS

Name of Microorganism	Amino Acid Added to Blood-Broth Medium	Broncho-spasm	Arterio-spasm	Histidine Converted Into Histamine	Tyrosine Converted Into Tyramine	Reaction After Incubation, P_H
6. Streptococcus lactis 339.......	Histidine	None	3+	None		5.0
	Tyrosine	None	2+		None	5.2
7. Streptococcus lactis 374.......	Histidine	None	None	None		5.4
	Tyrosine	None	None		70%	5.4
8. Streptococcus lactis 557.......	Histidine	None	None	None		6.6
	Tyrosine	None	None		None	5.8
9. Streptococcus inulinaceus 376.	Histidine	None	4+	None		5.2
	Tyrosine	None	2+		39%	5.2
10. Streptococcus cremoris 377....	Histidine	None	None	None		5.2
	Tyrosine	None	None		None	5.2
11. Streptococcus lactis 559.......	Histidine	None	None	None		6.0
	Tyrosine	None	None		None	5.8
12. Lactobacillus viscosis 337.....	Histidine	None	None	None		7.8
	Tyrosine	None	None		None	7.8
13. Vibrio tyrogenes 165...........	Histidine	None	None	None		7.4
	Tyrosine	None	3+		None	8.0
OTHER BACTERIA						
1. Alcaligenes abortus 727........	Histidine	2+	3+	None		7.0
	Tyrosine	None	None		None	7.8
2. Alcaligenes bronchosepticus 232	Histidine	None	None	None		8.0
	Tyrosine	None	None		None	7.8
3. Alcaligenes melitensis 739......	Histidine	None	None	None		
	Tyrosine	None	None		None	
4. Erwina aroidea 494............	Histidine	None	None	None		5.4
	Tyrosine	None	None		None	5.6
5. Erwina carotovora 495........	Histidine	None	None	None		6.0
	Tyrosine	None	None		None	6.2
6. Micrococcus conglomeratus 401	Histidine	None	None	None		7.2
	Tyrosine	None	None		None	7.5
7. Micrococcus flavus 140.........	Histidine	None	None	None		6.4
	Tyrosine	None	None		None	6.2
8. Micrococcus flavus 400.........	Histidine	None	None	None		6.8
	Tyrosine	None	None		None	7.3
9. Micrococcus ureae 408.........	Histidine	None	None	None		6.8
	Tyrosine	None	None		None	7.3
10. Hemophilus influenza 1........	Histidine	None	None	None		7.0
	Tyrosine	None	None		None	7.5
11. Hemophilus pertussis 777......	Histidine	None	None	None		
	Tyrosine	None	None		None	7.8
12. Pasteurella avicida 238........	Histidine	None	None	None		8.6
	Tyrosine	None	None		None	8.4
13. Pasteurella suiseptica 237.....	Histidine	None	None	None		6.0
	Tyrosine	None	None		None	7.4
14. Pasteurella pestis 87...........	Histidine	4+	None	None		7.8
	Tyrosine	3+	None		None	7.8
15. Pseudomonas aeruginosa 97..	Histidine	None	None	None		6.2
	Tyrosine	None	None		None	6.2
16. Proteus vulgaris 93............	Histidine	None	None	None		5.6
	Tyrosine	None	None		None	5.2
17. Sarcina flava 540..............	Histidine	None	None	None		7.8
	Tyrosine	None	None		None	7.8
18. Sarcina lutea 38a..............	Histidine	None	None	None		5.8
	Tyrosine	None	None		None	7.6
19. Sarcina lutea 38b..............	Histidine	None	None	None		7.2
	Tyrosine	None	None		None	7.6
20. Serratia marcescens 274.......	Histidine	None	None	None		4.4
	Tyrosine	None	None		None	4.4
21. Serratia pyoseptica 275........	Histidine	None	None	None		5.6
	Tyrosine	None	None		None	5.6
22. Spirillum rubrum 277..........	Histidine	None	None	None		
	Tyrosine	None	None		None	
23. Vibrio metchnikovi 163........	Histidine	None	None	None		6.0
	Tyrosine	None	None		None	7.0

PRODUCTION OF HISTAMINE, TYRAMINE AND BRONCHOSPASTIC AND ARTERIOSPASTIC SUBSTANCES IN PURE CULTURES OF MICROORGANISMS—*Continued*

HIGHER BACTERIA

Name of Microorganism	Amino Acid Added to Blood-Broth Medium	Broncho-spasm	Arterio-spasm	Histidine Converted Into Histamine	Tyrosine Converted Into Tyramine	Reaction After Incubation, P_H
1. Actinomyces bovis 549	Histidine	None	None	None		
	Tyrosine	None	None		None	
2. Nocardia macropodidarum 470	Histidine	None	None	None		6.4
	Tyrosine	None	None		None	7.0

MOLDS AND YEASTS

Name of Microorganism	Amino Acid Added to Blood-Broth Medium	Broncho-spasm	Arterio-spasm	Histidine Converted Into Histamine	Tyrosine Converted Into Tyramine	Reaction After Incubation, P_H
1. Aspergillus flavus 1004	Histidine	None	None	None		6.2
	Tyrosine	None	None		None	5.4
2. Aspergillus niger 1003	Histidine	None	None	None		5.8
	Tyrosine	None	None		None	6.4
3. Oidium albicans 569	Histidine	None	None	None		6.4
	Tyrosine	None	None		None	6.8
4. Penicillium roquiforti 528	Histidine	3+	2+	None		5.8
	Tyrosine	2+	None		None	6.4
5. Sporothrix schencki 353	Histidine	None	None	None		6.8
	Tyrosine	None	None		None	6.8
6. Blastomyces 352	Histidine	None	None	None		7.3
	Hyrosine	None	None		None	7.2
7. Torula (red) 917	Histidine	None	None	None		6.4
	Tyrosine	None	None		None	6.8

Histamine was not produced by any of the 129 microorganisms that do not belong to the colon-typhoid group. There were five tyramine producers, all were streptococci.

DISCUSSION

It will be noted that a given filtrate that is bronchospastic will usually be arteriospastic, and vice versa. This is not always true, however. There is no known theoretical reason why the smooth musculature of the artery and of the bronchi should not react with the same substance; and we are inclined to believe that it does. These variations may be accounted for by the individual differences in sensitiveness of various muscle preparations, and by quantitative differences in the concentrations of the active substance.

These experiments have all been performed with one cc. portions of the total concentrated filtrate. This fraction is eight times as concentrated as the original bacterial filtrate. A complete bronchial spasm is invariably obtained with 0.5 cc. of a highly active original filtrate; so the dose employed is nearly 16 times as great as would be required to give the maximum response with a highly active filtrate. The values do not, therefore, give quantitative data as to the amount of active substance present, excepting, perhaps, in those few cases in which the response was not maximal. The minimal effective dose and that required to give a maximal response are, moreover, not very different. For example, a filtrate that gives a maximal response with 0.7 cc. will give a 2 + reaction with 0.5 cc., and no reaction with 0.3 cc. Thus two filtrates that do not contain very much of the spastic substance might contain almost the same amount, and still the one might give a 3 + or a 4 + reaction, while the other might give no reaction.

Guinea-pig bronchi and hog arteries vary considerably in sensitiveness. Thus one pig may give a 4 + reaction with 0.7 cc. of filtrate, and a 2 + reaction with 0.5 cc. of filtrate, whereas another will give no reaction with 0.5 cc. of this same filtrate, and only a 2 + reaction with 0.7 cc. It is entirely possible that many of our 4 + reactions may have been borderline reactions for a given preparation and have been less than the minimal effective dose for another preparation. In this way it is possible to explain the discrepancies between bronchospasms and arteriospasms as well as the fact that positive reactions were obtained with the histidine broth and not with the tyrosine broth, or vice versa, in some cases. Our results indicate that the amino acids added are not responsible for the production of the spastic substances, excepting in those rare cases where histamine is produced. The amino acids may, however, have produced differences in growth and, in such cases in which the amount of spastic substance produced is small, even under the best conditions, this difference in growth may have been sufficient to give a 4 + reaction with one fraction, and no reaction with the other.

The spastic substance, or substances, appears to be an amine. It can be extracted quantitatively from a 30% sodium hydroxide solution with amyl alcohol. It can also be extracted with ether or with chloroform; but the substance appears to be less soluble in these solvents and the extraction is not as quantitative as it is with amyl alcohol. The substance can be quantitatively extracted from any of these solvents with dilute sulfuric acid. The substance appears, therefore, to form a sulfate. We have also prepared the chloride, oxalate, picrate, and picrolonate. The chloride and oxalate have not been obtained in crystalline condition. Crystalline picrates and picrolonates of considerable activity have been prepared; but the products have not been purified sufficiently to warrant an analysis. This work is being continued. The spastic substance is dialyzable. We feel justified in concluding, from these data, that the spastic substance is an amine. It is not histamine, and it is not an imidazole. It is not identical with the poisons described by Branham,[7] or by E. E. Ecker and C. Rimington.[8]

The data presented in this paper do not warrant any conclusion as to the possible significance of the spastic substances in disease. The ability

7. J. Infect. Dis., 1925, 37, p. 291.
8. J. Hyg., 1927, 27, p. 44.

to produce spastic substances, although it is a common property of those bacteria that invade the alimentary tract, is not so common for other microorganisms. We have amply demonstrated [1] that histamine, which is one of the most powerful spastic substances known, is a normal constituent of the contents of the alimentary tract. It is absorbed; but it is destroyed in its passage through the intestinal wall. It is always conceivable, of course, that the intestine may become more permeable under certain conditions, but this has never been satisfactorily demonstrated. There is no good reason for supposing that the spastic substance of unknown composition should penetrate the intestinal wall any more readily than does histamine. Whether or not there is a causal relationship between the diarrheas that are associated with infections by certain members of the colon-typhoid group, and the ability of this group to produce spastic substances will, for the present at least, have to remain a matter of conjecture. The possible relationship of the spastic substances that might be produced in foci of infection to bronchial asthma, has been adequately discussed in the paper by Koessler, Lewis, and Walker.[2]

SUMMARY

This paper contains a report on the production of histamine, tyramine, bronchospastic, and arteriospastic substances by 223 microorganisms [9] grown on a blood-broth medium. Ninety-four are members of the colon-typhoid group. Nine of these convert histidine into histamine, and of these two belong to the Escherichia group, and seven to the Salmonella group. Five of the eight Salmonella morgani strains produce histamine. There were no tyramine producers in this group. The faculty for producing bronchospastic and arteriospastic substances, other than histamine, is highly developed in the colon-typhoid group: Salmonella, 49 studied, 38 produced spastic substances; dysentery Shiga, six studied, five were spastic; paradysentery, 12 studied, six were spastic; Escherichia, nine studied, nine spastic; typhoid bacilli, all spastic. Taken collectively, of the 94 representatives of the colon-typhoid group studied, 67 produced spastic substances.

Bronchospastic and arteriospastic substances are rarely produced by microorganisms other than those belonging to the colon-typhoid group. Histamine was not produced by any of the 129 microorganisms that are not members of the colon-typhoid group. Of these 129 microorganisms, five, all of them streptococci, were tyramine producers.

9. Obtained from the American Type Culture Collection of The John McCormick Institute for Infectious Diseases.

THE METABOLISM OF LEISHMANIA TROPICA

A. J. Salle and Carl L. A. Schmidt

From the Divisions of Biochemistry and Bacteriology, University of California Medical School, Berkeley

An extensive literature dealing with the metabolism of bacteria has accumulated, but so far, little work has been carried out on the metabolic activities of the protozoa. The protozoologist's inability to grow the latter for many generations, has been and still is one of the difficulties in the way.

The pathogenic protozoa that have been cultivated in pure culture with the greatest success are the hemoflagellates, or blood parasites, but the growth is scanty even after a number of days of incubation. Cultivation of Trypanosoma lewisi was carried out by McNeal and Novy [1] on a nutrient blood agar medium, and the same investigators [2] have also described methods for the growth of T. brucei, T. avium, T. laverani, and T. mesnili. Others who have worked in this field are Rogers,[3] Longo,[4] Nicolle,[5] Row,[6] Laveran and Pettit,[7] Mathis,[8] Thomson,[9] Ponselle,[10] Luna,[11] Noguchi and Lindenberg,[12] Kligler,[13] Leiva,[14] and Pedroso.[15] In no case, does it appear that the growth was sufficiently heavy for studies of metabolism. It was therefore necessary in our work to develop mediums not only for the preservation of stock cultures of Leishmania, but also for carrying out studies of the metabolism of the organism.

Received for publication, June 4, 1928.

1. Contributions to Medical Research, Ann Arbor, Michigan, 1913, p. 549.
2. J. Infect. Dis., 1904, 1, p. 1; ibid., 1905, 2, p. 256.
3. Lancet, 1904, 167, p. 215; ibid., 1905, 168, p. 1484; Proc. Roy. Soc., London, 1906, 77, p. 284.
4. Policlinico (sez. med.), 1910, 17, p. 643.
5. Bull. Soc. path. exot., 1908, T. 1; Compt. rend. Acad. d. sc., 1908, 146, pp. 498 and 842.
6. Quart. J. Micr. Sc, 1908, 53, p 747.
7. Compt. rend. Soc. de biol., 1910, 68, p. 114.
8. Ibid., 1906, 61, p. 550.
9. J. Hyg., 1908, 8, p. 75.
10. Ann. de Parasitol., 1923, 1, p. 155.
11. Pathologica, 1914, 6, p. 443.
12. Am. J. Trop. Med., 1925, 5, p. 63.
13. Am. J. Trop. Med., 1924, 4, p. 69; Tr. Roy. Soc. Trop. Med. & Hyg., 1925, 19, p. 330; abstr. Bact., 1925, 9, p. 18
14 Philippine J. Sc., 1922, 20, p. 179.
15. Am. J. Trop. Med., 1923, 3, p. 47; quoted in Wenyon, C. M.: Protozoölogy London, Baillière, Tindall & Cox, 1926.

MEDIUMS

Preliminary experiments indicated that, while it was possible to obtain fairly good growth of Leishmania in mediums which contained whole rabbit blood, the growth became progressively poorer when the amount of blood was increased much above 15 per cent. In the complete absence of hemoglobin, no growth took place. Replacement of whole blood by serum did not lead to growth. It was suspected that the inhibitory effects of increasing the amounts of the whole blood were due to the inhibiting action of the serum. Experiments in which washed red cells were added to the medium showed good growth. In fact, the organisms apparently grew better when the concentration of the cell suspension in the medium was increased to 35 or 40% than when the amount was limited to the quantity which, when whole rabbit blood was used, led to good growth. Growth was more rapid when hemolyzed red cells were added to the medium than when whole cells were used. Heating the blood-containing medium was followed by decidedly decreased growth. It was also demonstrated that whole proteins, such as casein, edestin, and gelatin, could replace peptone in the medium. On the other hand, when peptone was replaced by substances which are rich in the lower products of split protein, growth became less luxuriant. In other words, growth was better when the medium contained whole protein or the primary protein split products. This statement must be taken in a relative sense only, since by the addition of red cells, amino-acids were undoubtedly included. Growth on a medium containing gelatin was followed by liquefaction, indicating the presence of a gelatinase. It was not found necessary to add additional buffer to the mediums. The added hemoglobin probably contributed a sufficient amount of this factor.

On the basis of the rather extensive preliminary experimental work, a solid and a liquid medium were developed, both of which when inoculated with Leishmania yielded good growth. The liquid medium was used for the experiments to determine metabolism. Its composition was as follows:

Basic Medium.—Proteose peptone (Difco), 10 gm.; beef infusion, 250 cc.; salt, 3 gm.; distilled water to make 800 cc. The reaction was adjusted to P_H 7.2. The broth was not filtered.

Hemoglobin Solution.—Defibrinated rabbit blood was centrifugated, the serum was removed and the cells were washed several times with salt solution. The cells were hemolyzed with two parts of distilled water. Sterile precautions were unnecessary.

Finished Medium ("Standard Medium" in the Text).—To 800 cc. of the basic medium 180 cc. of the hemoglobin solution and 20 cc. of 50% glucose solution, were added, giving a volume of 1,000 cc. The whole was clarified by centrifugation and filtered through a sterile Mandler filter, according to the procedure described by Salle.[16] This finished medium was placed in sterile flasks. The flasks were inoculated from cultured slants and incubated at 22 C. for 6 days. In all experiments for the study of metabolism a control flask of sterile medium was similarly incubated. The culture of Leishmania tropica used in these experiments was obtained from Professor Novy.

The solid medium was essentially the same as the liquid medium. In the basic medium described under (a) were included 15 gm. of agar. The solution was filtered and distributed in amounts of 80 cc. to each flask. The flasks were sterilized for 30 minutes at 15 pounds pressure. For use the agar was melted and cooled to 50 C., and 2 cc. of sterile 50% glucose solution were added, together

16. J. Lab. & Clin. Med., 1927, 12, p. 1009.

with 18 cc. of hemoglobin solution, prepared as described, with the exception, however, that precautions had to be taken to keep it sterile. After these had been mixed, the blood agar was poured into sterile test tubes, which then were slanted and the medium allowed to cool. When it was firm, the tubes were placed in an upright position, to allow a few drops of water of condensation to collect. The inoculum was added to this water of condensation and the tubes were tilted so as to permit the liquid to run over the surface of the agar, after which they were incubated in an upright position. A fairly satisfactory solid medium for the preservation of stock cultures of Leishmania tropica was also made by substituting sterile, defibrinated rabbit blood for the solution of hemoglobin. In all other respects, the procedures would have been the same as given above.

EXPERIMENTS

The procedures of the experiments to determine the metabolic activities of Leishmania tropica were essentially the same as those employed by Kendall [17] in his study of bacterial metabolism.

Flasks were inoculated with the organism and incubated at 22 C. for 6 days, and the analytic results were compared with those obtained on sterile portions of the same mediums kept under identical conditions. For the estimation of ammonia, the Folin-Macallum [18] modification of the Folin air current method was used. Total nitrogen was determined according to the method described by Folin and Farmer.[19] The nonprotein nitrogen was estimated by the method of Folin and Wu [20] as modified by Kendall.[17] The colorimetric method of Folin [21] was used for the determination of the amino-nitrogen. Glucose was estimated according to the method of Folin and Wu.[20] The measurements of the hydrogen ion activity were carried out with the aid of De Eds and Hanzlik's [22] micro-electrode. Dyer's [23] method using steam distillation was employed for the estimation of the volatile acids.

The results of the experiments to determine the protozoan metabolism are given in tables 1, 2 and 3. It should be stated that the results are to be considered as semiquantitative, since it was not feasible to correlate the quantitative changes in the medium with the number of the organisms.

Table 1 summarizes the results which were obtained when the organisms were grown on the standard liquid medium (previously described) with and without added glucose. It may be seen that there was a distinct decrease in the sugar content of the mediums and an increase in volatile acids. There was likewise a slight decrease in hydrogen ion activity. The increase in the content of ammonia nitrogen

17. J. Infect. Dis., 1922, 30, p. 211.
18. J. Biol. Chem., 1912, 11, p. 523.
19. Ibid., 1912, 11, p. 493.
20. Ibid., 1919, 38, p. 81.
21. Ibid., 1922, 51, p. 377.
22. Ibid., 1924, 60, p. 355.
23. Ibid., 1916, 28, p. 445.

was indicative of the breaking down of protein. The data showed that, when glucose was omitted from the medium (experiment 3) considerably more ammonia was produced, indicating the breaking down of protein. Little change was noted in P_H due to the neutralization of volatile fatty acids by ammonia, and the amount of volatile acids was less than in experiments 1 and 2. In experiment 4 both glucose and beef infusion were omitted from the medium. It contained only traces of sugar. This came from the hemoglobin. The data showed a considerable increase in the content of ammonia and a rise in P_H. The increase in nonprotein nitrogen and the decrease in protein nitrogen indicated a

TABLE 1.—METABOLIC ACTIVITIES OF LEISHMANIA TROPICA ON STANDARD MEDIUM

(Glucose was omitted from the medium in experiment 3. Glucose and beef infusion were omitted in experiment 4)

Experiment	Total Nitrogen Mg.	Ammonia Nitrogen Mg.	Non-protein Nitrogen Mg.	Protein Nitrogen Mg.	Amino-nitrogen Mg.	Glucose Gm.	P_H	Volatile Acids, Cc. of 0.02 N Alkali
1............	417	13.1	309	108	19.2	1.09	6.37	13.2
Control....	417	12.4	309	108	18.9	1.19	7.02	7.3
2............	439	11.6	334	105	22.2	1.02	6.37	13.2
Control....	439	11.1	334	105	22.2	1.09	7.13	7.6
3............	431	22.0	282	149	24.7	....	7.64	9.1
Control....	431	18.0	285	147	24.7	....	7.68	6.0
4............	430	14.0	323	108	20.9	....	7.68	8.7
Control....	430	8.3	298	132	22.6	....	7.13	4.4

TABLE 2.—METABOLIC ACTIVITIES OF LEISHMANIA TROPICA ON MEDIUM CONTAINING GELATIN

(Glucose and beef infusion were omitted in experiment 6)

Experiment	Total Nitrogen Mg.	Ammonia Nitrogen Mg.	Non-protein Nitrogen Mg.	Protein Nitrogen Mg.	Amino-nitrogen Mg.	Glucose Gm.	P_H	Volatile Acids, Cc. of 0.02 N Alkali
5...........	410	11.6	385	24.7	11.5	0.68	6.42	11.5
Control...	410	11.0	385	24.7	11.4	0.85	7.10	6.9
6...........	290	8.2	249	41.0	5.9	....	7.56	2.4
Control...	290	7.0	249	41.0	3.8	....	7.13	1.4

splitting of the protein. The amount of volatile acids produced was less than in a medium containing glucose. The results indicated a protein-sparing action by the glucose. These results were in harmony with the observations of Kendall [24] and his associates (Farmer, and Day and Walker) with respect to bacterial metabolism.

Table 2 summarizes the data which were obtained when the organism was grown on a medium containing 5 gm. of gelatin instead of 10 gm. of peptone. The other ingredients were the same as in the standard medium. In experiment 6 glucose was omitted from the medium containing gelatin.

24. J. Med. Research, 1911-1912, 25, p. 117; J. Biol. Chem., 1912, 12, p. 13; ibid., 1912-1913, 13, p. 63; J. Med. Research, 1913, 28, p. 465; J. Infect. Dis., 1913, 13, p. 425.

The results were essentially the same as those recorded in table 1. They showed a protein-sparing action on the part of Leishmania in the presence of the carbohydrate. Omission of the carbohydrate was followed by decreased production of volatile acids, and an increase of ammonia, amino-nitrogen, and P_H.

A series of experiments was then undertaken in which casein or its split products were substituted for the peptone. The casein digest was prepared according to the method of Kristensen, Lester, and Jürgens.[25] In experiments 7 and 8, 100 cc. of casein digest were substituted for the peptone in the standard medium. The results were essentially the same as those which were obtained with other mediums containing carbohydrate. A decrease in the content of glucose was followed by a rise in the production of volatile acids and an increase in the acidity. The

TABLE 3.—METABOLIC ACTIVITIES OF LEISHMANIA TROPICA ON MEDIUMS CONTAINING CASEIN
(Glucose was omitted in experiments 9 and 11)

Experiment	Total Nitrogen Mg.	Ammonia Nitrogen Mg.	Non-protein Nitrogen Mg.	Protein Nitrogen Mg.	Amino-nitrogen Mg.	Glucose Gm.	P_H	Volatile Acids, Cc. of 0.02 N Alkali
7...........	341	14.5	293	47	25.7	0.85	5.82	13.2
Control..	341	11.6	293	47	25.0	0.96	6.83	5.0
8...........	331	13.4	287	44	26.4	0.87	5.66	11.7
Control..	331	11.3	287	44	24.7	0.97	6.86	5.0
9.	328	15.3	282	46	26.4	....	7.42	3.1
Control..	328	8.5	282	46	25.2	....	6.90	1.7
10...........	338	11.0	253	85	22.6	0.89	6.31	9.0
Control..	338	9.0	231	107	8.8	0.94	7.15	3.6
11...........	328	13.0	293	35	19.4	....	7.57	1.5
Control..	328	6.2	282	46	5.3	....	7.24	1.0

slight increase in the ammonia is indicative of catabolism of the protein. It was, however, not sufficient to affect the figures for protein and non-protein nitrogen. In experiment 9, glucose was omitted from the casein digest mediums. The results were characterized by a considerable increase in the ammonia and a rise in P_H. The amount of the volatile acids was decidedly less than in experiment 8. This experiment also showed increased utilization of protein in the absence of carbohydrate. Several experiments were carried out by growing the organism on mediums containing unsplit casein with and without added glucose. Five grams of casein were substituted for the peptone in the standard medium. When the organism was grown on a casein medium containing glucose (exper. 10), the data showed a slight increase in the amount of ammonia nitrogen, volatile acids, and acidity, and a decrease in the sugar content. There is also a decrease in the amount of protein

25. Brit. J. Exper. Path., 1925, 6, p. 291.

nitrogen and an increase in the nonprotein nitrogen and the amino-nitrogen, indicating splitting of the protein. The omission of glucose from the medium (exper. 11) is followed by an increase in the amount of ammonia, an increase in the alkalinity, and a smaller production of the volatile acids. The protein fractions likewise indicated a breaking down of the whole protein.

An experiment was also carried out to determine whether nitrogenous end products other than ammonia are formed by Leishmania tropica. The organism was grown on the standard liquid medium, from which glucose and beef broth were omitted. There was no indication of the formation of urea, uric acid, or creatinine.

It appeared from our work, as well as the work of others, that hemoglobin was necessary for the culturing of Leishmania tropica, as well as other hemoflagellates. The question as to the function of hemoglobin at once suggested itself. The possible functions are: to furnish the organism with a complex compound, necessary for building up its protoplasm; to serve as carrier of oxygen to the organism; and to afford some accessory growth factor, accompanying the hemoglobin, which was needed by the organism. Our experiments had shown that while it was possible to grow Leishmania tropica on mediums containing less hemoglobin than was used in our standard medium, the amount of growth was decidedly less. This seemingly eliminated the first-mentioned possibility, since, if hemoglobin itself was used for metabolic purposes, a much smaller amount than was found necessary should have sufficed. Moreover, it was not found possible to substitute chlorophyl, a substance which also contains pyrrol groups, for hemoglobin.

Experiments were undertaken to determine, if possible, whether the function of hemoglobin was that of a carrier of oxygen. Some work in this field had already been reported by Rogers,[3] Longo,[4] Luna [11] and Kligler.[13] Their opinions as to whether or not hemoflagellates could grow in the absence of oxygen, were not unanimous. A series of tubes containing standard liquid mediums were prepared. While the total amount of hemoglobin in all the tubes was the same, the amount of oxyhemoglobin was varied by substituting carbon monoxide hemoglobin for it in amounts which varied from 0 to 25% of the total hemoglobin present. The tubes were inoculated, stoppered, and incubated for 5 days. At the end of this time, the growth in all the tubes was practically the same. In another experiment, all the hemoglobin was converted into carbon monoxide hemoglobin. The organism likewise grew on this medium. While the amount of oxyhemoglobin was undoubtedly small, complete anaerobic conditions did not prevail, since the air above the liquid was not excluded. When special precautions were taken to exclude oxygen by saturating the medium with carbon monoxide, and placing the tubes in a jar containing both alkaline pyrogallol and an atmosphere of carbon monoxide, no growth was observed. A few organisms survived for a period of 3 days but eventually died on continued incubation. In another series of experiments, anaerobic conditions were maintained by the use of hydrogen. As a check for anaerobiosis, a culture of Clostridium botulinum was placed in the jar. As in the previous experiment, the hemoflagellates survived for several days but did not multiply and the culture soon became sterile. Good growth of Cl. botulinum was obtained. These experiments indicated that Leishmania tropica could not grow under complete anaerobic conditions. It could, however, grow under lower concentration of oxygen than that which was provided by the large amount of hemoglobin which the standard medium contained. While it could not wholly be denied that the function of hemoglobin might be that of an oxygen carrier, this function was shown not to be proportional to the amount of hemoglobin which was required for optimal growth. It seemed likely that we were concerned with an accessory factor. While our experiments pointed to this possibility, they did not bring proof of it. For this, the isolation of the accessory factor was necessary.

Studies on the metabolism of other protozoa are under way.

SUMMARY

A solid and a liquid medium were prepared for the cultivation of Leishmania tropica. The growth on the liquid medium was sufficient for the determination of the metabolic activities of Leishmania tropica. The organism was grown on the standard medium and on mediums in which certain described variations were made. The analytic data indicated that the metabolism of Leishmania tropica does not differ essentially from that of many bacteria. Carbohydrate exerts a marked sparing action toward the protein of the medium. The organism possesses marked proteolytic powers. Its utilization of protein was demonstrated by an increase in the ammonia content of the medium and a rise in P_H. Its utilization of protein was demonstrated also in an increase of split-protein products. Experiments showed that this organism cannot survive under anaerobic conditions. The function of hemoglobin in the medium may be to contribute an accessory food or growth factor.

INTRANASAL INOCULATIONS OF RABBITS WITH BACILLUS INFLUENZA

JOHN E. WALKER

From the Department of Immunology, School of Hygiene and Public Health, Johns Hopkins University, Baltimore, Md.

Bull and McKee [1] have shown that the rabbit can be infected with the pneumococcus by intranasal inoculation. This method of inoculation approximates natural infections much more closely than intravenous injections and extends considerably the use of the rabbit in the experimental investigation of respiratory disease. The work of Bull suggested the study of other pathogenic human organisms in the same way. Results obtained with Pfeiffer's bacillus (Bacillus influenzae) will be described in this paper. The method seemed to be especially desirable for the study of Pfeiffer's bacillus, since the effects of intravenous injection of this organism are produced usually by the primary toxicity of the culture, rather than by actual invasion and multiplication. Pfeiffer [2] himself called attention to the fact that dead cultures injected intravenously produce approximately the same effect as living cultures.

Technique.—Most of the experimental work was carried out with a strain of Pfeiffer's bacillus isolated at necropsy from the lungs of an infant which had died of bronchopneumonia following pertussis. An accidental human infection due to the same strain has already been described.[3]

For the inoculation of the rabbits 0.1 cc. of a 24-hour chocolate broth culture was allowed to run from a pipet into each naris. The nasal cultures were made according to the method described by Bull and McKee.[4]

The rabbits were cultured immediately before inoculation, and thereafter at intervals of 2 or 3 days until disappearance of the Pfeiffer bacilli. The cultures before inoculation invariably showed gram-negative cocci as the predominating organism. The animals were all free of nasal discharge at the time of inoculation. This complete absence of respiratory disease was due to the fact that the animals were supplied from a special breeding colony maintained for the express purpose of furnishing animals free of infections. It is doubtful whether ordinary stock laboratory animals are suitable for work of this nature.

Results.—The first animal was inoculated on October 15, 1927, 5 days after the isolation of the organism at necropsy, and 13 animals were

Received for publication, May 10, 1928.

1. Am. J. Hyg., 1927, 7, p. 627.
2. Ztschr. f. Hyg. u. Infectionskrh., 1893, 13, p. 357.
3. Walker, J. E.: Infect. Dis., 1928, LATER
4. Am. J. Hyg., 1927, 7, p. 110.

inoculated between this date and March 10, 1928. The results of nasal cultures following inoculation are shown in the table.

Rabbits 1 to 6 were inoculated within a period of 2 months after the initial isolation of the organism. In these 6 animals, implantation of the organism on the mucous membrane occurred. The organism was recovered by culture for a period of at least 4 days, and in one instance for as long as 15 days. The plates presented a very striking appearance, usually being crowded with several thousand colonies of Pfeiffer's bacillus to the almost total exclusion of other bacteria. When the organism disappeared, it was replaced either by gram-negative cocci or B. bronchisepticus, or by a mixture of these two organisms. The disappearance of Pfeiffer's bacillus was always sudden and complete, and seemed to be by a sort of crisis as indicated by the cultures.

NASAL CULTURES ON RABBITS FOLLOWING INTRANASAL INOCULATION WITH PFEIFFER'S BACILLUS

Number of Rabbit	Date of Inoculation	Days after Inoculation					
		2	4	6	9	12	15
1	Oct. 15	+	+++	+++	+++	0	0
2	Oct. 18	+++	+++	0	0	0	—
3	Oct. 27	+++	+++	+++	++	+++	+++
4	Nov. 24	++	+++	0	0	—	—
5	Nov. 30	+	+++	+++	+++	0	0
6	Dec. 10	+++	++	0	0	—	—
7	Jan. 9	0	0	0	—	—	—
8	Jan. 13	+	0	0	—	—	—
9	Jan. 20	+	0	0	—	—	—
10	Jan. 31	0	0	0	—	—	—
11	Feb. 29	0	0	0	—	—	—
12	Mar. 5	0	0	0	—	—	—
13	Mar. 10	0	0	0	—	—	—

The + signs refer to the relative abundance of Pfeiffer's bacilli as compared to other organisms, +++ signifying the complete or almost complete exclusion of other organisms. 0, Pfeiffer's bacilli absent. —, no culture made.

In rabbits 1 and 5 the first cultures after inoculation showed only a few colonies of Pfeiffer's bacillus, so few that they would have been overlooked except on very careful examination of the plates. Subsequent cultures showed an enormous increase in the number of Pfeiffer bacilli. The course in these two animals is analogous to observations made in the human infection, to which reference has already been made. In the human case, culture at the time of the first symptoms (1 day after inoculation) failed to show any Pfeiffer bacilli. Later cultures showed Pfeiffer's bacillus in preponderating numbers, exactly as in these two rabbits. The observation is believed to be of some importance in demonstrating that early cultures in respiratory infections may fail to reveal the causative organism. The causative organism may appear in later cultures under conditions that might lead one to consider it merely a secondary invader, while another agent, such as filtrable virus, is postulated as the primary cause of the disease.

All organisms recovered from the rabbits which gave the cultural reactions of Pfeiffer's bacillus were agglutinated by an antiserum to its full titer, namely, 1 : 1,280. There was no evidence of antigenic change, even in the strain recovered from rabbit 3 fifteen days after inoculation.

Symptoms.—None of the animals inoculated showed any fever. Blood cultures on several of them at intervals of from 1 to 4 days after inoculation were also negative. Two of the animals showed a serous nasal discharge: rabbit 3 between the 12th and 15th days, and rabbit 5 between the 6th and 9th days. The discharge was fairly profuse, and at times was slightly purulent. Nasal cultures during the period of the discharge showed Pfeiffer's bacilli in enormous numbers to the almost complete exclusion of other organisms. The symptoms in the human infection were rhinitis, conjunctivitis and bronchitis. The nasal discharge in these two rabbits corresponds with the human symptoms about as well as could be expected when the great dissimilarity in the two species is considered. The other rabbits showed no evidence of nasal discharge, even when Pfeiffer's bacilli were present in pure culture.

Immunity to Reinoculation.—Attempts to re-infect rabbits 1, 2 and 3, after nasal cultures on them had become negative for Pfeiffer bacilli, were unsuccessful. These experiments were carried out at the same time and with the same cultures used in inoculating animals 4, 5 and 6, the latter animals serving as controls of the ability of the organisms to infect normal animals. It was not possible to determine the duration of this resistance to further inoculation since the strain soon lost its power to attack even normal rabbits. Nor was it possible to determine whether this immunity extended against other strains of Pfeiffer's bacillus since no other strain of Pfeiffer's bacillus with this ability of attacking rabbits was available.

Agglutination Reactions.—Five of the first 6 animals inoculated were followed for the development of agglutinins. Before inoculation the serum of all 5 failed to agglutinate the organism in 1 :10 dilution. One week after inoculation agglutinins were demonstrable, the titer of the serum ranging 1 : 10 to 1 : 40. The titer increased to at least 1 : 80, and in one animal to 1 : 320 between the second and fourth weeks. Agglutinins were still present at the end of the seventh week. The two animals which showed nasal discharges did not show significantly higher agglutination than the other animals. The serum of the animals failed to agglutinate two other strains of Pfeiffer's bacillus.

The ease of the demonstration of agglutinins in the rabbits contrasts with the results obtained in the accidental human infection. In the latter, no agglutinins were demonstrable.

Skin Reactions.—An attempt was made to determine whether the nasal infection in the rabbits brought any change in the reaction to injection of products of the Pfeiffer's bacillus. For this purpose 0.1 cc. of a 7-day chocolate broth filtrate was injected intradermally. In normal animals this produced red areas about 1 cm. in diameter after 24 hours. Two of the 6 animals that had had nasal infections showed only this reaction. In the other 4, however, the red area was definitely larger, and was accompanied by edema extending over an area of 2 to 3 cm. in diameter. The results are considered as suggesting the development of an altered reaction to Pfeiffer's bacillus as a result of the infection. It is possible that the results would have been more definite if a stronger test solution, corresponding in strength perhaps to the pneumococcus autolysates of Zinsser and Grinnell [5] had been available. This feature of the work was interrupted by the loss of virulence on the part of the organism.

Loss of Virulence.—It is apparent from the table that after the organism had been cultivated for a period of about 3 months on artificial medium, it failed to attack rabbits (rabbit 7 and subsequent animals). While this change in the character of the organism interfered with what had been planned to be a much more thorough study of experimental Pfeiffer bacillus infections, it nevertheless adds stronger emphasis to the positive results obtained immediately after the organism was isolated. Retrospectively it seems probable that the invasiveness of the organism could have been maintained, and possibly increased, if the animals had been inoculated with strains obtained from the immediately preceding animal.

From the fact that the organism lost its invasiveness, it is obvious that all strains of Pfeiffer's bacillus will not attack the mucous membrane of the rabbit. Two other strains, one from bronchopneumonia and one from meningitis, failed to do so. The meningitis strain was a month old when tested. It is probable that loss of virulence may occur even when the organism is growing in or on animal tissues.

5. J. Bact., 1927, 14, p. 301.

The reverse change, namely, the acquisition of virulence by an avirulent strain has already been demonstrated by Blake and Cecil.[6]

DISCUSSION

With the exception of the lack of febrile response, there are points of resemblance between the results with rabbits and the results obtained by Blake and Cecil [6] with Pfeiffer's bacillus in monkeys. This work with animals and the now considerable number of accidental and experimental infections with the organism in human beings all demonstrate the ability of some strains of Pfeiffer's bacillus to produce primary respiratory infections of the cold-influenza type.

The rabbit experiments explain to some extent the failures to produce disease in human being through experimental inoculations with the organisms. These failures are apparently due to either one, or to a combination of two factors: immunity produced by a previous infection with the organism, and the use of an avirulent strain.

Whether the diseases produced correspond to epidemic influenza is difficult to answer, especially since epidemic influenza is a very protean disease in its clinical manifestations. Clinical and epidemiological observations lead one to suspect that its causative agent (a single causative agent being postulated) is subject to wide fluctuations in virulence and invasiveness, connected with similar wide fluctuations in the resistance of the host population. It seems to me that Pfeiffer's bacillus answers these requirements far better than any organism that has yet been described.

The serologic heterogeneity of the organisms as recovered from human beings is often considered as evidence that Pfeiffer's bacillus cannot be concerned with the etiology of epidemic influenza, despite the widespread prevalence of the organisms in the disease. But this heterogeneity is so marked that logical considerations lead one to believe that the strains must be related genetically. It is merely a question as to how rapidly the serologic changes take place. Although in my own work no serologic changes have been observed I am impressed with the reports of other authors, notably Fenyvessy and Kopp,[7] who have reported such changes.

SUMMARY

Following the intranasal inoculation of rabbits with a recently isolated strain of Pfeiffer's bacillus, it was possible to recover the organ-

6. J. Exper. Med., 1920, 32, p. 691.
7. Centralbl. f. Bakteriol., O. 1, 1928, 98, p. 477.

ism from the nasal cavities of the animals for periods of from 4 to 15 days. Two animals so inoculated showed a nasal discharge at the time when the organisms were most numerous. The inoculation was followed by the appearance of agglutinins in the blood stream. Animals once infected were immune to reinfection. After two months cultivation, the strain lost its ability to attack the nasal mucous membrane of rabbits. Two other strains of Pfeiffer's bacillus were tested and were found to be unable to produce infection. Failure to produce disease with Pfeiffer's bacillus is demonstrated experimentally to be due either to immunity of the host as a result of previous infection or to lack of virulence on the part of the organism.

The fluctuations in the virulence of the organism and in the resistance of the host fit in well with what would be expected of the etiological agent of epidemic influenza. These facts, together with the now well substantiated ability of the organism to produce primary respiratory disease of the cold-influenza type, are believed to relate Pfeiffer's bacillus to the etiology of epidemic influenza more closely than ever.

MICROORGANISMS OF LUNG ABSCESS AND BRONCHIECTASIS

Lucille H. Ermatinger

From the Department of Bacteriology and Public Health, Washington University School of Medicine, and Barnes Hospital, St. Louis, Missouri

Chronic and acute infections of the lung, other than pneumonia and tuberculosis, have assumed an important place in the field of medicine in the past few years. The recent literature abounds with many methods of treatment for these conditions, which are both medical and surgical, together with many case reports and statistical studies; but very little work has been devoted to the study of the microorganisms which invade these lesions, and which even may be the causative factor. The direct object of this study is to record and describe the microorganisms found in the sputum, pus and pathologic tissues from patients suffering with lung abscess and bronchiectasis. The patients were selected from the chest service of J. J. Singer and E. A. Graham at the Barnes Hospital.

Discussion has arisen as to the sterility of normal lungs during life. Many believe the lungs to be sterile normally, while others have demonstrated the presence of bacteria in the lungs of healthy men and animals. Jones [1] and others demonstrated bacteria in a large number of laboratory animals. These were chiefly saprophytes, probably inhaled with contaminated air or dust. The cilia and other protective factors conceivably may be inhibited by cold and other environmental conditions, and this may be a potent factor in the establishment of infection in the respiratory tract. Stillman [2] demonstrated that organisms may pass through the upper respiratory tract to the lower portion of the lungs by droplet infection. After spraying white mice broth cultures of pneumococcus, hemolytic streptococcus, staphylococcus and other bacteria, these organisms were recovered from the lower lobes of the lungs. Spand [3] believes that in many cases of lung suppuration lowered resistance gives the organisms already present, an opportunity to become pathogenic. Thus, the occurrence of "primary abscess," and the great variety of organisms in many suppurations may be accounted for.

Received for publication, May 13, 1928.

1. J. Exper. Med., 1922, 36, p. 317.
2. Ibid., 1923, 38, p. 117.
3. Am. J. Dis. Children, 1925, 29, p. 621.

Compared to abscesses in other organs, there are two significant facts concerning pulmonary abscess; first, that it has a marked tendency to be multilocular; secondly, that the abscess may have an external path of drainage by way of the bronchial tree. As in any infectious process, when the microorganisms have reached the tissues outside the bronchial tree and found conditions favorable for their growth the usual phenomena of inflammation follow.

EXPERIMENTAL WORK

Procedure.—Repeated bacteriological sputum collections were made routinely on all cases here recorded, and direct wound cultures were taken in all cases involving operation. In cases of thoracentesis, aspirating fluids were also examined. Nearly always the sputum was collected at the time of postural drainage, the specimen being collected in a sterile container towards the end of the treatment. This procedure was followed in order that there would be fewer contaminating mouth organisms, and that we could be sure that the material came directly from the lesion.

As a matter of routine, two smears of the fresh material were made on all specimens; one was stained by Gram's method, to determine the type of bacteria, and the other was stained with gentian violet or by Fontana's method, to determine the presence of spirochetes. Before culturing the specimen, it was examined macroscopically; the color, odor and consistency being recorded. A part of the sputum, that of thick tenacious purulent consistency, was placed in sterile physiologic salt solution and washed. Particles of this were then cultured both aerobically and anaerobically on 5% rabbit blood agar plates. The aerobic plates were incubated for 24 hours, and the anaerobic plates for 48 hours, before examination. For anaerobic cultures, two methods were used, Wright's pyrogallic method and phosphorus jar method, described by Varney.[4] After the plates were incubated the proper length of time, they were examined macroscopically for various individual colonies. Gram stains were made from each colony and the morphological characteristics of each variety recorded. To complete the identification of the various strains, soft agar medium containing an indicator and dextrose, lactose, sucrose and mannitol were inoculated, and their fermentation reactions noted. Other mediums such as Sabouraud's, ascitic fluid broth, horse serum, and gelatin, were used when the occasion demanded. Each colony found on the anaerobic plates was recultured aerobically to differentiate the facultative aerobes from the true anaerobic microbes. Further methods such as, bile solubility for pneumococcus, capsule stains, motility, etc., were used to help establish the identity of some individual or atypical organisms. All material was stained to determine the presence of tubercle bacilli by the Ziehl-Neilson method, or other methods to determine acidfast organisms. Tuberculous cases were excluded from this report.

The bacteriology of lung abscess and bronchiectasis is that of a very mixed group of pyogenic organisms. Morphologically and culturally, these organisms are similar to those found about normal and diseased teeth, and tonsils. It seems reasonable to assume, however, that when

4. J. Lab. & Clin. Med., 1927, 11, p. 1183.

the same microscopic picture is present from the same individual over a long period of time and upon repeated examinations, that the bacteria present have some relation to the clinical findings.

In very foul and gangrenous lesions, the flora consists of putrefactive organisms associated with pyogenic bacteria. Lambert and Miller [5] report from the study of the microorganisms, obtained directly from the wound, in ten cases of lung abscess, that anerobic organisms predominated. From our study of 16 cases, it was noticed that many organisms, such as, hemolytic streptococcus, pneumococcus, and B. mucosus-capsulatus, were facultative anaerobes; growing very little or some times not at all aerobically, on first culture. On further transplanting these cultures, the organisms would almost invariably grow aerobically as well as anaerobically. This was especially true of direct cultures from the wound. This peculiarity might be explained by the fact that in the necrotic mass in the abscess cavity, the oxygen supply is limited, and partial anaerobiasis results.

1. LUNG ABSCESS

Predisposing Factor	Microorganisms
Pneumonia	B. xerosis, Micrococcus catarrhalis, Pneumococcus, Staphylococcus aureus, Hemolytic streptococcus, bacillus (?)
Postoperative (cholecystectomy)	B. xerosis, Hemolytic streptococcus, Yeast, Micrococcus catarrhalis
Tonsillectomy	Hemolytic streptococcus, Staphylococcus aureus, Micrococcus catarrhalis
Foreign body (cockle burr)	Staphylococcus aureus, B. mucosus-capsulatus
Syphilis (gumma)	Staphylococcus aureus, B. xerosis
Tonsillectomy	Hemolytic streptococcus, B. xerosis, Micrococcus catarrhalis
Tonsillectomy	Hemolytic streptococcus, Pneumococci, Micrococcus catarrhalis, Fusiform bacillus
Tonsillectomy	Staphylococcus aureus, Micrococcus catarrhalis
Diabetes	Staphylococcus aureus, Hemolytic streptococcus, Pneumococcus
Pneumonia	Staphylococcus aureus, Hemolytic streptococcus, Micrococcus catarrhalis
Postoperative (cholecystectomy and appendectomy)	Hemolytic streptococcus, Staphylococcus aureus, B. xerosis, B. proteus, fusiform bacilli, Micrococcus catarrhalis, Staphylococcus albus
Pneumonia	Staphylococcus aureus, Hemolytic streptococcus, Micrococcus catarrhalis
Postoperative (cholecystectomy)	Staphylococcus aureus, B. mucosus-capsulatus, Micrococcus catarrhalis
Pneumonia	Staphylococcus aureus, B. xerosis
Pneumonia	Staphylococcus aureus, Hemolytic streptococcus, B. xerosis, B. mucosus capsulatus, Micrococcus catarrhalis
Postabortive (embolic)	Staphylococcus aureus, Staphylococcus albus, Hemolytic streptococcus, Micrococcus catarrhalis, Bacillus (?)

Tabulation 1 records the type of organism found in repeated cultures from the 16 cases of lung abscesses studied.

5. Arch. Surg., 1924, 8, p. 446.

In lung abscesses hemolytic staphylococcus aureus is the pyogenic organism most frequently found. In this series it was found in 80.75% of the cases. The percentage of incidence of other organisms is as follows: hemolytic streptococci 68.75%; Micrococcus catarrhalis 63.5%; bacillus Xerosis 43.75%; Pneumococcus 18.25% (type 4 most commonly found); Mucosus capsulatus 18.25%; fusiform bacilli 18.25% and Staphylococcus aureus 18.25%. This high percentage of incidence of staphylococcus aureus in lung abscess is in agreement with the findings of Hartwell.[6]

Tabulation 2 brings out the relations of the same factors as they occur in the condition of bronchiectatic abscesses. In this type of abscess hemolytic Staphylococcus aureus is found in 85.8% of the seven cases; Micrococcus catarrhalis 85.8%; hemolytic streptococcus 57.2%; B. mucosus-capsulatus 42.9%; and Streptococcus viridans 14.3%.

2. Bronchiectatic Abscess

Predisposing Factor	Microorganisms
Pertussis and measles	Staphylococcus aureus, Streptococcus viridans, Micrococcus catarrhalis
Foreign body (blade of grass)	Staphylococcus aureus, Hemolytic streptococcus, Micrococcus catarrhalis
Pneumonia	Staphylococcus aureus, B. xerosis, Micrococcus catarrhalis
Foreign body (broncholithiasis)	Hemolytic streptococcus, B. mucosus-capsulatus
Tonsillectomy	Staphylococcus aureus, Hemolytic streptococcus, Micrococcus catarrhalis
Postoperative (gastro-enterostomy)	Staphylococcus aureus, B. mucosus-capsulatus, Micrococcus catarrhalis
Pneumonia	Staphylococcus aureus, Hemolytic streptococcus, B. mucosus-capsulatus, Micrococcus catarrhalis

Tabulation 3 indicates the relations of the foregoing factors in the condition of bronchiectasis. Thus in bronchiectasis, Staphylococcus aureus was found in 60% of the cases; Micrococcus catarrhalis 90%; hemolytic Streptococcus 40%; B. mucosus-capsulatus 40%; Bacillus xerosis 30%; fusiform bacillus 10% and Pneumococcus 40%.

In addition to the organisms given in the foregoing tables, the sputum cultures often contained many saprophytes, such as yeast, spore formers, spirilla, etc. These organisms were not recorded. When sputum and wound cultures were both obtained, the wound organisms were compared with those found in the sputum. Both were usually found to contain the same organisms.

An unusual organism was isolated from lung abscess cases 1 and 16. The pus was obtained from the wound in each case. This organism

6. Ann. Surg., 1920, 72, p. 333.

grew rapidly on ordinary medium and had a tendency to spread, not evenly as Proteus but resembling more the frost on a window pane. The surface of the growth was dry, rather hard and somewhat waxy in appearance. The organism was a small thick bacillus, discolored by Gram's stain, nonacidfast, noncapsulated with a tendency towards bipolar staining. It fermented none of the ordinary sugars nor did it liquefy gelatin. On medium containing blood, methemoglobin was produced to a marked degree, giving the growth a greenish brown appearance.

An organism which was exceptionally large was found in the wound culture from the bronchiectatic abscess of case one. This organism was a gram-negative diplococcus with a very large capsule. It grew in symbiosis with Staphylococcus aureus, Streptococcus viridans and Micrococcus catarrhalis on original culture, but repeated attempts to isolate it were unsuccessful.

3. BRONCHIECTASIS

Predisposing Factor	Microorganisms
Foreign body (broncholithiasis)	Staphylococcus aureus, Micrococcus catarrhalis, B. mucosus-capsulatus
Influenza	Staphylococcus aureus, Hemolytic streptococcus, Micrococcus catarrhalis
Pneumonia	Staphylococcus aureus, Pneumococcus, Micrococcus catarrhalis, B. mucosus-capsulatus, B. xerosis
Influenza	Streptococcus viridans, Pneumococcus, Micrococcus catarrhalis
Pertussis and measles	Hemolytic streptococcus, Micrococcus catarrhalis, B. xerosis
Pneumonia	Hemolytic streptococcus, Micrococcus catarrhalis, Staphylococcus aureus
Bronchitis	Streptococcus viridans, Pneumococcus, Micrococcus catarrhalis
Pertussis and measles	Hemolytic streptococcus, B. mucosus-capsulatus
Pertussis and measles	Hemolytic streptococcus, B. mucosus-capsulatus, B. xerosis, Micrococcus catarrhalis, fusiform bacillus
Pertussis	Staphylococcus aureus, B. mucosus-capsulatus, Micrococcus catarrhalis
Tonsillectomy	Staphylococcus aureus, Pneumococcus

At the time that this work was done the importance of immediate staining for spirochetes was not realized. And because of this, although we found spirochetes in some of the cases, I have limited this report to the bacterial findings with the exception of case 11. The bacteriology of this case is given in detail, because of the unusual clinical features, the great variety of organisms found and the opportunity it afforded to study spirochetes recovered directly from the lung lesion.

This patient's symptoms began with a cold and cough. A cholecystectomy and appendectomy were performed (not at the Barnes Hospital), after which the cough became worse. At this time physical examination revealed a lung abscess in the base of the right lung. Several months later the cautery pneumectomy operation was performed,[7] and the patient's condition improved. Several months after leaving the hospital the patient returned in very serious condition with another abscess on the left side. Surgical drainage was established, this time in the left upper lobe. Eventually the left wound entirely healed, but a bronchial fistula continued to drain dark grayish-green foul smelling pus from the right lower lesion. This exudate, obtained directly from the right bronchial fistula, was extremely fetid and contained mucus, some fibrous tissue, epithelial cells and pus cells, and many large masses of bacteria and spirochetes. The material obtained from the left wound contained similar organisms, although they were fewer in number and the exudate was more purulent. By a Gram's stain of this material, the following could be demonstrated: gram-negative fusiform-bacilli, diplococci, spirilla, and short straight bacilli; gram-positive cocci, diplococci, cocci in long and short chains, bacilli and a very thick mycelial-like organism occurring in wavy matted masses.

The various organisms were very difficult to isolate in pure culture from the pus obtained from this patient's lung, due to the presence of a proteus-like organism which grew very rapidly and covered the entire plate. This particular bacillus proteus was atypical in its fermentation reactions, producing acid and gas in mediums containing dextrose with no fermentation reaction in the other common sugars. The pure cultures of this proteus had a foul odor, resembling somewhat the odor of the patient's wound and sputum. In an attempt to correct this foul odor, an autogenous proteus vaccine was prepared and given subcutaneously each week to the patient in increasing doses, for nearly three months. This had no apparent effect on the odor. The vaccine therapy was then discontinued.

A Fontana's stain of the exudate revealed a large variety of spirochetes, averaging between fifteen and twenty to a field. These spirochetes varied in length from 4 to 25 microns, and the number of spirals from 2 to 18. Some had even, closely coiled, spirals, while others had coarse and irregular ones. On dark field examination the movements were variable. Some were jerky and moved rapidly, others had slow snake-like movements.

To culture the spirochetes a medium of horse serum diluted one to five with physiological salt solution was used. This medium was prepared each time before inoculating. The salt solution was boiled to exclude the air, cooled to about 38 C. and the horse serum added. By means of a long capillary pipet, about 0.5 cc. of diluted pus was placed at the bottom of the tube. The tubes used for these cultures were prepared according to Kendall's method; viz., a narrowing of the lumen at the center of the tube over which a glass ball is placed immediately after the inoculation of the medium. (The medium should cover the ball.) In addition to this, pyrogallic acid and potassium hydroxide (5%) were added over an absorbent cotton plug to insure as complete anaerobiasis as possible and the tube tightly closed with a rubber stopper.

In examining the cultures, smears were stained by Fontana's method. Dark field examinations were always made to determine whether or not the spirochetes were living. The inoculated medium became very cloudy on incubation, and when opened had an extremely foul odor. Cultures were examined at 24-hour intervals for 18 days. The mobility of these spirochetes ceased after 14 days' incubation. Subculturing was tried repeatedly but was successful only in the first transplant from a young culture. This subculture showed actively motile spirochetes after 24 and 48 hours' incubation, respectively; but after 72 hours a tangling and matting together of the spirochetes resulted, with very little, if any, motility.

7. Graham, E. A.: Arch. Surg., 1925, 10, p. 392; J. Am. M. A., 1925, 85, p. 181.

The spirochetes in these cultures were morphologically quite constant. The great variety of forms noticed among the spirochetes in the material directly from the wound, was not present. It is probable that only one of the apparently many types present survived in the culture. This spirochete averaged about 9.5 microns in length and .65 microns in width. The spirals were even, close together, and fairly rigid, six being the average number present. It had a characteristic free-swimming movement on dark field examination. It moved moderately fast with a corkscrew-like motion and had an occasional semicircular bending of one or both ends. In old cultures where tangling had taken place, frequently one very active spirochete could be seen, apparently trying to become free from the others. In this case, the spirochete would exhibit very jerky movements, and tow the entire mass over many microscopic fields.

To classify this spirochete would be very difficult. It could not be obtained in pure culture because of the many accompanying bacteria. The pathogenicity, therefore, could not be determined. Morphologically, a marked difference can be seen between the spirochetes of the mouth origin, Spirocheta vincenti and those of the culture. According to Noguchi's classification [8] the bending of the ends, in the free-swimming spirochetes, would place them in the Leptospira group.

After a course of three injections of arsphenamine the number of these spirochetes so greatly diminished that they could be found only with great difficulty. Some months later, however, they were again abundant; and another series of injections of arsphenamine was followed by no noticeable diminution in their number. As a rule, pulmonary spirochetes can be made to disappear by injections of arsphenamine. For example, Kline and Berger [9] have recently reported gratifying results in 11 of 16 cases of spirochetal pulmonary gangrene treated with arsphenamine.

The fact that the predominating organisms in all of these cases has been Staphylococcus aureus (75% of cases), might be considered to lend some support to the idea that most pulmonary abscesses are embolic in origin rather than due to inhalation, and that in this respect they are analagous to abscesses of the bones. But nevertheless too much weight cannot be placed on such evidence. Holman [10] has recently reported his important experiments in which he was unable to produce lung abscess by the placing of infected foreign bodies in a bronchus but was able frequently to produce them by injecting infected emboli into a systemic

8. J. Exper. Med., 1918, 27, p. 575.
9. J. Am. M. A., 1925, 85, p. 1452.
10. Ann. Surg., 1926, 86, p. 240.

vein. More recently, however, Crowe, Allen [11] and others have shown conclusively that lung abscess can be produced experimentally by inhalation.

SUMMARY

The bacteriological examinations in 33 cases of chronic and acute lung abscess and bronchiectasis disclosed the pyogenic organism Staphylococcus aureus in 75.40% of the total number of cases, hemolytic streptococci in 55.30% and pneumococci in 19.40%. A spirochete, apparently falling into the Leptospira group, according to Noguchi's classification, was obtained from the case reported and was kept alive, in a mixed culture containing bacteria, for a period of 14 days.

11. Arch. Surg., 1928, 16, p. 179.

ABSENCE OF INFECTIVITY IN FILTERED URINE FROM DIABETIC PATIENTS

G. Harold Ettinger and Guilford B. Reed

From the Laboratories of Physiology and Bacteriology, Queen's University, Kingston, Ontario

Among the many theories as to the causation of diabetes mellitus, one attributes the condition to infection. While no specific organism has been cited, many clinicians have pointed out the frequency of its association with known infections as appendicitis, tonsillitis, pancreatitis, cholecystitis, arthritis, malaria, influenza, syphilis, typhoid, etc. Gundersen [1] describes a wave of diabetes in young people following an epidemic of parotitis which occurred three or four years previously. He suggests that the two have the same etiological virus, which may cause an immediately fatal pancreatitis, or structural changes manifest later on as a diabetes. Labbé and Debre [2] describe a case in the latter group who responded favorably to dietetic treatment. Patrick [3] describes a case in which a girl of eight years died in diabetic coma three weeks after contracting mumps. Barach,[4] on the other hand, in considering the previous illnesses of a group of 226 diabetics, finds a history of parotitis in very few cases, the most frequent previous infections being tonsillitis and typhoid. McLean [5] suggests that the onset of diabetes as a result of acute infection is due to a defect in the pancreas which is not revealed before this unusual strain.

Attempts have been made to produce a diabetic condition in animals by injections of bacteria known to cause infections with which diabetes is associated. Ricen,[6] by intravenous injection of Streptococcus hemolyticus and B. typhosus, produced inflammation of the gallbladder, liver and pancreas, with hyperglycemia and lowered sugar tolerance. Menten and Manning [7] and also Zeckwer and Goodell [8] injected other types of bacteria and demonstrated a hyperglycemia. Levine and Kolars [9]

Received for publication, May 28, 1928.

1. J. Infect. Dis., 1927, 41, p. 197.
2. Bull. et Mém. Soc. méd. d'Hôp. de Paris, 1921, 45, p. 1306.
3. Brit. M. J., 1924, 2, p. 802.
4. Arch. Int. Med., 1927, 39, p. 636.
5. Medical Annual, 1927, p. 106.
6. Northwest Med., 1926, 25, p. 191.
7. J. Infect. Dis., 1925, 37, p. 400.
8. J. Exper. Med., 1925, 42, p. 43.
9. Proc. Soc. Exper. Biol. & Med., 1926, 24, p. 36.

injected dead bacteria of various types intraperitoneally. They report three groups of bacteria which increase blood sugar, do not affect it, or depress the blood sugar, over a period of three hours. No report of late effects is given.

Recently Bergey,[10] acting on the assumption that the disease might be caused by a filtrable virus to which the kidney might be permeable, attempted to infect rabbits with the urine of diabetic patients, by intravenous injection. He reports positive results under the following conditions:

The fresh Berkefeld-filtered urine caused a glycosuria of an irregular periodicity in from 22 to 42 days. Two rabbits developed coma in 38 days, were killed and their urine showed a slight reaction with Benedict's. Filtered diabetic urine, cultured under aerobic conditions in serum broth for 56 days caused a glycosuria in 7 to 8 days. Anaerobic cultures caused a glycosuria in 16 days. Urine from an infected rabbit caused a glycosuria 7 days after inoculation. Filtered urine, placed in sterile ampules and kept for 9 months, caused a glycosuria in 7 to 11 days. This was irregular in its occurrence. These results of Bergey's are based on experiments with some 12 rabbits and the urine from two patients, whose history is not indicated. None of the rabbits at necropsy showed any striking changes in the pancreas. A diabetic condition was judged to be determinable by daily analysis of urine using Benedict's quantitative reagent. No blood sugar estimations were made. Bergey concludes that his experiments suggest that "Diabetes Mellitus is caused by a filtrable virus, that the disease can be transmitted to rabbits by intravenous administration of a single dose of 2 cc. of the urine of diabetic patients, passed through Berkefeld filters to remove bacteria; that the filtered urine of diabetic patients contains an ultravisible organism which multiplies in serum broth medium."

An attempt has been made to carry out a similar series of experiments using what is believed to be greater care in estimating pancreatic damage, viz., frequent and regular blood sugar estimations, combined with daily urinalysis. Eight diabetic patients were selected, ranging from a child to men and women of middle age with variable histories. Berkefeld-filtered urine and cultures of urine from the patients were inoculated into fourteen rabbits and seven dogs. Since all results were negative, it was not thought worth while to try urine kept in sterile ampules for months, and for the same reason no use was made of urine from the animals used in the experiments.

The urine was injected fresh from the patients, except in three cases in which a 12 to 24 hour interval elapsed between the time of collection and that of inoculation. Rabbits were given doses of 3 to 10 cc. Doses proportionate to body weight were given to dogs. Bergey's rabbits were given 2 cc. Control animals were given normal human urine.

10. Proc. Soc. Exper. Biol. & Med., 1926, 24, p. 229.

Cultures were made in 10% dog or rabbit serum in fresh beef infusion broth. Aerobic cultures consisted in shallow layers of the medium inoculated with 1% of Berkefeld filtrate of the urine. For the anaerobic cultures the broth was placed in deep narrow tubes, boiled, serum added and covered with an oil seal. In part of the series a piece of sterile rabbit kidney was also added. In both cases the tubes were incubated for two to three days and then inoculated near the bottom with 1% of the urine filtrate. The cultures were incubated at 37 C. for 25 to 63 days and injected into rabbits in 1 to 7 cc. amounts, and into dogs in amounts proportionate to body weight. Bergey's cultures were incubated for 56 days and administered to rabbits in 0.1 cc. amounts.

By Benedict's qualitative method, daily analysis was made of 24-hour specimens of the rabbit urine for periods extending over 3 to 10 weeks, in every case for a longer time than Bergey found necessary for the infection to be demonstrated. The morning urine was examined in the case of the dogs, since these were confined in cages for most of the day, where they retained their urine until allowed out in the morning. This amounted practically to a 12 to 20-hour specimen. Blood sugar analyses were made regularly at intervals of from a day to a week by the Schaffer-Hartmann method. The blood was drawn in the morning before the animals were fed, and so the sugar should represent the fasting level.

RESULTS

Fresh Filtered Urine.—Urine was obtained from 7 patients whose ages ranged from 12 to 64 years, and whose diabetic symptoms prior to the experiment ran from 3 weeks to 9 months. Three dogs and 7 rabbits were inoculated. Control animals were given normal urine. No change was observed in the blood sugar over periods of from 55 to 236 days. Sugar was never demonstrated in the urine of the dogs. Traces of reducing substances were detected irregularly in the urine from the control and three of the experimental rabbits but never in amounts measurable by Benedict's quantitative method.

Anaerobic Cultures of Urine.—Urine supplied by five patients was cultured for 25, 42, 50 and 62 days, and the cultures injected into 3 dogs and 6 rabbits. There was no change in the blood sugar over periods of from 21 to 63 days. Sugar was never demonstrated in the urine of the dogs. Traces of reducing substances were found occasionally in the urine from two of the rabbits.

Aerobic Cultures of Urine.—Urine supplied by one patient and cultured for 42 days was injected into one dog and one rabbit. There was no change in blood sugar over a period of 21 days. The urine of the dog was negative to Benedict's test, the urine of the rabbit showed traces of reducing substances on three occasions only.

Rabbit urine occasionally reduced Benedict's qualitative reagent, but in no case was the reduction sufficient to be estimated quantitatively by Benedict's method, and the reduction was hardly in excess of that caused by the urine from the control rabbit. It is possible that this reduction was caused by activity or excretions of mice, who wandered freely at night through the cages of the confined rabbits. In confirmation of this, washings from the floors of empty cages which contained remnants of food to which mice for a month had access, and from cages in which mice had previously been housed, reduced Benedict's qualitative reagent in about the proportion noticed with the rabbit urine. Additional reducing substances might accumulate through diastatic fermentation of grain in the wet cages.

SUMMARY

Fresh urine from diabetic patients, filtered (Berkefeld) and injected into 14 rabbits and 7 dogs, caused no appreciable change in the blood sugar percentage over periods of 55 to 236 days. Aerobic and anaerobic cultures had similar negative results during periods up to 63 days. Small amounts of reducing substances were found occasionally in the urine of some of the rabbits, but not in excess of amounts found in the control animals, and there was never any suggestion of interference with carbohydrate metabolism.

The urine was obtained from eight diabetic patients, ranging in age from 12 to 55 years and with histories of diabetes from 3 weeks to 15 months. It may be presumed that if the urine of a diabetic patient contains a causal organism it would be present within this period. The conclusion is that the filtered urine of a diabetic patient contains no organism which can reproduce the diabetic condition in dogs or rabbits.

ACTION OF BACTERIOPHAGE ON PSYCHROPHILIC ORGANISMS

A. Lawrence Elder and Fred W. Tanner

From the Department of Bacteriology, University of Illinois, Urbana

Additional species of bacteria which are susceptible to bacteriophagy are being reported from time to time, and the list at the present time appears to be far from complete. It seemed of interest, in view of the report of Koser [1] on transmissible lysis of a thermophilic bacterium to determine whether the same phenomenon would be evident in the group of psychrophilic organisms which are capable of growth at low temperatures. A preliminary communication regarding the action of the bacteriophage on psychrophiles has appeared [2] and additional data will be presented here.

The cultures selected for investigation were originally isolated from samples of diluted aerobic sewage which had been held at 2 C. for three weeks. Sixty cultures, all of which grew quite well at 4 C. but would not grow at 37 C. were included in this study. From the sixty cultures first selected six which appeared to grow more rapidly at 4 C. than any of the others were selected for bacteriophage experiments. Attempts were made to find an active lytic principle against each of these organisms by means of the method of alternate feeding and filtration. A lytic principle was obtained by incubation of a filtrate of sewage-polluted water with small amounts of the young culture 9 in broth. Beef infusion peptone broth, P_H 7.4 to 7.6, was used in all the experiments. Continued alternate feedings and filtrations failed to produce a lytic principle for any of the other five organisms.

The lytic principle for culture 9 developed rapidly. The third filtrate showed some evidence of lytic power and the sixth filtrate gave a complete clearing when a drop of the culture was brought in contact with an agar slant previously inoculated with the culture. The psychrophilic lytic principle was shown to be filtrable, produced lysis which was transmissible in series and produced plaques on agar; it therefore fulfilled the common requirements of bacteriophagy.

Received for publication, May 29, 1928.

1. J. Infect. Dis., 1927, 41, p. 365.
2. Proc. Soc. Exper. Biol. & Med., 1927, 24, p. 645.

Specificity of the Bacteriophage.—The action of the bacteriophage which produced lysis in culture 9 was tested on the other 59 stock cultures of psychrophiles. The 59 cultures were streaked on agar slants, and after growth was noticeable on the slant, one small drop of bacteriophage was allowed to run down the surface of the slant. The bacteriophage appeared to have no influence on the growth of these cultures. The same quantity of bacteriophage would have completely lysed the center of agar slant culture 9. The 59 cultures were also inoculated into tubes of broth and 1 cc. of the bacteriophage added to each. Growth appeared to be normal in every tube. 10^{-7} cc. of this bacteriophage completely cleared 48-hour broth cultures of 9. Continued alternate feeding and filtration of the 59 cultures in the presence of the bacteriophage active for culture 9 was not attempted as we were primarily interested in the immediate effects of the bacteriophage. This psychrophilic bacteriophage appears to be very specific in its action.

Microscopic Examinations.—Numerous microscopic observations were made of the effect of bacteriophage on the culture. The dark field observations correlated to some extent those reported by d'Herelle[3] in that the addition of bacteriophage caused the formation of many very large cells. Some of them were over twice the size of the normal cell. Some of the cells appeared to be lined with many small granules or nodules and many more of these nodules which appeared as pin points in the field could be noted when bacteriophage was present. Such small particles were rarely noted in normal cultures. It would appear that these small particles must be either pieces of disintegrated bacterial cells or corpuscles of bacteriophage. A lysed bacterial culture always showed numerous small particles when examined under the ultramicroscope. Although single cells in the presence of bacteriophage were followed numerous times for thirty minutes at a time, never were we able to see the actual bursting of a bacterial cell. It is possible that the higher temperature at which the dark field work was carried on completely destroyed the action of this low temperature bacteriophage.

Macroscopic Observations.—As we are not aware of any other records of bacteriophage active at a temperature as low as 2 C. on a true psychrophile it appeared advisable to keep a permanent record of the appearance of the effect of this bacteriophage on culture 9. Photographs were taken of agar slants, broth tubes and agar plates on

3. The Bacteriophage and Its Behavior, 1926.

which the action of bacteriophage was observable. Plate 1, tube 1, shows the normal culture. Tube 2 shows the effect of a drop of bacteriophage. A few resistant colonies are to be noted in the center of the tube. These resistant colonies were encountered from time to time on agar slants. Tube 3 shows an agar slant which was streaked with a dilution of 1 : 100,000 of the bacteriophage. Several plaques are to be noted in this tube. In broth tube 4 normal growth is noted, while tube 5 shows the effect after 48 hours of one loop of bacteriophage

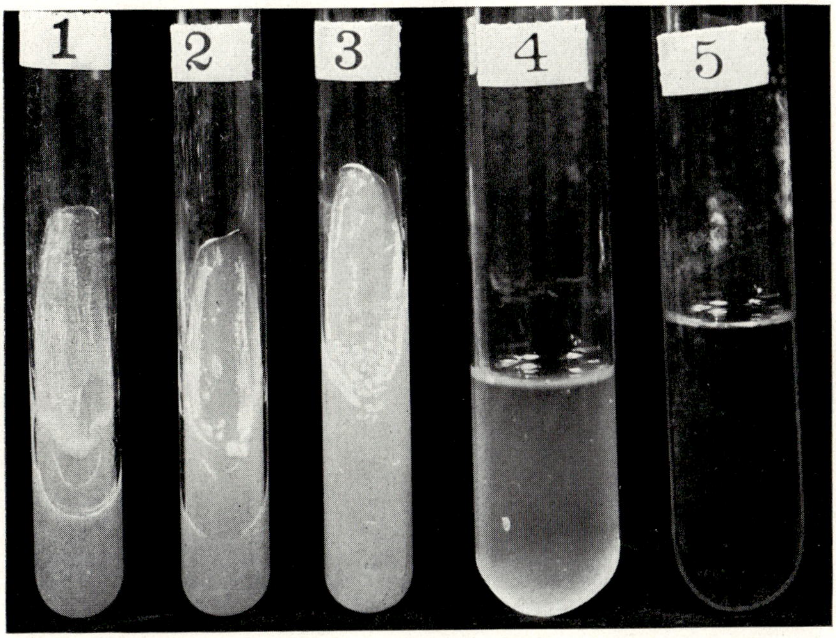

Normal cultures shown in tubes 1 and 4. Effect of bacteriophage on normal culture shown in tubes 2, 3 and 5.

to a tube of turbidity equal to that of tube 4. Photographs of agar plates were made which showed the result of varying quantities of bacteriophage. As these photographs were similar to the one shown (fig. 1) they were kept for reference and not included here.

Description of the Organism.—Although no attempt was made to completely identify the organism for which the lytic principle was obtained, some of the more prominent characteristics of the organism have been recorded. It readily fermented dextrose, lactose, sucrose and glycerol broths without production of gas. The P_H varied from less than 6 with dextrose to 7.6 with lactose. Litmus milk was turned slightly alkaline. A good top growth and some liquefaction was obtained with the gelatin stab. No nitrite was produced in nitrate broth. A floating growth was obtained with Koser's citrate medium. Lead acetate agar was slightly blackened. The organism is a short rod about 0.7 μ in diameter, not spore-forming, gram-negative, nonmotile, aerobic and non-chromogenic. The index number of the organism as determined thus far according to the 1925 descriptive chart of the Society of American Bacteriologists is 5000-u1100- 0222.

SUMMARY

A bacteriophage active for a psychrophile has been obtained. The specificity of the bacteriophage was quite pronounced as shown by the fact that it was not readily active on any of 59 other psychrophiles studied. Macroscopic observations of the lytic action confirmed all the usual characteristics of bacteriophagy.

MUCOSUS ORGANISM FROM SUPPURATIVE LESIONS OF RAT ON DIET DEFICIENT IN VITAMIN A

William L. Bradford

From the Department of Bacteriology, the University of Rochester School of Medicine and Dentistry, Rochester, N. Y.

Spontaneous infection of the upper part of the respiratory tract of the albino rat is not uncommon. In animals being used for experimental purposes, as well as among those kept in stock[1] one frequently encounters suppurative otitis media, purulent nasal sinusitis, and various types of pulmonary infections. As terminal events in the course of experimental avitaminosis in the white rat, such infections are frequent[2] and are instrumental in causing death. It is thought that deficiency of vitamin A causes such a reduction in cellular activity that it amounts to a deficiency of glandular activity[3] and that this, in turn, brings about secondary changes, bacterial invasion, and death.

Reviewing the literature, one is surprised to find that bacteriologic studies of these infections have not been extensive. For this reason, and because it was desired to find an organism in rats kept on diets deficient in vitamin A that might be suitable for use in the study of the relationship of vitamin deficiencies to infection, cultural studies of a group of animals dying from avitaminosis, were made.

Method of Culture.—By using ordinary skill one can obtain satisfactory cultures from the middle ears and the nasal turbinates of a rat by the following technique.

The lower jaw was removed with scissors and the middle ear bulbs exposed. These were seared, opened with a sterile, pointed knife, and the contents removed for cultures by means of a platinum loop. The head was then sectioned sagittally a little to one side of the midline. The nasal septum was carefully removed, and thus by sacrificing one side of the nasal cavity, the other could be exposed for the purpose of taking material for cultures. Cultures from pulmonary lesions, abscesses of the tongue and kidneys, etc., were made according to the usual post-mortem technique.

The cultures were inoculated into Douglas broth (P_H 7.4-7.6), from which blood agar plates were streaked. From these the various organisms found, were studied with a view to their identification. Anaerobic cultures were not made.

Received for publication, May 31, 1928.

1. McCordock, H. A., and Congdon, C. C.: Proc. Soc. Exper. Biol. & Med., 1924-1925, 22, p. 150.
2. Daniels, A. L.; Armstrong, M. E., and Hutton, M. K.: J. A. M. A. 1923, 81, p. 828.
3. Manville, I. A.: Arch. Int Med, 1925, 35, p 549.

THE ORGANISMS

Source.—The first group of animals studied, numbered 31. They were obtained from the Albino Supply Company, Philadelphia, and cultures were made immediately after their death from experimentally produced deficiency in vitamin A. Each animal presented marked signs of the disease. All had suppurative otitis media and purulent rhinitis. Six rats had abscesses of the kidneys. A few had abscesses of the tongue, lungs, and neck of the bladder. Cultures were taken only from the kidneys and from the ears, in this group.

In general, the organisms recovered were gram-negative. In 3 cases (all kidney cultures), Staphylococcus albus was isolated. A gram-negative, gelatin-liquefying bacillus, apparently belonging to the proteus group was found 6 times in the ears and 9 times in the kidneys. B. coli was isolated 8 times from the kidneys and twice from the ears. In 15 instances an encapsulated, gram-negative, coccoid bacillus, apparently belonging to the mucosus capsulatus group, was isolated. It was recovered twice from abscesses of the kidney and once from the lungs. In 5 cultures from the ears and in 6 from the kidneys no growth resulted. Except for 3 instances in which it was associated with the gram-negative spreader, the encapsulated coccoid bacillus was the only organism in the culture.

TABLE 1.—SHOWING THE NUMBER, SOURCE AND CONDITION OF THE RATS FROM WHICH CULTURES WERE MADE; THE OCCURRENCE OF SUPPURATION IN VARIOUS ORGANS; AND THE RELATIVE INCIDENCE OF RECOVERY OF THE ENCAPSULATED BACILLUS

			Ears		Nose		Tongue		Lungs		Kidneys	
Rats	Source	Condition	Pus	Encapsulated Bacillus	Pus	Encapsulated Bacillus	Pus	Encapsulated Bacillus	Pus	Encapsulated Bacillus	Pus	Encapsulated Bacillus
31	Albino Supply Co., Philadelphia	All animals died from vitamin A deficiency	31	12	—	—	—	—	1	1	8	2
17	Stock colony (Dept. of vital economics)	On an A-deficient diet	8	4	7	4	2	2	4	2	—	—
2	University of Iowa (Daniels)	On an A-deficient diet	2	0	1	0	0	—	1	0	0	—
13	Stock colony (Dept. of anatomy)	Normal; killed for cultures	3	0	1	0	0	—	0	—	0	—
3	Stock colony (Dept. of vital economics)	On a B-deficient diet; polyneuritic	0	0	1	0	0	—	0	—	0	—
9	Stock colony (Dept. of vital economics)	On a D-deficient diet; rachitic	3	0	0	—	0	—	0	—	0	—
10	Wild (brown) rats	Killed for cultures	0	0	0	1	0	—	0	—	0	—

Because this organism appeared in about one half of the ear cultures in this group of rats, it seemed of interest to make cultures from rats obtained from other sources and kept on various diets. Table 1 shows the relative incidence of recovery of the encapsulated organism from such animals.

Morphology and Staining.—The organism was a short, plump, pleomorphic coccoid bacillus, occurring singly and in pairs. In broth cultures longer forms were found and occasionally long threads. If these threads were stained with gentian violet they were found to be young forms in the process of division. The organism was gram-negative, nonmotile, and bore no spores. Gram stains from agar slants or from colonies revealed forms which closely resembled diplococci. Smears from young blood agar growth, from milk, and from the peritoneal fluid of an inoculated animal revealed definite capsules of moderate width. It stained well with the ordinary dyes: methylene blue, gentian violet, etc., and was not acidfast.

Cultural Characteristics.—Growth in broth (P_H 7.6) was slow during the first 6-8 hours but in 25 hours was heavy and produced a grayish white pellicle, which was broken up completely by shaking. Growth occurred in Douglas broth (P_H 5), though it was not heavy. At room temperature growth took place slowly in both Douglas broth and on plain 2% agar.

On plain 2% agar at 37.5 C. growth was profuse and mucoid in character. Under reduced oxygen tension growth occurred but was less profuse.

Colonies formed within a few hours on blood agar plates (10% rabbit's blood) and at 24 hours (37 C.) the colonies became 2-3 mm. in diameter, were round, smooth, elevated, yellowish white, and slimy. The growth resembled that of the Friedländer bacillus but was less stringy. Hemolysis occurred after 36 hours. A distinct ammoniac odor was obtained from the plate.

Gelatin (15%) was not liquefied. Along the stab-line, growth occurred, and also about the surface at the top of the stab, giving a nail-like effect.

Indol was not formed. Milk was slowly acidified (brom-cresol-purple) after 48 hours, and was coagulated after incubation at 37 C. for several days. Acid was formed slowly in 1% glucose broth (P_H 7.4). After 4 days the P_H was 5.2 and at 10 days it approached 6.8. Definite alkaline change was noted after 24 hours in mannitol, lactose, sucrose, maltose, levulose, and inulin. In lactose broth the P_H became 8.2 and after 10 days it was 8.4. No gas was formed in any of the sugars. Nitrates were not reduced. The Voges-Proskauer and methyl red reactions were negative. A strong production of ammonia was indicated qualitatively by the Nessler test. This was not determined quantitatively.

Table 2 summarizes the biochemical reactions of the organism as compared with those of other types of Friedländer bacilli. It also indicates the origin of the various strains studied.

Three strains, 6E, 48K, and 21E, were selected from the group for use as antigens in the production of agglutinating serums. After preliminary bleeding and tests for natural agglutinins, rabbits were regularly injected with killed and later with living organisms suspended in salt solutions of 24-hour old agar-slant growths. Ten days after the last injection the rabbits were bled and the serums preserved in a 0.5 per cent solution of phenol.

Against their homologous antigens the serums had the following agglutinating titers: 6E, 1:320; 48K, 1:1280; 21E, 1:1280. Agglutinating serum 6E was produced by intramuscular injections, while serums 48K and 21E were produced by the intravenous method.

The agglutination antigens were produced by suspending 24-hour agar-slant growths in salt solution, and were adjusted to a turbidity comparable to 4.5 on the McFarland nephelometer. The agglutinating serums were diluted in normal salt solution in proportions ranging from 1:10 to 1:2560. Controls in normal rabbit serum and in normal salt solution were had in each case. The tests were incubated 2 hours in the water bath at 55 C. The agglutinations were sharp, the clumped organisms forming a compact mass in the bottom of the tube with clear fluid above. Prozone reactions did not occur. Table 3 gives the results of the agglutination tests of the 3 serums against heterologous strains of the rat organism and also against other types of Friedländer-like bacilli.

TABLE 2.—ORIGIN OF STRAINS AND THEIR BIOCHEMICAL REACTIONS

Strains	Origin	Glucose	Mannitol	Lactose	Sucrose	Milk	Gelatin	Indol	Nitrate Reduction
6E, 21E, 43E, 39E, 46E, 13E, 37E, 29E, RGE, 47E, 4E, 27E, 23E	Isolated from middle ear exudate of vitamin-A-deficient rats	+	0	0	0	ca	0	0	0
48K, 36K	From kidney abscesses of A-deficient rats	+	0	0	0	ca	0	0	0
48L, RCL	From lung abscesses of A-deficient rats	+	0	0	0	ca	0	0	0
190N, 168N, 161N, RAN	From nasal exudate of A-deficient rats	+	0	0	0	ca	0	0	0
10WN	From nose of wild rat	+	0	0	0	ca	0	0	0
F10	Type C Friedländer bacillus (Julianelle)	(+)	(+)	(+)	(+)	a	0	0	+
F12	Group X Friedländer bacillus (Julianelle)	(+)	(+)	(+)	0	ca	0	0	+
SC	Type A Friedländer bacillus (Julianelle)	+	+	0	0	a	0	0	+
E	Type B Friedländer bacillus (Julianelle)	+	+	+	+	a	0	0	+
G8	Bacillus of granuloma (Julianelle)	(+)	(+)	(+)	(+)	ca	0	0	+
BRI	B. rhinoscleromatis (Am. Type Culture Coll.)	+	+	0	0	0	0	0	+
BR II	B. rhinoscleromatis (Univ. of Chicago)	+	+	0	0	0	0	0	+
P17, P51	Perez bacillus (Page)..........	(+)	0	0	0	a	0	+	+
FS, FA, FC	Stock cultures of Friedländer bacillus, isolated from human lungs	(+)	(+)	(+)	(+)	a	0	0	+

+ indicates acid production, indol production, or nitrate reduction; (+) acid and gas; a, acid in milk; ca, acid and coagulation in milk, and 0 = no reaction.

Specificity was proved for the serums by agglutinin absorption tests using both homologous and heterologous strains for absorption. The technic consisted, briefly, in incubating dilutions (1 : 10) of the serums with twice the minimal absorbing dose of the antigen 2 hours at 37 C. and then overnight in the ice box. Table 4 represents the results of agglutinin absorption tests carried out on the three agglutinating serums, 6E, 48K, and 21E, respectively. Various strains of other types of encapsulated bacilli were used as absorbing antigens but in no case were the agglutinins removed. In each case the absorbed serum was set up against the strain used for absorption as well as against the antigens 6E, 48K, and 21E. No agglutinations occurred with the antigens of the Friedländer-like group. Within the group of rat strains, however, the agglutinins were completely absorbed by both the homologous and the heterologous strain.

TABLE 3.—AGGLUTINATION REACTIONS

Bacterial Antigens	Serum Dilutions									Control
	1:10	1:20	1:40	1:80	1:160	1:320	1:640	1:1280	1:2560	
SERUM OF RABBIT IMMUNIZED TO 6E										
Strains from rats										
6E, 10WN, RGE, 4E	++++	++++	++++	++++	++++	+++	0	0	0	0
21E, 48K, 43E, 39E, 46E, 36K, 48L, 29E, 161N	++++	++++	++++	++++	++	0	0	0	0	0
47E, 23E, 13E, 37E, 190N, 168N, RCL, RAN, 27E	++++	++++	++++	++±	0	0	0	0	0	0
Other Friedländer types FS, FA, FC, F10, F12, SC, E, G8, BrI BrII, P17, P51	0	0	0	0	0	0	0	0	0	0
SERUM OF RABBIT IMMUNIZED TO 48K										
Strains from rats 48K, 39E, 10WN, 29E, RGE, 47E, 4E, 23E	++++	++++	++++	++++	++++	++++	++++	+++	±	0
21E, 43E, 36K, 13E, 37E, 48L, 190N, RCL, 161N, RAN	++++	++++	++++	++++	++++	++++	+++	0	0	0
6E, 46E, 168N	++++	++++	++++	++++	++++	++++	0	0	0	0
27E	++++	++++	++++	++++	++++	0	0	0	0	0
OtherFriendländer types FS, FA, FC, F10, F12, SC, E, G8, BRI, BRII, P17, P51	0	0	0	0	0	0	0	0	0	0
SERUM OF RABBIT IMMUNIZED TO 21E										
Strains from rats 21E, 48K, 13E, 48L, 190N, 10WN, 29E, RGE, 161N, 47E, 4E, 23E	++++	++++	++++	++++	++++	++++	++++	+++	±-++	0
6E, 39E, 36K, 37E, 168N, RAN	++++	++++	++++	++++	++++	++++	++++	0	0	0
43E, 46E, 27E, RCL	++++	++++	++++	++++	++++	++++	0	0	0	0
Other Friedländer types FS, FA, FC, F10, F12, SC, E, G8, BRI, BRII, P17, P51	0	0	0	0	0	0	0	0	0	0

In comparing the rat strains in regard to their physiologic and agglutinating properties, various strains of organisms of the encapsulated mucosus group were used. Four strains of the Friedländer bacillus representing types A, B and C and group X according to the classification of Julianelle[4]; 3 stock strains of the Friedländer bacillus; 1 strain

4. J. Exper. Med., 1926, 44, p. 113.

of the bacillus of granuloma; 2 strains of Coccobacillus foetidus ozaenae (Perez) and 2 strains of Klebsiella rhinoscleromatis comprised this group, as shown in table 2.

PATHOGENICITY

The organism possessed low virulence for rabbits, guinea-pigs, mice, and white rats when injected intraperitoneally or intravenously. Doses of from 0.5 cc. to 1.5 cc. of dilution 1:10 (24-hour broth growth)

TABLE 4.—AGGLUTININ ABSORPTION

Absorbing Antigen	Agglutinating Antigens	Serum Dilutions 1:10	1:20	1:40	1:80	1:160	1:320	1:640	1:1280	1:2560	Control
SERUM 6E											
Before absorption	6E, 48K, 21E	++++	++++	++++	++++	++++	++	0	0	0	0
6E	6E, 48K, 21E										
48K	6E, 48K, 21E	0	0	0	0	0	0	0	0	0	0
21E	6E, 48K, 21E										
Other Friedländer strains P17, E, F10, G8, SC	6E, 48K, 21E	++++	++++	++++	++++	++++	0	0	0	0	0
SERUM 48K											
Before absorption	6E, 48K, 21E	++++	++++	++++	++++	++++	++++	++++	0	0	0
48K	6E, 48K, 21E										
6E	6E, 48K, 21E	0	0	0	0	0	0	0	0	0	0
21E	6E, 48K, 21E										
Other Friedländer strains E, G8, F10, SC, BRI P17	6E, 48K, 21E	++++	++++	++++	++++	++++	++++	++++	0	0	0
SERUM 21E											
Before absorption	6E, 48K, 21E	++++	++++	++++	++++	++++	++++	++++	++	0	0
21E	6E, 48K, 21E										
6E	6E. 48K. 21E	0	0	0	0	0	0	0	0	0	0
48K	6E, 48K, 21E										
Other Friedländer strains E, F10, P17, BRI, FS, G8	6E, 48K, 21E	++++	++++	++++	++++	++++	++++	++++	0	0	0

when injected intraperitoneally failed to kill a rabbit weighing 1000 gm. Intravenous injection of 0.5 cc. of dilution 1:10 did not kill a rabbit weighing 500 gm. One cc. of a dilution of 1:10, given intraperitoneally, was not fatal in a guinea-pig weighing 350 gm.

White rats (100-120 gm.) were killed in about 50 per cent of the trials by doses of 0.4 cc. of a dilution 1:20 (24-hour broth growth) given intraperitoneally. Nasal instillations of the organism into normal and into rats on a diet deficient in vitamin A did not produce evidence of upper respiratory disease of the tract within a week. The serums of rats injected intraperitoneally with nonfatal doses of the organism agglutinated the homologous strain 10 days later in dilutions as high as 1:80. Serums of noninfected rats did not agglutinate the organism. In the case of the rat, the virulence was easily increased by passage through the animal.

Mice, weighing from 10 to 20 gm., were killed by doses of 0.2 cc. of a dilution 1:40 (24-hour broth growth) in 22 hours, and by the same dose of a dilution 1:160 in 6 days. They were protected when 0.6 cc. of a dilution of the immune serum 1:10 was injected 18 hours before a lethal dose of the organism was given (0.2 cc. of a dilution 1:50). Protection against the same dose of the organism was not given by 0.4 cc. of the serum. The filtrate of a 5 day growth of the organism in broth failed to produce death in mice when 0.6 cc. of a dilution 1:10 was injected intraperitoneally.

When a fatal dose of the organism was injected intraperitoneally, the rat, within a few hours, became acutely ill and lethargic, and the temperature became subnormal (34-36 C.). Food and drink were refused, the coat was distinctly roughened, diarrhea frequently occurred, and occasionally a bloody nasal exudate was seen. Death occurred within from 10 to 72 hours.

At necropsy I found a serous (if early) or (after 48 hours) a fibrinopurulent exudate within the peritoneal and sometimes within the pleural cavity. The spleen, liver, and kidneys were dark and enlarged, and in microscopic sections showed cloudy swelling. The intestines were hyperemic. The lungs were congested and frequently there was diffuse pneumonia. The bladder was often distended with blood-tinged urine. Smears of the exudate showed enormous numbers of the encapsulated bacillus and cultures from the heart blood were almost always positive for the organism.

DISCUSSION

Friedländer-like organisms have been isolated from various animals. Webster,[5] recently reported the isolation of a strain definitely responsible for an epidemic respiratory infection among mice. Edwards'[6] study of 25 strains of an encapsulated bacillus isolated from cases of metritis in mares showed them all to belong to a single, well defined type. He was not able to distinguish the equine strains from 3 cultures of human origin used in the comparative study.

5. J. Exper. Med., 1928, 47, p. 685.
6. J. Bact., 1928, 15, p. 245.

Strains were isolated from the rat by Skschivan,[7] Sachs,[8] Schilling,[9] and Toyama.[10] Aujenszky,[11] and later Xylander,[12] recovered encapsulated organisms from various organs of rats that died from a plague-like disease. None of these reports associates the organism with suppurative conditions of the upper part of the respiratory tract nor with the terminal infections of avitaminosis.

In a study of the gram-negative, capsulated organisms recovered from the bronchi in the human body at necropsy, Ball [13] found several strains capable of atypical reactions, among which were 2 that failed to produce acid or gas in any of the sugars. The various strains of the encapsulated mucosus group are so inconsistent in regard to their fermentative reactions that classification cannot be based on these reactions. Recently, Julianelle [4] has classified the organisms of the Friedländer group in 4 types on the basis of agglutination.

Using both methods of study, I find that the organism here described is different from representative strains of the 4 types of Julianelle. It likewise differs from other organisms of this group, for instance the bacillus causing granuloma, B. rhinoscleromatis, and the Perez bacillus. The 22 strains group themselves biochemically and by their agglutinations into a single definite type.

SUMMARY

By aerobic cultures from the suppurative terminal lesions in the white rat on a diet deficient in vitamin A, an encapsulated bacillus of the mucosus group has been isolated in about one-half the cases. From 50 rats on A-deficient diet, representing 3 different stocks, 21 strains were isolated. In 13 normal rats, 3 rats on B-deficient diets, and 9 rats on D-deficient diets, all without obvious infections, cultures from the ears and nose failed to reveal the organism. It was recovered once in a series of 10 wild (brown) rats from the nose. Although obviously more frequently present in the suppurative conditions of the animal on an A-deficient diet, it is probably a secondary invader of mucosa of the respiratory tract, made suitable for its invasion, by the dietary deficiency. The organism has been found to be suitable for use in a study of the relationship between vitamin deficiencies in diet and resistance to infection which will be reported.

7. Centralbl. f. Bakteriol., 1, O., 1902-1903, 33, p. 260.
8. Ibid., 1, O., 1902-1903, 33, p. 657.
9. Arb. aus dem Kaiserlichen Gesundh., 1902, 18, p. 108.
10. Centralbl. f. Bakteriol., 1, O., 1902-1903, 33, p. 273.
11. Ibid., 1904, 36, p. 603.
12. Arb. aus dem Kaiserlichen Gesundh., 1906, 24, p. 196.
13. J. Path. & Bact., 1925, 28, p. 674.

BIOLOGIC AND SEROLOGIC STUDIES OF STREPTOCOCCUS CARDIOARTHRITIDIS

William A. Kreidler

From the Bacteriological Laboratory of the Philadelphia General Hospital

Streptococcus cardioarthritidis was described as a new species by Small [1] in a report in January, 1927, which included the biologic reactions of 20 strains. Since this report appeared, I have collected 87 additional strains and have undertaken a study of the biologic and serologic reactions of the entire 107 strains. Of this group, 3 strains were obtained from blood cultures, 3 from cultures of feces and the remainder from throat cultures (table 1).

Isolation of Strains.—The blood cultures were made by adding from 3 to 5 cc. of blood to about 80 cc. of plain infusion broth (P_H 7.6). When the turbidity

Table 1.—Origin of the 107 Strains of Streptococcus Cardioarthritidis Included in This Study

Number of Strains	Source of Cultures	Diagnosis
3	Blood	Acute rheumatic fever
3	Feces	Chronic arthritis
51	Throat	Acute rheumatic fever
10	Throat	Chorea
26	Throat	Chronic arthritis
14	Throat	Miscellaneous *

* Obtained in throat culture from cases of myositis (2), vague rheumatic pains (6), acute nephritis (1), acute tonsillitis (3), and gonorrheal arthritis (2).

showing growth appeared (in from 4 to 17 days), the cultures were subcultured by streaking over the surfaces of blood agar plates. The colonies appeared after from 18 to 24 hours' incubation at 37 C. If growth was not apparent at the end of a month's incubation, a blood agar plate was streaked to verify the sterility of the culture before discarding it. Of 116 blood cultures, 3 (2.5%) yielded a growth of S. cardioarthritidis.

Cultures of feces were made by direct inoculation of light emulsions of the material on the surfaces of blood agar plates. At the same time, 3 tubes of plain infusion broth, containing varying amounts of acid fuchsin, were inoculated with a loopful each of the same emulsion. A loopful of the broth from each of these tubes, after from 18 to 24 hours' incubation, was seeded on the surfaces of blood agar plates. This latter indirect is the more reliable method since the interfering profuse growth of colon bacilli is suppressed by the fuchsin in the primary cultures.

The throat cultures were prepared by inoculation of material collected on sterile cotton swabs on the surfaces of blood agar plates. The colonies were studied after from 18 to 24 hours' incubation.

The strains isolated were grown in pure culture for from 18 to 24 hours in plain infusion broth. They were then tested for agglutination against an immune

Received for publication, May 9, 1928.

1. Small, J. C.: Am. J. M. Sc., 1927, 173, p. 101.

serum prepared from strain R1, in a manner similar to that by which the typhoid bacillus is identified by agglutination with its specific antiserum. The streptococcal antiserum agglutinated its homologous antigen in dilutions up to 1:20,000. For the identification of the newly isolated strains, it was used in a dilution of 1:2,000, that is, at 1/10 its full titer, a dilution not likely to pick up strains associated serologically in a group reaction.

BIOLOGIC REACTIONS

Table 2 presents the results of the action of 107 strains of S. cardio-arthritidis on the carbohydrates, on milk, and on gelatin, and the results of the tests for indol. The medium used for the study of the fermentation reactions was beef infusion broth to which 1% of the carbohydrate was added. To stimulate the growth of the streptococcus the gelatin was enriched by the addition of whey. The presence of indol was determined by the addition of Ehrlich's reagent to plain broth cultures of the strains. In control tubes containing plain broth, neither fermentation nor formation of indol occurred.

TABLE 2.—FERMENTATION OF CARBOHYDRATES, ACTION ON MILK AND ON GELATIN, AND FORMATION OF INDOL, BY 107 STRAINS OF STREPTOCOCCUS CARDIOARTHRITIDIS

Number of Strains	Glucose	Lactose	Sucrose	Mannitol	Inulin	Salicin	Raffinose	Gelatin	Milk	Indol
86 (80.4%)	+	+	+	0	+	+	+	0	+	0
21 (19.6%)	+	0	+	0	+	+	+	0	0	0

The remarkable constancy of the biologic reactions of the 20 strains reported by Small [1] was maintained by strains R 21 to 107. There was a noteworthy irregularity in the fermentation of lactose; 21 (19.6%) of the 107 strains were unable to attack this carbohydrate or to produce acid in milk. In spite of this irregularity, however, the action on carbohydrates is far more uniform than that of other types of streptococci. Most types of streptococci have difficulty in attacking inulin, but every strain of S. cardioarthritidis studied, fermented this carbohydrate with ease. Laboratory workers have found the fermentative reactions of streptococci so variable and so inconstant that they have been practically unable to classify them on this basis. This fact makes the uniformity of the corresponding reactions of the strains of S. cardioarthritidis the more significant. Such agreement suggests that these strains, obtained from 107 different persons, may represent a single species of streptococci.

AGGLUTINATIVE REACTIONS

Preparation of Immune Serum.—The immune serum used in the tests for agglutination was prepared by immunizing a horse against a single strain of S. cardio-arthritidis. The serum of the animal, before immunization was begun, agglutinated antigens of this streptococcus in a dilution of 1:20. Immunization was achieved as follows: Suspensions of heat-killed microorganisms were injected subcutaneously at intervals of from 2 to 4 days over a period of 1 month. The first dose consisted of 4 billions of killed microorganisms, and by the end of the month the dose had been increased to 48 billions. Then the killed microorganisms were injected intravenously, beginning with a dose of 3 billions. When a dose of 50 billions had been reached (after 5 weeks), 1 billion living bacteria were mixed with 50 billions of the killed microorganisms for the injection. Gradual additions of living bacteria and decreases of the killed ones were practiced in subsequent injections until finally only living bacteria were being injected. Twelve weeks after the beginning of the immunization, the serum of the horse agglutinated the homologous antigen in dilutions up to 1:20,480. The horse was then bled from the jugular vein. The serum was preserved with 0.5% phenol and stored for use.

Method of Tests for Agglutination.—The antigens consisted of 24 hour growths of the strains of S. cardioarthritidis in beef infusion broth (P_H 7.6). In determining the agglutinative titer of the immune serum prepared for strain R1 0.5 cc.

TABLE 3.—RESULTS OF TESTS FOR AGGLUTINATION OF STRAINS OF STREPTOCOCCUS CARDIOARTHRITIDIS WITH MONOVALENT (R1) ANTISERUM

	Dilution of Antiserum							
Number of Strains	20 to 1280	2560	5120	10,240	20,480	40,960	81,920	Control
R 1	+	+	+	+	+	0	0	0
5 (4.8%)	+	+	+	+	+	+	0	0
13 (12.6%)	+	+	+	+	+	0	0	0
32 (31%)	+	+	+	+	0	0	0	0
27 (26.2%)	+	+	+	0	0	0	0	0
19 (18.4%)	+	+	0	0	0	0	0	0
7 (6.1%)	+	0	0	0	0	0	0	0
8 S. viridans *	0	0	Control tests					
9 nonhemolytic streptococci †	0							

* Isolated from blood cultures in patients with ulcerative endocarditis.

† Nonhemolytic streptococci which in colonies on blood agar resemble S. cardioarthritidis, but which differ from S. cardioarthritidis in certain biologic reactions. These strains were isolated from patients with chronic arthritis.

of each antigen was added in turn to a series of tubes containing 0.5 cc., each of the immune serum in dilutions ranging from 1:20 to 1:81,920. The dilutions of serum were made in 0.85% sodium chloride solution. The tests were incubated in the water bath at 50 C. for 18 hours; then readings were made with the naked eye. The depth of the water in the bath was so adjusted that the level of the liquid in the agglutination tubes stood out somewhat above the surface of the water, thus bringing into play the slight convection currents within the tubes, which appear so effective in the development of sharp end results in the agglutination reaction.

The highest dilution of the antiserum of strain R1, which gave agglutination in the case of each antigen is shown in table 3. That different agglutinative titers were obtained with the different strains is apparent. The antiserum agglutinated its homologous antigen in dilutions up to and including 1:20,480. Five strains (4.8%) were agglutinated in dilutions higher than the highest that agglutinated the homologous antigen; 13 strains (12.6%) were agglutinated in dilutions just as high as the highest that agglutinated the homologous antigen; 32 strains

(31%) were agglutinated in dilutions up to half as high; 27 strains (26.2%) in dilutions to one fourth of the homologous titer; 19 strains (18.4%) in dilutions to one eighth, and 7 strains (6.1%) in dilutions to one sixteenth of the homologous titer.

As the antiserum diluted 1 : 1280 agglutinated every strain, there is little probability that group agglutinins are responsible for such reactions. This titer we believe is sufficiently high to justify regarding this collection of strains as a definite species of streptococci. The differences in agglutinin titer obtained, however, do suggest that there may exist within the species immunologic subtypes. Final decision on this question of subtypes will have to await the completion of tests for the absorption of the agglutinins. This work is well under way.

Antigens made from some of the strains studied have a tendency to clump spontaneously. This difficulty has been experienced by other

TABLE 4.—REACTIONS WITH R1 ANTISERUM, SHOWING VARIATIONS IN THE AGGLUTINATIVE TITER OF ANTIGENS AS INFLUENCED BY AGE OF THE ANTIGEN

Age of Antigen (Days)	Agglutinative Titer	
	Antigen R1	Antigen R2
1	1:5120	1:5120
2	1:5120	1:5120
3	1:2560	1:5120
4	1:2560	1:2560
5	1:1280	1:2560
7	1:2560	1:2560
8	1:1280	1:2560
9	1:1280	1:2560
10	1:1280	1:2560

workers with streptococci and is in a measure responsible for the different agglutinative titers obtained with the different strains. This factor is less difficult to control, however, with S. cardioarthritidis than with other types of streptococci because of a tendency of the former to grow diffusely in fluid mediums. Repeated transplants in infusion broth to which 1% glucose had been added, usually served to promote diffuse growth of any strains which previously had shown a tendency to clump. When these were later transferred to plain infusion broth for use in tests for agglutination, the tendency to clump has been practically eliminated. Although only antigens having a uniformly diffuse turbidity were used in the tests for agglutination, and although controls of the tests reported showed no clumping whatever, this tendency of different antigens to clump spontaneously cannot be ignored. For antigens showing this tendency to clump, were agglutinated by higher dilutions of immune serum and apparently with greater ease than those not exhibiting this tendency.

The age of the antigen is another important consideration. In table 4, are recorded the results of tests for agglutination in which the antiserum of R1 was used with antigens of varying age, prepared from strains R1 and R2. It will be noted that although the decrease in the agglutinative titer with age is not regular, there is a definite tendency in that direction. As it was impossible to perform all of the tests recorded in table 3 on the same day, the different ages of the antigens used evidently was a factor in the variation of the agglutinative titers obtained.

SUMMARY

The 107 strains of Streptococcus cardioarthritidis studied, exhibited a marked uniformity in their biologic reactions. All fermented glucose, sucrose, inulin, salicin, and raffinose; none, mannitol. Twenty-one strains (19.6%) failed to ferment lactose and failed to produce acid in milk. None liquefied gelatin or produced indol.

Antigens prepared from each of the strains were agglutinated by a monovalent antiserum of S. cardioarthritidis in dilutions high enough to indicate that these strains fall into a definite serologic group and that group agglutinins play but a small part in the results obtained.

When the foregoing facts are considered, there seems to be reason for the belief that these microorganisms biologically and serologically form a compact species of streptococci. The failure of some of the strains to ferment lactose and the difference in the agglutinability of the strains, suggest that there may exist, within the species, immunologic subtypes of Streptococcus cardioarthritidis.

THE APPROXIMATION OF THE TOXICITY OF DIPHTHERIA TOXIN IN VITRO

ARTHUR LOCKE AND E. R. MAIN

From the Henry Baird Favill Laboratory of St. Luke's Hospital, Chicago

A method is suggested, herewith, for the approximation of the L_0 equivalent of diphtheria toxin preparations by means of a modified flocculation titration.[1] The method comprises, in its essence, the estimation of the L_f unit and the unit flocculation time of the preparation according to the procedure described below, and the substitution of these values in an equation relating them to the L_0 equivalent.

Determination of the L_f Unit.—Graded volumes of a broth dilution of a quickly and specifically flocculating reference antitoxin, not exceeding 0.1 cc. in quantity, are measured into a series of 8 x 75 mm. test tubes with the aid of a micropipet, graduated in 0.01 cc. intervals. One-half cc. volumes of the toxin whose titer is to be measured are added, and the contents of the tubes immediately and carefully mixed. The mixtures are permitted to stand at room temperature until flocculation appears to be imminent. They are then centrifugated lightly and examined for the presence of a coherent sediment. Traces of this sediment are readily visible against a dark background when the tubes are shaken gently during illumination from below. An easily detected sediment is formed by the union of as little as 0.5 L_f units of toxin and antitoxin. The centrifugation is repeated, at intervals of 10 to 20 minutes, until flocculation appears to be complete. The readings are recorded in terms of completeness of flocculation. Incipient flocculation is expressed as tr, one-third flocculation as F, and complete flocculation as FFF.

The tubes in which coherent sediments are obtained first and in largest quantity are considered to contain the most nearly equivalent concentrations of toxin and antitoxin. If, for example, in a series of mixtures of 0.5 cc. of the unknown toxin with 4, 5, 6, 7, and 8 standard units of reference antitoxin, respectively, initial and maximum flocculation appears in the 6 and 7 unit tubes, the toxin titer is considered to be (6 to 7) /0.5 or 13 ± 1 L_f units per cc.

Received for publication, June 19, 1928.

1. An excellent bibliography and discussion of the literature of the Ramon flocculation titration method is given by S. Bayne-Jones in Newer Knowledge of Bacteriology and Immunology, edited by Jordan and Falk, 1928, p. 759. The Ramon procedure has been amended, as herein described, in order to permit an accurate timing of the appearance of first flocculation.

The L_f values obtained, under controlled conditions, are 85 to 95% accurate, and the flocculation times observed, under comparable conditions and for comparable toxin-antitoxin concentrations, are 80 to 90% reproducible.

Estimation of the Unit Flocculation Time.—The flocculation time t is reported as the interval required for a given toxin-antitoxin concentration n to become one-third flocculated at a temperature of 25 ± 1′C., as detected by the centrifugation procedure. The unit flocculation time t_1 is related to this value by the equation: $t_1 = t \cdot n^{3/2}$ (1)

The equation may be a special instance of the more general relation: $t = k/(n - x)^{3/2}$ .... (1A)
where x, the concentration of toxin-antitoxin already flocculated, has the specific value of n/3 by virtue of the definition of the flocculation time suggested above. The general relation becomes, upon differentiation, the velocity equation: $dx/dt = k' \cdot (n - x)^{5/2}$ (1B)
which may be of theoretical interest to students of the mechanism of the toxin-antitoxin combination.

The validity of the relation is demonstrated in table 1, where the flocculation times of a series of broth dilutions of toxin 6 vs. antitoxins 390, 500, and 503 are shown to reduce to identical unit flocculation times, characteristic of the respective reference antitoxins used.

The estimation of the unit flocculation time is further described in the following example:

Titration Assembled as Described in the Preceding Section

Cc. of antitoxin added	.06	.07	.08	.09	.10	
Cc. of toxin added	1.0	1.0	1.0	1.0	1.0	time set up:
Number of units of antitoxin in the mixture	6	7	8	9	10	11:00 a. m.
	Approximate size of the coherent centrifugation sediment:					times examined:
	---	---	---	---	---	12:45 p. m.
	---	tr	F	---	---	1:00
	---	F	FF	FF	---	:10
	tr	F	FFF	FF	tr	:30

Calculation:

Number of L_f units in the first flocculating mixture............... 8.0
Volume of the first flocculating mixture, cc........................ 1.08
"n," toxin concentration in the mixture, 8.0/1.08.................. 7.4
$n^{3/2} = (7.4)^{3/2} =$ 20
"t," interval elapsed before flocculation has become one-third complete, 11:00 a. m. to 1:00 p. m., hrs......................... 2.0
"t_1," unit flocculation time in hrs. $= t \times n^{3/2}$;
$= 2 \times 20 =$: 40
all estimated values subjected to a correction of ±7%.

Derivation of the Basic Equation.—The toxicity of a diphtheria toxin is assumed to be indicated by the avidity with which it tends to combine and flocculate with diphtheria antitoxin.[2] Defining the L_f unit as the unit of toxin substance, measurable as described, and the L_o unit as the unit of toxicity as measured by the standard Ehrlich-Behring procedure in guinea-pigs; expressing the toxicity per unit of toxin substance by the quotient of these values; and expressing the antitoxin binding avidity by A:

$$L_f/L_o = \text{fncn. } A \qquad (2)$$

TABLE 1.—THE RELATION OF FLOCCULATION TIME TO UNIT FLOCCULATION TIME

Reference Antitoxin	Concentration "n" of Toxin 6 in the Flocculating Mixture, L_f Units per Cc.	$n^{3/2}$	Flocculation Time "t" of Mixture, (Hours)	Unit Flocculation Time "t_1" Hours ($t_1 = t \cdot n^{3/2}$)
503	10.7	35	.45	16
	7.3	20	.85	17
	4.0	8.0	2.1	17
	2.0	2.8	5.3	15
	1.0	1.0	17	17
	.5	.36	42	15
Average:				16 ± 2
390	9.8	31	1.0	31
	7.3	20	1.5	30
	6.0	15	2.2	33
	4.3	9.0	3.4	31
	2.6	4.2	6.5	27
	1.7	2.2	15	33
Average:				31 ± 4
500	9.3	28	1.1	31
	7.0	19	1.7	32
	5.6	13	2.6	34
	4.0	8.0	3.8	30
	2.5	4.0	6.8	27
	1.5	1.8	16	29
Average:				30 ± 4

The avidity urging the combination of one L_f unit of toxin with one standard unit of antitoxin is measurable in terms of the time required for the combination to become one-third complete,[3] according to the relation:

$$A = k' \cdot (\log C - \log t_1) \qquad (3)$$

where k' is a reference coefficient, C a constant, equivalent to the unit flocculation time of a mixture of the reference antitoxin with a toxin preparation of approximately zero toxicity, and A and t_1 are the avidity and unit flocculation time as defined. Combining equations 2 and 3:

$$L_f/L_o = \text{fncn. } (\log C - \log t_1) \qquad (4)$$

2. Locke and Main: J. Infect. Dis., 1928, 43, p. 41.

3. Locke and Main: J. Infect. Dis., 1926, 39, p. 484. Locke, Main and Miller: ibid, 1927, 41, p. 32.

Calibration of the Reference Antitoxin.—Ten cc. samples of toxin 53 (unpreserved) were warmed at 49 C. for 0, 1.5, 3, 6, and 10 hrs., respectively. The L_0 titers of the respective samples, as determined in guinea-pigs, and the corresponding L_f titers and unit flocculation times as determined by titration with reference antitoxins 503 and 390, are recorded as preparations VII-XI in table 2 When the quotients of

TABLE 2.—THE VALIDITY OF THE PROPOSED METHOD FOR THE APPROXIMATION OF THE L_0 EQUIVALENT

Toxin Number	Source	L_f Titer Units per Cc.	Unit Flocculation Time in Hours vs. Antitoxins: 503	390	L_0 Titer as Calculated from the L_f Titer and the Unit Flocculation Time, Units per Cc. vs.: 503	390	L_0 Titer as Determined in Guinea-pigs, Units per Cc.	Correspondence Between L_0 Titers as Observed in Guinea-pigs and as Approximated in Vitro, %
	Produced by strains no.:							
I	R	0	...	...	0	0	0	..
II	4B	1.0	19	31	0.59	0.61	0.62	97
III	4703	1.0	19	31	.59	.61	.67	90
IV	170	1.25	24	41	.71	.73	.71	99
V	4172	2.25	18	30	1.35	1.37	1.25	92
VI	DT	3.5	14	26	2.2	2.2	2.3	96
VII	Park 8 (toxin no. 53)	12.5	19	32	7.4	7.5	7.1	(95)
	No. VII after a preliminary heating at 49 C. for:							
VIII	1.5 hours	11.0	26	49	6.3	6.2	6.3	(99)
IX	3.0	9.5	50	99	4.8	4.8	4.5	(94)
X	6.0	8.0	290	486	2.6	2.7	2.8	(95)
XI	10.0	6.5	750	1225	1.6	1.7	1.6	(97)
	Phenolized toxin 6 after a preliminary heating at 42 C. for:							
XII	0 hours	12.5	16	30	7.6	7.6	7.7	99
XIII	2.0	10.0	30	60	5.5	5.4	5.3	97
XIV	4.0	8.0	40	79	4.2	4.2	4.0	95
XV	8.0	6.5	220	380	2.3	2.4	2.5	94
	Mixtures of 50% of sample XII with 50% of sample:							
XVI	IV	6.9	19	32	4.1	4.1	4.2	98
XVII	V	7.4	20	34	4.4	4.4	4.5	98
XVIII	X	10.3	46	78	5.3	5.4	5.3	99
XIX	XI	9.5	49	76	4.8	4.9	4.7	97

the observed L_f and L_0 titers were plotted as ordinates against the logarithms of the observed unit flocculation times as abscissae, as is done in figure 1, it appeared that the locus of each set of values was a straight line characteristic of the reference antitoxin against which titration had been made. The line characteristic of antitoxin 503 intersected the axis of zero toxicity at a value of $\log t_1 = 3.98$ which defined, therefore, the value of log C for that preparation. The corresponding value of log C for preparation 390 appeared to be 4.25. The quotient of L_f/L_0 by (log C — log t_1) appeared to be a constant, identical for the two preparations and equal to 0.22. Equation 4 became simplified to:

$$L_f/L_o = 0.22(3.98 - \log t_1);\ \text{or:}$$

$$L_o \text{ titer} = L_f \text{ titer} \times 0.22(3.98 - \log t_1)^* \qquad (5A)$$

for use with reference antitoxin No. 503, and to:

$$L_f/L_o = 0.22(4.25 - \log t_1);\ \text{or:}$$

$$L_o \text{ titer} = L_f \text{ titer} \times 0.22(4.25 - \log t_1)^* \qquad (5B)$$

for use with reference antitoxin 390.

Application of the Equation to the Approximation of the L_o Equivalent.—The following examples illustrate the method used for the approximation of the L_o equivalents of the toxin preparations recorded in table 2.

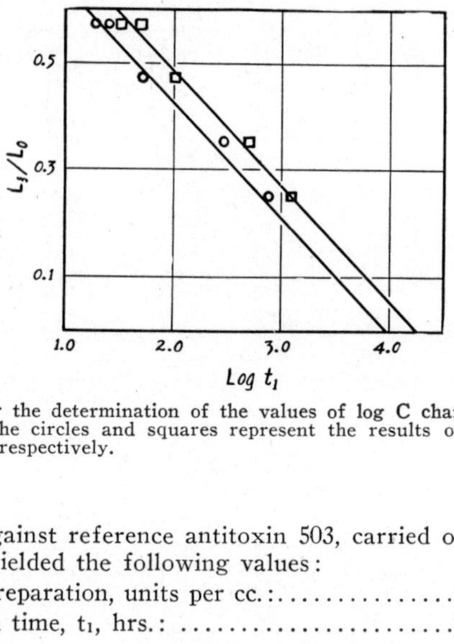

Graphical method for the determination of the values of log C characterizing reference antitoxins 503 and 390. The circles and squares represent the results of titration with reference antitoxins 503 and 390 respectively.

Sample IV:

(1) Titrations against reference antitoxin 503, carried out as described in the preceding sections, yielded the following values:

L_f titer of the preparation, units per cc.: 1.25
Unit flocculation time, t_1, hrs.: 24
Log t_1 = log 24 = : 1.38

Substitution of these values in equation 5A gave:

L_o titer = L_f titer x 0.22(3.98 — log t_1);
= 1.25 x 0.22 (3.98 — 1.38) = : 0.71

subject to a correction of ± 7%.

(2) Titrations against reference antitoxin 390 gave:

L_f titer of the preparation, units per cc.: 1.25
Unit flocculation time, t_1, hours: 41
Log t_1 = log 41 = : 1.61

Substitution of these values in equation 5B gave:

* The L_f and L_o titers are the respective reciprocals of the L_f and L_o units.

L_o titer $= L_f$ titer x $0.22(4.25 - \log t_1)$;
$= 1.25 \times 0.22(4.25 - 1.61) =$: 0.73
subject to a correction of $\pm$ 7%.

So soon as a standard antitoxin becomes universally available, tables can, of course, be constructed, from which the L_o equivalent may be read directly without recourse to the calculations suggested.

The correspondence between the L_o titer as observed in guinea-pigs and as approximated by the new method is indicated in the last column of table 2. It has appeared to us, for such preparations as we have examined, to equal the accuracy with which either unit may be determined under ordinary conditions. The method is naturally applicable, in its present form, only to the examination of toxin preparations similar in character to those used for the calibration of the reference antitoxins. Further studies are in progress concerning its applicability to the analysis of concentrated and formolized toxins and to the examination of toxins elaborated by other bacterial species.

SUMMARY

A simple, practicable method is reported, whereby the L_o titer of an unmodified diphtheria toxin may be predicted, in vitro, with an accuracy of 85 to 95 %. The method is based on the use of a formula correlating the properties of toxicity and antitoxin-binding avidity. It consists of a modified flocculation titration, wherein the latter property is evaluated in terms of L_f titer and "unit flocculation time;" the results being converted into toxicity units by reference to the basic formula.

ETIOLOGY OF DERMATITIS OF EXPERIMENTAL PELLAGRA IN RATS

W. D. SALMON, I. M. HAYS AND N. B. GUERRANT

From the Laboratory of Animal Nutrition, Alabama Polytechnic Institute, Auburn, Ala.

In May 1926, Goldberger and Lillie [1] described a pellagra-like condition in the albino rat. The animals in the experiment received a diet of purified casein, salt mixture, cod liver oil, vegetable fat, and cornstarch. To this basal diet there was added as a source of vitamin B, either a concentrated alcoholic extract of maize, or 0.5 to 1.0% of Seidell's "activated solid," which is the adsorbate obtained by treating a yeast extract with fullers' earth.[2] The rats that received such a diet for some weeks, developed the following symptoms: ophthalmia, alopecia, dermatitis, and stomatitis. There was a dried secretion on the margins of the eyelids with a tendency for the lids to adhere together. There was loss of hair "at the side or over the top of the head, the sides or front of the neck, or in the region of the shoulders." There was said to be almost complete denudation of the head, neck, and trunk in some cases. Some of the animals developed a dermatitis, with or without loss of hair, "at one or more of the following sites: ears, front of neck and upper part of chest, backs of forepaws or hindpaws and shins." The dermatitis on the paws, forearms, neck and ears was sharply outlined and bilaterally symmetrical. The condition was alleviated by the inclusion in the diet of 6% of an adsorbate prepared by treating an autoclaved extract of yeast with fullers' earth. Goldberger, Wheeler, Lillie, and Rogers [3] had shown previously that rats failed to grow on the diet described by Goldberger and Lillie, unless a further addition of autoclaved yeast was made.

Early in 1927 Salmon [4] reported the preparation of an adsorbate which was a potent source of a beriberi-preventive factor but which was devoid of growth-promoting action. He also obtained a preparation which was almost completely free of beriberi-preventive (antineuritic) action but which was an essential accessory of the beriberi-preventive factor for the support of growth. Rats on a vitamin B-free basal diet supplemented by a small amount of soy beans or by the beriberi-preventive preparation developed a condition similar to that described by Goldberger and Lillie. This condition was cured or prevented by the addition of either velvet bean leaves or the fraction containing the growth-promoting accessory.

Shortly afterward Chick and Roscoe [5] likewise reported the occurrence of the pellagra-like syndrome in rats receiving a vitamin B-free diet with a supplemental addition of a beriberi-preventive vitamin concentrate prepared by the Peters method. Under such a dietary regimen the rats failed to grow and some died after 6 to 8 weeks without any special external symptoms. In other cases the animals became thin and exhibited "rough coats, loss of hair, and red inflamed patches of skin on the nose and backs of the fore feet, which later became edematous." There was marked conjunctivitis and in some cases the ears became red and thickened.

Received for publication, May 17, 1928.

1. Pub. Health Rep., 1926, 41, p. 1025.
2. Seidell, Atherton: Pub. Health Rep., 1922, 37, p. 801; J. Am. Chem. Soc., 1922, 44 p. 2042.
3. Pub. Health Rep., 1926, 41, p. 297.
4. J. Biol. Chem., 1927, 73, p. 483.
5. Biochem. J., 1927, 21, p. 698.

The urine was often slightly blood-stained. Postmortem examination showed "an unhealthy condition of the whole alimentary tract, especially in the small intestine which was inflamed and often contained blood-stained mucus."

In these investigations it became apparent that by restricting rats to a vitamin B-free basal diet supplemented by certain sources of antineuritic or beriberi-preventing vitamin, a syndrome, radically different from the symptom-complex previously associated with a vitamin B deficiency, was produced. It was thus shown that the simple addition of the beriberi-preventing vitamin to an otherwise vitamin B-free diet did not render the diet adequate for growth or continued maintenance of the rat. The further addition of autoclaved yeast or of a fractionated extract (containing the substances not readily absorbed by fullers' earth) of plant leaves prevented the morbid changes and rendered the diet adequate for growth. These findings substantiated the conclusion of Funk and Dubin[6] and of Smith and Hendrick[7] that vitamin B is a composite. It was thus proven that at least two active factors are concerned in the action commonly attributed to vitamin B: one of these (the B-P factor) prevents experimental beriberi; the other, alone, has neither beriberi-preventing nor growth-promoting action but is an essential accessory of the B-P factor in the support of growth. Identical or associated with the growth-accessory factor is a substance (the P-P factor) which inhibits the onset of experimental pellagra in the rat.

One phase of the investigation of the vitamin B complex,[4, 8] now being conducted in this laboratory is a detailed study of the pathological and bacteriological features of experimental pellagra of the rat. It is the purpose of this paper to describe the gross pathological manifestations and to discuss the relation of a dietary deficiency and a concomitant infection as etiologic factors.

THE DERMATITIS ON STOCK RATS

In December, 1923, a peculiar dermatitis was observed on some rats which were receiving a vitamin B-free basal diet supplemented by velvet bean seed. During the following spring it was again noted among other rats on a similar diet; a severe case was developed by one of these rats that was receiving orange juice (4 ml. daily) in addition to the above test diet. Similar lesions were also found on some of the older individuals in the stock colony and have been observed from time to time ever since. Our stock rats receive diet 14 A, consisting of yellow maize 25, wheat 25, linseed meal 10, peanut meal 10, dried meat 14, skim milk powder 10, cod liver oil 3, and dried yeast 3 gm.; to each 100 gm. of the mixture are added $CaHPO_4$, 0.50 gm.; $CaCO_3$, 0.75 gm.; NaCl, 1.0 gm.; KI, 0.0004 gm., and ferric citrate, 0.0496 gm. A liberal supply of whole milk is given daily; orange juice is supplied twice a week and

6. Proc. Soc. Exper. Biol. & Med., 1921, 19, p. 15.
7. Pub. Health Rep., 1926, 41, p. 201.
8. Salmon; Guerrant and Hays: J. Biol. Chem., 1928, 76, p. 487.

fresh lettuce once each week. The diet supports excellent growth, reproduction, and lactation; litters usually reach an average weight of 45 gm. at 25 to 26 days of age. Although special measures of cleanliness and sanitation are practiced in the animal colony, a parasitic infestation was suspected to be the etiologic factor of the dermatitis. Careful examinations at different times, however, failed to reveal the presence of a causative parasite. Neither were systematic local treatments of various kinds effective.

The Lesions.—The lesions as found on the stock rats (fig. 1) are somewhat circumscribed, brownish-red eschars ranging in size from 1 to 4 mm. in diameter. They first make their appearance in the form of minute multiple vesicles. A pruritus often accompanies the appearance of the vesicles and the animal lacerates the small area affected, resulting in the formation of the dry, hemorrhagic eschar. If the vesicles are not disturbed they eventually rupture, forming the same type of lesion. This heals and disappears in from 4 days to 2 weeks, unless the animal continues to lacerate the lesion. New lesions are continually forming as the old lesions heal and disappear. When the eschar is completely formed, it is somewhat elevated and quite superficial without any nodule formation in the deeper layers of the skin. When the naked lesion is exposed by a careful lifting of the eschar, a small pit is seen in the center and the margin appears slight elevated. Lymph readily exudes from the granulating surface.

The sites usually affected are the shoulders, neck, and masseteric region but are not entirely confined to these regions. There is a marked tendency toward bilateral symmetry in the distribution of the lesions but this rule likewise is not invariable.

The dermatitis in the stock rats produces no alopecia, the hair remaining in an apparently normal condition up to the margin of the lesion. However, if an animal be clipped over the affected region, the hair fails to grow and the short stubs remain as they were clipped.

THE DERMATITIS AND OTHER SYMPTOMS IN RATS ON VITAMIN B-FREE BASAL DIET

The production of a pellagra-like syndrome as mentioned in our previous papers [4, 8] has been referred to in the introduction. Young rats weighing 45 to 50 gm. receive diet 2B (purified casein, 20%; salt 186, 3.7%; agar, 2%; Argo corn starch, 67.3%; cod liver oil, 2%, and butter fat, 5%) for a preliminary depletion period of 2 weeks. They then

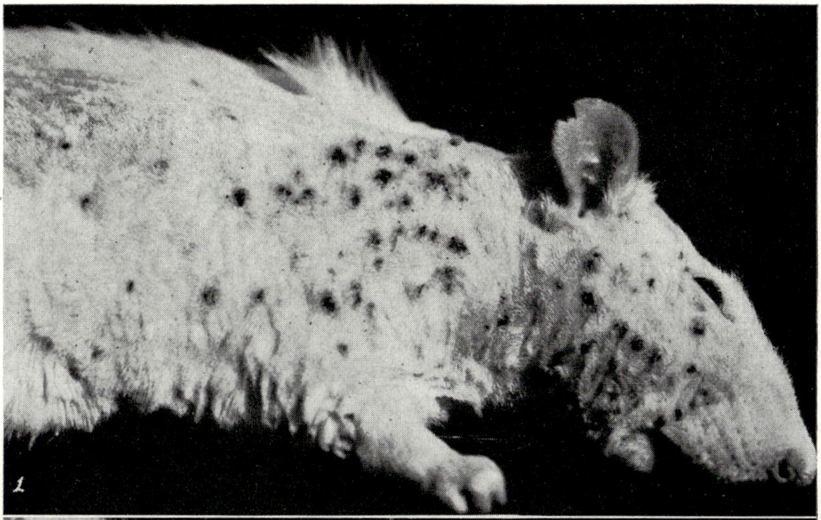

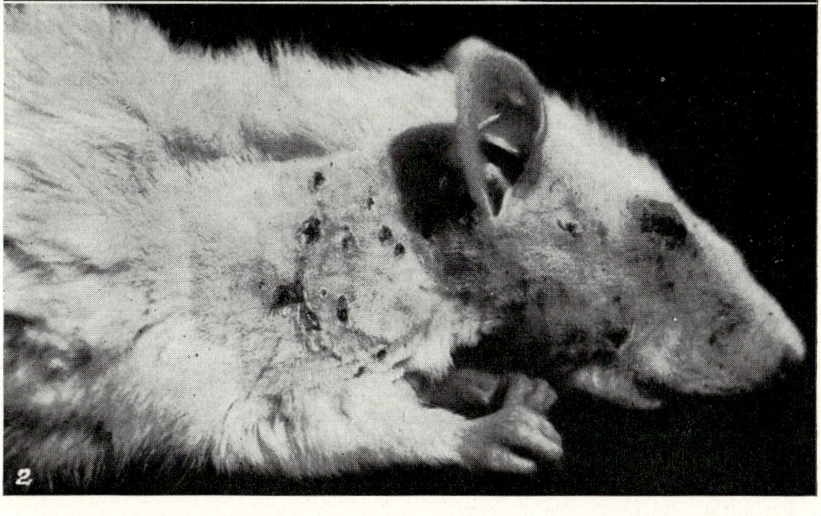

Fig. 1.—Dry eschars on stock rat 12, male, on diet 14A developed a severe case of the mild form of dermatitis. Hair clipped over affected region; ether anesthesia for photograph Feb. 21, 1928.

Fig. 2.—Dry eschars and ophthalmia on rat 35, male, on diet 2B and B-P solid, with 10 ml. suspension of coccus per day. Hair clipped over affected region; ether anesthesia for photograph Feb. 21, 1928.

receive an addition of 0.03 gm. daily of B-P solid 25, which furnishes an ample supply of the B-P factor (beriberi-preventive or antineuritic). This solid is the adsorbate obtained by extracting white maize with 80% (by weight) alcohol, concentrating the extract by vacuum distillation, removing the precipitated protein, and finally adsorbing the B-P factor from the concentrated extract by English fullers' earth at P_H 4.0. The usual precautions that are necessary in the study of vitamin B are observed; these are individual caging on raised screens, careful cleaning of cages, daily feeding and watering in clean vessels, use of distilled drinking water, and quantitative weighing of extracts.

Under such a regimen the rats make little or no increase in the weight shown at the end of the depletion period. With the exception of a general unthriftiness and a gradual roughening of the hair coat and in a few cases a slight alopecia, no particular symptoms are apparent before 2 to 4 weeks following the preliminary period of 2 weeks. The condition described below then gradually develops.

Symptoms and Lesions.—The animal becomes somewhat emaciated, the eyelids droop, the ears appear thin, wrinkled and usually anemic. Alopecia areata is often seen and the hair is not usually regained. An ophthalmia, originating as a mild conjunctivitis, appears and a hemorrhagic exudate gathers in the inner canthi. The flow of lacrimal fluid is increased and very soon the margins of the lids are covered with a film of yellowish-red exudate; the lids are found to adhere together early in the morning but separate later in the day. Eventually the lids remain permanently closed and are under some tension from the retained secretions. Alopecia is quite marked around the eyes. If the lids are forced open, the eyeball is found to be opaque, the opacity centering in the vitreous humor but sometimes affecting the crystalline lens. The cornea is rarely involved.

As the ophthalmia progresses, a stomatitis appears. The oral commissures become hardened and fissured; there is a profuse salivation which continues throughout the course of the disease. Rarely, small vesicular formations or pseudo-membranes are found on the surface of the tongue.

There also develops, in most cases, a dermatitis. Two general types of the dermal lesions are common, a dry form and a wet form. The dry form is characterized by eschars identical with those found on the stock rats. The emaciated animals apparently show less tendency to lacerate the lesions; as a result the eschars are often light brown in color instead of hemorrhagic as are the usual lesions on the stock rats. In some cases the dry lesions coalesce and the superficial layer of epithelium sloughs off, leaving a large, patchy, moist lesion. In other cases small bullae form in a denuded area; the epithelium cracks and erodes, leaving the surface bathed with lymph. These lesions sometimes become progressive, advancing with a sharply marginated periphery behind which healing may occur.

The front feet (and occasionally the hind feet) become dry, scaly and often cracked and hyperemic. An arthritis, involving the articulations of the toes, frequently develops and eventually becomes so severe that the feet are useless for grasping.

In the late stages of the disease, there is marked cachexia; constipation, which has previously been quite marked, often gives way to diarrhea; incontinence of urine

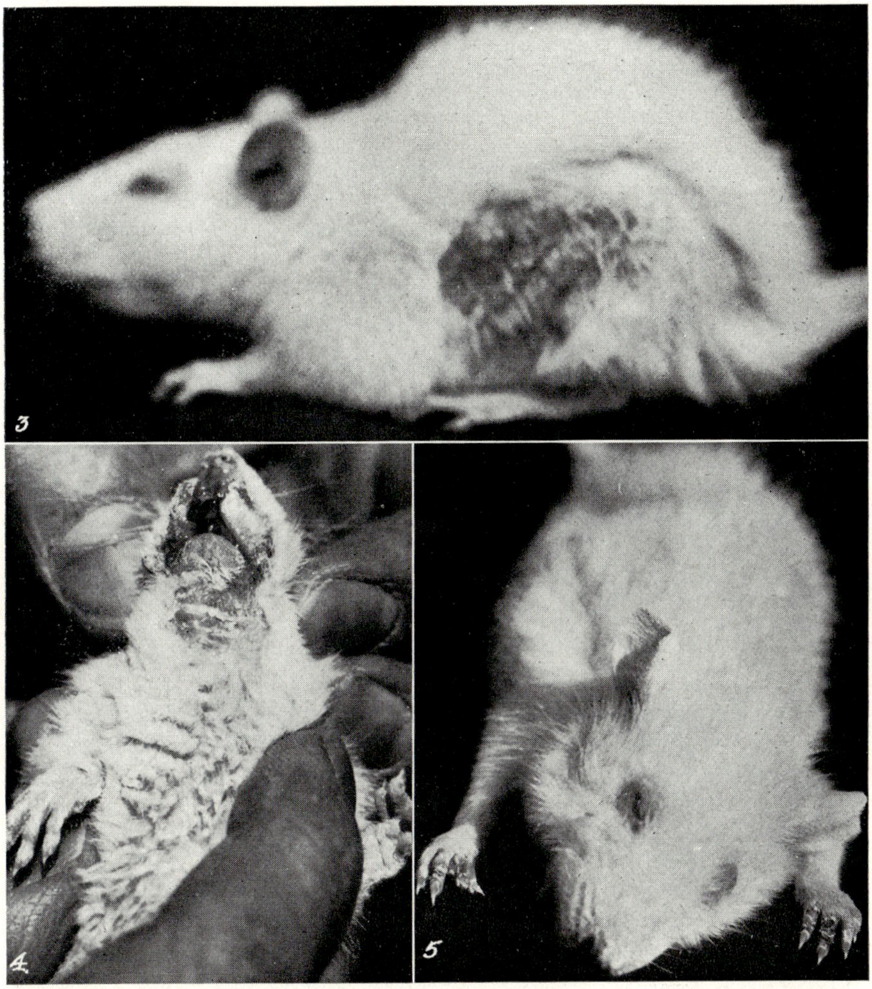

Fig. 3.—Alopecia and moist dermal lesion on experimental rat 28, female, on diet 2B and B-P solid. An irregular elevataion of light brown epithelium first appeared in denuded area; the surface of the elevation then eroded leaving a moist lesion which became progressive. Bilaterally symmetrical lesion was present on other side and both eyes were closed when photo was made. Photographed April 4, 1927.

Fig. 4.—Alopecia on chin and throat, and stomatitis of experimental rat 57, male, on diet 2B and B-P solid. Photographed April 7, 1928.

Fig. 5.—Ophthalmia, also arthritis and dermatitis on toes of front feet. Male 1139 on diet 2B and B-P solid with 10 ml. suspension of coccus per day. Ether anesthesia for photograph Feb. 21, 1928.

is common; hemoglobinuria is rarely observed. The length of life of the test animals varies through a period of 8 to 18 weeks from the end of the preliminary period.

The whole combination of symptoms does not occur in every case. Some of the test animals die without having external signs except emaciation and debilitation; such a case, however, is rare. As a rule one or more forms of external lesion are present, becoming intensified as the disease progresses. Figures 2, 3, 4, 5 show typical pellagrous lesions on animals of the experiment.

Internal Lesions.—Many rats have been chloroformed at various stages of the disease. The necropsy records show a rather definite group of internal lesions which have been characteristic, in varying degrees of intensity, of all the cases studied. The most striking condition is a gastro-enteritis which may involve the digestive tract from the stomach to the cecum. When gastritis is present, the chief lesion is hemorrhage in the submucosa; rarely, a suffusion is seen between

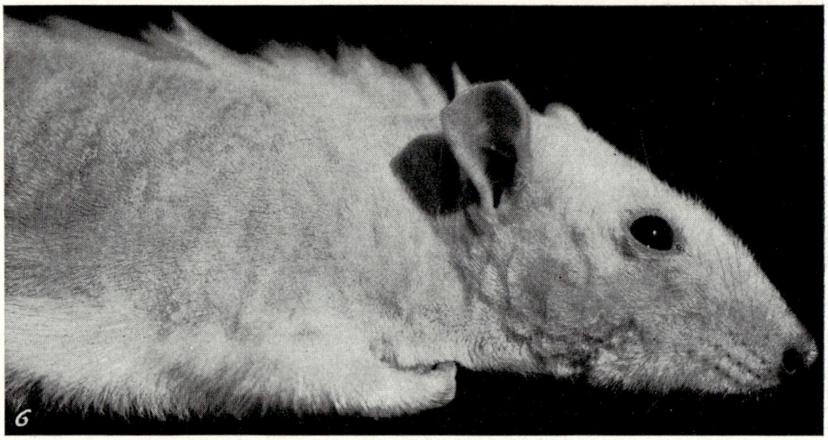

Fig. 6.—Results of prophylactic action of P-P factor. Male, 40, on diet 2B supplemented with both B-P solid and fraction 2. Rat received 10 ml. suspension of coccus per day. Compare with fig. 2 showing litter-mate which did not receive fraction; both animals same distance from camera. Ether anesthesia for photograph Feb. 21, 1928.

the peritoneum and the muscular layers. The stomach is usually distended with free gas but if food residues are present, they are infiltrated with gas, forming a frothy mass. The mucosa is covered with a layer of grayish, catarrhal exudate. In those cases where only a portion of the intestines is involved, the seat of localization is invariably the ileum. In cases that have gone to completion the enteritis frequently involves all the small intestine; when the abdomen is opened, the affected intestine often appears to be a reddish-brown, gelatinous mass; the walls are very thin and flabby, possessing no tonus; if one coil is lifted, the whole mass adheres. In these severe cases the intestinal content is frothy and reddish-brown in color, the red color being due to the presence of whole blood. The wall of the intestine contains many hemorrhages of varying size, and the mucosa is covered with a dark red exudate.

An atrophy of the spleen is always observed. Fatty degeneration of the liver is common. In some cases the kidneys are infiltrated with fat and the bladder contains a fine, granular, grayish-colored material. Secondary complications, the most common of which is pneumonia of both the fibrinous and the catarrhal type, are sometimes found.

Rat 6, Male.—Started on Diet 2B July 27, 1927: wt. 47 Gm.; August 3: wt. 59 Gm.; August 10: wt. 62 Gm.; 0.05 Gm. B-P solid and 0.20 Gm. dried leaves of Pueraria thunbergiana given daily after August 10; weekly wts. to September 14: 76, 90, 102, 116, 130 Gm.

September 13: first symptoms appear, drooping eyelids, secretion in inner canthi; September 21: eyelids thickened, wt. 144 Gm.; September 28: wt. 162 Gm.; October 5: secretion in eyes, a few eschars on neck, wt. 163 Gm.; October 12: eschars persist, wt. 176 Gm.; October 19: eschars persist, eyeballs opaque, wt. 179 Gm.

October 27: dry eschars more numerous, salivation, stomatitis, severe conjunctivitis, incontinence of urine, rat appears weak, wt. 184 Gm.; November 2: eschars more numerous, eschars appearing around mouth, conjunctivitis more severe, wt. 175 Gm.

November 17: wt. had remained unaltered from November 2 (wts. November 9: 175 Gm. November 17: 175 Gm.) animal killed for necropsy.

Necropsy Report: Stomach inflated with gas, severe catarrhal enteritis, no tonus to intestinal walls, intestines contain dark-brown frothy fluid; liver enlarged and yellowish in color, spleen atrophied. Pure cultures of the coccus of rat pellagra were obtained from the liver and spleen.

Rat 7, Female.—Started on diet 2B Aug. 10, 1927: wt. 48 Gm.; August 17: wt. 59 Gm.; August 24: wt. 55 Gm.; rat received addition of 0.05 Gm. B-P solid per day after August 24; weekly weights August 31 to October 5, inclusive: 55, 59, 61, 65, 60, 63 Gm.

October 4: first marked symptoms, emaciation, eyelids anemic, secretion along margins of lids; October 12: cachexia, wt. 61 Gm.; October 19: cachexia, eyelids drooping, wt. 62 Gm.

October 26: salivation, incontinence of urine, moist lesions between toes and on tops of feet, wt. 63 Gm.

November 2: arthritis of the phalangeal articulations on fore feet, fierce stomatitis, conjunctivitis in both eyes, right eyeball opaque, wt. 60 Gm.; November 9: lesions more severe, rat very debilitated, wt. 55 Gm.; killed for necropsy.

Necropsy Report: Catarrhal pneumonia in left lung, fatty infiltration of liver, spleen atrophied, enteritis centered in ileum which is flabby and gelatinous and contains dark red frothy material. Coccus of rat pellagra obtained from liver, spleen and lung.

Rat 8, Male.—Started on diet 2B Aug. 20, 1927: wt. 44 Gm.; August 27: wt. 52 Gm.; September 3: wt. 52 Gm.; rat received addition of 0.10 Gm. B-P solid per day after September 3; weekly wts. September 10 to October 15, inclusive: 61, 65, 60, 65, 67, 63 Gm.

October 15: no previous symptoms except slight emaciation and eyes somewhat prominent; October 22: cachexia, eyes hyperemic, wt. 64 Gm.; October 29: no change, wt. 65 Gm.; November 5: cachexia, abdomen slightly distended, wt. 64 Gm.; November 8: wt. 62 Gm., rat killed for necropsy.

Necropsy Report: Marked enteritis, intestinal wall flabby and gelatinous, small tumor in wall of intestine, fatty infiltration of liver.

BACTERIOLOGIC EXAMINATION

The inability to find parasites in the dermal lesions on the stock rats led to bacteriological examinations of these lesions. Smears and cultures, taken from the deeper part of the eschars, revealed a large coccus. Many cases were examined and in every instance, this organism was present, usually in pure culture. The same organism was isolated later, not only from the eschars, but from the moist dermal lesions, the parenchymatous organs, the intestinal submucosa, and the involved joint cavities of many cases of experimental pellagra; in fact typical pellagrous lesions have been found invariably to contain the organism.

Isolation of the Organism.—The skin lesions present perhaps the best source from the standpoint of the greatest number of organisms. The hair is clipped or shaved up to the margin of the lesion; the surface is cleaned with a light swab of 60% alcohol (the alcohol should not penetrate beneath the eschar) ; the eschar is carefully lifted with sterile pincers; the skin containing the lesion is raised and gently squeezed until droplets of serum appear on the surface; the serum is then transferred with a sterile loop to a slant of common agar medium. As a rule a practically pure culture may be obtained by this method. The organism has been isolated from the liver and spleen of every advanced case of experimental pellagra examined. It has also been found in the walls of the intestine and in the mesenteric lymph glands. With careful technique pure cultures are very frequently obtained from the liver and spleen of such cases. With the exception of two cases the organism has not been isolated from the blood stream.

The organism is a gram-positive coccus, about 1 micron in diameter. It is very uniform in size and is distinctly spherical in shape. There is no regular grouping.

Pathogenicity.—This organism under ordinary conditions is not pathogenic; even when favorable conditions for its growth are created, it is apparently not highly pathogenic until great numbers have accumulated.

Heavy suspensions of the organism, removed from agar medium with sterile physiologic salt solution, have been injected into rats. Varying doses of the suspension were injected, intraperitoneally, intramuscularly, intradermally, and subcutaneously. In no case have typical pellagrous lesions been produced. The intramuscular injections sometimes produced local abscesses and the intradermal injections frequently caused small skin lesions which readily healed and did not appear again.

Daily doses of 1 ml. of the suspension were next supplied (in the drinking water) to rats receiving diet 14A. Negative results were obtained. The dosage of suspension was increased to 10 ml. daily; on this dosage the animals began to develop eschars in 10 days to 3 weeks after the feeding of the suspension was begun. The lesions were identical with the eschars which sometimes occur on the stock rats; the organism was recovered from the lesions in all cases. The coccus was then grown in nutrient broth; 20 ml. of the broth culture were given each rat daily, no drinking water being supplied; this likewise produced the characteristic dermatitis on the test animals. Some animals appeared to be very resistant to the infection; about 80 to 85% of the test animals were readily susceptible and the remainder eventually developed symptoms. All the rats that received large dosages of suspension or broth culture were unthrifty, developed harsh coats, and eventually became somewhat emaciated.

In later tests white maize meal replaced diet 14A. This shortened the incubation period and increased the susceptibility of the animals.

ACTION OF THE P-P FACTOR

The pellagra-preventive and growth-promoting actions of our fraction 2 from leaves of the velvet bean (Stizolobium deeringianum) have been described elsewhere.[8] A similar preparation was obtained by a slightly modified procedure from kudzu leaves (Pueraria thunbergiana). The method of preparation was as follows:

40 L. of tap water were placed in a steam-jacketed kettle and brought to 90 C.; 4 kilos of air-dried kudzu leaves were added and allowed to steep for 1 hour; the decoction was drawn off and the extraction was repeated with 32 L. of water; the leaves were then pressed out in a fruit press; the extract was filtered through heavy muslin and concentrated in an enamel-lined vacuum still. When the volume had been reduced to 6 L., the solution was allowed to cool and the reaction brought to P_H 3.0 with H_2SO_4; it was then treated with 30 Gm. of English fullers' earth, agitated for 30 minutes and the adsorbate removed by a supercentrifuge; the centrifugate was again treated with 40 Gm. of English fullers' earth as before; sufficient NaOH was then added to the extract to bring it to P_H 5.7, the original reaction of the concentrated extract; the volume of the solution was made up to 8 L., and 12 L. of 93% (by weight) alcohol were added; the flocculent precipitate was removed by a supercentrifuge and discarded; the centrifugate was returned to the vacuum still and concentrated to 1 L.; 10 L. of 93% (by weight) alcohol were added, which threw down a dark viscous mass; this precipitate was macerated in absolute alcohol, the alcohol decanted, and the precipitate dried in an electric oven at 60 to 70 C.; the precipitate was ground into a powder which was light brown in color and somewhat hygroscopic; a total yield of 554.85 Gm. was obtained from the 4 kilos of leaves. This product was the fraction 2 used in the following tests.

In order to test the prophylactic action of fraction 2, 8 rats were placed on diet 2B, Nov. 14, 1927. After the two-week depletion period, each rat received 0.05 gm. daily of B-P solid 25, diet 2B being continued. Four of these received a further addition of 0.30 gm. daily of fraction 2 as a source of the P-P factor. All 8 rats received 10 ml. daily of a heavy suspension of the coccus of rat pellagra as the sole source of water.

The 4 rats receiving the B-P solid 25 as the sole vitamin concentrate developed severe cases of pellagra in 4 to 8 weeks, not including the preliminary depletion of 2 weeks. Three of these died after 14, 14, and 16 weeks, respectively. All 4 showed ophthalmia; three developed both dry eschars and moist dermal lesions, while the fourth showed a marked arthritis of the second phalangeal articulations, accompanied by a tendovaginitis; stomatitis was quite marked in all 4

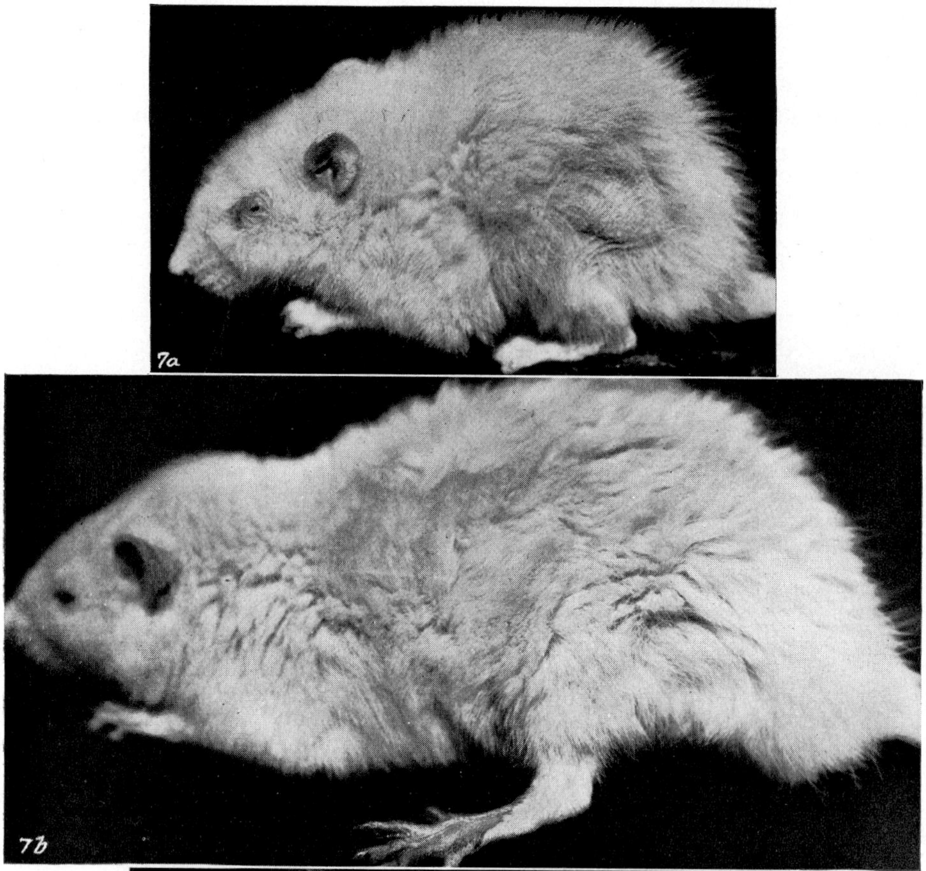

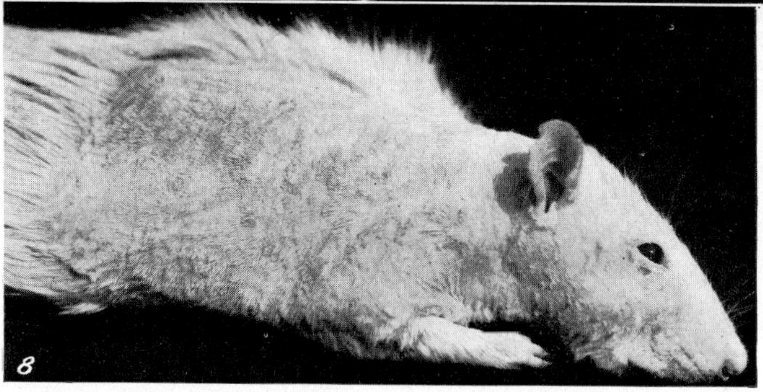

Fig. 7.—Results of prophylactic action of P-P factor when injected. Female 56 (*7a*), on diet 2B and B-P solid; note ophthalmia, alopecia and dry wrinkled condition of skin. Male, 53 (*7b*), litter-mate, on same diet but 53 received 0.30 Gm. of fraction 2 by intraperitoneal injection on alternate days. The hair is soft and dense and rat is below normal in size but no pellagrous lesions are visible. Both animals photographed April 7, 1928, at same distance from camera.

Fig. 8.—Cure of dermatitis by injection of P-P factor. Rat 12, male (see fig. 1), was completely free from eschars after 5 injections (of 0.50 Gm. each) of fraction 2. Ether anesthesia for photograph March 20, 1928. Animal farther from camera than in fig. 1.

cases. The internal lesions of the 3 fatal cases were the same as those previously described. One rat was in the advanced stages of pellagra at the end of the seventeenth week. A daily dose of 0.50 gm. of the fraction 2 concentrate was then supplied, the diet remaining otherwise unaltered and the feeding of the organism being continued. Although this animal had steadily declined in weight for 4 weeks before the addition of fraction 2, the weekly gains following this addition were as follows: 1.0, 11.0, 28.5, 22.0, and 20 gm. At the end of the third week the ophthalmia and the dermatitis had completely cleared up; a full coat of hair had been grown and the rat appeared normal in every respect. In the fifth week, however, this animal suddenly began lacerating the sides of his face and two hemorrhagic eschars about 15 mm. in diameter appeared. The lacerations are being continued and the outcome is not yet apparent.

The 4 rats which received the 0.30 gm. of fraction 2 per day from the start of the test, made almost normal gains. No abnormal symptoms, except perhaps somewhat roughened hair-coats, were manifest until the thirteenth week of the test proper. At this time one rat developed a few small eschars over the shoulder. The dosage of fraction 2 was then increased to 0.50 gm. per rat daily. The dermatitis completely subsided in two weeks and no further symptoms have yet appeared (22d week of test).

Some studies of the prophylactic action of fraction 2, when injected, have been made. Four depleted rats receiving diet 2B plus 0.05 gm. per rat daily of B-P solid 25, were injected intraperitoneally on alternate days with 0.30 gm. of fraction 2 in sterile solution. The injections produced a transitory debilitating effect. The rate of growth was considerably below normal but the animals maintained a fair general condition. At the end of the thirteenth week of the test no symptoms of pellagra were apparent. Three litter mates as controls on the same diet, but not injected, died in 8 to 10 weeks, showing typical symptoms and lesions of experimental pellagra.

Curative Action.—The curative action of the fraction 2 concentrate of the P-P factor on one rat was discussed above. Numerous tests have demonstrated that this preparation, either fed or injected, has marked curative properties.

In the few cases which appear among the older rats of the stock colony, the animals are apparently normal except for the dermatitis; such cases apparently respond more readily to injections of the P-P factor. Injections of a sterile solution containing 0.50 gm. of fraction 2 per rat on alternate days usually results in a complete clearing up of these dermal lesions within 10 days (fig. 8). This form of dermal lesion responds quite readily to such injections, even though the animal may be receiving rather large doses of the organism. In cases which develop on diet B where a marked deficiency of the P-P factor exists and an enteritis is well established, there is a more favorable response to feeding of the fraction 2 than to its injection.

Rat 10, Female.—Started on diet 2B Aug. 20, 1927; received daily dosage of 0.05 Gm. B-P solid after two weeks, in late stage of pellagra in tenth week of experiment. At this point (October 29) 0.50 Gm. of fraction 2 was added to diet; November 8: rat has made only slight improvement, laparotomy performed and severe enteritis found in ileum which was filled with reddish-yellow, frothy material; November 22: recovery apparently complete, no pellagrous lesions visible, autopsy shows no enteritis or other abnormalities.

Rat 11, Male.—Rat taken from growth experiment Nov. 9, 1927, and placed on stock diet 14A.

December 1: started on 10 ml. daily of a heavy suspension of the coccus of rat pellagra, diet 14A continued; December 15: large red eschars appearing in region of head and shoulders; January 15: a severe pruritus developed and animal lacerated head until whole frontal region was covered by a hemorrhagic scab.

January 17: animal injected intraperitoneally with 0.50 Gm. of fraction 2 on alternate days; January 24: lesions had shown considerable improvement, but animal lacerated frontal region again today until a considerable area of skin is destroyed, injections of fraction 2 continued.

February 15: animal almost completely recovered from dermatitis; March 6: no evidence of dermatitis. The animal had received 10 ml. of the suspension of organisms during the entire experiment.

Rat 12, Male.—Feb. 21, 1928: rat in stock colony has severe dermatitis (see fig. 1); 0.50 Gm. of fraction 2 in sterile solution injected intraperitoneally on alternate days; March 4: dermatitis completely cleared up after 5 injections (see fig. 8).

Effect of P-P Factor on Organism in Culture Mediums.—The results reported in the preceding pages seemed to prove that the characteristic lesions of experimental pellagra in the rat are caused by a specific organism. Nevertheless, the injection or the feeding of sufficient P-P factor prevented or cured the disease. It was evident either that the lack of an essential substance indirectly affected the resistance of the animal to invasion of the organism or that the P-P factor had a direct effect on the organism itself.

Preliminary studies showed that fraction 2 had an inhibiting action upon the growth of the organism in nutrient broth. In further work upon the purification of the P-P factor a fraction was obtained by electrodialyzing fraction 2 until all the cations and the readily diffusible anions had been removed; this left a residue of nonelectrolytes and a small amount of organic acids which were neutralized by NaOH; the solution was concentrated under diminished pressure and finally dried in an air-oven at 60 to 70 C. Tests on rats showed the resulting product to be a very potent source of the P-P factor. A series of tubes each containing 20 ml. of nutrient broth and varying percentages of this product was prepared. The reaction was adjusted to P_H 6.30 (by the hydrogen electrode). The tubes were then inoculated with a standard loopful of the coccus of rat pellagra and the inoculates incubated at 37.5 C. The results are shown in table 1.

It is evident that the P-P factor has a significant inhibiting action upon the growth of the organism. Where growth did occur in the mediums containing the smaller percentages of the dialyzed product, there was a marked tendency for the organisms to agglutinate and cling in clumps to the sides of the tubes.

DISCUSSION

In the preceding pages there is described a syndrome characterized by symptoms and lesions which are strikingly similar to those found in human pellagra. The condition has, therefore, been referred to as experimental pellagra of the rat. In some of its aspects, the disease resembles those morbid states which are usually termed deficiency diseases. The tendency of the disease to develop among animals that are restricted to certain diets has been noted previously by the investigators cited in the introduction. Goldberger and associates led in presenting the view that a deficiency of factor P-P, believed to be a vitamin-like substance, is the etiologic factor.

TABLE 1.—EFFECT OF P-P CONCENTRATE (ELECTRODIALYZED) ON GROWTH OF ORGANISM OF RAT PELLAGRA

Nutrient broth, PH = 6.30, temperature 37.5 C.

Content of Concentrate, %	Growth	Time for Turbidity to Appear, Hours
0 (check)	+	10
0 (check)	+	11
.05	0	..
.05	+	11
.10	+	14
.10	+	33
.20 and .30 (2 tubes each)	0	..

Our studies have shown, however, that the etiology of rat pellagra can not be explained on the basis of a simple deficiency. It seems beyond question that an organism is the direct cause of the dermatitis which characterizes the disease. Whether the whole pathological picture can be ascribed to the organism or its products, is not yet certain; there are significant indications of the validity of such a view; the possible influence of other factors, however, can not be overlooked.

The effect of concentrates of the P-P factor upon the causative organism in culture medium indicates that the protective substance has a direct etiotropic action. It seems to be impossible to infect a rat with the organism of experimental pellagra, if the animal has a sufficient supply of the P-P factor. The amount required for complete protection depends to some extent on the number and virulence of the organisms ingested by the animal; the amount required is also in large measure dependent upon individual susceptibility of the animal. The ability of rats to resist invasion by the organism apparently varies greatly even among animals of uniform age that are receiving the same diet. Different age groups present even more striking differences in resistance to the infection; the dermatitis has never been found among the young groups in the stock colony; when it appears, it is invariably on mature rats and usually on only a few of the oldest individuals in the colony. Even in the experiments where large doses of organisms are fed, it is noticeably more difficult to produce the dermatitis on young rats than on mature rats. However, when the diet is lacking in the P-P factor and the animals' reserve of this substance becomes depleted, the young rats eventually succumb to the infection, most of them readily, all of them eventually; furthermore, the degree of deficiency seems, in a large measure, to determine the intensity of the reaction to the infection.

Whether the protective principle has any function in the metabolism of the animal other than the protection against the pellagra-producing organism, is not yet apparent. Rats, restricted to diet B with an addition of only the B-P (beriberi-preventive) factor, fail to grow. The further addition of potent sources of the P-P factor, is followed by marked growth; however, the correlation between the degree of protection against the infection and the rate of growth is not always good; this has been especially marked in recent experiments where some rats have continued to gain even after all the external lesions of pellagra, dry eschars, moist lesions, stomatitis, and ophthalmia, have become quite pronounced. Moreover, the results on stock diet 14A have shown that a diet which supports excellent growth is not always adequate for complete protection against the organism. Such results seem to afford significant indications that the P-P factor and the growth-promoting accessory factor of the vitamin B complex are not identical. Special efforts to effect a separation of these factors are now being made.

SUMMARY

The external symptoms of experimental pellagra of the rat are alopecia, dermatitis, stomatitis, ophthalmia, and arthritis, and usually cachexia. The internal lesions of advanced cases are hemorrhagic gastroenteritis, atrophy of the spleen, fatty infiltration or degeneration of the liver, cloudy swelling of the kidneys, and often cystitis. There is a relation between the character of the diet and the occurrence of the syndrome. A mild dermatitis has been found among mature rats receiving a diet which is adequate for excellent growth and reproduction. The severe form has been produced only on restricted diets.

A gram-positive coccus has been found constantly associated with the disease. This organism has been isolated (often in pure culture) from skin lesions, arthrtic lesions, parenchymatous organs, and walls of the intestines of pellagrous rats. With two exceptions the organism has not been obtained from the blood stream. The organism has been fed to rats and the characteristic lesions, from which the organism has been recovered, have been produced.

Concentrates of a protective principle (P-P factor) which cure or prevent the occurrence of the disease have been prepared from Pueraria thunbergiana. A relatively low concentration of these preparations in nutrient broth inhibits the growth of the causative organism.

OBSERVATIONS ON SNUFFLES IN RABBITS

F. Rene Van de Carr and Kathleen J. Kilgariff

From the Department of Bacteriology, University of California, Berkeley

The etiology of snuffles, a disease of the respiratory tract of rabbits, which seriously interferes with many laboratory studies, and frequently becomes epidemic, has not been established conclusively, despite the numerous observations recorded by McCartney and Olitsky,[1] Webster,[2] De Kruif,[3] Tanaka,[4] and others, recently reviewed by Meyer.[5] In the majority of instances in which careful bacteriologic studies were conducted, two organisms, Bacillus bronchisepticus and Bacterium lepisepticum, were isolated from the nasal passages, sinuses, and respiratory tree. Although it is definitely established that B. lepisepticum alone is invariably associated with pleuropneumonia, pericarditis, septicemia, sinus, and middle ear infection; differences in opinion seem to exist between Tanaka [4] and Bull and McKee,[6] on one hand, and Webster [2] on the other hand, concerning the causative organisms in acute snuffles.

In the light of these differences, we thought it would be of interest to conduct further studies on this respiratory infection, which had developed in the animal house of the department of bacteriology.

The investigations were carried out during the months from September to December, 1927. The animals under observation were stock rabbits, raised in the department. Among them snuffles had been endemic for some time. Many of them had been used by the class in medical bacteriology and therefore represented all types of experimental inoculations; the rest were socalled normal stock animals. Routine examinations were conducted on the series as follows: clinical examination; isolation of suspected colonies from field cultures and classification of them according to biochemical reactions and according to their morphology in staining with Gram's stain and toluidin blue; serologic tests for agglutination; allergic tests; detection of carriers by the use of silver nitrate; and postmortem examinations.

Received for publication, June 4, 1928.

1. J. Exper. Med., 1923, 38, p. 591.
2. Ibid., 1924, 39, p. 837.
3. Ibid., 1922, 35, pp. 561 and 621.
4. J. Infect. Dis., 1926, 38, p. 389.
5. Newer knowledge of bacteriology and immunclogy, 1928, p. 607.
6. Am. J. Hyg., 1925, 5, p. 530.

OBSERVATIONS

Bacteriologic Examinations.—For the isolation of the organisms of the nasal passages a sterile swab was passed well into the nasal fossa. The mucoid material was then thoroughly streaked on freshly prepared, 6% defibrinated rabbit blood beef infusion agar, and the plate incubated 24 hours. Colonies were picked and studied further in their biochemical reactions. It was found that certain strains of B. lepisepticum, when successively transplanted to plain agar, lost fermentative power; but if they were replanted on freshly prepared, defibrinated blood agar, after two or three subcultures they would again react characteristically with the carbohydrates; B. lepisepticum fermented glucose, mannitol, and sucrose, while B. bronchisepticus (also known as Alkaligines bronchisepticus) failed to attack the sugars.

The type of colonies of B. lepisepticum which were looked for on the plates were small, fluorescent, slightly raised colonies, with round, even borders and with centers sometimes opaque; similar colonies with somewhat irregular borders; and the same general type of colony, but more opaque and mucoid.

From 5 to 10 suspected colonies were picked from each swab culture. These were transplanted to freshly prepared, defibrinated rabbit blood agar plates and incubated 24 hours. Transplants to sugars, and smears, were made from these growths. Considerable experience was required to recognize these colonies of the flora of the rabbit respiratory tract on plate cultures. De Kruif's[3] observation that typical colonies of B. lepisepticum disintegrated when touched with the loop was confirmed in every case, and proved to be helpful. B. bronchisepticus and B. lepisepticum could not be distinguished morphologically. Both were gram-negative, bipolar rods. Sometimes they were short and coccoid; sometimes, fairly large and slender, resembling diphtheroids. They frequently were arranged in chains, and then were streptothrix-like. In order that the data might be dependable, the nasal passages of the rabbits were not considered free from B. lepisepticum or B. bronchisepticus until from 3 to 5 independent swab cultures, taken at different intervals, had been analyzed.

A total of 108 animals were studied together with approximately 500 cultures. Clinically the rabbits of this series could be divided into two groups: rabbits with typical snuffles—marked by nasal discharge, matting and loss of hair on the four paws and around the head, coughing and sneezing, and, in a few cases, torticollis, as a result of middle ear infection; and clinically healthy rabbits either carrying B. lepisepticum or B. bronchisepticus in the nares or free from these organisms, as revealed by cultures. It is possible, of course, that in some cases one or both of the organisms were present in the nasal passages, but escaped detection even after repeated examinations. The results, as recorded in table 1, indicated that in the 57 rabbits with clinical cases of snuffles, as well as in the 41 carriers, the two organisms B. lepisepticum and B. bronchisepticus were present in approximately equal numbers. Only 10 (10.8 %) of the animals were normal.

Serologic Tests.—Recent papers on the relation of B. lepisepticum and B. bronchisepticus to "snuffles," failed to indicate that serologic tests had been used to detect infected animals. In this study tests for agglutination were carried out with polyvalent serums obtained from the same series of rabbits.

For antigens, several 24 hour cultures of B. bronchisepticus grown on beef infusion agar, were pooled and washed 5 times in sterile, distilled water. The suspension used for the tests was standardized in distilled water to prevent spontaneous clumping. A similar antigen was made from pooled 24 hour cultures of B. lepisepticum grown on 6% defibrinated blood, beef infusion agar, the blood being obtained from a normal rabbit. The antigen was made as before, but was suspended in salt solution. After the suspensions had been added to the dilutions of serum they were allowed to stand in a water bath at 52 C. before being read.

TABLE 1.—THE RELATION OF BACTERIOLOGIC OBSERVATIONS IN SNUFFLES TO ITS CLINICAL INCIDENCE

Result of Bacteriologic Examinations	Animals Showing Clinical Symptoms 57	Animals Showing No Symptoms 51
B. lepisepticum	17 (29.83%)	12 (23.5%)
B. bronchisepticus	17 (29.83%)	15 (20.5%)
B. lepisepticum and B. bronchisepticus	23 (40.35%)	14 (27.5%)
Absence of B. lepisepticum and B. bronchisepticus	0	10 (19.5%)

TABLE 2.—CORRELATION BETWEEN THE SERUM AGGLUTINATION AND THE BACTERIOLOGIC FINDINGS IN RABBITS WITH SNUFFLES

Antigens	Incidence of Agglutination in Serum Dilutions of 1:10 to 1:80	Bacteriologic Observations in the Rabbits from Which Serums Were Drawn: B. Lepisepticum	B. Bronchisepticus	B. Lepisepticum and B. Bronchisepticus	Animals Free from Organism	Correlation, %
B. lepisepticum	63 present	21	16	26	0	74.6
	35 absent	8	16	11	0	45.7
B. bronchisepticus	64 present	19	21	24	0	70.3
	34 absent	12	10	12	0	35.3

The failure of a number of the serums from rabbits that yielded the organisms in bacteriologic examination to agglutinate the organisms, may be explained by the fact that the rabbits, in some cases, were probably in a state of incipient infection. It is reasonable to assume that a somewhat prolonged state of infection was necessary before antibodies against B. lepisepticum and B. bronchisepticus might be demonstrated. The distribution of the agglutination is shown in table 3.

In general, the observations indicated that in the case of infections with B. lepisepticum and B. bronchisepticus, systemic reactions occurred of varying intensity, as expressed by the agglutination reactions. From the observations it may be concluded that both organisms are sufficiently pathogenic to excite a general response to the nasal infection.

Allergic Tests.—It seemed desirable to have criteria other than agglutinations to demonstrate the systemic response to the invasion of the respiratory tract by B. lepisepticum and B. bronchisepticus. Therefore, cutaneous allergic tests were used in these studies, because of their wide applicability in the detection of a general body reaction to bacterial infection.

For the allergens, the organisms were grown in the same manner as for the agglutination tests, were washed 5 times in physiologic salt solution, and a 6th time in distilled water, and each was alkalinized to approximately P_H 8. They were then placed in a water bath at 52 C. for 3 days. The suspensions were then brought back to neutrality with acid. Tricresol, in 0.3% solution, was added to preserve the allergens, and these were kept at 37 C. for one week. Tests for sterility showed no growth at the end of this time in subculture. These autolysates were kept on ice until needed.

TABLE 3.—THE DISTRIBUTION OF THE AGGLUTINATIONS IN THE SEROLOGIC TESTS IN SNUFFLES

		Reactions in Dilutions of			
Antigens	No Reaction	1:10	1:20	1:40	1:80
B. bronchisepticus	34	8	23	13	20
B. lepisepticum	35	14	17	9	23

TABLE 4.—THE CORRELATION BETWEEN SKIN REACTIONS AND THE AGGLUTINATION

	Reaction of Skin		Reaction of Serum		
Antigens	Positive	Negative	Positive	Negative	Correlation, %
B. bronchisepticus....	69	..	49	20	71.0
	..	29	12	17	58.7
B. lepisepticum........	75	..	55	20	73.3
	..	23	9	14	60.8

Intracutaneous injections of 0.2 cc. of each allergen were made on the shaven side of each animal in widely separated areas. The results were read at 24, 36 and 48 hours. A reaction was considered positive when it showed an indurated, inflamed area, with a central necrotic zone.

Since from the nature of the study no animal could be considered normal "a priori," the rabbits which gave negative results served as controls. Tables 4 and 5 show the correlation between skin reaction, the agglutination, and the bacteriologic observations.

Although the skin reactions checked closely with the serologic reactions, it was impossible, without further study, to evaluate them other than as indications of a systemic response to the respiratory infection with the organisms of which the allergens were composed.

Subsequent to the completion of these studies, Hanger[7] reported observations, in which he noted that Berkefeld filtrates of 72-hour cultures of B. lepisepticum, B. bronchisepticus, B. influenzae, B. coli, and Meningococcus all individually call forth reactions when injected intracutaneously into rabbits exhibiting clinical snuffles. He concludes that skin reactions to gram-negative organisms are nonspecific.

In subsequent experiments we failed to substantiate Hanger's observations, using autolysates of B. paratyphoid B, B. coli, B. aertrycke, and B. enteritidis. These autolysates were prepared by the same method as the allergens with B. lepisepticum and B. bronchisepticus.

TABLE 5.—THE CORRELATION BETWEEN SKIN REACTIONS AND THE BACTERIOLOGIC FINDINGS

	Number of Rabbits with Positive Skin Reactions	Bacteriologic Observations: B. Lepisepticum	B. Bronchisepticus	B. Lepisepticum and B. Bronchisepticus	Correlation, %
To B. lepisepticum	69	22	19	28	72.5
To B. bronchisepticus	75	24	24	32	74.6

TABLE 6.—THE BACTERIOLOGIC FINDINGS AFTER TREATMENT OF THE RABBIT'S NOSTRILS WITH SILVER NITRATE

Condition of Rabbits	Number of Animals in Which Organisms Were Present: Before Silver Nitrate 44	After Silver Nitrate 22
B. lepisepticum	36.5%	0
B. bronchisepticus	34.0%	64.0%
B. lepisepticum and B. bronchisepticus	7.0%	36.0%
Negative for both organisms	23.5%	0
Clinical snuffles	0	54.0%

Detection of Carriers.—Silver nitrate (Freund[8]) was used with the principle in mind that by lowering the local resistance of the mucous membranes of the nasopharynx, a chronic infection with B. lepisepticum could be changed into an acute condition which would manifest itself clinically. About 2 cc. of a 2% solution of silver nitrate was introduced into each nostril with an eye-dropper, care being taken not to transmit the infection from animal to animal; the droppers were sterilized in alcohol and rinsed in sterile salt solution each time. The results are shown in table 6. At this time 12 rabbits (54%) presented clinical snuffles, while 10 (46%) were still healthy. The results tended to confirm the

7. Proc. Soc. Exper. Biol. & Med., 1927, 35, p. 230.
8. Ztschr. f. Hyg. u. Infectionskrankh., 1926, 106, p. 627.

value of silver nitrate in the demonstration of a carrier state in clinically healthy animals.

SUMMARY

A systemic response of the rabbit to infection of the respiratory tract with B. lepisepticum and B. bronchisepticus, was demonstrated by serologic and allergic reactions. The serologic and allergic reactions correlate with the bacteriologic findings to a high degree: the allergic reactions to a higher degree than the serologic reactions. The allergic reactions were apparently specific. They may prove to be a simple, more direct method of detecting infected or immune rabbits.

B. lepisepticum or B. bronchisepticus, or both, were demonstrated in every case of clinical snuffles in this study. B. lepisepticum or B. bronchisepticus, or both together, may be responsible for snuffles in rabbits. In manifestations of acute snuffles, such as bronchopneumonia, pleurisy, pericarditis, and septicemia, B. lepisepticum alone was demonstrable.

A 2% solution of silver nitrate was found to be useful in separating the carriers from the uninfected animals in a group of clinically healthy rabbits.

SENSITIZATION AND IMMUNIZATION WITH BACTERIOPHAGE IN EXPERIMENTAL PLAGUE

ARTHUR COMPTON

From the Public Health Laboratories, Alexandria Municipality, Egypt.

High mortality rates still characterize bubonic plague among the native population of Egypt. In Alexandria, for instance, the death-rate from this disease during the past twelve months stands at the formidable level of 55%. Recently we have been investigating the relative merits of various specific methods of therapy in experimental plague, working with mice * and plague bacilli isolated from cases of the disease at Alexandria. Our object has been to obtain information which might lead to better control and treatment of the disease in man. The present paper records the results arising from the application of antiplague bacteriophage in the experimental disease.

D'Herelle[1] conceived and initiated the treatment of bubonic plague by bacteriophage. It was natural that the question should interest him in view of his other brilliant therapeutic applications of phage, particularly in avian typhosus, in hemorrhagic septicemia of the buffalo and in bacillary dysentery. As concerns plague, after first assuring himself of the innocuity of the clear filtrate resulting from the bacteriophagy of a suspension of B. pestis by inoculating a guinea-pig therewith, and later inoculating himself, he felt justified in applying it to the treatment of plague in man. Four cases of bubonic plague were treated by him at Alexandria in 1925—the antiplague phage being injected directly into the bubos in 1 cc. quantities—with 100% successes.

Doorenbos[2] treated, with like results, 4 experimentally infected rats by the subcutaneous injection of phage simultaneously with the injection of plague bacilli.

Since d'Herelle's publication, however, little in the way of confirmation has appeared. In fact, it soon became evident from private reports,[2a] more particularly from India, that while in many cases of bubonic plague temporary improvement resulted following the treatment, such improvement was not long sustained, and the patients eventually succumbed to the disease. Before such facts the conclusion was reached that the phage employed was probably not of sufficient potency, or virulence, and pending the obtention of a phage of maximum virulence, so energetically insisted on by d'Herelle as concerns therapeutic phages in general, phage treatment in plague had better be suspended, owing to the possible risk of the development in vivo of phage-resistant bacteria.

Received for publication, June 2, 1928.

* These animals were the offspring of English stock recently introduced into Egypt, and presumably untainted hereditarily by any previous plague contact.

1. The bacteriophage and its behavior, 1926, pp. 567-576.
2. Ned. Tid. v. Hyg. Microbiol. et Serol., 1926, 1, p. 278.

2a. Personal communication to the author.

EXPERIMENTS

The phage used in the experiments which follow was a strain originally placed at my disposal by d'Herelle. It was not a strain of "maximum virulence," in the sense, as arbitrarily defined, of being able to lyse completely in 4 to 5 hours at 37 C. a 1 to 2 thousand million suspension of B. pestis in broth; it nevertheless possessed a virulence such that a few drops added to a broth tube lightly seeded with B. pestis completely inhibited growth of the latter. Further when added to a 24 hour broth culture of B. pestis, diluted 1:2 with fresh broth at the moment of the phage addition, it led to clarification of the culture in 24 to 36 hours.

A sufficient stock of the phage was prepared by this latter method for the present investigation. The clarified broth cultures resulting from the lysis after 24 to 36 hours of a number of strains (nine in all) of B. pestis were mixed, filtered through an infusorial-earth impregnated filter and then through a L2 Chamberlain candle. This filtrate remained indefinitely sterile and showed a constant lytic activity to the power mentioned.

BACTERIOPHAGE INOCULATIONS BEFORE AND AFTER PLAGUE INFECTION

Exper. 1.—To test the therapeutic effect of the phage, 6 adult mice of average weight 30 gm. were experimentally infected with B. pestis (laboratory strain 39N from a fatal case of bubonic plague in man), receiving subcutaneously in the right groin 0.1 to 0.2 cc. of a 24-hour broth culture diluted 1:2 immediately before use. Then each animal in turn received respectively 1, 2, 3, 24, 48 and 48 hours later 0.5 to 1.0 cc. of antiplague bacteriophage subcutaneously in the rump.

The animals succumbed on the 3rd, 2nd, 3rd, 2nd, 3rd and 3rd day respectively with the typical lesions and bacteriological findings of experimental plague.

This experiment established that, following experimental infection with virulent plague bacilli, the subcutaneous injection of the specific phage in question was without any curative effect. We shall see later that it was actually sensitizing.

Exper 2.—To test if the phage were capable of any prophylactic action, 6 mice similar to the above were inoculated subcutaneously with 0.5 cc. of antiplague phage, and 4 days later [3] all were infected experimentally with B. pestis (same culture and infecting dose as in exper. 1). The three phage-inoculated animals died on the 2nd, 4th and 9th day following infection; the three controls on the 3rd, 3rd and 4th day. The animal surviving 9 days lived twice as long as the longest surviving control, and during most of this time, during several days following the death of its fellows, it appeared perfectly fit and looked as if it would

3. An interval of time decided upon as sufficient to provoke a beginning of antibody formation, by analogy with bacterial antigens (Madsen: Harben Lectures, J. State Med., 1922 31, p. 52), and at the same time as being possibly insufficient for complete elimination of the phage.

survive. It succumbed, however, on the 9th day, after a sudden indisposition first noticed on the 8th day; and the necropsy, as reported later, showed that it died of plague.

This experiment is interesting because of the survival time of two of the animals in the phage inoculated series: one succumbed early, on the 2nd day; one late, on the 9th day, as compared with the survival period of 3 to 4 days for the controls. This suggests both sensitization and immunization occurring as a result of the phage inoculation.

In view of the foregoing result, and the possibility which it indicates of securing prophylaxis by phage inoculations, it was felt desirable to investigate the effect of phage when used at a considerably longer time interval before infection; also, at the same time, the effect of 2 interspaced injections of the phage instead of one.* As a control to this study, another

TABLE 1.—SUMMARY OF EXPERIMENT 3

Mouse No.	Prophylactic Inoculations (Subcutaneous)		Experimental Infection	Day of Death
	Nature	Dose		
1	Phage	0.25 and 0.5 cc. in two successive weekly doses	10 days after last inoculation	2nd
2				4th
3				7th
4				Survival
5				Survival
6	Vaccine	0.25 and 0.5 cc. in two successive weekly doses	10 days after last inoculation	3rd
7				3rd
8				3rd
9				4th
10				4th
11				4th
12	—	—	(Controls) 16 days from the beginning of the experiment	3rd
13	—	—		5th
14	—	—		7th
15	—	—		8th

series of animals received 2 corresponding subcutaneous inoculations with a recognized antiplague vaccine.

Exper. 3.—Sixteen mice of average weight 25 to 27 gm. were divided into 3 groups of 6, 6 and 4 animals. To the first group, a subcutaneous injection of 0.25 cc. of antiplague bacteriophage was given in the right groin; while the second group was inoculated with 0.25 cc. of a recent stock antiplague vaccine "Hoechst." Six days later the respective groups were given a repeat inoculation of 0.5 cc. of phage and 0.5 cc. of vaccine. Nine days subsequently one of the animals in the phage inoculated series died; the necropsy revealed a tapeworm cyst of the liver as the only cause to account for its death, thus leaving 15 animals. The 3rd group of 4 animals received neither phage nor vaccine, and constituted the control. On the 16th day from the beginning of the experiment, i. e., on the 10th day from the second inoculation, all the remaining animals were given an infecting dose of virulent plague bacilli: 0.1 to 0.2 cc. of a 24-hour broth culture diluted 1:2 before use, being injected subcutaneously in the right flank. Table 1 summarizes this experiment and the results obtained with the 15 mice finally taking part in it.

* This latter by analogy with current practice in securing protection by vaccines against infectious diseases, e. g., typhoid-paratyphoid vaccination, etc.

Table 1, column 5, shows that all the animals succumbed to the experimental infection in from 2 to 8 days, with the exception of mice 4 and 5, both of which survived indefinitely and were quite fit and well 57 days later. That these two mice were really immune was further proved by giving them another infecting dose of B. pestis on the 57th day. This, they in turn survived; four controls dying of septicemic plague, each on the 4th day.

If now, from the data set out in table 1, we estimate the percentage survivors in each group during the few days following the experimental infection, and plot percentage survivors against survival time in days, we get the curves set forth in the accompanying figure.

Examination of this figure shows that the general aspect of the phage curve is quite different from that of either the vaccine treated or the

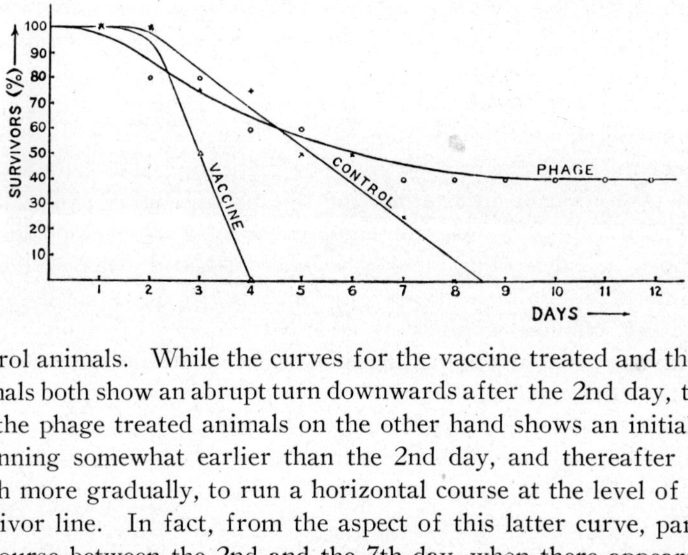

control animals. While the curves for the vaccine treated and the control animals both show an abrupt turn downwards after the 2nd day, the curve for the phage treated animals on the other hand shows an initial descent beginning somewhat earlier than the 2nd day, and thereafter descends much more gradually, to run a horizontal course at the level of the 40% survivor line. In fact, from the aspect of this latter curve, particularly its course between the 2nd and the 7th day, when there appears the dip or upward concavity there impressed upon it, it becomes evident that its terminal portion should never reach the abscissae line, but instead should become horizontal or asymptotic, as in reality it does from the 10th day onwards.

This curve, then, records an entirely different mechanism as being at work in the experiment which it portrays than in the experiments portrayed by the other two curves. That mechanism can hardly be anything else but the immunity, or resistance to plague infection, conferred on the animals taking part in the experiment by the two previous injections of the weak phage employed. And, interesting fact, even though a certain percentage of the animals succumbed early in the phage experiment, e.g. on the second day, that event in its contribution to the general shape of the curve would seem to indicate that they also, in this unforeseen way, came under the influence of the general immunity reaction which enabled 40% of their fellows ultimately to survive permanently.

This, however, is a point of such general importance, and even philosophic significance, that, although established pretty definitely in this particular study—and already suggested in both experiments 1 and 2—it will require to be worked out still more fully, and confirmed on a much larger scale, before being finally accepted. As occurring here, it is allegorically an illustration of the true case of martyrs: the sacrifice of certain individuals in witness of the truth and for the common weal. Whatever the cause may ultimately turn out to be, of this hypersusceptibility to infection of certain of the animals: whether a function of phage dosage, which is possible, or to be attributed to some other cause, are matters for subsequent investigation.

Further, this phage curve of figure 1 indicating the definite percentage of protection of 40%, following the use of a weak phage, there is every reason to hope that, by the employment of a stronger phage and manipulation of the other factors concerned—the phage dosage and the interspacing of the doses—a curve portraying a still higher percentage of immune animals should be possible of achievement, with a terminal portion running at a higher level, say, in the neighborhood of the 90 or 100% survivor line. This experiment will be attempted, as soon as a stronger antiplague phage has been met with in nature or has become available. In spite of repeated bacterial passages it was not possible to increase the virulence of the present strain of phage.

Turning now to the vaccine curve it is seen that the mechanism at work among these animals is in its general aspect the same as for the controls: from the 2nd day onwards the respective curves proceed directly in straight lines to meet the abscissae line, thus affording no indication of the intervention of any resistance mechanism of the nature alluded to. Compared, however, to the curve relating to the controls,*

* It is noteworthy that the controls here survived on the whole longer than is usual in the case of the mouse; but no doubt the explanation of this is that the strain of B. pestis employed may have undergone some slight attenuation during its successive passages on agar since its isolation some 2½ months previously, or that the animals were peculiarly fit and in good condition; they were slightly older. But this in no way invalidates the general findings, since in reality the controls all died of septicemic plague.

figure 1 establishes that the vaccinated animals were definitely more susceptible to the experimental infection than the controls, in that the former on the whole succumbed earlier.

This finding is in agreement with that of other workers. Thus, Calmette [4] surmised from laboratory experiments that protection with a plague vaccine is not attained for some days, and in the interval susceptibility to infection is increased; also, Besancon [5] states in the case of man that he is more susceptible than his fellows to plague infection when in the period of immunization.

ISOLATION OF PHAGE-SUSCEPTIBLE B. PESTIS FROM A PARTIALLY PROTECTED ANIMAL

Necropsy Findings.—That the death of the animal in experiment 2, considered as an instance of "partial protection," was due to plague and not to some intercurrent disease was established by necropsy.

At the site of inoculation a subcutaneous pocket of cheesy, necrotic material was seen, containing a few bipolar coccobacilli, which yielded B. pestis on culture. A neighboring, slightly enlarged, congested gland ("bubo") showed in direct films B. pestis, which was confirmed by culture. The spleen was enlarged, without showing any miliary abscesses; direct films were crowded with B. pestis, and culture was positive. The liver was friable, showed whitish, necrotic areas ("creamy mottling"), was crowded with B. pestis, which was recovered by culture. The kidneys appeared normal; no direct films were made, but culture revealed B. pestis. The heart blood gave a pure growth of B. pestis.

Studies in Phage-Susceptibility of the B. pestis Isolated.—The seven strains of B. pestis, recovered from the site of inoculation, the bubo, the spleen, the liver, the kidney, the lung and heart blood were tested as to phage-susceptibility with the phage employed for the prophylactic inoculation of the animal. Two series of broth tubes were seeded from a 24-hour agar culture of each strain; and to one of the series was added a few drops of phage, the other series serving as controls. Complete inhibition of culture resulted in the series with the added phage.

The phage used for treatment was, therefore, perfectly able to inhibit growth in vitro of the various strains of B. pestis recovered from the organs and tissues of the animal. In other words, the microbes recovered were not phage-resistant. This finding is of importance in that it eliminates at once any such hypothesis as that the animal succumbed from the development of resistant forms of plague bacilli.

4. Hewlett, R. T.: A manual of bacteriology, 1921, p. 475.
5. Precis de microbiologie, 1920, p. 317.

IMMUNITY IN THE PHAGE-PROTECTED ANIMALS: SEARCH FOR INJECTED PHAGE

The Partially Protected Mouse of Exper. 2.—Was the prolongation of life and partial protection observed of bacteriophagic origin or not? Since it might also be explained in terms of a simple vaccine response, the bacteriophage filtrate being known to contain the entire products of disintegration of the plague bacillus, the question is important. From the 3rd day onwards after infection, data fortunately were collected relating to the presence or absence of specific phage in the excreta and blood of this animal which permits of an answer. Since phage manifestations are, as a rule, at a maximum during convalescence—and the animal seemed at the time to have passed into that category—any evidence, if obtained, of the elimination of phage would, by indicating a superabundance thereof, afford reasonable grounds for assuming a cause and effect relation between its presence and the animal's well-being.

Some seven specimens were examined: 4 of feces, collected on the 3rd, 4th, 5th and 6th days following infection; 1 of urine of the 5th day; 2 blood specimens (from tail) of the 4th and 6th days.

The actual search was carried out as follows. The seven specimens were each incubated for 24 hours at 37 C. in 5 cc. of nutrient broth of P_H 7.4, then diluted 1:2 with fresh broth and filtered successively through an infusorial earth impregnated filter and an L2 Chamberlain candle. A series of 9 broth tubes were next lightly seeded from a 24-hour agar slope culture of B. pestis after which, to the first seven tubes respectively were added a few drops of one of the corresponding 7 filtrates. To the 8th tube was added a like quantity of a known antiplague phage, to constitute a positive control; while to the 9th tube nothing was added in the way of filtrate, or phage, thereby constituting a negative control. After incubation overnight at 37 C., the tubes were inspected for inhibition of growth. Also, the seven filtrates were at the same time incubated to verify their sterility.

No inhibition of growth was found in any of the experimental tubes; only the positive control showed inhibition. In other words, all seven specimens proved negative as concerns the presence of any active phage for the strain of B. pestis employed to infect the animal.

It is seen, therefore, that this animal showed no evidence of the presence of any antiplague phage in its circulatory system or in its alimentary tract between the 3rd and 6th day after infection, when clinically it appeared resistant.

This raises the question: where had the antiplague phage previously injected gone? We will consider this presently in the discussion.

The Completely Protected Mice 4 and 5 of Exper. 3.—A search was made from the 7th day onwards in specimens of feces, urine and blood for the presence of specific phage against four different laboratory strains of plague bacilli (all strains from cases of bubonic plague in man). Completely negative results were obtained.

It follows then, that the intestinal tract, the urinary tract, and the circulatory system of these animals showed no sign of the presence of phage at the end of 1 week and of 2 weeks after infection, at a time when it was reasonable to suppose that the animals were in full convalescence, and phage, if operative, would have been expected to be found.

DISCUSSION

That absolute protection from experimental plague can be attained by prophylactic injections of antiplague bacteriophage, is definitely established in experiment 3. Without that definite proof one might perhaps be tempted to explain the case of the animal surviving nine days in experiment 2 as one of chronic plague infection—in which the animal survived in virtue of an exceptional individual resistance—rather than as an instance of partial protection. Mace [6] defines chronic plague as that form seen in an animal surviving from one to several weeks after experimental infection, succumbing in a pronounced cachectic state, giving the impression of an intoxication, the bacillus frequently not being found in the organs. This definition provides two additional reasons, which I esteem, for considering the case referred to as one of partial protection: it differed from the foregoing picture of chronic plague in the absence of any marked cachectic state before death, and the presence of plague bacilli in abundance in the organs at necropsy; it occurred in a phage-treated, not a normal, animal, and on that account the possibility of some protective mechanism being at work cannot be overlooked.

Failure to recover injected phage, in the early days following experimental plague infection, from the excreta, urine, and blood of protected animals is significant. It indicates that the direct cause of the resistance can hardly be attributed to the operation of active phage. And still more is this borne out when it is recalled that innumerable phage-susceptible bacilli were found at necropsy in the tissues of the animal showing partial protection, without any evidence of the development of phage-resistant bacteria.

It becomes reasonable, then, to suppose that the immunity was due to some other cause: probably to antibody formation consequent on the injection of the phage lysates, rich in the products of disintegration of plague bacilli. Unfortunately, mice being animals which do not lend

6. Traite pratique de bacteriologie, 1913, p. 311.

themselves to the collection of blood, and the search therein of such antibodies as amboceptors, agglutinins, etc., it was not possible to confirm this view in the present work, but the formation of such antibodies after phage injections is well known, as established by the work of several investigators.[7]

It further follows from this absence of phage in the excreta of protected animals, and from the failure of phage to cure when injected in the early hours following infection (exper. 1), that a weak antiplague phage, such as that experimented with, when inoculated subcutaneously, tends, within a very short time to disappear or be suspended. We must, I think, look for the cause of this in vivo suppression in the tissues, rather than in the specific infecting bacteria multiplying in them; for, the multiplying bacteria being phage-susceptible, as demonstrated, their contact with any free phage should result theoretically either in their destruction and lysis, or in their getting the upper hand of the phage and becoming phage-resistant, neither of which occurs. Would a stronger phage have dominated matters and resisted being neutralized by the tissues in the presence of susceptible bacilli? That is a question for future investigation to settle. It is worthy, however, of remark in passing to recall the suppression effect recorded by Flexner and others in regard to the brain and corneal tissues of the rabbit and guinea-pig towards the ultramicroscopic virus of herpes-encephalitis. Flexner[8] states that weak strains of herpes-encephalitis virus are suppressed while strong strains can be passed indefinitely, so that the brain tissue of these animals can serve to distinguish grades of virus according to strength or virulence. It is possible that the suppression of a weak phage in vivo may be but a particular instance of the more general suppression of weak ultraviruses by tissues, thereby bringing the phage into line with the ultramicroscopic viruses in general, and incidentally confirming the living and ultravirus nature of the Protobios bacteriophagus of d'Herelle.

SUMMARY

Treatment of experimental plague by subcutaneous injection of a weak phage after infection is without any curative effect. The prophylactic use of such a phage, however, is occasionally attended by a partial protection, sufficient to prolong life but insufficient to save the animal. The partially protected animal does not die of phage-resistant, but of ordinary phage-susceptible plague bacilli. Better prophylaxis

7. Ref. 1, p. 397.
8. J. Exper. Med., 1928, 47, p. 36.

results from two interspaced subcutaneous inoculations of antiplague bacteriophage than from one. Actually, after two inoculations of phage, at 6 days' interval, 40% of such highly susceptible animals as mice showed absolute immunity. No immunity whatever, but instead increased susceptibility to infection followed the prophylactic use of stock vaccine under similar conditions. Marked hypersensibility to infection—sensitization—attends a limited proportion of the animals undergoing phage immunization, their early deaths being apparently part of a process whose end-result is the establishment of absolute immunity among a certain other proportion of the animals.

Weak phage, subcutaneously inoculated, is apparently suppressed by the tissues, in this respect recalling the suppression of a weak herpes-encephalitis virus by the brain tissue of the rabbit or guinea-pig. Failure to detect the presence of any active phage in the excreta and blood of animals exhibiting absolute immunity after phage inoculations, leads to the tentative conclusion that the immunity in question is probably fundamentally antibacterial rather than protobiotic in nature.

THE PROTEUS HEMOLYSIN

John F. Norton, Elizabeth Verder
and
Catherine Ridgway

From the Department of Hygiene and Bacteriology, the University of Chicago

The production of a hemolysin by organisms belonging to the proteus group was demonstrated by Kraus and Clairmont [1] in 1900. Later reports have been made by Glaessner and Roscules,[2] Bachrach and Grafe,[3] Kostrzewski,[4] Shuster,[5] Baerthlein,[6] Bach,[7] Braun and Choa Shi-Tsing [8] and Ecker and Brittingham.[9] Only in rare instances does hemolysis occur when the organisms are grown on blood agar plates. Such an instance has been reported by Kline.[10] The hemolysin, when present, is found in the medium, such as broth, used for culturing. Braun and Choa Shi-Tsing have shown its presence in highest concentration in 6-hour broth cultures. Ecker and Brittingham used 24-hour synthetic medium cultures. According to the latter investigators the hemolysin is heat labile, filtrable, is neutralized by proteus antiserums and is independent of the life of the organism. On the other hand Braun and Choa Shi-Tsing believed that the hemolytic activity was dependent on the active growth of the organism and were unable to demonstrate the presence of the lysin in filtered cultures.

We have studied the production and properties of the proteus hemolysin formed by 26 cultures of organisms of the proteus group obtained from several sources. The series included 20 strains designated as Proteus vulgaris, three Proteus X strains, one labelled Proteus mirabilis, and one Proteus zenkeri. Only 6 of these strains, 4 Proteus vulgaris and 2 Proteus X, produced a demonstrable amount of lysin when first tested. As will be shown later, it was possible to cause all but one of the 26 strains to form hemolysin, and we believe that this lytic

Received for publication, June 19, 1928.

1. Wiener. klin. Wchnschr., 1900, 3, p. 49.
2. Ztschr. f. exper. Path. u. Therap., 1906, 3, p. 314.
3. Arch. f. Hyg., 1909, 70, p. 1.
4. Centralbl. f. Bakteriol., 1. O., 1911, 58, p. 263.
5. Dissertation (Geissen), 1911.
6. Centralbl. f. Bakteriol., 1. O., 1914, 74, p. 201.
7. Ibid., 1921, 85, p. 305.
8. Ibid., 1922, 89, p. 139.
9. Am. J. Hyg., 1925, 5, p. 662.
10. Ibid., p. 656.

agent is a characteristic product of the so-called proteus group of bacteria.

Nutrient meat broth and liver broth at a P_H of 7.0 gave maximum hemolysin production in 6 hours. This confirms the observations of Bach and of Braun and Choa Shi-Tsing. We also used the synthetic medium of Melick,[11] as suggested by Ecker and Brittingham. On this medium maximum hemolysin production occurs in 24 hours. The difference in time is due to a less rapid multiplication of organisms in the synthetic than in the meat extract and liver mediums. Anaerobic conditions had no effect on the amount of hemolysin formed. This confirms the observations of Bach. The lysin is present in the washings from agar slant cultures.

We were unable to demonstrate the presence of hemolysin in filtrates from Berkefeld N filters. The supernatant liquid from centrifugated cultures contained the lysin. The lysin is therefore independent of the organisms but is adsorbed by filters.

The observations of Ecker and Brittingham on the effect of heat on the hemolysin were confirmed and extended. Centrifugated broth cultures were stored in an incubator and daily tests made for the presence of the lysin. The concentration was gradually reduced until after 4 days only traces were found. In 5 days the hemolysin had completely disappeared. A 30-minute exposure to 45 C. greatly weakened the lytic power of the broth, while at 56 C. there was complete destruction. At 10 C. the hemolytic power remained unimpaired for eight days and then gradually declined. After 20 days' storage the lysin had disappeared.

The hemolysin was destroyed by 0.5% phenol and 0.3% tricresol. Our observations were made after storage for 24 hours in the ice chest. This confirms the observations of Kostrzewski.

The formation of a hemolysin during growth appears to be a characteristic of organisms of the proteus group. As stated, only 6 of our 26 strains produced a lysin when first tested. The non-lytic strains were planted in blood broth and daily transfers made to fresh tubes containing blood broth. After five successive transfers 11 strains produced a hemolysin and after 15 daily transfers all but one strain formed the lysin. This strain differed in no other respect from the others.

The proteus group is known to be immunologically heterogeneous. Serums obtained from immunization of rabbits will agglutinate only a few strains other than the homologous ones. We have prepared serums

11. J. M. Res., 1922, 43, p. 405.

from seven strains, including two Proteus X organisms. These were tested for their agglutinative properties against our series of cultures. No significant grouping of strains was observed. The serums were then tested for their ability to prevent lysis of red blood cells by the hemolysin produced during the growth of the organisms. In all cases lytic action was inhibited independently of the relation between the serum and culture used. Normal rabbit serum did not prevent lysis.

Bacteria of the proteus group are pathogenic for white mice on intraperitoneal injection. Centrifugates of 6-hour cultures are as effective in causing the death of mice as are the whole cultures. If, however, an antiserum is mixed with the centrifugate the mice survive. An heterogeneous serum is as effective as an homologous serum. The same relation exists as in the prevention of the lytic activity toward red blood cells.

SUMMARY

The production of an agent which is lytic for red blood cells is characteristic of the proteus group of bacteria. The agent is heat labile, is formed during the first few hours of growth in a culture, is rapidly destroyed by phenol disinfectants, is absorbed by a Berkefeld N filter and is neutralized by both homologous and heterologous antiserums.

THERMOPHILIC BACTERIA IN CANNED FOODS

Myrtle Shaw

From the Laboratories of Agricultural Bacteriology of the University of Wisconsin, Madison

Thermophilic bacteria have been known since 1879, when Miquel described the first member of this group. Since then they have been isolated from such sources as hay, water, snow, hot springs, soil, milk, the intestinal tract of man and the lower animals, and from canned foods. Their ability to produce spores resistant to heat and desiccation enables them to withstand the canning process and, under favorable temperature conditions in storage, to cause undesirable changes in the food products. They are generally associated with the production of "flat sours."

Sound canned goods are not necessarily sterile, as the work of Cheney [1] (1919), Weinzirl [2] (1919), and Savage [3] (1923) showed. Thermophiles isolated in Weinzirl's investigation of over 1,000 cans of food constituted a very small percentage of the total number of organisms obtained. Cheney found thermophiles in canned crab and lobster only. Savage found thermophiles widely present in canned foods but considered them of little significance as a cause of spoilage, since "none of them possessed any fermentative properties and only a few any proteolytic ability. Direct inoculation experiments failed to cause decomposition." The data that he gave did not include any observations on canned vegetables.

Barlow [4] (1913) and Donk [5] (1920) reported thermophiles in spoiled canned corn. Barlow's organism differs from most of those described by others in not forming spores. Cameron and Esty [6] (1926) studied bacteria isolated from spoiled, as well as sound, canned foods to determine the types significant in the production of "flat sours." Their work indicated that 2 large groups are responsible for this type of spoilage, facultative thermophiles and obligate thermophiles, the latter being those which grow at 55 C. or above, but not at 37 C.

Received for publication, June 8, 1928.

1. J. M. Research, 1919, 40, p. 177.
2. Ibid., 1919, 39, p. 349.
3. Canned foods in relataion to health, 1923.
4. A spoilage of canned corn due to a thermophilic bacterium, 1913.
5. J. Bact., 1920, 5, p. 373.
6. J. Infect. Dis., 1926, 39, p. 89.

Wyant and Tweed [7] (1923) described organisms involved in the production of "flat sours" in peas. These differ from the organisms described by Cameron and Esty [6] and those to be described in this paper in the degree of temperature below which they do not grow and in their relative lack of resistance to heat.

SOURCES OF MATERIAL AND METHODS EMPLOYED

The organisms described in this paper were isolated in the examination of 65 cans of food, including normal and spoiled corn, sound and "flat sour" peas, tomatoes, beans, pumpkin, meats, fish, evaporated milk, processed cream, and "swelled" canned fruits.

The sound material was obtained from the local stores, the spoiled material from that discarded by the university dormitories and commons and sent to the Laboratory of the State Dairy and Food Commission for examination.

The apparently normal cans, purchased on the market, were incubated at 55 C. for from 4 days to a week before culturing. The cans that were "swelled" and those which were sent to the Laboratory of the State Dairy and Food Commission as being "flat sours" were sampled without preliminary incubation.

The top of the can was moistened with alcohol, flamed, then covered with a layer of sterile absorbent cotton, through which a hole was punched in the can with a sterile can opener. In the case of the more compact foods, such as corn and pumpkin, untapered pipets of large bore were used for sampling.

In the earlier part of the work, a number of mediums under various conditions were used for culturing the sample. Later, the observations were limited to dextrose agar shake cultures, dextrose agar plate cultures and cultures in flasks of dextrose broth in 75 cc. amounts. These were used for mass inoculations of 5 to 10 cc. of material for enrichment purposes. The flasks were inoculated in pairs, 1 of each set being covered with a layer of sterile vaseline, to favor anaerobes, if present. The test tube cultures and plates were incubated in moist chambers to prevent evaporation.

When the material was sampled, the physical appearance and odor were noted, the P_H was determined, and a stained smear was made of the contents. The P_H was determined with the LaMotte testing set devised by Brown. The smears were stained by Gram's method. Sterling's gentian violet was used as a staining agent, prepared according to the laboratory methods of the United States Army.[8] 95% alcohol was used as a decolorizer.

With the exception of the broth, the mediums used were prepared according to the methods outlined by the Society of American Bacteriologists in the manual of methods for the study of bacteria in pure culture.[9] Beef infusion broth was used instead of standard beef extract broth. For the study of the carbohydrate fermentations, beef infusion fermented with Bacillus coli was used as a basis for the broth, adjusted to P_H 7.2. Saturated aqueous solution of bromcresol purple was added at the rate of 2 cc. per liter, the broth was tubed in definite amounts, and enough of a sterile 10% solution of the carbohydrate was added to give a final concentration of 1% of the test substance. The final P_H of the culture medium

7. Tech. Bull. 59, Michigan Agricultural College Exper. Sta., 1923.
8. Medical War Manual No. 6, Laboratory Methods of the United States Army, 1919.
9. Manual of methods for pure culture study of bacteria, 1926.

was determined after sterilization, which generally lowered the P_H by 0.2 or 0.3. Tests on cultures were read after 48 hours, as results were not changed by a longer period of incubation.

P_H determinations were made on some of the carbohydrate broth cultures. For this work, a medium of the same type was employed, with the bromcresol purple omitted.

Dunham's solution was used for the determination of indol. Bactopeptone was used in this and in all other mediums in which peptone was used. Both the Ehrlich and Vanillin tests were made. The hydrogen sulphide test was made with Kligler's lead acetate agar as outlined in the manual. For nitrate reduction, broth containing 0.1% of potassium nitrate was used in Durham tubes. Trommsdorf's reagents were used in the test for nitrites. Liquefaction of gelatin was determined by the resolidifying of the culture on being placed in ice water after incubation at 55 C. for 1 week and 2 weeks.

All Gram stains recorded in the descriptions of the cultures were made from standard agar slants not more than 18 hours old.

Flagella stains were made by the method described by Plimmer and Paine.[10] Capsules were looked for in moist India ink preparations. Pathogenicity was tested by inoculating guinea-pigs intraperitoneally with 1 cc. of a 48 hour broth culture. 7 strains were tested. The strains selected were representative of the various types isolated, in respect to both source and cultural characteristics.

DESCRIPTION OF CULTURES

Twenty-three cultures were isolated and studied in detail. These cultures were obtained from market corn and peas incubated at 55 C., from "flat sour" peas, and "swelled" cans of pumpkin. The remaining cans of normal and spoiled foods did not yield thermophiles. Weinzirl[2] (1919) and Savage[3] (1923) reported isolating thermophiles from canned fruits, but no such results were obtained in this study.

The cultures fell into 2 groups: 21 apparently closely related and probably identical strains; and 2 that corresponded with each other but not with the majority of those isolated. The description of the 2 groups follows:

Group 1 (21 Cultures).—Morphology: On plain agar, these microorganisms appeared as straight rods, with rounded ends, 1 by 3.5 or 4 microns in size, generally occurring singly, occasionally in pairs (see fig. 1).

Staining: They were gram-positive. A granulated appearance was often noted in stains of old cultures or of smears direct from contents of cans.

Spores: These were terminal or subterminal, oval, and produced some bulging of the rod. Sporulation appeared within 18 hours. The germination of the spores was polar, wherever it was observed.

Motility: The organisms were motile in young broth culture, some being sluggish, other strains showing active movement.

Flagella: Flagella were few, and these were peritrichiate (see fig. 2).

Capsules: None.

Relation to Oxygen: The thermophiles were facultative anaerobes.

Nutrient Broth: In this, the growth appeared as a moderate turbidity. Generally, no surface growth was obtained, though several cultures showed a delicate surface membrane. No sediment was observed in 24 hours. After several days, the broth became clear with a distinct sediment, which had to be shaken up if successful subcultures were to be made from the broth.

Nutrient Agar Slant: In this, growth was moderate, beaded, white, opaque, glistening.

Agar Colonies: They were circular, 1 to 2 mm. in diameter, the edge entire to undulate, granular, with sometimes a rather filamentous appearance.

10. J. Path. & Bact., 1921, 24, p. 286.

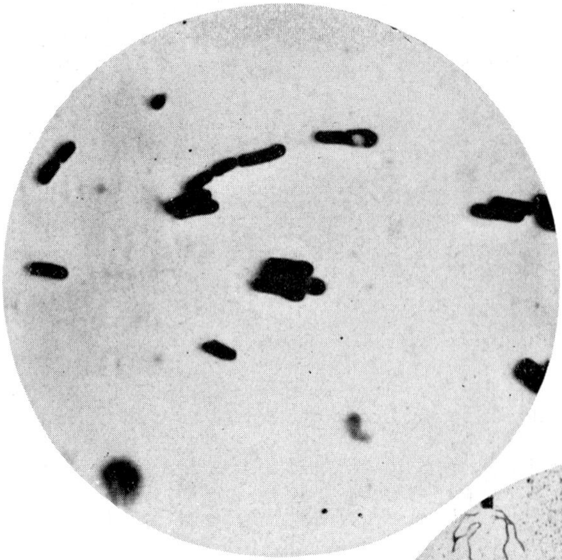

Fig. 1.—Culture 22, group 1; isolated from canned peas, plain agar, 18 hours at 55 C.; Gram stain. × 1866.

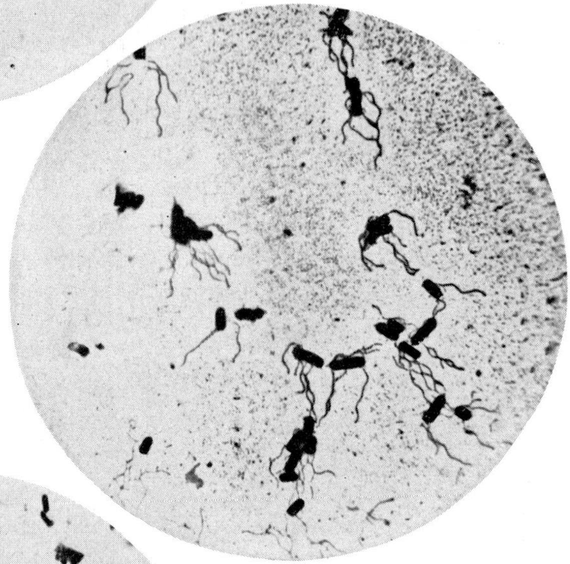

Fig. 2.—Culture 7, group 1; isolated from canned peas, plain agar, 8 hours at 55 C.; stained for flagella by Plimmer and Paine method. × 1000.

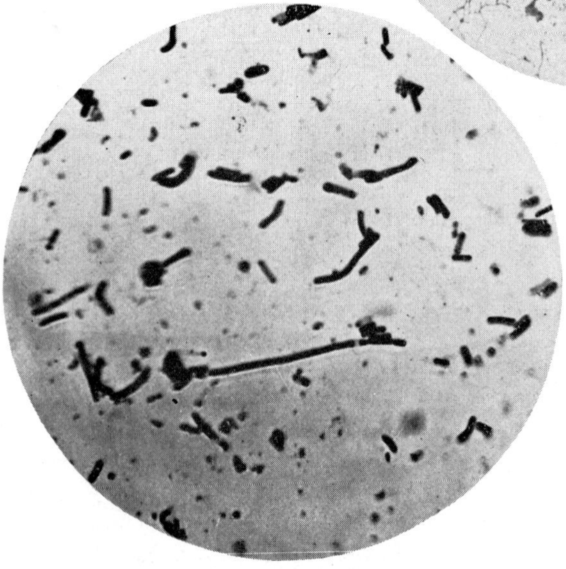

Fig. 3.—Culture 9, group 2; isolated from canned pumpkin, plain agar, 18 hours at 55 C.; Gram stain. Note variation in length. × 650.

Litmus Milk: In this, a rennet curd was generally formed after an incubation of from 5 days to a week. This was followed by some digestion of the curd. The PH of the curd was 6.1 or 6.2.

Potato Slants: No growth was observable on the surface of the potato slant. However, the liquid below the potato became turbid. This would indicate that growth had occurred, but because of the nature of the surface of the slant and because of the usually moderate, beaded growth of the organism, it was invisible. Potato slants were then made, to which a few drops of an aqueous solution of brom-cresol-purple were added. This gave a purplish green color to the liquid, which color was also imparted to the potato on sterilization. When these slants were inoculated with the organisms, the indicator turned yellow, indicating that growth had occurred.

Gelatin: Thermophil action on it was variable, but generally gave rise to some liquefaction in 1 week.

Nitrates: These were reduced to nitrites or ammonia.

Indol: None.

Hydrogen Sulphide: The amount produced was very slight.

Blood Serum: Most of the strains showed no digestion of blood serum; 2 strains seemed able to produce slight liquefaction.

Starch Agar: This showed strong hydrolysis.

TABLE 1.—ACTION OF DIFFERENT STRAINS ON CARBOHYDRATES

Reaction in beef-infusion broth, PH 7.0, containing 1% test substance with bromcresol purple as indicator. Tests read at end of 48 hours.

Number	Dextrose, Levulose Sucrose, Maltose Galactose	Mannitol, Lactose, Inulin	Salicin	Rhamnose	Raffinose
1	+	0	+	+	+
2	+*	0	+ sl	0	+
3	+	0	+ sl	0	+
4	+*	0	+ sl	0	+
5	+	0	+ sl	0	+
6	+	0	+ sl	0	+
7	+*	0	+ sl	0	+
8	+*	0*	+	0	+
9	+	0*	+	0	+
10	+	0	0	0*	+
11	+	0	0	0	+
12	+	0	0	?	+
13	+	0	+	0	+
14	+	0	+	0	0
15	+	0	+	0	0
16	+	0	+	0	0
17	+	0	+	0*	0
18	+	0	+ sl	0	0
19	+	0	+ sl	0	0
20	+	0	+	0	0
21	+	0	+ sl	0	0
22	+	0	0	0	+
23	+	0	+	0	+

* 8 and 9 slightly positive in mannitol; 10 and 17 slightly positive in rhamnose; and 2, 4, 7 and 8 only slightly positive in galactose.

Temperature Relations: As determined in broth of PH 7.0, the maximal temperature (no growth) was 70 C., the minimal temperature was 42 C., and the optimal temperature was from 55 to 62.5 C.

Pathogenicity: The organisms were nonpathogenic.

Carbohydrate Fermentations: All fermented dextrose, levulose, saccharose, maltose, and galactose. Most of them fermented raffinose and salicin. Few fermented lactose, mannitol; inulin or rhamnose. Xylose and arabinose were also tested but the results were doubtful inasmuch as the indicator changed rapidly to a brownish red color, even in the control tubes, so that PH changes could not be detected and even turbidity due to growth seemed slight. When PH determinations were made with no indicator present in the broth, the change was as great in the control as in the inoculated tubes. No gas was formed in dextrose broth in fermentation tubes. The carbohydrate fermentations of all the strains are given in table 1.

Group 2 (2 Cultures).—These strains vary considerably in morphological and cultural characteristics from the previous group.

Morphology: On plain agar, the microorganisms appeared as long rods, varying in length from 3 microns to threadlike forms 20 microns in length, as shown in figure 3.

Staining: They were gram-positive.

Spores: The spores were terminal, producing bulging.

Motility: The thermophiles were nonmotile.

Capsules: None.

Relation to Oxygen: They were facultative anaerobes.

Nutrient Broth: In this, the turbidity was not marked; surface growth was absent; the sediment was viscid.

Nutrient Agar: In this, growth was abundant, white, moist, glistening, slimy.

Agar Colonies: These were round, 3 mm. in diameter, with edge entire, and they appeared to be formed of concentric rings with a dark central spot. The inner circle had a finely granular to wavy or curled appearance, with radiations extending to the outer circle.

Litmus Milk: The litmus was reduced so that the milk became yellow on continued incubation. There was no coagulation. Milk became slimy and "strung off" on the loop. After two weeks, a slight peptonization was observed.

Potato: No growth was apparent on the surface and no color change of bromcresol purple appeared, but some turbidity was evident in the liquid below the potato.

Gelatin: The liquefaction was slight.

Nitrate Broth: Gas was formed in the fermentation tubes. Probably this was nitrogen, as the broth did not react to tests for nitrate, nitrite, or ammonia.

Indol: None was formed.

Hydrogen Sulphide: A considerable amount was produced.

Blood Serum: In this medium the organism formed light yellow colonies. No digestion was observable.

Starch Agar: In this the thermophiles revealed a weak diastatic action. With the usual test, the results seemed negative. However, when a culture was first washed off by means of a stream of water and then the plate flooded with iodine, a clear streak appeared in the area where the culture had been, indicating hydrolysis, but this zone did not extend beyond the limits of the culture.

Carbohydrate Fermentations: They fermented dextrose, levulose, saccharose, maltose, salicin, galactose, raffinose, and mannitol. They did not ferment lactose, inulin, or rhamnose. With xylose and arabinose the same difficulties were encountered as when these carbohydrates were tested with the other strains. Gas was not formed in dextrose broth in the fermentation tubes.

Pathogenicity: They were nonpathogenic.

Temperature Relations: As determined in nutrient broth of P_H 7.0, the maximal temperature (no growth) was 70 C.; the minimal temperature was 42 C., and the optimal temperature was from 55 to 62.5 C.

EFFECTS OF P_H ON THE GROWTH OF THERMOPHILES AT DIFFERENT TEMPERATURES

Temperature relations were determined in broth adjusted to P_H 7.0. In such a medium, growth failed to occur at 37 C. although some cultures were kept for several weeks at that temperature, and transfers made from them at the same time were always successful at higher temperatures. At 55 C. and 62.5 C. cultures were incubated in a moist chamber to prevent evaporation. Morrison and Tanner [11] suggested that the temperatures at which thermophiles will grow vary with the medium, and that in growth at low temperatures a time element is involved; canned goods stored at ordinary temperatures might spoil if kept for a sufficiently long time. Cameron and Esty,[6] however, kept some canned corn, inoculated with a thermophil, at 37 C. for 3 years without spoilage. It seemed possible that the P_H would bear a relation to the temperatures limiting growth, and an experiment was instituted to test the relation between P_H and temperature. Beef infusion broths were prepared, ranging in P_H between 5.0 and 8.2. At least 3 different broths of varying P_H on either side of neutrality were used in the study of each organism. Since all 23 strains were not studied at the same time, the actual P_H varied with the different cultures. Four tubes of each broth were inoculated from a 24-hour culture grown at 55 C., a Pasteur pipet being used in order to give the same amount of inoculum to each tube. These tubes were kept at temperatures of 37, 43, 55, and 62.5 C., respectively.

11. J. Bact., 1922, 7, p. 343; Bot. Gazette, 1924, 77, p. 171.

Some of the results are shown in table 2. Growth was not obtained in broths of P_H 5.4 or below at any temperature. Growth occurred in broths from P_H 5.8 to P_H 8.2. In general, within this range, growth occurred within 18 hours at 55 C. regardless of the reaction. No turbidity in the broth was ever noticed at 37 C. At 43 C., the growth

TABLE 2.—TABLE SHOWING GROWTH OF THERMOPHILES IN BROTH OF VARYING PH AND VARYING TEMPERATURE

Culture	Temperature C.	Days After Which Growth Appeared in Broth of Varying P_H						
		(P_H 6.1)	(P_H 6.3)	(P_H 6.5)	(P_H 7.0)	(P_H 7.4)	(P_H 7.6)	(P_H 8.0)
1	37	0	0	0	0	0	0	0
	43	11	7	1	1	11	2	7
	55	1	1	1	1	1	1	1
	62	1	1	1	1	2	2	1
2	37	0	0	0	0	0	0	0
	43	6	10	2	1	2	2	1
	55	1	1	1	1	1	1	1
	62	1	1	1	1	1	1	1
3	37	0	0	0	0	0	0	0
	43	9	6	1	1	1	1	2
	55	1	1	1	1	1	1	1
	62	1	1	1	1	1	1	1
4	37	0	0	0	0	0	0	0
	43	0	6	1	1	4	9	2
	55	1	1	1	1	1	1	1
	62	1	1	1	1	2	1	1
5	37	0	0	0	0	0	0	0
	43	6	6	2	1	0	2	2
	55	2	1	1	1	1	1	1
	62	1	1	1	1	1	1	1
6	37	0	0	0	0	0	0	0
	43	0	4	2	6	6	4	2
	55	1	1	1	1	1	1	1
	62	1	1	1	1	1	6	1
7	37	0	0	0	0	0	0	0
	43	0	4	2	1	4	1	2
	55	1	1	1	1	1	1	1
	62	1	1	1	1	1	1	1
8	37	0	0	0	0	0	0	0
	43	6	6	1	1	11	1	—
	55	1	1	1	1	1	1	—
	62	2	1	1	1	1	1	—

0 indicates no growth, a — indicates no tests.

occurred within 18 hours when the P_H ranged around 6.5 to 7.0. Outside of that range, growth did occur but only after a day or two or even a week, and usually the more alkaline tubes showed a turbidity earlier than the more acid ones. The temperature of 62.5 C. was almost as favorable to growth as 55 C. It seems possible that the retarding of growth at the lower temperatures, except at the neutral point, might be of some practical significance, as most vegetables are on the acid side of neutrality.

RELATIONS OF GROWTH TO TEMPERATURE UNDER AEROBIC AND ANAEROBIC CONDITIONS

Rabinowitsch [12] found that the minimal temperature for her strains was lower under anaerobic conditions than under aerobic. She stated that "under aerobic conditions the minimum was above 42 C., but under anaerobic conditions the minimum fell to 34 C." De Kruyff [13] (1910) did not find this to be true of the strains that he studied. Inasmuch as the ability to grow at a lower temperature under anaerobic conditions would be of practical importance in the case of organisms that are of the types that cause spoilage in canned foods, I studied the 23 strains in this regard. An experiment was carried out, with duplicate inoculations in dextrose broth, heated before being inoculated, with one of each set then covered with sterile vaseline. Growth did not occur at 37 C. in either set but growth obtained in both sets at 43 C. and above, and there was no difference in the amount of growth under the 2 conditions, judged by the turbidity of the cultures.

EFFECT ON GROWTH OF STANDING AT ROOM TEMPERATURE

One point most noticeable about the broth cultures of these organisms was that they cleared up rapidly after once becoming turbid, and subsequent inoculations from the broth were not always successful. An opinion had been stated that both standing at room temperature and long continued incubation have a lethal effect on thermophiles. To determine whether these factors were the cause of clearing the broth, several experiments were instituted. Broth cultures were made from 7 strains; these were incubated at 55 C., and then held at room temperature. At the end of 2, 4, and 6 weeks, subcultures were made. At that time the supernatant liquid was clear but the sediment was shaken into the liquid before inoculations were made. At the end of 6 months at room temperature, broth was added to the residue, and transfers were made to fresh broth and incubated. In all cases, the secondary broth cultures became turbid within 24 hours.

To test the effect of continued high temperatures, platings were made daily for 7 days from a broth culture kept at 55 C. There seemed to be no decrease in the number of colonies that appeared on the plates. It seems probable that the spores, which form readily, settle to the bottom of the tubes leaving the liquid clear, and thus cause the failure

12. Ztschr. f. Hyg. u. Infectionskrankh., 1895, 20, p. 154.
13. Centralbl. f. Bakteriol., Abt. II, 1910, 26, p. 65.

to get subcultures unless the sediment is shaken up. This clearing up of the broth cultures is probable evidence that the protoplasm of thermophiles differs from that of most organisms in being of higher specific gravity. The greater density may explain the ability of thermophiles to grow at a high temperature without coagulation of the protoplasm.

EFFECT OF DEXTROSE ON THE GROWTH AND SPORULATION OF THERMOPHILES

The turbidity of the broth cultures gave evidence that the addition of dextrose was favorable to the growth of the organism. But it was also noticed that sporulation took place much less readily in the dextrose mediums. Smears made from dextrose broth and agar showed few spores, while cultures made at the same time in plain broth had innumerable spores. Only in a few cases were spores noticed in smears made directly from spoiled canned goods. Subcultures were obtained, however, from 1-week cultures in dextrose broth that had been boiled for 10 minutes, and from dextrose agar slant cultures that had been refrigerated for 10 months, although no spores were detected in stained smears made from these cultures in dextrose mediums.

TABLE 3.—THE PRODUCTION OF ACID FROM CARBOHYDRATES BY THERMOPHILES (INDICATED BY PH IN 48 HOURS)

Culture	Dextrose	Levulose	Levulose-Dextrose Mixture	Sucrose	Maltose	Mannitol	Salicin	Lactose
1	5.4	5.6	6.9	5.4	—	—	—	6.6
2	5.6	5.5	6.9	5.6	5.6	6.8	6.2	7.0
3	5.8	5.8	5.6	5.5	5.6	6.8	6.2	7.0
4	5.6	5.5	6.9	5.6	5.6	6.8	6.3	7.0
5	5.8	5.8	5.6	5.6	5.6	6.8	6.4	7.0
6	5.7	5.6	5.7	5.7	5.6	6.8	5.8	7.0
7	5.7	6.0	5.7	5.6	5.6	6.8	6.4	7.0
Control	7.0	6.9	6.9	7.1	6.8	6.8	6.8	7.0

CARBOHYDRATE FERMENTATIONS

All these strains fermented dextrose with the production of acid but not gas. They also formed acid from various other carbohydrates. The change in hydrion concentration brought about by the growth of some of these strains in carbohydrate broths is given in table 3. The failure of some of the strains to ferment the mixture of dextrose and levulose was noted and checked and the same results were obtained. No explanation is offered for these results.

It was interesting to note that the broth did not become as acid as the "flat sours" from which the organisms had been isolated nor as acid as the foods which had been soured by the inoculation of these strains. This difference in their production of acid was shown not only by a difference in P_H but also in the titratable acidity.

ACTION OF CRYSTAL VIOLET ON THE GROWTH OF THERMOPHILES

Since the work of Churchman [14] (1921) had shown a parallelism between Gram's stain and the bacteriostatic action of crystal violet, it seemed well to check up on the Gram reaction of organisms described in this paper, by means of Churchman's divided plates. Considering the well known variability of the results obtained in the use of Gram's stains, depending on technic used, it was not surprising that supposedly gram-negative thermophiles obtained from other sources were gram-positive when stained in accordance with the technic described in this paper. These strains, as well as the 23 strains isolated in this study, were checked as to their reaction to crystal violet on Churchman's divided plates.

Standard beef extract agar, to which was added 1 per cent of dextrose, and crystal violet in dilutions ranging from 1 : 50,000 to 1 : 1,000,000 was used as a medium. Gram-negative organisms, as of the colon group, are not inhibited by such dilutions of crystal violet. Streak inoculations were made on plates containing plain dextrose agar on one half of the plate and, on the other half, crystal violet dextrose agar. The loop was drawn across the crystal violet agar then over the dextrose agar, so that if there were growth on the control side, failure to grow on the crystal violet dextrose could not be laid to the lack of sufficient inoculum.

Growth of all the cultures was inhibited by the crystal violet, even in the dilution of 1 : 1,000,000. At that dilution after several days' incubation, a few colonies would appear on the crystal violet agar, but never as profuse a growth as appeared on the control. The supposedly gram-negative cultures reacted in the same way to the crystal violet as did my gram-positive cultures, indicating that probably all should be considered as gram-positive. The same results were obtained when plain nutrient agar was used instead of dextrose agar.

RESISTANCE OF THE THERMOPHILIC SPORES TO HEAT

The resistance of the spores of thermophiles to heat is a factor which enables them to withstand the processing of canned goods and

14. J. Exper. Med., 1921, 33, p. 569.

to remain viable in the can. Bigelow and Esty [15] (1920) showed the relation of time and temperature, of the number of the spores present, and of the P_H of the medium to this resistance of the spores. Morrison and Tanner [11] (1924) tabulated the thermal death points of thermophiles as reported by various investigators. These varied from 3 or 4 minutes to 20 hours at 100 C.

In this study an attempt was made to find the length of time during which the spores could withstand the temperature of boiling water. 8 strains were tested. Week old cultures of the organisms in broth of P_H 7.0 were used. The number of spores present per cc. was determined by plating. The culture was shaken to get an even suspension, then 0.1 cc. amounts were drawn into a series of Pasteur pipets by means of a pipetometer. The ends were sealed and the tubes placed in a rack in a bath of boiling water. A set of tubes filled in the same way with sterile broth were placed in the rack at the same time. At the end of a given time, varying from 15 minutes to 17 hours, 1 of the tubes of each set was removed, cooled, and placed aside. When all the tubes were out, the controls were also removed. To determine whether living spores remained, the pipets were wiped with mercuric chloride, flamed, the tips broken off and sterile broth drawn into the bulbs of the pipets and the tips resealed. Each pipet was filled from a separate test tube of broth and the corresponding tube and pipet were so labelled. These tubes were incubated, as well as the broth-filled pipets, to check on possible contamination. Growth in the test tubes might be due to contamination from outside or to the escape of material from the pipet into the tube. Sterility of the broth in the test tubes would indicate that any growth in the pipets was due to living spores in the pipet and not to contamination from handling or from the outside of the pipet.

Of 150 test tubes, 10 showed growth, whereas all 150 of the pipet cultures became turbid on incubation, while the controls remained clear, indicating that 17 hours at 100 C. was not sufficient to destroy the spores in the given medium with the given concentration of spores, which varied from 36,000 to 500,000 per cc., as determined by the plate method.

INOCULATION OF CANNED FOODS WITH PURE CULTURES OF THERMOPHILES

Large-mouthed bottles were filled with corn or peas, plugged either with cotton or corks, and sterilized at 15 pounds pressure for 45

15. J. Infect. Dis., 1920, 27, p. 602.

minutes. These were then inoculated with strains of group 1, each strain being tested on peas and on corn under both aerobic and anaerobic conditions, the latter being attained by sealing over the corks with sealing wax. The bottles were incubated at 55 C. The contents of all the bottles became sour, having a P_H of 4.7 to 5.5 as shown in table 4.

The juice on the peas became cloudy. The corn darkened and had a more or less watery layer on top, probably due to the diastatic action of the organism. The darkening may well have been due to the carmelization of the sugars at the high temperature of incubation, for sterile carbohydrate mediums show a similar change on incubation.

Smears were made from all the bottles and the organisms re-isolated by plating. The smears showed gram-negative organisms, very granular in appearance. Smears from colonies and from slant cultures of the

TABLE 4.—THE CHANGE IN PH IN CANNED CORN AND CANNED PEAS INOCULATED WITH STRAINS OF THERMOPHILES

		Cotton Stoppered (Aerobic Conditions)		Sealed (Anaerobic Conditions)	
Cultures	Source	Peas	Corn	Peas	Corn
1	Corn	5.0	5.0	5.4	5.5
2	Peas	4.7	5.0	5.2	*
5	Peas	4.7	5.0	5.2	5.2
7	Peas	4.7	5.4	5.2	5.2

Controls	Before Incubation	After Incubation
Peas	6.1	6.1
Corn	6.5	6.3

* Seal broke and contents became dry.

organisms isolated were gram-positive, as were the cultures which had been used for inoculation.

IDENTIFICATION OF ORGANISMS

Bergey [16] describes no thermophil which corresponds exactly with either of these two groups. Group 1 corresponds most nearly with Bacillus stereothermophilus Donk, with the correction made by Cameron and Esty [6] as to the motility of this culture. There are certain discrepancies; although some of them may be more apparent than real and due merely to a difference in technic. The cultures described here differ from B. stereothermophilus Donk in being gram-positive, in showing evidence of growth on potato, in the production of a rennet curd in litmus milk, and in the liquefaction of gelatin by most members of the group. Inasmuch as results with Gram's stain vary with the method, it is possible that these cultures and B. stereothermophilus Donk would be found identical in this regard if the same technic were used.

16. Bergey, D. H.: Manual of Determinative Bacteriology, 1925.

The growth on potato shows an apparent discrepancy as the strains herein described also do not have any visible growth on potato, and only by the use of bromcresol purple can it be shown that growth has occurred. The production of a rennet curd in litmus milk is similar to the action in this respect of group 100 of Cameron and Esty,[6] who considered their group identical with B. stereothermophilus. The organisms of my group 1 do not liquefy gelatin within 3 days, and this checks with the description given by Donk, but they do liquefy when incubated for a longer period.

No organism corresponding with group 2 has been found described in the literature. Its distinctly viscid character renders it different from other thermophiles recorded. This sliminess appeared in milk cultures and in the character of the surface growth on agar slants and starch agar plates. Apparently, this is a new species, and, as it has been isolated from pumpkin, the name Bacillus pepo is suggested as suitable.

DISCUSSION

It was shown by a number of investigators that sound canned foods are not always sterile, that sometimes they contain viable spores, which develop under suitable conditions of oxygen supply and temperature. The work of Cameron and Esty [6] showed that thermophiles, either facultative or obligate, are responsible for the "flat sour" type of spoilage of canned foods.

In the material I examined, corn and peas seemed to contain thermophiles much more frequently than the other vegetables studied. Fruits and acid vegetables, such as tomatoes, yielded negative results. In the case of several "swelled" cans of pumpkin, direct smears showed no bacteria; yet subsequent mass inoculations in dextrose broth yielded cultures. It seems likely that in such cases the organisms isolated are not the ones causing the spoilage, since they are not formers of gas. They are due to dormant spores, which were not destroyed in the process of sterilization.

A study of the descriptions of strains in the literature shows these descriptions to be frequently inadequate and incomplete. With variations in technic, such conflicting results have been obtained that possibly identical cultures have been made to seem distinctly different.

The observation made in this study that the reaction of the organism to Gram's stain varies with the medium and the age of the culture, bears out the work of Stearns and Stearns [17] on the effect of P_H in

17. J. Bact., 1924, 9, p. 463.

causing variation in the reaction to Gram's stain. In dextrose mediums or in direct smears from "flat sours," the organisms were always gram-negative, whereas in young cultures on nutrient agar slants they were gram-positive.

When the action of the thermophil was weak or difficult to determine, special variations of standard technic were devised. This was necessary in the case of the potato slants, in which the nature of the surface of the slant was probably the cause for the culture's not being visible. Addition of bromcresol purple to the water below the potato and subsequent sterilization, which caused the potato plug itself to be colored by the indicator, was necessary to show that growth had occurred and that the starch had been hydrolyzed and acid formed.

Group 2, the diastatic action of which was weak, gave results seemingly negative with the usual methods; the presence of the culture masked the light streak where hydrolysis had taken place. When the culture was washed off with a stream of water and the plate flooded with iodine, the clear streak could be seen.

If newly isolated organisms are to be checked against species already recorded, the conditions of growth of the known species and the technic used in demonstrating their characters must have been given in the literature about them. Otherwise a satisfactory correlation cannot be expected.

SUMMARY

Twenty-three strains of obligate thermophiles were isolated from sixty-five cans of fruits and vegetables, and classified in two groups. Twenty-one were so nearly identical as to be considered of the same species, all but one of which were obtained from corn and peas which were "flat sours," as indicated by the hydrogen ion concentration. This would indicate a fairly homogeneous group responsible for this type of spoilage. Two cultures were obtained from swelled cans of pumpkin. These cultures seemed unlike the above cultures and unlike any previously described in the literature. They were considered a new species and named Bacillus pepo.

Facultative thermophiles were not found.

Two variations of standard technic were devised and used in the determination of reactions which, with the use of standard methods, were weak or indefinite. These were variations in the use of potato slants and starch agar plates.

THE USE OF PECTIN IN FERMENTATION TESTS

Elizabeth McCoy and W. H. Peterson

From the Departments of Agricultural Bacteriology and Agricultural Chemistry, University of Wisconsin, Madison

In the course of a study on the fermentation reactions of some anaerobic, butyric acid-forming bacteria, the fermentability of pectin was given special attention. It was of interest because of a recent paper by Weyer and Rettger [1] in which pectin is listed as fermented by the butyl organism, Cl. acetobutylicum, Weizmann. Furthermore, the anaerobic bacteria of retting described by Winogradsky,[2] Störmer,[3] Beijerinck and Van Delden,[4] and more recently by Carbone [5] are undoubtedly members of the great anaerobic, butyric acid-forming group. One might then expect to find some pectin-fermenting cultures in a collection of 45 butyl and butyric anaerobes, although in 1904 Beijerinck and Van Delden clearly stated that most of their Granulobacter cultures "did not attack pectin at all."

There are few citations in the literature on the fermentation of pure pectin. Beijerinck and Van Delden report only Granulobacter pectinovorum and Granulobacter urocephalum able to attack it. Donker [6] in 1926 found only one culture (his strain 6) in 4 isolations of Beijerinck's retting organism, which fermented pectin in the laboratory.

EXPERIMENTAL METHODS

In the present investigation 45 cultures of butyric and butyl anaerobes were studied. A description of these organisms is reserved for another paper. At present it is sufficient to consider them representatives of the anaerobic, butyric acid-forming group. Of the predominantly butyric acid-forming division there are 33 cultures: Cl. Pasteurianum type, no. 1-7; B. saccharobutyricus type, no. 8-28; Plectridia, no. 29-33. Of the butyl alcohol-forming division there are 12 strains—all of Cl. acetobutylicum, Weizmann.

Received for publication, July 2, 1928.

1. J. Bact., 1927, 14, p. 399.
2. Compt. rend. Acad. Sci., 1895, 121, p. 742.
3. Mitt. deut. Landw. Gesell., 1903, 18, p. 193.
4. Arch. Neerlandaises Sci. Exactes et Naturelles, ser. 2, 1904, 9, p. 418.
5. Faserforsch., 1922, 2, p. 163.
6. Bijdrage tot de kennis der Baterzuur-, Butyl-alacohol-, en Acetongistingen, 1926.

Four samples of pectin were used: (1) a commercial grade of apple pectin, (2) purified apple pectin from a chemical supply house, (3 and 4) two samples of commercial lemon pectin. Fermentation tests were made on 1% of these pectins in the following synthetic medium:

The tubes containing 10 cc. of medium were inoculated with 3 drops of 24 hour corn mash cultures of the organisms in question and were immediately stratified with vaseline. The vaseline layer served both as an anaerobic seal and as a means of trapping the gas produced by the cultures. The approximate amount of gas, as shown by the rise of the vaseline plug, and the final titratable acidity were taken as criteria of fermentation. Both of these measures are subject to error from the initial fermentation of the organic matter in the inoculum. The very fact, however, that initial growth is provided for is a distinct advantage. When positive fermentation follows, there is no doubt of it because of the large volume of gas and degree of acidity produced. When there

K_2HPO_4	0.5 gm.	$FeSO_4$	0.01 gm.
KH_2PO_4	0.5 gm.	$MnSO_4$	0.01 gm.
$MgSO_4$	0.2 gm.	Peptone	5.0 gm.
NaCl	0.01 gm.	Water	1000.0 cc.
Reaction	PH 7.0		

In order to avoid, as far as possible, hydrolysis of the pectin, a 2% solution was made which after sterilization was added to the nutrient solution to make medium of 1% strength.

is no fermentation as shown by no gas production after the first 12 to 24 hours, there is assurance that the negative result is not due to lack of growth. From figures for the amounts of gas and acid produced in a control series consisting of the same inoculum in the basal medium without pectin, the fermentation data may be properly evaluated. Such a control series including all 45 cultures has given the following average figures for the amounts of gas and acidity: gas—2.6 cm. rise of plug; acidity—1.75 cc. 0.1 N acid in 10 cc. of culture. For a positive reaction therefore the amounts of gas and acid must be well above these control figures. For example, glucose which is known to be fermented by all of the organisms gives an average rise of plug of 21.8 cm. and an acidity of 3.3 cc. 0.1 N acid per 10 cc. of culture.

EXPERIMENTAL RESULTS

Fermentation tests of all 45 butyric and butyl cultures on the 4 samples of pectin are summarized in table 1. Pectin 1, the commercial apple pectin, gave 3 to 5 times as much gas as did the control series with inoculum in basal medium with no pectin. The titratable acidity was also higher than the controls (average 3.2 cc., as compared with

1.75 cc.) and approximately equal to the final acidity in a glucose series (average 3.2 cc., as compared with 3.3 cc.) Pectin 2, purified apple pectin, gave less than twice as much gas as the control and slightly higher titratable acidity (average 2.3 cc., as compared with 1.75 cc.), thus indicating slight fermentation. The two lemon pectins, 3 and 4, gave gas from a trace to 1 cm. rise of plug and acidity averaging only 1.6 cc. of 0.1 N acid in 10 cc. These values are negative—even slightly less than the average of controls, a result which may be due to poor growth and

TABLE 1.—FERMENTATION TESTS ON THE PECTIN BEFORE PURIFICATION

Cultures		10 Cc. of Medium Containing 0.1 Gm. of Pectin.							
		Gas Production Rise of Plug in Cm.				Titratable Acidity 0.1 N Acid in 10 cc. of Culture			
		Apple Pectin		Lemon Pectin		Apple Pectin		Lemon Pectin	
Type	Number	1	2	3	4	1	2	3	4
A. Butyric Acid									
Cl. Pasteurianum..	1	7.0	3.0	0.5	1.0	3.6	2.2	1.4	1.8
	4	4.0	4.0	0.5	tr*	2.5	1.2	1.3	1.4
Other cultures......	2,3,5–7								
Limits	..	4.0-7.0	1.0-4.0	tr -0.5	tr–1.0	2.3-3.8	1.9-2.3	1.3-2.0	1.3-2.2
Average	..	5.2	3.0	0.5=	0.5	2.9	2.1	1.6	1.6
B. saccharobutyricus	10	9.0	3.5	0.5	tr	3.1	2.2	2.1	1.4
	20	9.0	4.0	1.0	tr	3.4	2.1	2.1	1.5
Other cultures......	8,9,11–19 21–28								
Limits	..	5.5-9.5	3.0-6.0	tr -1.0	tr	2.6-4.1	1.8-2.9	1.2-2.4	1.2-1.9
Average	..	7.5	3.7	0.6	tr	3.2	2.4	1.8	1.6
Plectridia	29	5.0	4.0	0.5	tr	2.4	2.9	1.6	1.6
	33	5.0	3.5	tr	tr	3.4	2.8	1.6	1.7
Other cultures......	30–32								
Limits	..	5.0-7.5	3.5-4.0	tr -0.5	tr	2.4-3.8	1.9-2.9	1.6-2.0	1.5-2.2
Average	..	5.6	3.7	0.5=	tr	3.4	2.5	1.7	1.6
B. Butyl Alcohol									
Cl. acetobutylicum	7	13.5	5.0	tr	tr	3.4	2.6	1.7	...
	5	10.0	4.5	tr	tr	3.6	2.1	1.9	...
Other cultures......	1-4,6, 8-12								
Limits		7.0-13.5	3.5-5.0	1.0-1.5	1.0-2.0	3.6-4.9	2.1-3.5	0.8-1.9	1.4-1.9
Average	..	9.7	4.2	1.3	1.6	4.2	2.8	1.3	1.5
Uninoculated medium.	..	...	...	...	...	1.1	1.1	1.3	1.5

* tr = trace—less than 0.5 cm. rise of plug.

incomplete fermentation even of the material of the inoculum in medium of initial titratable acidity of 1.3 to 1.5 cc. 0.1 N acid. For such results there are two possible explanations—difference in the fermentability of the 4 pectins or fermentable impurities in the two. The first explanation could not account for the opposing results on the two apple pectins. Therefore it seemed more probable that the pectins were impure; unless especially purified the apple pectins might be expected to contain sugar from the apple fruit. Two methods of analysis were therefore applied to test for reducing sugar in the 4 pectins. First, one gram of each was extracted 3 times with 50 cc. of 80% alcohol (heated on the steam bath one-half hour each time), and filtered. The combined filtrates were evaporated nearly to dryness to remove the alcohol; the residue was made up to a definite volume and sugar determined by the Shaffer-Hartmann micro method upon appropriate aliquots. The second method consisted of analyses upon aqueous pectin solutions. Direct tests showed more or less flocculent precipitate suggesting a reaction between the pectin itself, or some decomposition product of it, and the sugar reagent. The pectin was therefore removed from solution by precipitation with lead acetate, the clear supernatant liquid filtered off, deleaded, and sugar analyses run upon aliquots of it. By these two methods the following amounts of sugar calculated as glucose were obtained.

Table 2.—Sugar Content of Pectins. Analyses of Alcohol Extracts and Clarified Aqueous Solutions

		Glucose per Gm. of Pectin	
Number	Sample of Pectin	In Alcoholic Extract Mg.	In Aqueous Solution Mg.
1	Apple pectin (commercial)	142.4	119.2
2	Apple pectin ("purified")	8.2	7.0
3	Lemon pectin (commercial)	1.6	1.4
4	Lemon pectin (commercial)	1.3	1.2

Table 3.—Fermentation Tests on Repurified Apple Pectin

Cultures		Gas Production	Titratable Acidity
Type	Number	Rise of Plug, Cm.	0.1 N Acid in 10 Cc.
A. Buytric Acid.			
Cl. pasteurianum	1	trace	1.45
	4	trace	1.50
B. saccharobutyricus	10	2.5	1.80
	20	2.0	2.00
Plectridia	29	2.0	1.80
	33	2.5	2.00
B. Butyl Alcohol			
Cl. acetobutylicum	7	2.5	2.0
	5	1.5	2.0
Uninoculated medium	..	...	1.1

It is evident that both apple pectins contained sugar and that in sufficient quantities to account for the positive and slightly positive tests, while the lemon pectins contained practically none and gave no fermentation.

To prove that the positive tests were due to the sugar impurity and not to difference in the fermentability of apple and lemon pectins, the "purified" apple pectin was repurified by dialysis in colloidion sacs for 48 hours in distilled water. From the aqueous solution in the sacs the pectin was precipitated with 70% alcohol, filtered off, redissolved in water, and reprecipitated with 95% alcohol. The precipitate was pressed as dry as possible, washed in ether, pressed, and finally dried in a hydrogen desiccator over $CaCl_2$. These precautions were necessary to prevent serious darkening, probably by oxidation, during drying. The recovered pectin was entirely free from sugar as shown by micro-analyses of the pectin directly and of an alcohol extract of a portion of it.

With this repurified pectin new fermentation tests were made. The gas production in these averaged only 2.2 cm. rise of plug and the acidity 1.57 cc. 0.1 N acid per 10 cc. of culture. Some of the fermentation data from which these averages were obtained are given in table 3. For comparison the same cultures, representatives of each physiological group, are given in detail as in table 1. These figures, of course, indicate no fermentation and show that the positive results in the first trial were due to impurity and not to inherent qualities of apple pectin. In other words, none of the 45 butyric and butyl organisms were able to ferment pure pectin.

DISCUSSION

Such results indicate the pitfalls in the general use of pectin in testing the fermentation reactions of an organism. Unless carefully purified until free from sugar, pectin may carry enough carbohydrate impurity to give false and misleading reactions. Tests on impure pectin may account for the positive fermentation by Cl. acetobutylicum reported by Weyer and Rettger since the 12 strains of Cl. acetobutylicum here studied gave no fermentation of pectin.

The fact that the known retting organism, Cl. pectinovorum of Beijerinck, did not show fermentation here is not unusual since Donker emphasizes the weakness or complete inactivity of certain strains. This lack of activity on the part of laboratory strains is a second argument against the use of pectin in test cultures, for failure under laboratory conditions and with pure pectin may be no indication of inability to cause retting under natural conditions.

CONCLUSIONS

In order to avoid false reactions, pectin for fermentation tests must be of known purity. Laboratory cultures even of retting organisms may not ferment pure pectin under laboratory conditions.

RELATIONSHIP BETWEEN CHRONIC INTESTINAL STASIS AND ANEMIA

PAUL R. CANNON

From the Department of Pathology and the Otho S. A. Sprague Memorial Institute, the University of Chicago

Chronic intestinal stasis has long been regarded as a possible cause of certain types of anemia. Although the evidence for this view is inconclusive and conflicting, the frequent association of the two conditions warrants further investigation of the idea. Particularly in pernicious anemia, gastrointestinal disturbances have been prominent, and the socalled "gastrointestinal theory" of the origin of this disease is based on the hypothesis that undue bacterial activity in the gastrointestinal tract may lead to the formation and absorption of hemolytic substances with a resultant anemia. The demonstration that in most instances the achlorhydria precedes the development of the anemia serves to strengthen the idea through the favoring of increased bacterial action throughout the digestive tract. Before this hypothesis can be accepted, however, it must be proved, first, that there is an unusual formation of hemolytic and neurotoxic substances within the intestines of patients with pernicious anemia and, second, that there is an increased absorption of these materials.

The recent review by Cornell [1] summarizes the evidence thus far collected as to the possibility of a toxin absorbed from the bowel being the cause of the disease. Only contributions not discussed by him will be mentioned, in the main, in this paper.

Briefly, it may be stated that there are two principal views as to the hypothetical gastrointestinal origin of pernicious anemia, viz., the toxemic and the infectious. The former implies that hemolytic and neurotoxic poisons or toxins are formed within the bowel, are absorbed and in time lead to symptoms and clinical findings of pernicious anemia. The other view is that chronic infection of the wall of the gastrointestinal tract by various bacteria may lead to the absorption of hemolytic and neurotoxic poisons from the foci of infection and thus cause pernicious anemia.

Most investigators are agreed that in pernicious anemia there is, with few exceptions, a preceding achlorhydria of long duration and an abnormal intestinal flora with undue numbers of proteolytic bacteria, both aerobic and anaerobic, in the upper gastrointestinal tract. Inasmuch as many of these organisms form both hemolytic and neurotoxic substances in vitro, it is tempting to assume that such substances may be absorbed and cause pernicious anemia. It must be recognized, however, that this abnormal bacterial flora may be merely secondary to the achlor-

Received for publication, June 26, 1928.

1. The etiology of pernicious anemia, Medicine, 1927, 6, p. 375.

hydria, itself, and that the bacterial products may not be absorbed to any marked degree at all. Test tube experiments cannot solve this problem by demonstrating the presence of hemolytic substances. These or their effects must be demonstrated within the body, and there is no conclusive evidence that any such are present in the blood or tissues of patients with pernicious anemia, although the recent work of Macht [2] and of Horrall and Buchman [3] suggests that such may be the case. The logical way to decide this question is to simulate the conditions above mentioned in experimental animals, but thus far no satisfactory method of securing a permanent achlorhydria, other than by total gastrectomy, has been devised. Kahn and Torrey [4] have recently approached the problem from this angle. By injuring the mucosa of the stomach of a monkey with sodium fluoride, and then feeding cultures of B. welchii, they secured, in two instances, an anemia with a concomitant leukopenia. No immunity, such as that obtained in previous experiments by the intravenous injection of B. welchii toxin, resulted.

As stated by Cornell, most of the work has centered around B. welchii and its toxic products, but the results to date are conflicting and unconvincing. Recently, Draper and Barach [5] have reported an extended series of experiments in which they injected B. welchii toxins into rabbits, in several instances over a period of two years. Although they at times obtained a secondary type of anemia there was always an immunity developed with a subsequent return to normal. No spinal cord changes were found. These workers concluded that there is no essential similarity between pernicious anemia and experimental Welch bacillus anemia in the rabbit.

The problem has also been studied by the injection of extracts of various bacterial cultures, stool extracts from patients with pernicious anemia, etc. Lepehne [6] lists the outstanding European contributions on this phase of the subject up to 1925. Among these, the work of Seyderhelm [7] has attracted the most attention. He claimed to have produced a pernicious anemia-like blood picture in rabbits by the injection of certain extracts of stools from patients with pernicious anemia, and also with extracts from especial bacteria. Nyfeldt [8] makes similar claims. He injected autolysates of various bacteria into rabbits and obtained a blood picture which he thought was identical with that of pernicious anemia. There is much evidence, however, at variance with these findings. In Europe, Busson and Kosian [9] Autor,[10] and Moses and Warschauer [11] and in this country, Draper and Barach [4] were unable to confirm them. Sapinoso and Jobling [12] injected into rabbits the Berkefeld filtrates of cultures from the growth of stools from patients with and without pernicious anemia and obtained only a secondary type of anemia.

In our laboratory, Duerfeldt [13] studied the effects of long continued injections of "products" obtained from the growth of bacteria from the stools of patients with pernicious anemia. Nine dogs were injected intravenously at almost daily

2. J. Am. M. A., 1927, 89, p. 753.
3. Arch. Int. Med., 1928, 41, p. 482.
4. Proc. Soc. Exper. Biol. & Med., 1927, 24, p. 413.
5. J. Clin. Invest., 1927, 4, pp. 507, 529, 539; Proc. Soc. Exper. Biol. & Med., 1927, 24, p. 411.
6. Med. Klinik, 1925, 21, p. 205.
7. Engebn. d. inn. Med. v. Kinderh., 1922, 21, p. 301; 36 Kong. f. inn. Med., 1924, p. 152, cited by Lepehne.[6]
8. Compt. rend. Soc. de biol., 1926, 94, p. 608.
9. Ztschr. f. d. ges exper. Med., 1921, 25, p. 199.
10. Deutsch. med. Wchnschr., 1923, 49, p. 80.
11. Klin. Wchnschr., 1923, 2, p. 581.
12. Proc. Soc. Exper. Biol. & Med., 1926, 24, p. 734.
13. A study of experimental anemia produced with bacterial filtration, 1927.

intervals with these products for a period of fifteen months. A secondary anemia resulted, being more pronounced in the case of animals injected with the aerobic than with the anaerobic growth products. The amount of tyramine and histamine in the injections had no bearing on the degree of anemia produced. Experiments according to the methods of Seyderhelm also failed to produce anything but a secondary type of anemia. Chemical studies of the fraction considered most potent by Seyderhelm showed it to be an achrodextrin and Duerfeldt suggests the possibility of anaphylactoid reactions from the injection of this material being the cause of the blood changes in the animals studied by Seyderhelm.

INTESTINAL STRICTURES

Faber [14] first called attention to the presence of strictures of the small intestine in certain patients dying from pernicious anemia. These were healed fibrous tuberculous ulcers in most cases. Since then, Meulengracht,[15] Haden,[16] Zadek,[17] Kretz [18] and Deutsch [19] have reported similar cases. Faber assumed that a stricture of the ileum may lead to stagnation of the intestinal contents above this point and that abnormal bacterial action might in time lead to pernicious anemia.

Seyderhelm, Lehmann and Wichels [19a] put this idea to the experimental test by making intestinal strictures in ten dogs by means of fascial strips and reported that two of the animals developed the blood picture of pernicious anemia with many megaloblasts, a color index of 1.5 to 1.7, marked anisocytosis and with much urobilin in the urine. Above the stricture they found a dilated bowel full of bacteria resembling those of the large intestine. There was a high grade hemosiderosis of the liver and spleen and in the latter the reticulo-endothelial cells were stained intensely by the iron reaction. However, in the other dogs, the contents above the stricture were germ free.

Seyderhelm [19b] carried his ideas further by performing ileostomies in ten patients with pernicious anemia. The opening was made from ten to twenty centimeters above the ileocecal valve. Seyderhelm states that for twenty-four hours the fecal material coming from this could not be distinguished from that of the large bowel. Concomitantly with the clinical improvement there was a change in the character of the fecal material, which became more yellowish, more acid, less foul in odor and had a diminished bacterial content. In cases in which there was no clinical improvement, the material from the fistula remained unchanged. Seeland (quoted from Lepehne [6]), however, performed an ileostomy on four patients with pernicious anemia, with early death in two cases and with no improvement in the others.

The other view of the gastrointestinal origin of pernicious anemia is that a chronic infection is present which, over a period of years, may give rise to a marked hyperchromic anemia. This idea has been particularly advocated in England, being first advanced by William Hunter as early as 1889. Hunter suggested that infection of the tongue, teeth, sinuses, stomach and intestine led to the absorption of hemolytic toxins by the digestive tract. More recently Hurst [20] has maintained a similar view, and is convinced that pernicious anemia is due to

14. Hosp. tid. Købenk., 1895 (4 R), 3, p. 601; Berlin klin. Wchnschr., 1897, no. 30.
15. Arch. f. Verdauungskr., 1921, 28, p. 216.
16. J. Lab. & Clin. Med., 1926, 11, p. 454.
17. München. med. Wchnschr., 1926, 73, p. 2165.
18. Med. Klinik, 1926, 22, p. 886.
19. Deutsch. med. Klinik, 1926, 22, p. 1145.
19a. Klin. Wchnschr., 1924, 3, p. 1439.
19b. Ibid., p. 568.
20. British M. J., 1924, 1, p. 93.

achlorhydria, either of congenital or familial cause, or to an aquired gastritis which allows hemolytic bacteria, mainly streptococci, to pass through the stomach and cause an infection of the intestine, gall bladder, appendix, etc. He has demonstrated a hemolytic streptococcus in the duodenum of ten patients with pernicious anemia and in five with subacute combined degeneration of the spinal cord, and hypothesizes that this organism has both a hemolytic and a neurotoxic action. In a later paper Hurst [21] deals with an analysis of 28 cases of pernicious anemia and 72 cases of subacute combined degeneration of the cord in which Hurst states that in 77.5% of 28 cases of Addison's anemia and twelve of subacute combined degeneration of the cord, Streptococcus longus was found in the duodenum as compared with 20% of 145 controls. More recently, Knott [22] has examined 37 patients with pernicious anemia with particular reference to the bacteriologic findings in the duodenum and has found a high percentage of hemolytic coliform bacilli and streptococci in the duodenum. He feels that pernicious anemia may result from the absorption of hemolysins from various organisms, the absorption possibly being facilitated by the catarrhal state resulting from the passage of septic material through the stomach or by ascent from below. In either case, he thinks that the oral administration of hydrochloric acid will have an inhibiting bacterial effect.

Warfield [23] cites several cases of infected gallbladders with a blood picture of the pernicious anemia type with recovery after removal of the focus of infection. Maynard and Sturton [24] and Coates [25] have also reported cases of pernicious anemia with ulcerative colitis and the latter suggests that hemolytic toxins may penetrate an abraded or ulcerated surface more easily than through a normal one. Reiche [26] also reports the occurrence of pernicious anemia as a consequence of very protracted typhoid ulcerations of the bowel.

The present investigation was undertaken primarily to determine whether or not a chronic intestinal obstruction in the presence of a proteolytic intestinal flora will lead to excessive blood destruction. For this purpose adult white rats, 12 to 18 months of age, in most cases from the Wistar strain, were used. Strictures were produced in the colon immediately distal to the cecum as follows.

The serosa was scarified and a strip of sterile vegetable sausage casing [27] about 5 mm. wide and 7 cm. long was wrapped around through a hole in the mesenteric attachment, and then anchored with sutures. By smearing blood on the casing while wrapping it around the bowel, the surfaces tended to adhere and, later, to become organized by connective tissue, thus causing an obstruction of a partial degree. After operation, the animals were put on a diet which has been shown by many investigators to lead to a predominance of proteolytic organisms. The accumulation of fecal material in the cecum soon leads to incompetency of the ileocecal valve under these conditions and fecal material is then retained in the lower ileum. This fact was determined by exploratory operations at certain intervals, by palpation and by postmortem examination. The results of various diets will be given.

21. Brain, 1925, 48, p. 218.
22. Guy's Hosp. Rep., 1927, 77, p. 1.
23. New York State J. Med., 1925, 25, p. 147.
24. British M. J., 1921, 2, p. 685.
25. Ibid., 1923, 1, p. 677.
26. Arch. f. klin. Med., 1926, 152, p. 1.
27. Henderson, W. F., and H. E. Dietrich: Indust. & Eng. Chem., 1926, 18, p. 1190.

The degree of the stricture was determined in the following ways. The fecal pellets were counted daily for some time before the operation; thus, the change in this count after operation would indicate the degree of stenosis produced. Usually an average daily excretion of about twenty-five pellets decreased following production of the stricture, to from five to ten per day or less. The abdominal circumference, measured at the time of the operation gradually increased; and the distended cecum and, at times, the ileum could be palpated.

Red and white cell counts, hemoglobin determinations and smears were taken before and at intervals following the operation. Blood smears were stained routinely with Giemsa's blood stain.

Animals with these strictures lived for various lengths of time after operation. At death, examination was made of tissues from the bone marrow, liver, spleen, lungs, kidneys and, in some cases, suprarenals and lymph nodes, which had been fixed for from 18 to 24 hours in Zenker's fluid without acetic acid, embedded in paraffin and sectioned at from six to eight microns. The tissues were stained with hematoxylin and eosin and by the potassium ferrocyanide-hydrochloric acid method to demonstrate hemosiderosis.

RESULTS

Series 1.—Twelve rats were placed on a diet which was a modification of that used by Steenbock [28] as a maintenance diet for albino rats, This consists of

	Gm.		Gm.
Yellow corn	76.0	Sodium chloride	0.5
Linseed oil meal	16.0	Calcium carbonate	0.5
Crude casein	5.0	Milk and water, ad lib.	
Ground alfalfa	12.0		

In this experiment approximately 20 grams of fresh ground beef was substituted for the casein, and butter ad lib. was furnished instead of the milk. Such a diet, high in animal protein, has been shown uniformly to lead to a proteolytic intestinal flora in the white rat. The adequacy of this diet is shown by the fact that rat 35, after being on it for 82 days, had a normal blood picture and later histologic examination gave no evidence of any significant abnormality.

Only the animals which lived as long as 21 days after operation are included in this summary. The longest period of survival was 109 days; the average, 49 days. The general course of events after operation was as follows: the abdomen gradually became distended, defecations were scanty and infrequent and the animals appeared sick. Postmortem

28. Science, 1923, 58, p. 449.

examinations revealed the cecum greatly enlarged, frequently measuring 5 cm. by 2 cm. In addition the ileum was distended by fecal material, many times having a diameter of from one to two centimeters for a distance of from 15 to 20 cm. above the ileocecal valve. The contents of the cecum and ileum were foul smelling, alkaline in reaction, and the flora was predominantly of the coliform type. Indol was constantly present. In spite of these conditions of marked ileal stasis in the presence of a proteolytic flora, no significant anemia developed in any case uncomplicated by infection. For example, rat 19 at the end of the period of observation had a red cell count of 7,240,000 per cm. and a hemoglobin content of 10.9 gm. per 100 cc. of blood. Postmortem examination, however, revealed an abscess of the lung. Rat 25 developed an anemia two weeks after operation. The chart shows the course of events

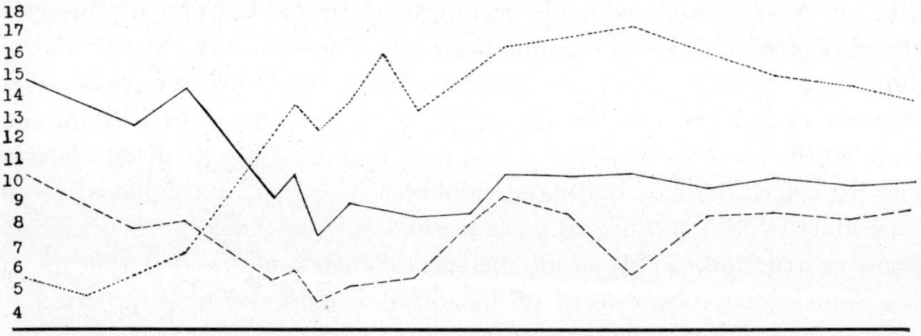

——Hemoglobin in grams per 100 cc. - - - - -Erythrocytes in millions per cmm. ......White blood cells in thousands per cmm.

in this case. The fact that as the obstruction gradually became more marked the anemia became less, speaks strongly against the idea that the anemia had been caused by hemolytic poisons of intestinal origin. This rat was from a strain in which tape worm cysts of the liver are extremely common, and the postmortem examination showed a small red nodule in the liver, which appeared to be the remnants of an old tape worm cyst. It may be that intraabdominal pressure caused the death of this tape worm larva with the liberation from it of hemolytic substances, followed later by blood regeneration in spite of the increasing degree of intestinal stasis. The rising leukocyte count, however, may indicate an intercurrent infection which later showed no traces of its previous existence. In any event, one cannot feel that hemolytic poisons from the bowel were absorbed and caused the anemia, inasmuch as the bone marrow at death was essentially normal in spite of the increasing ileal stasis during the last few weeks of life.

Series 2.—Eleven animals are included in this series, the period of survival ranging from 18 to 49 days after operation, with an average survival period of 30 days. This group was given a mixture of cooked ground beef and whole eggs with milk ad libitum in order to furnish optimal conditions for the promotion of intestinal putrefaction. This is essentially the type of diet used by Kendall [29] in some of his early studies on the transformation of the intestinal flora.

Only one animal, rat 32, will be mentioned in detail. He had a very effective obstruction for 49 days, as proved by the fact that during this time the average daily fecal excretion was less than one pellet. The initial abdominal circumference of 15.5 cm. increased to 16.5 cm. two days after operation and then gradually became greater until a few days before death it was 21.5 cm. Coincidently there was marked tympany with an enlarged and palpable cecum and ileum. In spite of this continued obstruction, blood examinations five days before death showed no significant variation from the initial readings, the blood smears showing only an occasional polychromatophilic cell. Postmortem examination revealed the cecum and lower five cm. of ileum filled with fecal material with a marked odor of hydrogen sulphide. Sections of the liver, spleen, bone marrow and suprarenal were normal with no evidence of increased blood destruction. This is all the more remarkable in that the animal lost approximately one-third of its initial weight during the period of obstruction.

In none of the other animals was there evidence of increased blood destruction, as shown by direct counts, stained smears or histologic examination.

Series 3.—Eight rats were placed on the meat and egg mixture plus a daily addition of from five to ten grams of saccharose in order to determine the effect of increased gas formation from fermentation. This diet caused a marked tendency to diarrhea. The shortest period of survival was 24 days; the longest, 68 days, and the average, 42 days. Rat 48, which survived for 68 days with increasing abdominal circumference and decreasing fecal output, showed the following blood picture:

	Red Cells	White Cells	Hemoglobin (Gm. Per 100 Cc.)
Initial	9,040,000	11,900	15.4
Terminal	9,620,000	11,000	12.3

At death, the ileum had a diameter of 15 mm. and was filled with fecal material for a distance of 7 cm. above the ileocecal valve.

29. J. Biol. Chem., 1908, 7, p. 203.

In the case of rat 44, an anemia developed during the last two weeks of life as follows:

	Red Cells	White Cells	Hemoglobin (Gm. Per 100 Cc.)
Initial	8,800,000	12,750	15.3
Terminal	6,970,000	23,200	10.1

Postmortem examination revealed a generalized plastic peritonitis with an abscess of the lung.

Rat 42 survived for 39 days. His blood picture was as follows:

	Red Cells	White Cells	Hemoglobin (Gm. Per 100 Cc.)
Initial	8,240,000	7,050	14.6
Terminal	4,850,000	20,550	9.6

Histologic sections from this animal showed infiltrations of polymorphonuclear leukocytes and lymphocytes in the lungs and under the capsule in the kidneys. This fact, together with the leukocytosis, indicates an infection as the probable cause of the anemia.

Smears from the contents of the ileum in the rats of this series were predominantly gram-negative with, however, many plump gram-positive bacilli of the B. welchii type. In spite of these conditions, in none of the animals was there any significant anemia in the absence of an evident infection.

Series 4.—Six rats were then placed on an alternating diet of meat, eggs, and milk ad lib. one day with the same plus from five to ten grams of saccharose the following day. Here again, the purpose was to attempt to create optimal conditions for the development of B. welchii in the intestinal tract. The unoperated control on this diet was observed for 69 days; his blood picture at the end of this period was essentially unchanged. None of these animals showed any anemia of any degree as the result of the treatment. Rat 112 survived for 82 days. His abdominal circumference at the time of operation was 13.5 cm.; during the six weeks preceding death it was 18.5 cm. and the fecal output was extremely scanty. The blood picture was:

	Red Cells	White Cells	Hemoglobin (Gm. Per 100 Cc.)
Initial	9,520,000	15,200	15.5
Terminal	8,060,000	23,100	14.8

Series 5.—Three rats were fed the grain mixture for ten days after operation and were then put on the diet used for series 4. This was done in order to get more residue in the cecum and thus encourage an earlier incompetency of the ileocecal valve. The longest period of sur-

vival was 51 days, in the case of rat 82. This animal showed no anemia at the end of 31 days although the abdominal circumference had increased from 14.5 cm. to 19.0 cm. During the last two weeks a leukocytosis developed with a concomitant decrease in the erythrocyte count and hemoglobin readings. However, at death it was found that the ligature had slipped down to the lower sigmoid region with a resulting peritonitis. The other animals had normal blood pictures throughout the period of observation.

Series 6.—Five rats which had been splenectomized were operated upon in order to see if the absence of the spleen would help to produce an anemia. Rat 58 was splenectomized seven weeks before the obstruction was made. He was placed on the alternating diet of meat, eggs and sugar. He survived for 91 days in spite of the fact that the abdominal circumference increased from 14.5 cm. to 19.5 cm., and that there was practically no fecal output for the last 60 days. The blood picture remained virtually unchanged. The same general course of events occurred in the case of the other four animals.

DISCUSSION

It is evident from these experiments that the gastrointestinal tract of the albino rat possesses to a marked degree the ability either to detoxify or to prevent the absorption of hemolytic substances from the lumen of the bowel. The experiments of Koessler and Hanke [30] on the absorption of histamine from the intestinal lumen suggest that the intestinal epithelium under normal conditions can render certain poisons inert during their passage through the intestinal wall. The experiments of Dragstedt and his associates [31] have also emphasized the importance of a normal intestinal mucous membrane in preventing the absorption of poisonous substances from the bowel. It is, of course, possible that under certain conditions, such as vitamin deficiency, atrophy, ulceration, etc., this normal protective mechanism may be impaired. It is also possible that in man the condition that leads to the achlorhydria may also affect the functional activities of the intestinal epithelium. Certainly that point cannot be studied experimentally until a method can be devised for producing an achlorhydria of long duration.

It may at least be concluded that under the conditions of these experiments it has been demonstrated that intestinal stasis of marked

30. J. Biol. Chem., 1924, 49, p. 889.
31. J. Exper. Med., 1919, 30, p. 109.

degree with a proteolytic type of intestinal flora may exist within the small bowel of the albino rat for several months with no significant effect upon the hemopoietic system. In that connection it might be added that recently the writer made a postmortem examination of a man who, for eighteen years, had had symptoms of chronic intestinal obstruction with vomiting spells at almost weekly intervals. The necropsy revealed a well marked stenosis of the ileum about fifteen centimeters above the ileocecal valve, due to a kinking of the bowel by fibrous adhesions. He showed no evidences of anemia and the bone marrow at the middle of the femur was yellow and fatty.

In this series of experiments there was no case in which chronic intestinal obstruction was followed by an anemia with leukopenia. Whenever anemia occurred, it was accompanied by a leukocytosis and postmortem evidences of acute infection. Tissue examinations of the spinal cord were not made but in no rat were there evidences of spinal cord involvement observed. From experiments with animals one certainly cannot accept evidence that an anemia is the result of increased absorption of hemolytic poisons from the intestinal lumen until one has excluded the presence of infection elsewhere.

SUMMARY

Chronic intestinal obstruction with resulting stasis in the ileum has been produced in 45 albino rats. Diets favoring the development of proteolytic bacteria have been fed to such animals in an attempt to determine whether or not hemolytic substances may be formed and absorbed and thus lead to an anemia.

In most instances, no significant anemia occurred; whenever it did develop under these conditions, it was possible to demonstrate evidences of a concomitant acute infection.

Chronic ileal stasis in the albino rat, with a proteolytic intestinal flora, may be present for several weeks with no significant increase in blood destruction, provided an intercurrent infection does not supervene. Consequently from experiments one cannot conclude that an anemia is due to the absorption of hemolytic substances from the lumen of the bowel until all evidences of acute infection have been eliminated by bacteriologic and histologic procedures.

A HEMOLYTIC SUBSTANCE IN PNEUMOCOCCUS CULTURE BROTH

G. M. Sickles and J. M. Coffey

From the Division of Laboratories and Research, New York State Department of Health, Albany

In previous studies reports have been made on the effect of type 1 pneumococcus culture broth on the protective action [1] and on the phagocytic action [2] of type 1 pneumococcus serum. During these experiments a hemolytic substance was noted in the broth of young, actively growing pneumococcus cultures. The hemotoxin described by Cole [3] and later by Avery and Neill,[4] Neill,[5] Fleming and Neill,[6] and Neill, Fleming and Gaspari [7] was contained within the bacterial cells and was reported to be set free by their dissolution.[7a] This paper records the results of experiments which were undertaken to investigate the nature of the hemolytic substance.

The strains of pneumococci selected varied in type and in degree of virulence. In addition to the standard type 1 strain used in the previous studies (type 1, 5) the virulence of which is such that 0.000,000,01 cc. kills a mouse within 48 hours, another type 1 strain, 124, of approximately the same virulence was used; also, a group 4 strain 107, isolated from the same case of lobar pneumonia as strain 124, comparatively avirulent in its present form but capable of having its virulence exalted by animal passage; and, an atypical pneumococcus strain 189 isolated from a horse which died during immunization with the standard type 1 strain 5 and which is completely avirulent for mice, rats, and rabbits.

Tests were made on cultures grown in different mediums and incubated for varying periods of time, to determine the conditions under which the most potent lytic substance was produced. The mediums used were the routine beef-infusion

Received for publication, June 18, 1928.

1. Sickles, G. M.: J. Infect. Dis., 1927, 40, p. 369.
2. Wadsworth, A. B., and Sickles, G. M.: J. Immunol., 1927, 14, p. 321.
3. J. Exper. Med., 1912, 16, p. 644; 1914, 20, p. 346.
4. J. Exper. Med., 1924, 39, p. 745.
5. Ibid., 1927, 45, p. 105.
6. Ibid., 1927, 46, p. 755.
7. Ibid., 1927, 46, pp. 735, 777.

7a. Since this paper went to press we have seen a report of hemolysis of sheep cells by broth culture of pneumococci in: Cotoni, L.; C. Truche and A. Raphael: Pneumococcus and Pneumococcal Affections (translation by Page, D. S., and Morton, E.), 1924, p. 16.

pneumococcus broth,[8]* this broth plus 25% of normal horse serum, beef-infusion broth,[9] beef-infusion broth plus 1% dextrose, beef-infusion broth plus 1% dextrose plus calcium carbonate and the infusion-free peptone medium of Wadsworth and Wheeler.[10]

The length of incubation was 4, 8, 12, 16, 20, 24, 48 and 72 hours, and three weeks. Each medium was dispensed in flasks and in tubes to observe the effect of the difference in area of surface exposed. Each tube and flask of culture after incubation was tested for the presence of peroxides by the benzidin-potato test[11] and the hydrogen-ion concentration was determined by the colorimetric method.[12]

To test hemolysis, varying amounts of the culture broth from 1.0 cc. to 0.01 cc. were added to 1 cc. of washed 1% sheep cells. These tubes were then incubated for one hour at 37 C., production of methemoglobin noted by color change; then centrifugalized, and the amount of hemolysis read. In the preliminary tests whole culture was used. Later, the culture was centrifugalized to remove as many organisms as possible. At present the Berkefeld filtrate is used.

With all of the mediums more hemolytic activity was demonstrated when the pneumococci were grown in tubes than when grown in flasks. The hemolysin was present after from four to twelve hours' incubation, depending on the medium and the strain.

The titer of the lytic substance as indicated by the amount of broth culture required to produce an appreciable amount of hemolysis in 1 cc. of 1% sheep cells was greatest with most strains after from 16 to 24 hours' incubation. All of the strains used produced lytic substance in plain routine pneumococcus broth in tubes. Strain 107 was the only culture which produced hemolysin in this medium in flasks. Normal horse serum added to the medium inhibited the production of the lytic substance. No lysis was obtained with any of the cultures grown for 24 hours in pneumococcus broth to which 25% normal horse serum had been added.

In plain beef-infusion broth strains 124 and 107 only, grown for 16 hours in flasks and from 16 to 48 hours in tubes, caused hemolysis. The presence in the medium of 1% dextrose, however, greatly increased the amount of lytic substance produced by the pneumococci. After the addition of the dextrose all strains grown in both tubes and flasks produced the hemolytic substance. The titer of the lysin in the tubes was higher than that of the flask cultures.

8. Standard Methods of the Division of Laboratories and Research of the New York State Department of Health, 1927, p. 87.

* The infusion used for this medium is adjusted before heating, while that used in the ordinary routine beef-infusion broth is heated before adjustment. The hydrogen-ion concentration and the manner and period of sterilization also differ from those of the routine beef-infusion broth. To broth poor in muscle sugar, very small amounts of dextrose are added to effect a satisfactory growth of the pneumococcus.

9. Ibid., p. 84.

10. J. Infect. Dis., 1928, 42, p. 179.

11. Morgan, H. J.: J. Exper. Med., 1924, 39, p. 565.

12. Clark, W. M., and H. A. Lubs: J. Bact., 1917, 2, pp. 109, 191.

The hydrogen-ion concentration of some of the cultures in beef-infusion broth plus 1% dextrose was high enough to account for part of the hemolysis present. When this broth was adjusted to P_H 5.8 it hemolyzed washed red cells slightly and when adjusted to P_H 5.0, 0.1 cc. caused 25% hemolysis of 1 cc. of 1% sheep cells. The reaction of the pneumococcus cultures ranged from P_H 5.0 to P_H 5.6. The addition of calcium carbonate to the broth containing 1% dextrose kept down the hydrogen-ion concentration and did not inhibit the formation of the lytic substance by the pneumococci. The pneumococci grown in this medium produced lysin in from 4 to 8 hours. The most potent substance was obtained after from 12 to 24 hours. As with the other mediums, the tube cultures were more lytic than the flask cultures.

Some difficulty was experienced in obtaining growth in the infusion-free peptone medium but when growth was obtained the hemolytic substance was present.

The tests for the presence of peroxides indicated that cultures when grown in tubes, where a small surface was exposed to the air, did not with most mediums produce peroxides unless incubated for 48 hours or longer. The tube cultures contained the most potent lytic substances. Traces of peroxides were found in the tube cultures of strains 5, 107, and 189 after incubation periods of four, eight, and twelve hours in beef-infusion broth plus 1% dextrose, plus calcium carbonate. These broth cultures were actively hemolytic during the time the peroxides were demonstrated and continued to be so when the peroxides had disappeared after longer incubation periods. When peroxides were present in large amounts, the titer of the lytic substance was low.

That the ability of a strain of pneumococcus to produce methemoglobin was related in any way to the production of the lytic substance was not demonstrated. In many of the titrations the change to methemoglobin did not take place in the tubes containing the smaller amounts of culture broth while marked hemolysis was present. The ability to produce methemoglobin often appeared earlier than the lytic substance and persisted after the hemolysin had disappeared. Color change was the criterion by which methemoglobin production was determined. No spectroscopic readings were made.

With none of the mediums tested did any hemolysis occur in the uninoculated controls.

Tests were also made to determine the active part of the whole broth culture. With the supernatant fluid after centrifugalization, the amount of hemolysis was approximately the same as with the whole culture. The organisms resuspended in broth also produced hemolysis in red cells but less in amount. The results with the Berkefeld filtrate varied. Some candles held back practically all of the hemolytic substance while others held back very little, even though subcultures of 1.0 cc. of the filtrate in broth showed that the candle was not defective.

Since the most potent lytic substance was produced by pneumococci which had grown for from 12 to 24 hours in beef-infusion broth plus 1% dextrose plus calcium carbonate, with a small surface exposed to the air, the hemolysin used in the remaining experiments was obtained by growing the pneumococcus strains in this medium for 18 hours, and filtering through a Berkefeld N filter.

PROPERTIES OF THE HEMOLYTIC SUBSTANCE

Heating at 45 C. for 30 minutes lessened to some extent the hemolytic activity of the culture filtrates of all strains except 124. After 30 minutes at 50 C., culture broth from type 1 strain 5 was no longer hemolytic, while after 30 minutes at 55 C. no hemolysis was produced by the culture broth of any of the strains.

The activity of the hemolytic substance is diminished by standing at cold-room temperature. After one week in the cold room in a rubber-stoppered bottle, a noticeable lessening of the hemolytic property had occurred. After two weeks the lytic action on red cells was still less but had not completely disappeared. Tests were not made after longer intervals of time. After standing for 24 hours in a warm room at approximately 37 C. in a rubber-stoppered tube, the hemolytic substance in the culture broth had lost much of its activity.

Absorption of the hemolytic substance by red cells was almost complete. The usual amount of red cells, 1 cc. of a 1% suspension, was added to amounts of culture broth, from 1.0 cc. to 0.01 cc., and left at cold-room temperature for one hour. Slight hemolysis had taken place in the 1.0-cc. and 0.1-cc. tubes. The cells and supernatant broth were then separated. No further hemolysis took place at 37 C. when fresh cells were added to the tubes of absorbed culture broth, while the amount of lysis of the red cells used to absorb the substance when resuspended in salt solution and incubated at 37 C. approximated very closely that in the unabsorbed culture broth.

Stroma of red cells also completely absorbed the hemolytic substance from the culture broth. Stroma from 25 cc. of horse blood were used to each 2 cc. of culture broth and incubated at 37 C. for one and a half hours. Before absorption 25% hemolysis of 1 cc. of 1% sheep cells was caused by 0.05 cc. of type 1 strain 5, 25% with 0.02 cc. of strain 124, 25% with 0.05 cc. of strain 107, and 50% with 0.02 cc. of strain 189. After absorption with stroma there was no hemolysis with 1.0 cc. of the culture broth of any of the strains.

Leukocytes obtained by the injection of aleuronat in the peritoneal cavity of guinea-pigs were also used to absorb the hemolytic substance. The small number of red cells present were removed as completely as possible. Aleuronat alone under the same conditions did not absorb the substance from the culture broth. The culture filtrate before absorption contained sufficient hemolytic substance to cause 25% hemolysis of 1 cc. of 1% cells with 0.05 cc. of filtrate. After absorption no hemolysis was obtained with 1.0 cc.

The hemolytic substance was also absorbed by shaking with animal charcoal and with alumina. Shaking alone, however, greatly reduced the lytic titer of the culture broth.

Normal horse serum actively inhibits the lysis of red cells by the culture broth. In a dilution of 1 : 10 the hemolytic property of 1.0 cc. of the culture broth was completely inhibited, while traces of inhibition were still found with a dilution of 1 : 400. The inhibitory effect of pneumococcus immune serum, however, is very much greater. A dilution of 1 : 1000 completely inhibited the hemolytic activity of 1.0 cc. of culture filtrate. An immune horse serum produced against type 1 strain 5 was used. This serum proved nearly as effective with the group 4 and with the atypical organism as with its homologous strain.

From the limited number of tests made with a heterologous serum it would appear that the inhibitory effect is species rather than type specific.

SUMMARY

There is present in the culture broth of pneumococcus strains of different types and degrees of virulence, a substance which has a lytic action on red blood cells. This substance was produced when pneumococci were grown in several different mediums and appeared after from 4 to 12 hours' incubation depending on the medium and the strain. The most potent substance was obtained when the pneumococcus strains were grown in beef-infusion broth plus 1% dextrose, plus calcium carbonate with a small surface exposed to the air.

The hemolytic substance is thermolabile and is destroyed by heating for thirty minutes at 55 C. Its activity is diminished by standing at cold-room temperature and, in a shorter time at 37 C. The hemolytic substance may be absorbed from the culture broth by sheep red cells, horse stroma, guinea-pig leukocytes, animal charcoal, and alumina.

Normal horse serum has an inhibitory effect on the hemolytic power of the substance while pneumococcus immune serum has a much more marked effect.

STUDIES ON BOTULINUS TOXIN

5. INFLUENCE OF NITROGENOUS AND LIPOID COMPOUNDS ON THE POTENCY OF BOTULINUS TOXIN

E. WAGNER SOMMER AND H. SOMMER

From the George Williams Hooper Foundation for Medical Research, University of California San Francisco

It has been frequently observed that animals succumb to injections of a mixture of botulinus toxin and nonspecific antitoxin in a shorter time than animals receiving the toxin alone. The same effect has been observed also when normal serum (Leuchs,[1] Bitter,[2] Coleman,[3] Bronfenbrenner,[4] Jensen [5] or leukocytes (Coleman [3]) have been inoculated simultaneously with the toxin. These observations tend to show that the addition of certain substances to botulinus toxin may increase its potency. In fact, Leuchs and Amako [6] demonstrated a similar adjuvant action on the poison by peptone, and Bronfenbrenner [4] found that its toxicity was enhanced by ordinary broth.

No quantitative tests were recorded by the workers mentioned. We undertook therefore to measure the increase in potency of botulinus toxin, type A, on the addition to it of various nitrogenous and lipoid compounds. We were also interested to ascertain whether the enhancing action occurred immediately or only after incubation; temperatures of 28 and 37 C. were chosen. Dernby and Walbum [7] had found that the titer of diphtheria toxin was increased after its contact with an equal amount of broth for 5 hours at 37 C., so that the MLD of 0.006 cc. was reduced to 0.001 cc. Dilution of the poison in 4% peptone solution and subsequent incubation of the mixture for 6 hours decreased the lethal dose from 0.005 cc. to 0.002 cc. Determinations after 18 hours showed a loss in potency. On the basis of these and earlier experiments Dernby and Walbum had formulated the protoxin and toxinase theories, explaining the formation of diphtheria toxin. These hypotheses will be discussed in connection with the results of the experiments with botulinus toxin reported in this paper.

Received for publication, June 29, 1928.

1. Ztschr. f. Hyg. u. Infectionskrankh., 1910, 65, p. 55.
2. Ergebn. d. allg. Pathol. u. Path. Anat., 1921, 19, p. 781.
3. J. Infect. Dis., 1924, 34, p. 614.
4. Proc. Soc. Exper. Biol. & Med., 1924, 21, p. 318.
5. J. Infect. Dis., 1926, 39, p. 413.
6. Kolle-Wassermann: Handb. d. pathog. Mikroorg. 1912, 4, p. 943.
7. Biochem. Ztschr., 1923, 138, p. 505.

EXPERIMENTS

Sources of Toxin.—Toxins 1, 2 and 3 were beefheart peptone cultures of strain 97 Cl. botulinum, type A, which had been incubated for from 14 to 15 days, filtered through paper, and stored in the icebox with phenol as a preservative. Toxin 1 was passed through an F Chamberland filter. Toxin 4 was a purified dry product prepared according to E. W. Sommer, H. Sommer, and K. F. Meyer.[8]

Toxin Measurements.—Each sample was tested by injecting intraperitoneally, into mice and guinea-pigs, from 3 to 5 different dilutions of the toxin; that dilution of the poison which in a given amount (1 cc.) killed a mouse in 48, or a guinea-pig in 96 hours was considered the MLD. Since the titers frequently had to be judged from only 2 animals, the values in the charts are to be considered approximate.

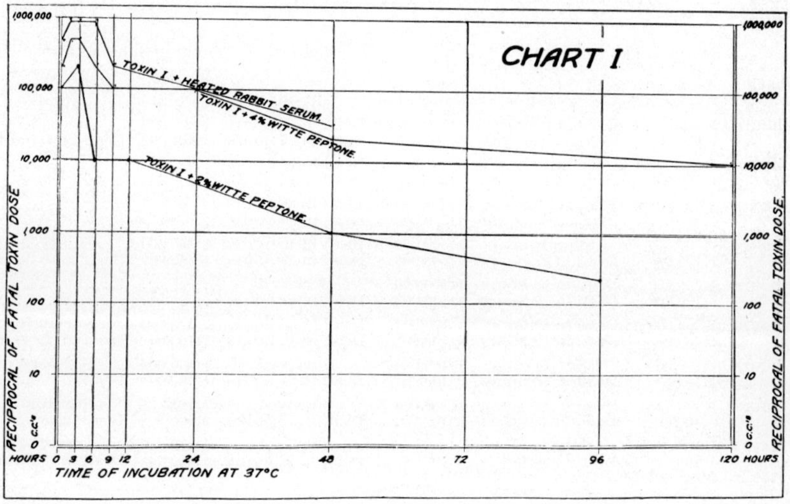

Exper. 1.—Equal parts of toxin 1 and a 2% solution of Witte's peptone * were mixed and incubated at 37 C. and samples of the mixture removed at intervals, as indicated in chart 1. For tests of the toxicity of the mixture various dilutions of the samples were made in salt solution. Results: Before the incubation, 1 cc. of the toxin-peptone mixture in the dilution of 1:100,000 fatally intoxicated a mouse in 36 hours, whereas the animal receiving 1 cc. of the mixture in dilution of 1:200,000 survived. After 3 hours' incubation, the titer increased so that the dilution of 1:200,000 killed in less than 36 hours while a dilution of 1:500,000 was not lethal. In subsequent determinations

8. J. Infect. Dis., 1926, 39, p. 345.

* If necessary the peptone and the "Aminoid" solutions were adjusted to neutrality before mixing with the toxin.

(at 6, 12 and 20 hours) the potency was found to have decreased until it was far below the original titer.

The toxin was next diluted with a 4% solution of Witte's peptone and incubated. One cc. samples of these dilutions were inoculated so that the mice uniformly received 1 cc. each of the 4% peptone solution. Results: The initial titer of the mixture was 1: 200,000. After 1½ hours' incubation, it was 1: 500,000 (causing death in 30 hours). After 3 hours' incubation, the titer was exactly 1: 500,000.

In order to test the effect of serum on botulinus poison, dilutions of toxin 1 were made with fresh rabbit serum and incubated. Before the

TABLE 1.—THE INCREASED POTENCY OF BOTULINUS TOXIN INCUBATED WITH HORSE SERUM

	Toxin + Horse Serum		Toxin + Horse Serum Heated		Toxin + Salt Solution	
Incubation at 37 C.	Dilution Inoculated *	Result	Dilution Inoculated	Result	Dilution Inoculated	Result
0 hours	1:500,000	Symptoms	1:1,000,000	Dead in 48 hours	1:500,000	Survived
	1:100,000	Dead in 24 hours	1:500,000	Dead in 22 hours	1:100,000	Dead in 30 hours
1½ hours	1:1,000,000	Dead in 48 hours	1:1,000,000	Dead in 72 hours	....	....
	1:500,000	Dead in 24 hours	1:500,000	Dead in 72 hours	....	....
3 hours	1:1,000,000	Symptoms	1:1,000,000	Dead in 36 hours	....	....
	1:500,000	Dead in 36 hours	1:500,000	Dead in 36 hours	....	....
6 hours	1:500,000	Symptoms	1:500,000	Dead in 40 hours	1:500,000	Survived
	1:100,000	Dead in 27 hours	1:100,000	Dead in 36 hours	1:100,000	Dead in 80 hours
9 hours	1:500,000	Dead in 63 hours	1:500,000	Survived	....	....
	1:100,000	Dead in 22 hours	1:100,000	Dead in 63 hours	....	....
14 hours	1:100,000	Dead in 36 hours	1:100,000	Dead in 36 hours	1:100,000	Survived
	1:10,000	Dead in 10 hours	1:10,000	Dead in 12 hours	1:10,000	Dead in 60 hours
24 hours	1:100,000	Survived	1:100,000	Survived	1:100,000	Survived
	1:10,000	Dead in 30 hours	1:10,000	Dead in 24 hours	1:10,000	Dead in 48 hours
48 hours	1:100,000	Dead in 72 hours	1:100,000	Survived	1:1000	Survived
	1:10,000	Dead in 48 hours	1:10,000	Dead in 72 hours	1:100	Dead in 48 hours
7 days	1:1000	Survived	1:1000	Survived	1:100	Survived
	1:100	Dead in 44 hours	1:100	Dead in 72 hours	1:10	Dead in 28 hours

* Three or four mice were injected for the determination of 1 MLD. Only the results in the 2 that gave the most significant ones are recorded in the table.

dilutions were tested they were further diluted with salt solution to such an extent that each inoculum contained only 0.1 cc. of serum. Results: At the start of the experiment 1 cc. of the serum-toxin mixture in a dilution of 1: 500,000 killed a mouse in 32 hours. After 1½, 3, and 6 hours' incubation at 37 C., it killed in less than 20, 19, and 24 hours, respectively, while 1 cc. of the mixture in a dilution of 1: 1,000,000 invariably produced severe symptoms for several days, after which the animals recovered. A value of 1: 750,000 was chosen as an approximate MLD (chart 1).

Exper. 2.—The effect of horse serum on toxin 2 was tested in the following series: 30 cc. toxin + 30 cc. horse serum; 30 cc. toxin + 30 cc. horse serum heated ½ hour at 60 C.; and 30 cc. toxin + 30 cc. salt solution. The samples were removed and after proper dilution were injected at the intervals indicated in table 1 and chart 2. Results: The original saline-toxin titer, >200,000 mouse MLD per cc., was immediately increased by the addition of the serum. In subsequent tests the titer of the toxin held in heated and unheated serum was higher (at 3, 6, and 9 hours) and equal to that of the original salt dilution (at 14 hours).

A similar experiment made with normal rabbit serum and toxin 2 also showed a definite increase of potency in this mixture over that of the saline control (chart 2B).

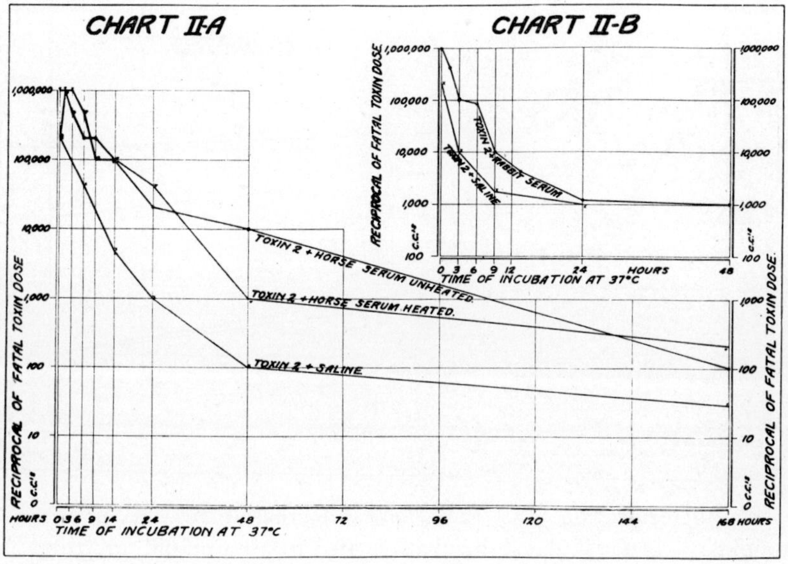

Exper. 3.—Toxin 2 and toxin 3 were incubated each with an equal amount of a 25% solution of aminoids (a commercial protein hydrolysate, biuret free). The control contained a corresponding amount of salt solution. The data of these experiments are shown in chart 3.

Results: There was an increase in potency of toxin 2 in aminoids over that of the salt control. The drop in titer on the 3rd and 6th hour of incubation may be more apparent than real, since the mice receiving the dilutions of 1 : 500,000 had marked symptoms in both cases and those inoculated with a dilution of 1 : 100,000 died in less than 48 hours. On the 9th and 15th hour the toxin dilution of 1 : 500,000 killed in 40 and 36 hours, respectively. The chart also shows that one of the salt solution controls acquired a slight rise in toxin titer. This behavior of the control is the only example of its kind which has been encountered in the numerous tests with an unfiltered toxin. It may, in all probability, be explained by the variable susceptibility of the test animals.

There was no apparent increase in the potency of toxin 3 plus aminoids prior to incubation; however, an indication of a slight rise in titer was observed on the 14th and 24th hour; mice receiving 1 cc. of a dilution of 1 : 100,000 at these time intervals died in 20 and 26 hours, respectively, whereas those inoculated in the first four determinations died in 48 hours.

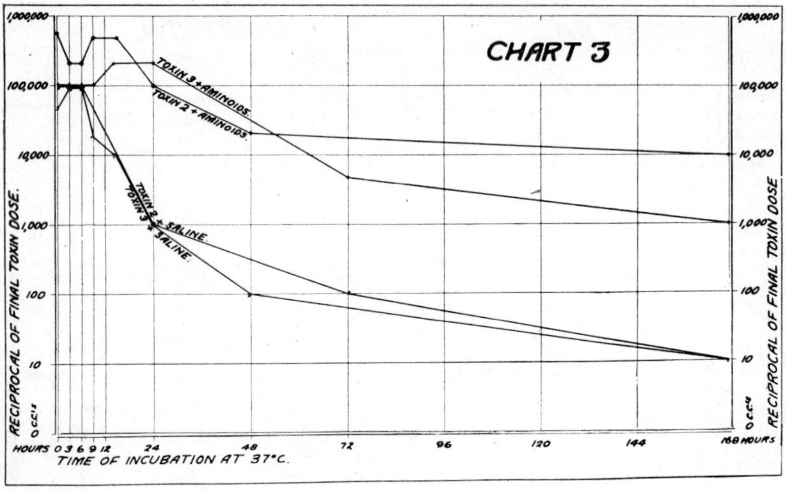

The deterioration was remarkably decreased by the presence of aminoids. After 7 days' incubation the toxin-aminoid mixtures had titers of 1 : 10,000 and 1 : 1000, while the potency of the saline controls had dropped to 1 : 10.

Exper. 4.—In order to eliminate as far as possible the nonspecific substances of the culture fluid, a purified dried toxin was used in the next series. Twenty mg. of toxin 4 were dissolved in 10 cc. of salt solution and dilutions of 1 : 10 and 1 : 100 were made in normal horse serum, 4% Witte's peptone solution, and salt solution. Incubation took place at 28 C. The tests were made on guinea-pigs. Results: The addition of serum and peptone caused an immediate increase in potency of the purified toxin. Prolonged incubation for 96 hours intensified the toxicity of the serum-toxin mixture, while the peptone retarded the rate of deterioration.

Exper. 5.—Experiments were made to ascertain the effect of incubating a purified toxin with lecithin (acid and neutral), sodium oleate, sodium stearate, and sodium ricinoleate, with acid and basic phosphates and salt solution as controls.

0.1 gm. of lecithin (Digest Ferment Company) was dissolved in from 1 to 2 cc. of hot alcohol and stirred into 100 cc. of salt solution. This emulsion had a P_H of 4.0 to 4.5; part of it was adjusted to neutrality with sodium phosphate. 1% solutions of the sodium salts of oleic and stearic acid were prepared and as much of the excess base was neutralized with HCl as was possible without causing a precipitate of the free fatty acids. The P_H values were then 9.0 and 7.8 for the stearate and the oleate, respectively. Sodium ricinoleate in a 1% solution gave a P_H of 7.4.

TABLE 2.—THE INCREASED POTENCY OF BOTULINUS TOXIN (PURIFIED DRIED FORM) WHEN INCUBATED WITH PEPTONE AND WHEN INCUBATED WITH HORSE SERUM

	Toxin + Peptone		Toxin + Serum		Toxin + Salt Solution	
Incubation at 28 C.	Dilution Inoculated *	Result	Dilution Inoculated	Result	Dilution Inoculated	Result
0 hours	1:750	Dead 60 hours	1:750	Dead 72 hours	1:500	Dead 72 hours
	1:500	Dead 50 hours	1:500	Dead 26 hours	1:200	Dead 40 hours
12 hours	1:1,000	Dead 8½ days	1:1,000	Dead 60 hours	1:500	Survived
	1:750	Survived	1:750	Dead 72 hours	1:200	Dead 84 hours
	1:500	Dead	1:500	Dead 42 hours	.....	....
24 hours	1:750	Dead 96 hours	1:750 †	Dead 48 hours	1:500	Survived
	1:500	Dead 86 hours	1:500	Dead 48 hours	1:200	Dead 36 hours
48 hours	1:500	Survived	1:750 †	Dead 36 hours	1:200	Dead 48 hours
	1:200	Dead 36 hours	1:500	Dead 36 hours	1:100	Dead 36 hours
96 hours	1:500	Survived	1:1,000	Dead 96 hours	1:200	Survived
	1:200	Dead 96 hours	1:750	Dead 90 hours	.....	....
10 days	1:200	Survived	1:750	Dead 5 days	1:100	Survived
	1:100	Dead 5 days	1:500	Dead 96 hours	1:50	Dead 24 hours

* Three or four mice were injected for the determination of 1 MLD.
† Not tested in higher dilution.

Results: Chart 5 records the results. Only lecithin in acid and neutral solutions had a slight enhancing effect on the toxin. On the other hand, it may be seen in chart 5 that the P_H value is of primary importance for the deterioration of botulinus toxin. In an acid medium (P_H 4.3) the titer of the toxin stays fairly constant for several days at 37 C., while a P_H of 8.0 destroys most of the potency in 24 hours. The action of the stearate and oleate may be explained on the same assumption. The detoxifying action of sodium ricinoleate on the poison is not immediate but is distinctly more rapid than would be predicted from the slight alkaline reaction. These observations confirm the statement of Larson and Nelson.[9]

9. Proc. Soc. Exper. Biol. & Med., 1924, 21, p. 278.

DISCUSSION

In summarizing the results of the experiments presented, it may be stated that when the botulinus toxin was mixed with serums its potency was increased 2-10 times over the initial titer. When the toxin was mixed with Witte's peptone instead of with rabbit or horse serum, its toxicity was approximately doubled (3 experiments), while, when it was combined with aminoids, its potency showed at 2 and 6 fold increase. Lecithin raised the potency 1.5 times in 2 experiments. No adjuvant action was observed with soaps. In this connection, it must be stated

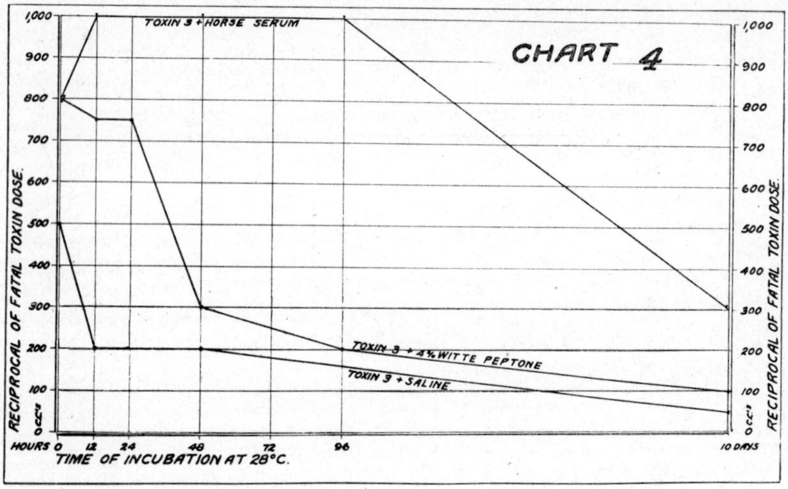

that 1 of the 8 saline and phosphate controls doubled its potency during the first 3 hours of incubation.

Before the adjuvant effect of the nitrogenous and lipoid compounds is discussed, it is advisable to consider the rate of destruction which takes place in a solution of botulinus toxin on incubation at 28 and 37 C. After 24 hours at 37 C., 5 toxins diluted in salt solution (charts 2, 3 and 5) contained only from 1 to 10% of the original MLD value; the sample incubated at 28 C. (chart 4) decreased to 40%. The stability of the toxin at different P_H values is well illustrated in chart 5. At a P_H of 4.3 the decrease was approximately 50%, and at P_H 8.0 it was approximately 98%. These and other observations tend to show that the maximal stability of the poison lies between P_H 4.0 and 5.0. The determination of an exact toxin destruction curve would naturally necessitate the sacrifice of a large number of animals and was not undertaken.

These results compared with the data recently published by Walbum[10] for the toxin of diphtheria indicate that botulinus toxin incubated at 37 C. is much more labile than the poison of the diphtheric bacillus. It is well known that the latter at neutrality deteriorates slowly, a condition certainly not found for the botulinus toxin.

By comparison of the curves representing the mixtures of the toxin with serum, peptone, aminoids, and lecithin with that of the toxin diluted in saline solution, three distinct effects may be noted:

1. Serum and lecithin as well as peptone immediately enhance the toxin titer. The increase in potency on the addition of serum and pep-

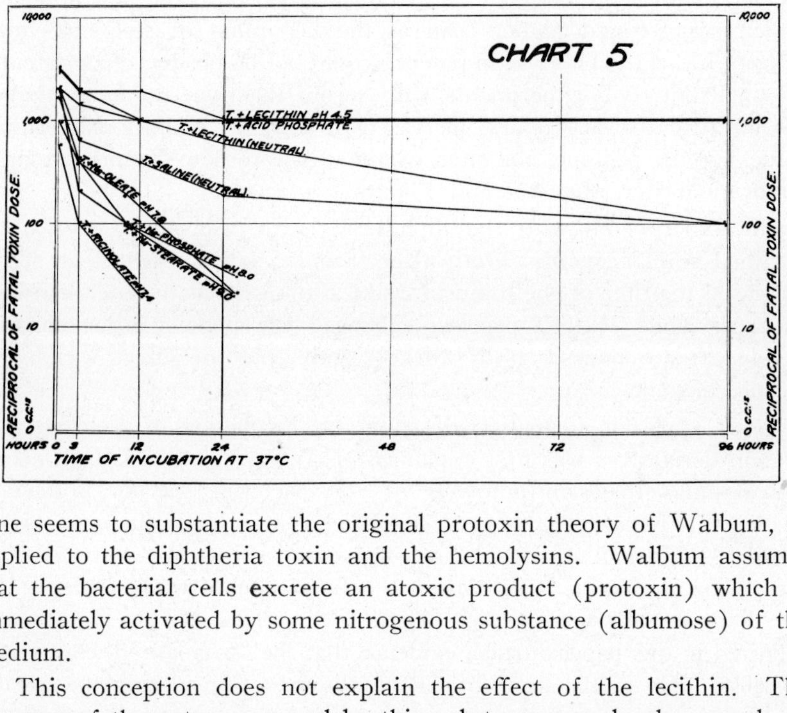

tone seems to substantiate the original protoxin theory of Walbum, as applied to the diphtheria toxin and the hemolysins. Walbum assumes that the bacterial cells excrete an atoxic product (protoxin) which is immediately activated by some nitrogenous substance (albumose) of the medium.

This conception does not explain the effect of the lecithin. The increase of the potency caused by this substance may be due merely to the solvent action of the lipoid. Many years ago De Waele[11] found that small concentrations of lecithin enhanced diphtheria toxin when injected subcutaneously, and he attributed this effect to the increased permeability of the cells for the poison. On intraperitoneal injection of

10. Kolle, Kraus, and Uhlenhuth: Handb. d. pathog. Mikroorg., ed. 3, 1928, 2, p. 535.
11. Ztschr. f. Immunitätsforsch. u. exper. Therap., O., 1909, 3, p. 478.

the toxin-lecithin mixture, however, he noted a retarding action of the lecithin, which obviously is at variance with the results obtained with botulinus toxin.

As a possible explanation of the adjuvant effect, the direct action of the foreign protein on the animal body could be considered. Such a mechanism is, however, unlikely since identical results were obtained with widely variant and relatively small amounts of serum and peptone, which had been inoculated along with the toxin.

2. Aside from an immediate increase in toxin titer, serum and peptone in several series had a second distinctly different effect on the potency of the poison. After an incubation period of several hours the toxicity was found higher than at the beginning of the experiment (charts 1, 2, 4). This rise in potency could not be produced consistently, but in 2 out of 5 experiments with serum the titer, on incubation of the mixture for 1½ hours, increased to 1.2 and 5 times the original value. With peptone, the titer of the toxin rose to 2 and 2.5 times the original titer, after 1½ and 3 hours' contact.

In experiments with the diphtheric toxin, Dernby and Walbum obtained similar results; broth after 9 and 5 hours' contact at 37 C., increased the titer of the toxin to 2 and 5 times what the titer had been at first; while Witte's peptone enhanced the potency approximately 2 fold after 6 hours. Both workers state that the effect was by no means constant.

This apparent formation of toxin on incubation of a toxin with protein derivatives was first explained on a theoretical basis by Dernby. He assumes that, on autolysis of the bacteria, specific proteolytic enzymes (toxinases) are set free, which act on the albumose of the medium to form the toxin. Since he assumes that the destruction of the poison is enzymatic in nature, the formation of toxin is dependent on 2 processes working in opposite directions. The experiments reported in this paper furnish evidence that the "toxinase" theory might possibly apply to the toxin of Cl. botulinum. Considering the greater proteolytic activity of the anaerobe, one is not surprised to find the maximal toxicity developed after a shorter period of incubation in the botulinum than in the diphtheric solution. In view of the fact, however, that a rise in the titer of botulinus toxin occurred on the addition of a 25% aminoid solution (2 experiments are detailed in chart 3), the toxinase theory cannot find universal application. More detailed experiments are necessary to elucidate this point. The ultimate verification of the toxinase theory for botulinus toxin or any other toxin can only be accomplished when the poison is once separated from the proteolytic enzymes. Thus far the samples used in the tests reported in this paper, inclusive of the dry toxin, contained gelatinase and peptidase.

There is a remote possibility that a uniform explanation may hold for the increase in toxin before and after incubation. Since the potency was not measured at shorter intervals than 1½ to 3 hours the experiments are not sufficiently complete to allow final conclusions.

The composition of the toxic fluid may be of primary importance for the attainment of a high adjuvant effect. The toxins used for the experiments had a high titer and had been produced in protein-rich mediums containing peptones. It is not unlikely that the latter had already had an additive effect and that consequently the toxin could not be activated much more. The same holds true for the dried toxin, since it had been produced from a similar base. On the other hand, the increase in potency may well be due to a reactivation of an aged toxin. The samples which served in these experiments were fresh and had been stored for a short period. It is barely possible that a weak toxin, aged for a considerable period of time, may be more readily subjected to a greater activation.

3. A third effect which the protein derivatives exert on the botulinus toxin is the retardation of its spontaneous destruction. This protection is pronounced when the poison is diluted in 25% aminoid solution (chart 3). It is doubtful whether the serum or the peptone, in the dilutions used, had a similar protective effect. If it is assumed that the toxin is altered by an enzyme—possibly peptidase—the retarded destruction can readily be explained by the fact that a high concentration of protein split products (amino acids) inactivates the peptolytic ferments. The protection of the toxin in an acid environment is probably due to the same factor, since the enzymes of Cl. botulinum thus far investigated (gelatinase, peptidase, and lipase) are practically inactive at P_H 4.0.

SUMMARY

On incubation of neutral botulinus toxin in salt solution at 37 C. a decrease in potency of 90 to 99% occurred in 24 hours. The deterioration was accelerated in alkaline mediums, but was greatly retarded at P_H 4.3. The addition of serum caused an immediate increase in toxicity; in several samples a further rise in the titer of the toxin was observed on incubation. Witte's peptone showed the same influence as serum but in a less marked degree. Dilution in a 25% aminoid solution greatly stabilized the toxin. The addition of lecithin slightly increased the initial titer of the toxin. No effect was observed with sodium stearate and oleate. Sodium ricinoleate caused rapid though not immediate inactivation of the poison.

The results are discussed in the light of the protoxin and toxinase theories.

A POISON PRODUCED BY BACTERIUM ENTERITIDIS AND BACTERIUM AERTRYCKE WHICH IS ACTIVE IN MICE WHEN GIVEN BY MOUTH *

SARA E. BRANHAM, LUCILE ROBEY AND LOIS A. DAY

From the Department of Hygiene and Bacteriology of the University of Chicago

The occurrence of toxic materials in cultures of bacteria of the paratyphoid group has been recognized ever since Gaertner isolated the first known member, Bact. enteritidis, in 1888. The effect of these so-called toxins on laboratory animals has received considerable study, undoubtedly because of the frequent association of certain members of this group with food poisoning. Apparently the symptoms that characterize intoxication with these substances (viz., an incubation period of about 45 minutes followed by dyspnea, diarrhea, prostration, and often convulsions and death) are produced only when the materials are given intravenously. Injection by other routes and feeding have rarely seemed to produce noticeable effect.

During recent years two reports have presented some evidence that these bacteria contain within themselves something that affects the mucosa of part of the gastrointestinal tract when they are fed to certain animals. Savage and White [1] have reported that both living and heat killed suspensions of Bact. enteritidis and Bact. aertrycke have an irritating action upon the stomach and duodenum of rabbits, causing marked congestion, which could be noted when these animals were killed a few hours after being fed the preparations. Arnold and Singer [2] have found a marked diminution in the secretion of acid in the stomachs of dogs fed both unheated and heated cultures of Bact. enteritidis. Bact. enteritidis and Bact. aertrycke are undoubtedly the members of the paratyphoid group that are most commonly involved in food poisoning.

This paper presents the results of experiments in which bacteria of these 2 types, and their products, were given by mouth to animals that are susceptible to spontaneous infection by this route with these organisms. Mice were chosen. Their susceptibility to Bact. enteritidis and to Bact. aertrycke is high, and spontaneous epidemics among them are

Received for publication, July 7, 1928.
* This work was aided by a grant from the National Canners' Association.

1. Med. Res. Council, Special Rep. Series, no. 91, 1925.
2. Proc. Soc. Exper. Biol. & Med., 1927, 24, p. 833.

frequent. Due consideration was given to the fact that mice are sometimes carriers of these bacteria.

Seventeen strains of these types which were either actually involved in food poisoning outbreaks, or else isolated from rodents, were obtained from Professor Jordan's collection. These were as follows:

E E 52:—Bact. enteritidis. Received by Johns Hopkins Pathological Laboratory from the laboratory of Dr. Herbert Durham, University of Cambridge, England, in 1900. Sent from Johns Hopkins to Prof. Jordan in 1902. Is probably a very old strain.

E 137:—Bact. enteritidis. From the spleen of a rat fed "Azoa."

E 228:—Bact. enteritidis. This is the famous Limerick strain isolated in 1909 by Dr. McWeeney, School of Medicine, University College, Dublin, Ireland.

E 272:—Bact. enteritidis. Isolated by Savage and Forbs from the spleen of a fatal case of food poisoning in Brighton, 1917. Received from Dr. Savage, 1919.

E 343:—Bact. enteritidis. "126-Newcastle." Isolated by Prof. Hutchens from milk that caused food poisoning, 1910. Received from the Lister Institute, 1922.

E 396:—Bact. enteritidis. Isolated in 1921 from feces of a food poisoning case, by Dr. W. D. O'Kelly, University College, Dublin.

E. 397:—Bact. enteritidis. Isolated in 1921 by Dr. O'Kelly, University College, Dublin, from the intestinal contents of a mouse which died from having been fed meat from a sick cow.

B 152:—Bact. aertrycke. From organs of a fatal food poisoning case, isolated in 1908 by Savage and Gunson. Received from Dr. Savage in 1914.

B 180:—Bact. aertrycke. Isolated from a pie mixture involved in an outbreak in Westerly, R. I., 1915, by Dr. Bernstein.

B 222:—Bact. aertrycke. Isolated from a fatal case of food poisoning in Dublin, Ireland, by Prof. McWeeney in 1916.

B 275:—Bact. aertrycke. Isolated in 1918 by Delepine in a food poisoning outbreak at a place near Manchester. Received from Dr. Savage, 1919.

B 355:—Bact. aertrycke. Isolated from food poisoning in man, Newcastle, 1911. Received from the Lister Institute, 1922.

B 356:—Bact. aertrycke. Isolated by Lieut. Col. Martin from blood in a case of food poisoning in France. Received from the Lister Institute, 1922.

B 379:—Bact. schotmülleri. Isolated by Dr. J. C. Geiger in 1922 from a meat sandwich during a food poisoning outbreak in Birmingham, Ala.

B 388:—Bact. aertrycke. Isolated from a case of food poisoning caused by eating infected mutton. Received from Dr. G. D. Dawson, Manchester Univ., 1922.

B 391:—Bact. aertrycke. Isolated in 1922 from feces of a food poisoning case. Received from Dr. C.-E. A. Winslow.

B 409:—Bact. aertrycke. Isolated from ice cream in Hollywood, 1919, in an outbreak involving 60 persons. Received from Washington State Board of Health, Seattle, in 1923.

First the actual pathogenicity of these strains for mice was determined. With each strain, normal mice, in quadruplicate, were given one 0.5 cc. dose of a 24-hour veal infusion broth culture intragastrically by stomach tube. A small silver eustachian tube catheter was used for this purpose. Each of these mice was kept in a separate compartment of a wire cage, and maintained on the usual laboratory diet of bread, carrots, and grain. Typical paratyphoid infection developed in all mice. The minimum incubation time among those mice given Bact. enteritidis was 3 days; and among those given Bact. aertrycke, 5 days. The greatest number of deaths occurred between the 4th and 9th days. On the whole, they showed no marked symptoms of illness until shortly before death. One hundred per cent of the mice died. The curve (chart 1) is comparable to those obtained with mice by Webster and by Pritchett [3] in

3. Webster, L. T.: J. Exper. Med., 1923, 37, p. 231; 38, pp. 33 and 45; 1924, 39, p. 879; 1925, 42, p. 1. Webster, L. T., and I. W. Pritchett: ibid., 1924, 40, p. 397; Pritchett, I. W.: 1925, 41, pp. 195 and 209.

their studies of these same members of the paratyphoid group of bacteria, differing chiefly in the higher percentage of mortality occurring in our experiments. These workers have shown that a definite variation in susceptibility to these bacteria occurs among mice, due to the breed and to dietary and seasonal factors.

At necropsy of these mice very few changes were apparent in heart, lungs, liver, spleen, kidneys and alimentary tract. Bact. enteritidis and Bact. aertrycke were regularly isolated, most commonly from the blood and spleen, but often from the intestines also. Blood and intestinal contents were plated on Endo or Simmon's citrate medium,[4] usually both; and blood and spleen cultures were made in veal infusion broth. These

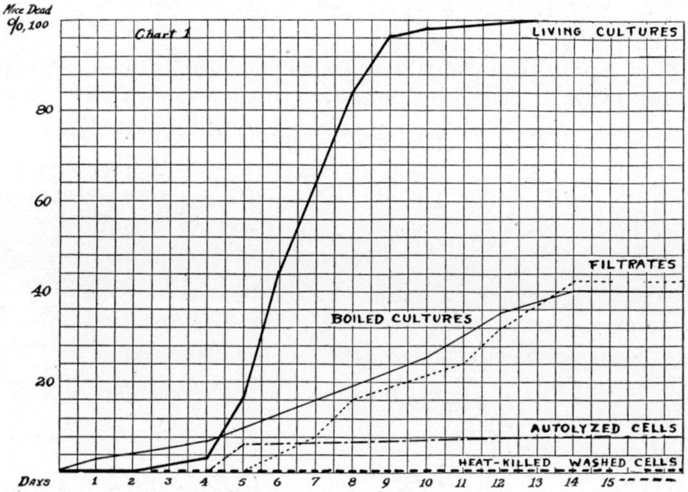

Chart 1.—Mortality curves obtained by feeding to mice varieties of 24-hour broth cultures of Bact. enteritidis and Bact. aertrycke or their products.

broth cultures were later plated on Endo agar or Simmon's citrate agar. Colonies from these plates were inoculated into Russell's double sugar medium, and these strains subsequently identified as the same types that had been fed by their cultural behavior, including their reaction with sodium d-tartrate medium, and by agglutination and absorption agglutination tests. The one strain of Bact. schottmülleri that was fed was not recovered, though the mice fed with this type died and an unagglutinable paratyphoid strain was isolated from one of them. Bact. aertrycke was recovered from one mouse that was fed Bact. enteritidis.

The pathogenicity of these 17 food-poisoning strains for mice having been established, other series of mice, in triplicate, were fed, intra-

4. J. Infect. Dis., 1926, 39, p. 209.

gastrically, one dose of 1 cc. of the three following preparations obtained from the same strains: heat-killed broth cultures; autolyzed suspensions; and Berkefeld N filtrates of broth cultures. As in the preliminary experiments, these mice were kept in separate compartments on a diet of bread and carrots and grain. The heat-killed cultures were prepared by boiling 24-hour broth cultures for 15 minutes. The heavy autolyzed suspensions were made by suspending 24-hour agar surface growth in sterile 0.8% salt solution, adding a little chloroform, and incubating at 37 C. for 2 weeks. Any chloroform remaining was driven off by gentle heating just before use. The filtrates were prepared by passing 24-hour veal infusion broth cultures through Berkefeld N filters. The sterility of all of these materials was checked by poured plate cultures.

Of the mice fed with the heat-killed broth cultures, 40% died—46% of those given Bact. aertrycke as contrasted with 33% of those given Bact. enteritidis. Bact. aertrycke was isolated from 7 of these mice, one of which had been given Bact. enteritidis and another Bact. schottmülleri. Bact. enteritidis was not recovered from any animal in this series. In three of the 7 mice yielding Bact. aertrycke there was evidence of diarrhea, in one case for three days, before death. Necropsy of these mice revealed nothing noticeably different from the findings in the mice fed with living organisms.

When autolysed suspensions were fed, only 8% of all the mice died, 4% having been given autolysates of Bact. enteritidis, and 4% autolysates of Bact. aertrycke. Most of these died on the 4th and 5th days after feeding. Bact. enteritidis was isolated from one mouse that had been fed an autolysate of Bact. enteritidis. Otherwise no paratyphoid organisms could be isolated from blood, spleen, peritoneal cavity, or intestines.

As a result of being fed with filtrates, 41% of all mice died between the 5th and 14th days—44% of those given filtrates of Bact. aertrycke and 40% of those given filtrates of Bact. enteritidis. There was some evidence of diarrhea in these mice before death. No paratyphoid bacteria could be recovered from any animals in this series.

A superimposition of all mortality curves obtained by feeding these materials may be seen in chart 1. Of the mice fed with the living broth cultures, 100% died. The greatest mortality was between the 4th and 9th days after feeding. Deaths among the mice fed with the autolyzed suspensions were only 8% of the total number. The curves obtained with boiled broth cultures and with filtrates of broth cultures were strikingly similar. Approximately 40% of both of these series of mice died. The greatest number of deaths here occurred between the 7th and 14th days; in the latter part of the period during which the infected mice died.

The common factor in the materials yielding these similar curves was broth in which the bacteria had grown. The chief difference between the filtrates and the boiled broth cultures was the presence in the latter of heat-killed cells. The rôle of these cells was investigated by feeding series of mice, by the usual technique, with salt solution suspensions of washed bacteria killed by heat in the same way, viz., boiling for 15 minutes. There were no deaths among these mice in the four weeks' period during which they were under observation. The filtrate and boiled broth culture curves suggested the possibility that thermostable toxic products were formed in broth by the bacteria, and that the relatively slow action of these is usually masked by the more rapid course of infection with living organisms in these animals.

To determine this point more than 300 mice were given 1 cc. of filtrates of cultures grown in the following mediums: plain meat extract broth, veal infusion broth, veal infusion broth aerated during incubation, liver broth, chopped liver medium, chopped meat medium, and beef heart medium. These mediums were used in 100 and 200 cc. amounts in liter flasks, and were inoculated with 24-hour broth cultures of the strains chosen. Samples were removed from these cultures after the desired incubation time, filtered through Berkefeld N or W filters, and the sterility checked by broth cultures and poured plates. Control series of mice were fed with the uninoculated mediums. Some were fed with filtrates that were boiled.

The results of feeding these materials varied according to the medium in which the bacteria were grown. Occasionally there were lots of medium which produced filtrates that seemed entirely nontoxic. In veal infusion broth the mortality usually varied from 10% to 40% according to the batch of medium or the age of the culture. In a similar medium aerated during incubation the hightest mortality was 20%. In veal infusion broth containing ground liver the highest rate was 30%. With filtrates of beef heart cultures the mortality ranged from 10 to 40%. Boiling the filtrates for 10 minutes did not lessen the mortality. No deaths occurred in any series fed with the uninoculated mediums.

Necropsy of these mice revealed few changes. The most uniform and striking feature was marked cloudy swelling of the kidneys. No paratyphoid bacteria could be isolated from any of these animals.

There seems, unquestionably, to be something present in many filtrates of cultures of these microorganisms that is toxic for mice when taken by mouth. Is this poison formed in greater abundance as the culture grows older, or is it destroyed during extended incubation? To answer this question samples were removed from veal infusion broth cultures after 1, 3, 7, and 14 days of incubation, filtered, and fed to mice in the usual manner. The younger cultures were found to be the most toxic, The percentage of mortality among the mice fed 24-hour filtrates was 40%; that among those fed 3-day filtrates of the same culture was 20%; that among those fed 7-day filtrates 10%. There were no deaths among the mice given the 14-day filtrates.

The idea occurred to us that some of the toxic principle might be absorbed by the filter candles used in preparing the filtrates. Therefore, some of the beef heart cultures were divided into 3 parts: 1 part was filtered, 1 part was boiled for 10 minutes, and the third portion was autoclaved at 10 pounds for 10 minutes. Mice were then fed with these materials. A catheter could not be used conveniently with these cultures because of the particles of heart muscle, so the mice were made to fast for a half day, and were then given the material in a watch glass while they were hungry. They ate these cultures readily.

The unfiltered material proved to be much more toxic than the filtered. Among the mice fed with the unfiltered boiled materials 40 to 100% died, the proportion varying with different cultures. Among those fed the autoclaved whole cultures 70% to 95% died. Not only did autoclaving fail to destroy the poison, but in some cultures it seemed to be even more potent after subjection to these high temperatures. Charts 2 and 3 show the mortality curves obtained with the filtered, boiled, and autoclaved portions of 2 different lots of 24-hour beef heart cultures of the microorganisms used. In chart 2 the autoclaved materials are seen to have produced a combined mortality of 70%; whereas the same set of cultures boiled resulted in a mortality of 40%, and, filtered, gave only 10%. Greater toxicity of the autoclaved material is not evident in the curves of chart 3, where the autoclaved material is represented by a mortality of 95%, the boiled material 100%, and the filtrates 10%. The mice that were given the whole beef heart cultures showed the same pathological picture at autopsy as those that were fed the filtrates. Mice that were fed the uninoculated medium were not affected in any way. No paratyphoid bacteria were found in any animals of these series.

It seemed possible that this greater toxicity of the unfiltered cultures might be due to the presence of the heat-killed bacterial cells. Consequently a number of mice were fed with suspensions of the same strains prepared as follows: the growths from 24-hour agar slant cultures were suspended in 0.8% NaCl solution, centrifugated, and resuspended. Part of each suspension was boiled 10 minutes; part was autoclaved 10 minutes at 10 pounds. None of the mice in these series died.

DISCUSSION

Apparently there is often something produced in broth, chopped meat, and beef heart cultures of Bact. enteritidis and Bact. aertrycke that is toxic for mice when given by mouth. This conclusion has been drawn from experiments in which approximately 1,000 mice have been fed

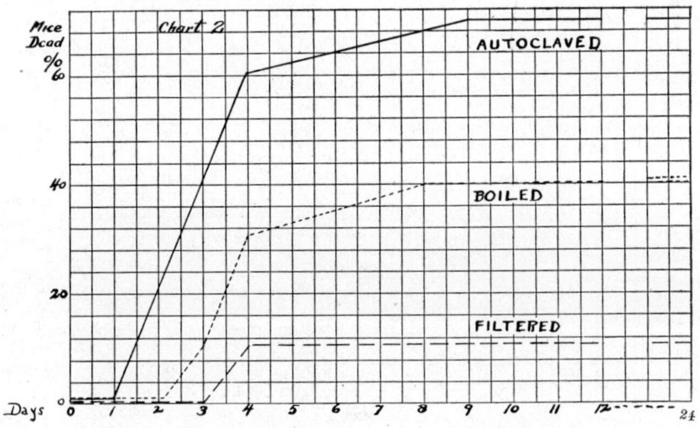

Chart 2.—Mortality curves obtained by feeding to mice filtered, boiled and autoclaved beef-heart cultures of paratyphoid organisms (lot 1).

living, boiled, autoclaved, and autolyzed washed cells, as well as whole unaltered, boiled, autoclaved, and filtered fluid cultures of 17 food-poisoning strains. Whenever living cultures were fed, infection developed in a high percentage of the animals, and the same types of paratyphoid bacteria were regularly recovered at necropsy. When materials that apparently contained no living cells were given, these types could not be isolated from the animals that died, although the mortality in some of these series was as great as in the group fed with the living bacteria. Control mice fed with uninoculated medium, or merely kept under identical conditions were unaffected. There was no great difference in the pathological picture presented at necropsy by the mice receiving living cells or sterile materials derived from them. In the mice given filtrates and heated beef heart cultures cloudy swelling of the kidneys was more marked. The greatest mortality among the mice fed living cells, and from which the organisms were recovered, was between the 4th and 9th days; whereas among the mice fed with other materials, and from which no paratyphoid bacteria could be isolated, it was between the 7th and 14th days.

The fact that one mouse fed Bact. enteritidis yielded Bact. aertrycke at necropsy and that 7 of those given autolysates yielded Bact. aertrycke, no matter which type had been fed to them, is of epidemiological interest, but does not arouse surprise, since Bact. enteritidis and Bact. aertrycke are characteristically rodent types, and mice are sometimes carriers of

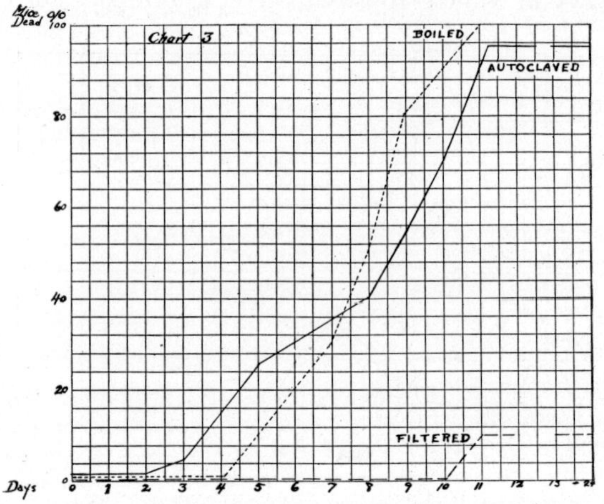

Chart 3.—Mortality curves obtained by feeding to mice filtered, boiled and autoclaved beef-heart cultures of paratyphoid organisms (lot 2).

them. Many bacteriologists consider that infection of food by these rodents is responsible for food poisoning outbreaks in which these types are involved.

The poison described in this paper is not injured by boiling or by ordinary autoclaving; this remarkable thermostability suggests the other toxic substances which have been described as occurring in this group of bacteria. But the resemblance apparently ceases here. The toxic substances which have been usually described are active only when given intravenously, after a brief incubation period of 40 to 50 minutes; and such evidence as has been presented for the existence of gastro-enteric irritants in the bacterial cells themselves indicates very prompt action and recovery. The action of the poison described in these experiments is relatively slow, the greatest number of deaths among the mice occurring between the 7th and 14th days after feeding. This delayed effect may be easily masked by the more rapid action of the living bacteria.

The poison seems to be produced by the growth of the bacteria in the medium, but the evidence accumulated does not show whether it is secreted as such by the bacteria, or whether it is formed by the action of the microorganisms on the constituents of the medium.

The fact that there are poisonous products in fluid cultures of these bacteria which may be fatal to mice when they are given by mouth is undoubtedly worthy of attention, although these experiments offer no evidence that the poison has any relation to the occurrence of food poisoning in man.

SUMMARY

Seventeen strains of paratyphoid bacteria, isolated from foods, or rodents, or from persons infected during food poisoning outbreaks, produced fatal infection in 100% of mice to which they were fed. These strains included 7 of Bact. enteritidis, 9 of Bact. aertrycke, and 1 of Bact. schottmülleri.

When boiled broth cultures and Berkefeld N and W filtrates of broth cultures of these strains were fed similarly to mice, a mortality of approximately 40% occurred.

When whole unfiltered cultures in beef heart medium are boiled or autoclaved, and then fed to mice, the mortality is often from 40% to 100%.

Feeding autolyzed, boiled, or autoclaved suspensions of the washed bacteria had little, if any, effect. Filtrates of 24-hour cultures produced a higher mortality than those from cultures which were incubated for longer periods of time.

In its remarkable heat stability this poison resembles the other toxic materials which have been described in the paratyphoid group, but its surprisingly long incubation period seems to separate this toxic substance quite definitely from that responsible for the violent gastrointestinal symptoms occurring in man after eating foods containing these bacteria, and from any other toxic product of these bacteria that has yet been described.

Further investigation will be necessary before it can be determined whether this toxic principle is a product of the bacterial cells or a chemical poison formed by the action of the microorganisms on the constituents of the medium.

NEISSERIA SUBFLAVA (BERGEY) MENINGITIS IN AN INFANT *

Harriet Benson, Rose Brennwasser
and
Dorothy D'Andrea

From the Henry Baird Favill Laboratory and the Pediatric Service of St. Luke's Hospital, Chicago

Pathogenicity among the organisms of the gram-negative diplococci designated Neisseria (Bergey [1]) is generally limited to the intracellularis (meningococci), and to the gonorrhea organisms. Neisseria catarrhalis, Neisseria sicca, and the three species of flava group are considered to have only a limited or no pathogenicity as far as human hosts are concerned. Yet even among these N. catarrhalis has been found associated with disease and has been regarded as the causal agent. Endres [2] and Schilf [3] have recorded the clinical and bacteriological features respectively of an infection in a man (47 years of age) from whose blood during life N. catarrhalis was recovered. After having a septic fever six weeks, he died and the postmortem examination disclosed a thromboulcerative endocarditis of the anterior mitral leaflet. The inability of the isolated organism to ferment sugars indicates that it was N. catarrhalis, although the results of the agglutination reactions recorded in the report are rather unsatisfactory. A polyvalent antimeningococcus serum caused some flocculation of the organism in the dilution 1 : 100, a reaction considered to be nonspecific. An immune serum (titer 1 : 5000) prepared in a rabbit with an N. catarrhalis strain obtained from the Pfeiffer Institute did not agglutinate strains from the patient. No comment was made of the difficulties of spontaneous agglutination of the N. catarrhalis such as Elser and Huntoon [4] encountered, nor is mention made of specific absorption tests with members of the Neisseria group. Nagell [5] recently has recorded the clinical progress of a man 19 years old having a sepsis caused by N. catarrhalis. He recovered in three months. During his illness the organism was

Received for publication, July 10, 1928.

* Aided by the Winfield Peck Memorial Fund.

1. Manual of Determinative Bacteriology, 1923.
2. München. med. Wchnschr., 1925, 72, p. 723.
3. Ibid., 1925, 72, p. 724.
4. J. M. Research, 1909, 20, p. 371.
5. München. med. Wchnschr., 1928, 75, p. 124.

isolated four different times from the blood, and in histological preparations of a skin lesion, organisms in morphology like those in the cultures were found. The cultured bacteria did not ferment maltose, levulose, or dextrose. The results of agglutination or absorption tests are not mentioned. Penetration of N. catarrhalis into the cerebrospinal tissues causing a suppurative meningitis has been reported a number of times, most often in children. Mayerhofer-Lateiner [6] related the clinical course of the illness of a child six months old that came under observation five days after the onset of fever and rigidity of the neck. Cultures of the spinal fluid obtained by lumbar puncture contained N. catarrhalis. The spinal fluid obtained on the tenth day of observation was almost clear and was sterile in cultures. The child improved rapidly, and when seen several times after the acute illness, apparently remained well. Mayerhofer-Lateiner said that in 1911 she reported a pyothorax in which N. catarrhalis was associated with the influenza bacillus. Cot and Robert [7] in 1921 reported meningitis in a young man from whose spinal fluid N. catarrhalis and an enterococcus were isolated. They stated that at the January meeting of the society of pediatrics, Henri Lemoine gave an account of cerebrospinal meningitis induced by N. catarrhalis in two nurslings, and at the same meeting Cassoute made a report of meningitis caused by the same organism in a child three years old. In the next year Reuss [8] published the clinical, bacteriological and postmortem observations of meningitis in a boy eight and one-half years old. He described the organism found in the spinal fluid as "like" a meningococcus. Three spinal fluids obtained during life, and exudate from tissues obtained after death contained an organism which varied in several respects from the meningococcus. These as listed by the author were variability in staining according to the Gram method, prompt growth on plain agar, growth at 22 C., failure to ferment maltose and dextrose in young cultures (although maltose was split in old cultures and one strain fermented dextrose in 14 days), failure to agglutinate with antimeningococcus serum, failure of homologous immune serum to agglutinate meningococci, and increased resistance to certain extraneous agents such as heat, and prolonged viability on plain and ascitic agar mediums. Reuss made no further suggestion on the classification of this organism excepting to refer to a number

6. Wiener klin. Wchnschr., 1918, 31, p. 1107.
7. Paris Medical, 1921, 11, p. 318.
8. Centralbl. f. Bakteriol., 1, O., 1922, 87, p. 532.

of reports of atypical meningococci. In 1923 Garland[9] reported a meningitis caused by N. catarrhalis in a girl five years old. Death occurred 108 days after the onset of symptoms but no postmortem examination was made. Garland quoted a personal communication from J. B. Neal that she had observed cerebrospinal meningitis caused by N. catarrhalis in a child seven weeks old, and that the infant died the following month.

Although most of these reports are based on the bacteriological results of clinical material and although only a limited number include additional information gained by postmortem examinations which would help greatly in determining whether N. catarrhalis was the actual causal agent, or was only an accidental saprophyte accompanying a pathogenic organism, there is some basis for believing that the organisms of the group Neisseria other than the intracellularis and gonococcus may cause disease.

There is, however, practically no mention of pathogenic invasion of human hosts by members of the flava group. Elser and Huntoon have arranged these gram-negative cocci into three divisions on the basis of the fermentation reactions with dextrose, maltose, levulose, and sucrose, on the results of agglutination tests, and especially, by specific absorption. Elser and Huntoon were primarily interested in establishing differentiating characters of the gram-negative cocci present in the nasopharynx and found the agglutination tests with certain of these organisms, especially N. catarrhalis, quite unsatisfactory because of the instability of the bacterial suspensions in physiologic salt solution. Among the sixty strains of N. catarrhalis there were only two that formed stable suspensions. Some difficulty was encountered also with the flava organisms. They found, however, that absorption tests served to differentiate the various groups of gram-negative cocci from each other in a way not possible by agglutination.

Intracellular and extracellular gram-negative diplococci found in spinal fluids removed from patients having symptoms of meningitis generally are considered to be meningococci. The accuracy of this interpretation in all of these patients becomes questionable when one is encountered in whom the illness is clinically mild and protracted, and it becomes more questionable when the gram-negative diplococci grown in cultures of the spinal fluid are atypical for N. intracellularis. Such difficulties arose in connection with an investigation into the illness of a male child 7 months old who was admitted to Isaac Abt's pediatric service at St. Luke's Hospital, February 8, 1928. A statement was

9. Am. J. Dis. Child., 1923, 26, p. 600.

made by the mother that the baby, born at full term, had gained rapidly in weight until it was five months old when an infection of the left eye and a discharge from the left ear were noted. In a few days tremor of the right hand and foot, and persistent projectile vomiting appeared. The statements recording the physical examination at the time of admission mention a large head with tense open fontanelles, a vertical squint, enlarged left cervical lymph nodes, pale drum membranes of both ears, without bulging or perforation, opisthotonos, marked spasticity of the muscles of the right side, and positive Kernig and Brudzinski reflexes. A tentative diagnosis of hydrocephalus and brain abscess was made. The spinal fluid removed on the day following admission was turbid, opalescent, and contained 3000 cells (chiefly polymorphonuclear leukocytes) per c.mm. In the cultures, only gram-negative diplococci were isolated. The left drum membrane was incised and a small amount of gray exudate was drained from this ear. This exudate was not received for culture. The leukocyte count of the blood varied between 10,500 and 13,500 per c.mm. The temperature ranged between 98.6 and 103 F., averaging about 99 to 100 F. The child continued to lose weight, and the muscular rigidity became more pronounced. Spinal fluid was withdrawn from time to time, and as a last resort mercurochrome was given intraspinously. The child died 27 days after admission to the hospital, 3 months after the onset of symptoms. The postmortem examination (by Edwin F. Hirsch) was made on the same day after about 14 hours. Permission was obtained for examining the head and trunk only, not the neck and spinal canal.

The pertinent features of the anatomic diagnosis are as follows: bilateral suppurative otitis media; chronic suppurative leptomeningitis; marked internal hydrocephalus; pressure (?) necrosis of the inferior portion of the cerebellum and upper part of the spinal cord; hypostatic hyperemia and edema of the lungs; acute emphysema of the lungs; cloudy swelling and fatty changes of the liver and kidneys; hyperplasia of the mesenteric lymph glands; mercurochrome staining of the cerebrospinal fluid; etc.

The scalp tissues were moderately moist. The lining of the superior longitudinal, the right and the left lateral, and the right and the left sigmoid sinuses of the dura was smooth and unchanged. The convolutions of the brain were markedly flattened and there was a huge internal hydrocephalus. In removing the brain the left lateral ventricle was ruptured and a large quantity of spinal fluid stained with mercurochrome escaped. (See further description of formalin-hardened brain). In each middle ear there was a thick viscid secretion. There were no gross changes in the hypophysis, the sphenoid, ethmoid, and frontal sinuses of the cranium.

The routine examination of the chest and abdomen followed. This included an examination of the right and left axillary fossae, the general condition of the peritoneal, pleural, and pericardial spaces, the thymic gland (weight 8 grams), the azygos veins, the lining of the aorta and its large branches, the ductus arteriosus, the periaortic lymph glands, the esophagus, the trachea and main bronchi, the pulmonary veins and arteries, the heart including the leaflets, lining, etc., the cavae, the lungs, the kidneys and ureters, the suprarenal glands, the liver, bile ducts, portal and splenic veins, the pancreas, spleen, stomach, bowel, urinary bladder, and testes.

There were no noteworthy changes in these tissues except as mentioned in the cranium and brain, and noted otherwise in the anatomic diagnosis. The body was examined carefully for tuberculous lesions. No additional information was obtained by the microscopic examination of sections of the lymph glands, lungs, bowel, stomach, suprarenal glands, kidneys, pancreas, hypophysis and liver.

The cultures of fluids such as the heart blood, pericardial fluid, spinal fluid, right middle ear, and left middle ear were markedly contaminated by a variety of organisms probably due to the length of time (15 hours) after death that the fluids were obtained. For this reason, the results of these cultures were unsatisfactory.

Brain.—The formalin-hardened brain without the dura weighs (4-28-28) 651 grams. The cerebral hemispheres are normally symmetrical except for slight misshaping in the fixing solution. The right lobe is 13 cm. long, 5.7 cm. wide and in the temporal region is 8.3 cm. thick. The left lobe is 13.5 cm. long, 6.2 cm. wide and in the temporal region 8 cm. thick. The convolutions of the cerebrum are markedly flattened and the sulci are narrow, shallow grooves. The blood vessels along the sulci are compressed and thin-walled. The leptomeninges covering the convolutions of the cerebrum are closely adherent to the brain. They are thin, transparent, and along the Sylvian fissures and elsewhere are without opacities. The tip of the left olfactory bulb is torn but otherwise there are no gross changes in the contour of these structures. The optic chiasma is pushed forward and away from the base of the brain. Directly behind it, bulging and markedly dilated into a vesicle-like structure, is the tuber cinereum, 1 cm. long and 1.2 cm. wide. The attachment of the stalk of the infundibulum, now torn away, is an opening 2 mm. in diameter just behind the center in the midline of this dilated structure. The structures behind the tuber cinereum to the posterior margin of the pons, on both sides of the midline as far as the temporal lobes of the cerebrum are hidden by an opaque white thickening of the leptomeninges. The basilar artery is but faintly visible through this membrane. The upper part of the spinal cord has the appearance of having been wedged into the base of the brain. On both sides of the upper part of the brain stem, narrow in front and widening toward the back, is a depressed tissue defect on the inferior surface of the cerebellum, irregular in outline, slightly wider on the left side than on the right side of the midline. In front on the left side it is 1 cm. wide and just behind the spinal cord it is 3.5 cm. wide, while on the right side the corresponding dimensions are 7 mm. and 1.5 cm. The maximum length of this place on the inferior surface of the cerebellum is 4.5 cm., and the widest place just behind the spinal cord is 5 cm. The base, depressed 1.2 cm., is covered by a thick (0.5 mm.), opaque, white membrane stained with mercurochrome, continuous all around with the leptomeninges covering the cerebellum. The margins of the tissue defect rise sharply from the base to a rounded edge on a level with the surface of the cerebellum. The leptomeninges covering the superior surface of the cerebellum and for a narrow region around the tissue defect mentioned are moderately thickened and dull. The outside of the upper 4 cm. of the cord attached to the brain is red granular and these tissues seem to have been included in the lesion causing the tissue defect on the base of the cerebellum.

On surfaces made by cutting the cerebrum in a coronal (frontal) plane on a level through the descending fibers of the internal capsule there is a marked widening of all the ventricles of the brain. The right lateral is 2.5 cm. wide and 2.1 cm. high, the left is 3 cm. wide and 3.2 cm. high, and the third is 2.5 cm. wide and 2.5 cm. high. On each side the opening between the lateral ventricle and the third ventricle is 1.5 by 1.2 cm. The lining of the ventricles is stained pink-red with mercurochrome and the surfaces are finely granular. The choroid plexus in both lateral ventricles is markedly flattened forming on the right side at the level mentioned a mass 2 by 4 mm. and 1 mm. thick, on the left, a mass 3 by 4 mm. and 1 mm. thick. It is firmly adherent to the floor of the ventricles and the surface is rounded over and smooth as though the individual villi were fused by an organized exudate.

Tissues for histological examination were taken from five different places along the border of the tissue defect on the inferior surface of the cerebellum, from the floor of both lateral ventricles, and from the choroid plexus in several places. For routine study these were stained with hematoxylin and eosin, and with phosphotungstic acid hematoxylin.

The floor of the depressed region on the inferior surface of the cerebellum is a layer of pia arachnoid tissue thickened to a width of 0.5 mm. by newly grown, collagenic fibrous connective tissue, some moderately dense, some edematous and having, between the parallel fibrils, singly distributed plasma cells and polymorphonuclear leukocytes, in no large numbers. As a narrow border along the surface is a zone of large mononuclear cells (monocytes), polymorphonuclear leukocytes, necrotic cells, and granular detritus. Even in the hematoxylin-eosin stained preparations, both intra and extracellularly, are groups of organisms in pairs and tetrads arranged like intracellular meningococci. The cerebellar tissues have been pushed away so that the arrangement of the various cortical and medullary layers is not disturbed. Extending between the folds of the cerebellum is a thin pia without any or with similar moderate inflammatory changes. At the margin the thickened tissue is continuous on the one hand with an edematous pia arachnoid, modified slightly by a chronic inflammation and on the other hand with a layer of equally wide fibrous and granulation tissue, identical in width and structure as though there had been a fusion with the dura to hold an encepsulated exudate. The cells of this exudate still present are about equally polymorphonuclear leukocytes and monocytes. Among these, both intra and extracellularly, are bacterial masses as mentioned. Over 500 sections from various regions were examined. The changes are essentially as has been mentioned, and in none did these lesions in any way resemble tuberculosis. In thin sections stained overnight with Loeffler's methylene blue, paired diplococci, some in groups of four, were found (fig. 1).

Genu Inferior (Left Lateral Ventricle): 150 sections examined. There is a slight edema of the subependymal tissues.

Genu Inferior (Right Lateral Ventricle): 168 sections examined. Much of the ependymal lining is absent. Along this edge is a narrow zone of edematous subependymal tissue in which there are aggregates of monocytes and plasma cells (chiefly), and a few polymorphonuclear leukocytes arranged concentrically about small blood vessels. These cell aggregations about the blood vessels lying close to the ependymal surface have made small elevations like hummocks that project from the margin and correspond grossly to the fine granulations already noted. On the surface of these is an exudate of monocytes and polymorphonuclear leukocytes, in places continuous into the subenpendymal tissues a short distance. Around the blood vessels somewhat deeper in the tissues there is a similar perivascular exudate of plasma cells and monocytes.

Right Choroid Plexus: 119 sections examined. Covering the outside of the choroid plexus like an envelop and fusing together the distal portions of the individual villi is a mass of healed and healing chronic granulation tissue, as thick as 1 mm. The deeper healed portions are dense bands of collagen fibers wrapped around the outside of the choroid plexus, enclosing within them some of the villi, while the more superficial portions are newly grown collagenic connective tissue cells loosely held together, and in the meshes are many plasma cells, a smaller number of monocytes, and a few polymorphonuclear leukocytes. Although the fusion of the villi of the choroid plexus by the granulation tissue is limited largely to the more peripheral portions, there are a few extensions from this capsule between the individual villi toward the base portions. The interstices not so filled with chronic granulation tissue have a granular amorphous precipitate, a few threads of fibrin, and an occasional leukocyte or monocyte. The subependymal

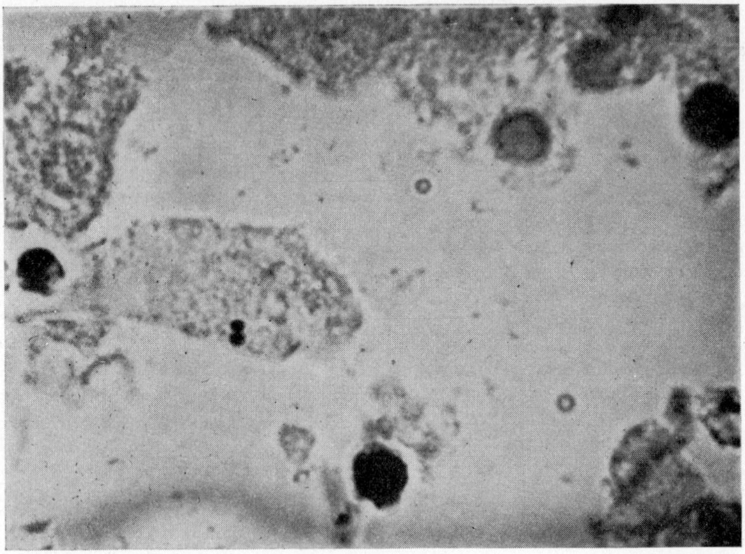

Fig. 1.—Photomicrograph of stained organisms in the tissues. × 1580.

blood vessels are surrounded by a zone of plasma cells, monocytes, and a few polymorphonuclear leukocytes, all held in a loose stroma of coarse collagen fibers.

Right Choroid Plexus and a Small Piece of Adjacent Brain Tissue: 181 serial sections, 7μ thick examined. The ependymal cells are markedly flattened so that the transverse dimension is 2 or 3 times the length. Around the blood vessels are aggregates of monocytes and polymorphonuclear leukocytes, those close under the ependyma forming small hummocks. Along the superior portion of the capsule over the choroid plexus is a monocytic and polymorphonuclear leukocytic exudate.

Left Choroid Plexus and Adjacent Brain Tissue: 280 sections examined. They are essentially like the right.

Bacteriology.—Spinal fluid removed Feb. 9, 14, 20, and 24 was cultured on blood agar. Colonies of only one variety grew in these cultures. Transferred to dextrose agar they formed at the end of

24 hours mucoid, raised, rough-edged colonies 1 mm. and less in diameter with a faint yellow-green pigment. The pigment was more definite in older cultures. On blood agar the colonies grew to considerable size. They were moist, viscid, gray-white, and were characterized by ragged edges, smooth raised tops, and well defined high centers. The growth was modified by heat, cold, and drying. In stained preparations the organisms contained in these colonies were gram-negative cocci, of uneven staining qualities, arranged in paired diplo-forms, tetrads, and masses. Those of older cultures contained many forms in stages of dissolution. Though acting slowly on sugars when first isolated, two strains in 48 hours fermented dextrose and maltose in Huntoon's semi-solid sugar medium, and in 5 days in infusion sugar broths. Levulose, lactose, sucrose, salicin, mannitol, and inulin were not fermented, and gelatin was not liquefied.

Serum from the child did not agglutinate the organisms. At intervals of several days two rabbits were given six intravenous injections of living cultures without manifesting ill effects and 10 days after the last injection the blood serum was tested for agglutinins. The homologous organisms were agglutinated by these serums in dilutions as high as 1 to 640 and 1 to 1280. A known strain of N. catarrhalis (835 of the American Museum Type Collection), four strains of N. intracellularis from the same source (992, type 1; 923, type 2; 924, type 3; and 925, type 4) and seven different strains of N. gonorrheae were not agglutinated by these serums. The suspension of the N. catarrhalis strain was unstable, a difficulty not fully appreciated when the first agglutination tests were made.

Absorption experiments were then carried out by adding to a volume of each immune serum diluted 1 to 100 in separate containers, a heavy suspension of N. catarrhalis, N. intracellularis (polyvalent including types 1, 2, 3 and 4), N. gonorrheae (331 of the American Museum Type Collection), and the homologous organism. After two hours incubation at 37 C. each of the containers was centrifugated and the clear supernatant liquid, in dilutions, was mixed with a suspension of the homologous organism. There was no loss of the agglutinin titer in those fluids treated with N. catarrhalis, N. intracellularis, and N. gonorrheae, whereas all of the agglutinin titer had been removed by contact with the homologous organisms.

The results of these tests indicate quite clearly that the gram-negative diplococcus is not N. intracellularis, N. gonorrheae, or N. catarrhalis. Gram-negative diplococci that produce a yellow-green pigment when cultured on dextrose agar belong, according to the present classification, in the flava group of organisms. On the basis of the results of the fermentation reactions along with the production of pigment, the organism described in this report is N. subflava.

SUMMARY

This report describes the clinical progress, the bacteriology, and the results of the postmortem examination, including an extended account of the alterations in the brain, of a chronic meningitis in a child 7 months of age from whose spinal fluid N. subflava was repeatedly isolated. Anatomically there was a marked internal hydrocephalus and a pressure displacement by a circumscribed abscess of the tissues of the inferior portion of the cerebellum and the upper part of the spinal cord.

The prolonged mild course of the illness continuing for about 3 months was a notable clinical feature. Gram-negative diplococci observed in stained preparations of spinal fluid commonly are considered to be meningococci. This conclusion cannot be safely made without careful study of the organisms in culture mediums and by serological tests. Although the members of the flava group as well as N. catarrhalis and N. sicca have little pathogenicity in human hosts they seem to be able to produce disease in susceptible persons.

Note.—Since the submission of this paper for publication, a report of meningitis caused by Micrococcus catarrhalis has been published by F. P. Moersch in the Proceedings of the Staff Meetings of the Mayo Clinic, 1928, 3, p. 238.

THE OPSONIFICATION TEST FOR THE RAPID IDENTIFICATION OF THE STREPTOCOCCUS OF SCARLET FEVER

Katharine M. Howell and Marie Werner

From the Philip and Emma Stein Fund for Clinical Research of the Michael Reese Hospital and the Nelson Morris Institute for Medical Research, Chicago

The opsonification test described by Tunnicliff [1] for the rapid identification of the streptococcus of scarlet fever has been tried with a number of streptococci isolated from patients with scarlet fever and from patients with a variety of other diseases, in order to study further the efficiency of the test in the diagnosis of scarlet fever.

The opsonic technic used in the test was the modified method employed by Tunnicliff. The phagocytic leukocytes were obtained by mixing equal parts of normal human blood and 2% sodium citrate in physiologic salt solution. The streptococci under examination were either picked directly from the first blood agar plate or from subcultures on blood agar slants, and were suspended in physiologic salt solution. The serums used in the test were serum of horse immunized against scarlet fever streptococcus, and normal horse serum. Equal parts of serum, citrated blood, and streptococcus suspension were mixed in capillary pipets and incubated 25 minutes at 36 C. Each mixture was smeared on a glass slide and stained with Wright's blood stain; 50 polymorphonuclear leukocytes were counted, and the number taking part in phagocytosis was noted (phagocytic index). The phagocytic index of the immune serum divided by the phagocytic index of the normal serum constituted the opsonic index. A high opsonic index would indicate that the streptococcus under examination was probably of scarlatinal origin, and a low index would indicate that the strain of streptococcus was nonscarlatinal.

Certain difficulties arose from time to time in the performance of the opsonification tests. One immune serum had a tendency to agglutinate the citrated blood that was ordinarily used in the test. Whenever it was necessary to use new serum, a preliminary test was made mixing equal parts of serum and citrated blood and incubating the mixture. If agglutination resulted, the citrated blood of this person was not used again. A few of the cultures that grew with difficulty

Received for publication, July 17, 1928.

1. J. Am. M. A., 1926, 87, p. 625.

on blood agar medium were subcultured in ascites dextrose broth. Luxurious growths of streptococci resulted, but the organisms were phagocytosed to a marked degree with both the normal and the immune serums. Whether the ascitic fluid contained opsonin for the scarlet fever streptococcus, or whether the ascitic fluid decreased the virulence of the strain, or whether some other factor was involved, was not determined; nor was it possible to rule out a previous scarlet fever in the patient from whom the ascitic fluid was obtained. After this experience blood agar cultures were used exclusively. The person whose blood was used for the opsonic test developed an acute coryza, and his leukocytes during this period had almost no phagocytic activity in the presence either of normal or of immune serums. In order to study further the influence of the use of different leukocytes, we ran 20 opsonic tests (4 or 5 a day) in duplicate, with the exception of the citrated blood. Although the leukocytes of the one person were always more phagocytic than those of the other person, this occurred in the presence of both normal and immune serums, with the result that the opsonic indices were almost identical in the two sets of tests. Fifty of the opsonic tests were done independently by 2 persons using identical constituents. There were slight variations in the resulting indices, but in no instance enough to change a low index to a high index, or the reverse. It would appear, therefore, that the opsonic index is not subject to great variation whether performed by different trained persons or with different materials. The opsonification test could be of practical use in any general laboratory.

The streptococcus strains from scarlet fever were obtained from 2 hospitals for contagious diseases (Durand Hospital of the McCormick Institute of Infectious Diseases, and the Municipal Contagious Disease Hospital, Chicago). The streptococcus strains used as controls were obtained in the bacteriologic department of a general hospital (Michael Reese Hospital, Chicago). Although the cultures from both the hospitals for contagious diseases were made by skilled physicians, the blood agar plates from the two institutions showed such variation in bacterial flora that they will be taken up as 2 groups.

Twenty-two cultures were received from one of the hospitals for contagious diseases. All the strains of streptococci were of the beta hemolytic type. Eight strains were on blood agar plates; they showed typical wide zones of hemolysis about the colonies and they were in almost pure culture. The other 14 strains were subcultures made from similar colonies. All the cultures had been obtained from typical cases of scarlet fever. Most of them were taken early in the course of the disease. The opsonic indices in this group varied from 2 to 12.5, with an average index of 4.8. The indices were as follows: 7, 2, 3, 5, 2.5, 6, 5, 6, 6, 2.5, 8, 3, 6.4, 12.5, 5, 4.4, 2.5, 3, 5, 2, 4.5, 3.

Ninety-eight throat cultures streaked on blood agar plates were received from the other hospital for contagious diseases. All were taken from patients with clinicaly typical scarlet fever, some in the early stage of the disease, during the rash, others in the desquamating stage. The blood agar plate cultures revealed in most instances mixed bacterial flora. A few blood agar plates resembled those from the other hospital for contagious diseases, revealing almost pure cultures of wide zoned hemolytic streptococcus colonies. Other blood agar plates, however, contained hemolytic streptococcus colonies surrounded by very narrow zones of hemolysis. A few blood agar plates contained both varieties of streptococci. Most surprising of all, 24 blood agar plates contained anhemolytic streptococci only. The histories of the patients from whom these cultures had been taken, and the clinical observations made on them, were carefully re-examined; all the patients apparently had typical cases of scarlet fever. The cultures from 9 of them had been taken during the rash and from 15 of them while desquamation was in progress. It is possible that some of the 15 patients may have had the hemolytic type of streptococcus in their cultures during the early period of the disease; for it has been observed by many investigators that the scarlatinal streptococcus disappears in the 2nd or 3rd weeks of the disease, and that it is replaced by the streptococcus strains found in normal throats; for example, in our series, cultures were taken from 2 patients' throats in 3 successive weeks. The opsonic results with the cultures from the 1st patient were as follows: the unusually high index of 17 the 1st week, an index of 15.3 the 2nd week, and an index of 1.2 the 3rd week. The cultures from the 2nd patient had an opsonic index of 7 the 1st week, with a hemolytic streptococcus; in the 2nd and 3rd weeks no hemolytic streptococci appeared on the blood agar plates.

Most of these plates containing anhemolytic streptococci were discarded. However, after such plates were repeatedly obtained, opsonic indices were made with 3 of the anhemolytic streptococcus strains. A culture taken from a patient during the rash (5th day) gave an index of 2.9. The 2nd culture taken on the 11th day, when the rash was fading, gave an index of 3. A 3rd culture, taken from a patient in the desquamating stage, gave an index of 3.

Four blood agar plates showed only streptococci with very narrow zones of hemolysis about the colonies. Indices made on these 3 cultures were as follows: 2, 0.5, and 0.5.

Of the blood agar plates from the 2nd hospital for contagious diseases, 7 were selected that contained both the wide and the narrow zoned hemolytic streptococcus colonies. Indices were made with each type of streptococcus; the results as shown in the accompanying chart indicate that the indices were lower with the narrow zoned hemolytic streptococci than with the typical wide zoned hemolytic streptococci of scarlet fever.

Seventy of the wide zoned hemolytic streptococci obtained from the 2nd hospital for contagious diseases were examined. Forty-four were cultures taken in the first week of scarlet fever and 26 in the later stages

Cultures	Opsonic Index Using Wide Zoned Hemolytic Streptococci	Opsonic Index Using Narrow Zoned Hemolytic Streptococci
1	17	7
2	4	3
3	2	1
4	4	1
5	14	14
6	2	2
7	2	0.6

of the disease. In the group of 44, five indices were less than 2. Three were 1.5, one 1.6, and one 1.8. The patients from whom the 3 cultures giving the latter indices were obtained had mild cases of scarlet fever. The other 41 indices varied from 2 to 17, the average being 4.8. Of the 24 hemolytic streptococcus strains obtained from patients in the later stages of scarlet fever, 17 gave indices from 2 to 15.3, an average of 5.6. Seven gave indices less than 2; for example 1.6, 1, 1, 1.1, 1.2, 0.7, and 0.5. It seems probable that here, too, the scarlatinal streptococci had been replaced by the hemolytic streptococci found in the throats of normal persons.

The group of streptococci used as controls comprised 16 strains of hemolytic streptococci. Four taken from blood cultures gave the following indices: 16, 0.8, 0.3, and 1.4. Five of the strains were obtained from throat cultures; the indices on these were 0.4, 0.4, 1, and 4.2. The index of 4.2 was obtained from a culture from the throat of a nurse who had been on duty in a hospital for contagious diseases; this suggests that she was probably a carrier of a scarlatinal strain of streptococcus. Two of the controls were obtained from ground tonsillar tissue, and each gave an index of 1.5. One strain obtained from pus was not phagocytosed. Two strains cultured from spinal fluid gave indices of 2 and 0.1. A culture from a mastoid had an index of 4; no history of a previous attack of scarlet fever could be obtained in the case of this patient. An index of 12 was obtained with a culture from a suppurating gland; the patient from whom it was taken had peeling of the soles of the feet and palms of the hands. A physician from a hospital for contagious diseases made the comment that if he had not known the history of the case, he should have supposed the patient was in the desquamating stage of scarlet fever. The opsonic index of this group, therefore, varied from 0 to 16. Four high indices occurred: an index of 16 with a culture from a terminal septicemia; an index of 4.2 with one from a probable carrier of scarlet fever; an index of 4 with a culture from a mastoid; and an index of 12 with one from an infection in which there was desquamation resembling that occurring in scarlet fever. It seems probable that the 2nd and the 4th were strains from scarlet fever.

When it became apparent that a considerable number of the blood agar plate cultures from patients with typical scarlet fever contained anhemolytic streptococci only, we decided to include 4 anhemolytic streptococcus controls. Three of these strains were obtained from blood cultures and had the following indices: 3, 1.6, and 1.8. The 4th was isolated from spinal fluid and gave an index of 0.3. These indices were lower than the 3 obtained on anhemolytic streptococci isolated from patients with scarlet fever.

While we were working on this series, a number of cultures from cases suspected of being scarlet fever were brought in for examination. Most of these streptococci were hemolytic, and all gave low indices; in no instance was scarlet fever diagnosed. One case is worthy of note; a child, six months old, had a throat typical of scarlet fever, but an atypical rash. Repeated cultures revealed anhemolytic streptococci only. The child became progressively worse, and convalescent scarlet fever serum was administered, with immediate improvement. The opsonic index with this anhemolytic streptococcus was 4.

SUMMARY

The opsonification test for the identification of the streptococcus of scarlet fever can be completed within 24 hours, when the streptococcus from the suspected material is in pure culture, and within 48 hours, when there is a mixed bacterial flora necessitating subcultures from picked colonies.

The opsonification tests are practical for use in any general laboratory, since there is only slight variation when the tests are performed independently by two persons or when different leukocytes are used.

Of the 94 strains of hemolytic streptococci cultured from patients with scarlet fever, 80 (85%) gave indices over 2.

Of the 16 hemolytic streptococci from sources other than scarlet fever, 4 gave indices over 2. However, at least 2 of these strains were probably scarlatinal streptococci.

Streptococci surrounded by narrow zones of hemolysis appeared on many of the blood agar plate cultures from patients with scarlet fever. This strain of streptococcus appeared alone or in conjunction with the typical wide zoned hemolytic streptococcus associated with scarlet fever. The opsonic indices with the narrow zoned hemolytic streptococcus, were, for the most part, lower than those with the typical scarlatinal strains.

Twenty-four of the 118 cultures examined, revealed anhemolytic streptococci exclusively, although these 24 cultures were taken from cases of clinically typical scarlet fever. Opsonic indices made on a few of these cultures, and also on anhemolytic streptococcal cultures from other sources used as controls, tended to be lower than those with hemolytic scarlatinal streptococci.

CONCLUSION

Although the opsonification test for the identification of scarlet fever streptococci is not absolutely specific in our series, it nevertheless offers a rapid, valuable aid in the diagnosis of scarlet fever.

THE UNITS OF PROTECTIVE ANTIBODY IN ANTI-PNEUMOCOCCUS SERUM AND ANTIBODY SOLUTION *

LLOYD D. FELTON

From the Department of Preventive Medicine and Hygiene, Harvard Medical School, Boston

Just what method should be used for standardization or estimation of the protective strength of antipneumococcus serum is a problem. The method of choice to date is the mouse protection test which has been developed by the work of Neufeld, Avery, Chickering, Cole, Dochez, Wadsworth, and others,[1] and applied as a practical standard by the Hygienic Laboratory.[2] The test consists of the protection of two out of three mice from 0.1 cc. of a highly virulent 18-hour serum broth culture by 0.2 cc. of serum. In our work on pneumococcus antibody in which fairly accurate comparison of antibody content of various serum fractions was essential, it was soon seen that 0.1 cc. of culture was too large a dose. This was especially true with type 2 and type 3 organisms. Consequently from time to time dosages of organisms varying from 0.05 cc. to 0.0005 cc. were tried against varying dilutions of serum. The change to a smaller dose of organism proved successful for a two-fold reason: first, because it minimized the zone effect, that is, the death of the animals receiving large amounts of serum or antibody solution while those receiving less survived; and second, because the endpoint became more definite. Many serums have been studied which not only passed the standard of the Hygienic Laboratory, but also were found to contain from two to four times as many protective units when estimated with dilute culture as they did when the 0.1 cc. dose of culture was the standard. For example, one lot of serum, some 70 liters, shipped to our laboratory for experimental purposes because of failure to pass the government standard, when tested by dilute culture, had 600 protective units per cc. However, in view of the possible antagonistic

Received for publication, Oct. 6, 1928.

* This is one of a series of studies carried out in part under a grant by the Influenza Commission of the Metropolitan Life Insurance Company.

1. Neufeld, F., and L. Händel: Ztschr. f. Immunitätsf. u. exper. Therap., Orig., 1909, 3, p. 159; Berl. klin. Wchnschr., 1912, 49, p. 680; League of Nations, Health Org. Serological Investigations, 1923, p. 74. Avery, Chickering, Cole, Dochez: Rockefeller Inst. for M. Research, monograph 7, 1917. Wadsworth, Kirkbride and Gilbert: Arch. Int. Med., 1919, 23, p. 269. McCoy, G. W.: In the Newer Knowledge of Bacteriology and Immunology, ed. by Jordan & Folk, 1928, p. 958. Cotoni, I.: League of Nations, Health Org. Serological Investigations, 1923, 123, p. 56.
2. U. S. Public Health Report, Nov. 21, 1919, p. 2663; Enlows, E. M. A.: Hyg. Lab. Bull., 1923, 134, p. 45.

substance present in immune serum, which in fact may be the cause of the zone effect, the Hygienic Laboratory method for standardization of serum has practical usefulness, inasmuch as serums exhibiting this antagonistic effect would thus be eliminated. Its limitation lies in the failure fully to measure the actual number of protective units in a given serum.

Before presenting the experiments it might be well to interpret the Hygienic Laboratory standard in the terms of the units that have been used in this laboratory for the last four years. The unit as advocated by us [3] as well as recently by Park and Cooper,[4] is that dilution of antibody or serum which will protect against 1,000,000 MLD of virulent pneumococci. In the actual test 100,000 to 500,000 fatal doses of pneumococci are used against varying dilutions of antibody in series, and from the dilution protecting, the amount that should protect against a million doses is estimated. Virulence of the test culture is such that 3 to 10 organisms kill a mouse in 36 to 48 hours. On the other hand, the Hygienic Laboratory standard requires the protection of two out of three mice injected simultaneously with 0.1 cc. of a virulent culture and 0.2 cc. of serum. If, as shown by plating out experiments, 0.5 cc. of 1 : 100,000,000 dilution of a virulent 18-hour culture contains from 3 to 10 organisms and will kill a mouse in from 36 to 48 hours, then in 0.1 cc. of undiluted culture there would be $\frac{200,000,000}{10}$ or 20,000,000 lethal doses. Consequently in 1 cc. of serum which passed the standard test there would be 5 x 20 or at least 100 units of protection. This is in reality a weak protective serum; most of the type 1 serum that has been tested in our work contained from 200 to 1,000 units per cc. averaging perhaps 300; in other words, of such potency that 0.2 cc. of serum should theoretically protect against 0.3 cc. of 18-hour culture of maximum virulence.

The attempt in our study to estimate quantitatively the antibody content of the various serum fractions involved three definite problems, all well known, first the virulence of the organism, second the susceptibility of the test animal, and third the dose of the organisms when of maximum virulence. The first two variables are too interdependent from the standpoint of our present purpose to admit separation. The problem in virulence is the percentage of mice susceptible to a fatal infection from a minimum dose of organisms. In the first place, it should be stated that

3 Felton, L. D.: Boston M. & S. J., 1924, 190, p. 819.
4. J. Am. M. A., 1928, 90, p. 1349

it has been found possible to maintain the virulence of types 1, 2, and 3 pneumococci to such a degree that the injection of 3 to 10 organisms (perhaps 1) becomes invariably fatal for as many as 100 mice, the individual susceptibility of some of the animals seemingly having no influence other than causing a slight delay over the usual 36-hour survival time.

EXPERIMENT 1.—INFLUENCE OF VIRULENCE ON FATALITY RATE IRRESPECTIVE OF DOSE OF ORGANISMS

The point of practical importance is how much will a dose of slightly less virulent organisms influence the number of fatal infections of a relatively large number of mice. The answer to this question is given in one experiment illustrative of many. To obtain cultures of varying virulence a highly virulent type 1 organism was grown in an automatic transfer machine [5] on ordinary broth and transfers taken on the first, second, and third days. Counting the original strain (A) these four cultures were of supposedly different virulence, namely B, C, and D in order of the number of transfers. Dilutions were made from each culture in a logarithmic series from 10^{-2} to 10^{-7} and ten mice injected intraperitoneally with each. The results are given in table 1. Leaving out for the present the discussion of virulence and animal susceptibility, it is at once apparent from the practical standpoint that consistent results may be expected only with pneumococci of maximum virulence. Thus from the results here shown, by the use of a culture of fair degree of virulence (B) the chances of two mice out of ten being resistant toward a relatively dilute culture are good. This is true not only for a dilution of 10^{-7}, but even for dilutions containing 10, 100 or even 1,000 times more organisms. On the other hand, with a less virulent culture, (D) for example, there were only three possibilities out of ten that the mice would die when injected with 14 organisms, four with 140 organisms, six with 1,400. This experiment is given, not to show the relation of virulence to susceptibility in a general way, but rather as an example to emphasize the importance of maintaining test organisms at maximum virulence for standardization of pneumococcus serum and antibody.

EXPERIMENT 2.—TITRATION OF PROTECTIVE ANTIBODY SHOWING VARYING SUSCEPTIBILITY OF MICE

That maximum virulence is not the only essential variable in estimating antibody content with the mouse method has been observed many times in our study. Noteworthy variations have occurred when large doses of organisms were used. For example, in table 2 are given the

5. Felton, L. O., and Daugherty, K. M.: J. Exper. Med., 1924, 39, p. 137.

TABLE 1.—INFLUENCE OF VIRULENCE ON FATALITY RATE IRRESPECTIVE OF DOSE OF ORGANISMS

	Hours of Survival	Dilutions of Culture 10^{-2}	10^{-3}	10^{-4}	10^{-5}	10^{-6}	10^{-7}	Number of Organisms in Dilution 10^{-7}
A	24	6*	5	3	2	1	..	6
	36	4	3	4	6	8	..	..
	48	..	2	3	1	1	6	..
	72	..	..	..	..	..	1	..
	96	..	..	..	..	..	2	..
	120	..	..	..	..	..	..	..
Total	...	10	10	10	9	10	9	..
B	24	4	2	..	..	..	..	9
	36	4	6	6	3	..	..	..
	48	..	2	4	4	4	5	..
	72	2	..	..	3	3	2	..
	96	..	..	..	..	1	..	..
	120	..	..	..	..	..	1	..
Total	...	10	10	10	10	8	8	..
C	24	3	..	..	..	..	..	12
	36	4	4	3	1	..	..	..
	48	3	4	4	3	1	..	..
	72	..	1	1	..	1	..	..
	96	..	..	..	1	2	2	..
	120	..	..	..	1	..	1	..
Total	...	10	9	8	6	4	3	..
D	24	..	..	..	..	..	..	..
	36	7	9	4	2	..	..	14
	48	..	..	1	2	1	..	..
	72	..	1	1	1	2	1	..
	96	1	..	..	1	..	..	..
	120	..	..	..	..	1	2	..
Total	...	8	10	6	6	4	3	..

* Indicates number of mice dying in number of hours specified.

TABLE 2.—TITRATION OF PROTECTIVE ANTIBODY SHOWING VARYING SUSCEPTIBILITY OF MICE

TYPE 1 LOTS

Lot	Number Survived Out of Six Mice Injected. Dilutions of Antibody 1 : 100	1 : 200	1 : 300	1 : 400
21	6	2	3	.
23	5	3	2	.
24	6	6	1	.
25	3	5	.	2
26	5	6	.	3
27	5	2	.	0
28	5	2	.	3
29	5	6	.	3
30	6	0	.	1
31	6	3	.	4
32	{ 5	{ 6	.	{ 2
	{ 5	{ 3	.	{ 1
33	3	4	.	3
35	{ 5	{ 6	.	{ 3
	{ 6	{ 6	.	{ 4

Culture: 0.5 cc. of an 8-hour broth culture of such virulence that 0.5 cc. of a 1 : 10,000,000 (3 to 5 organisms) killed in 36 hours.

results of the estimation of units in type 1 antibody concentrate using 0.5 cc. of a 1: 10 dilution of an 8-hour culture and 0.5 cc. of the varying dilutions of antibody solution. Six mice were used for each dilution of antibody and all were injected as nearly as possible with the same technique under identical conditions. The results show great variation in susceptibility of the individual mice. Thus, if 3 survivals out of 6 be used as the criterion what would be the units of no. 28? Should the

TABLE 3.—TITRATION OF PROTECTIVE ANTIBODY SHOWING VARYING SUSCEPTIBILITY OF MICE

POLYVALENT LOTS

	Type 1 Dilutions of Antibody			Type 2 Dilutions of Antibody		
	1 : 6000	1 : 8000	1 : 10000	1 : 2000	1 : 4000	1 : 6000
Lot 12	36	36	84	84	36	60
	66	36	84	S	36	84
	S	36	S	S	36	18
	S	S	S	S	S	36
	S	S	S	S	S	36
Lot 13	36	36	36	S	36	36
	36	S	60	S	36	36
	S	S	S	S	36	S
	S	S	S	S	S	S
	S	S	S	S	S	S

S indicates survival, and numbers refer to hours of survival.

TABLE 4.—TITRATION OF PROTECTIVE ANTIBODY SHOWING VARYING SUSCEPTIBILITY OF MICE

Type II

	Dilutions of Antibody			
	0.5*	1 : 100	1 : 200	1 : 400
Lot 18	36	S	S	S
	36	S	S	S
	20	S	S	S
	S	S	36	S
	36	S	84	S
	36	84	22	S

S indicates survival, and numbers refer to hours of survival.
* Indicates 0.5 cc. injected undiluted.

calculation be based on the dilution of 1: 200 or 1: 400, a mere 100% variation? If 4 out of 6 is taken, the same difficulty occurs with no. 31. Five out of 6 would surely be the safest estimate, but would it be necessarily correct?

That the problem of varying susceptibility is not limited to a relatively large dose of organism is shown by a titration of two polyvalent lots of antibody using a culture dilution of 1: 500, as shown in table 3. With both lots the titration of the type 2 antibody gave consistent results, but with the type 1 protective substance it is rather difficult to determine whether the number of units in no. 12 or no. 13 is 1,200 or 2,000.

Again in table 4 are given the results of the titration of a lot of type 2 antibody. It is of interest to note that only one mouse out of 6 survived when 0.5 cc. of the undiluted material was used against 0.5 cc. of a 1 : 100 dilution of culture, whereas 6 out of 6 mice lived when the same dose of culture was used against 1/400 as much of the protective material, a typical zone effect. Here, also, the estimation of the endpoint is doubtful. These three experiments were carried out with what seemed to be organisms of maximum virulence, the control animals all dying when

TABLE 5.—INFLUENCE OF MASSIVE DOSES OF CULTURE

POLYVALENT 24—TYPES 1 AND 2

Culture Dilutions	Dilutions of Antibody					
			Type 1			
0.5 cc. *	1 cc.*	0.5 cc.*	1 : 2.5	1 : 5	1 : 10	
	18	18	18	S	18	
	18	18	18	S	18	
	0.5 cc.	1 : 2.5	1 : 5	1 : 10	1 : 20	
1 : 2.5	18	S	18	18	20	
	18	S	18	36	36	
	1 : 2.5	1 : 5	1 : 10	1 : 20	1 : 40	
1 : 5	36	S	S	S	60	
	S	S	S	S	S	
	1 : 5	1 : 10	1 : 20	1 : 40	1 : 80	
1 : 10	36	S	S	S	S	
	S	S	S	S	S	
			Type 2			
	1 cc.	0.5 cc.	1 : 2.5	1 : 5	1 : 10	1 : 20
0.5 cc.	18	18	19	18	18	18
	18	18	18	18	36	36
	0.5 cc.	1 : 2.5	1 : 5	1 : 10	1 : 20	1 : 40
1 : 2.5	19	18	18	20	19	18
	18	18	36	S	S	60
	1 : 2.5	1 : 5	1 : 10	1 : 20	1 : 40	1 : 80
1 : 5	18	20	S	S	60	36
	19	36	S	S	84	72
	1 : 5	1 : 10	1 : 20	1 : 40	1 : 80	1 : 160
1 : 10	20	60	S	60	S	S
	S	S	S	S	S	S

S indicates survival; numbers refer to hours of survival
* indicates 0.5 cc. and 1 cc. injected undiluted.

injected with less than 10 organisms, thus indicating that in spite of the large dose of organisms, the irregularity in death of mice in serum titration is due at least in part to the individual variation in susceptibility.

EXPERIMENT 3.—INFLUENCE OF MASSIVE DOSES OF CULTURE

In spite of the difficulties encountered in estimating the unit protective strength of serum or of antibody solution, there can be no doubt that a method of estimation sufficiently accurate for therapeutic purposes can be developed. The problem of the proper dilution of culture is taken up in the following experiments. The first point is the effect of large doses of culture against a fairly potent polyvalent lot. The doses of culture used were 0.5 cc. undiluted, and dilutions 1 : 2.5, 1 : 5, and

1 : 10. The experiment as given in table 5 is self-explanatory. The results are quite definite. That is, for both type 1 and type 2 any dose of culture larger than 0.5 cc. of a 1 : 5 dilution is too large inasmuch as all mice receiving these doses, regardless of the amount of antibody solution succumbed. In the case of the type 2 antibody there was a pronounced zone effect when using 1 : 5 dilution of culture. These results are representative of those obtained from other experiments where the culture is of maximum virulence.

EXPERIMENT 4.—INFLUENCE OF SMALL DOSES OF CULTURE

In this experiment the titration was carried out with culture of different dilutions, the variation of the dilutions of the culture as well as of

TABLE 6.—INFLUENCE OF SMALL DOSES OF CULTURE

POLYVALENT 24—TYPE 1

Culture Dilutions	Dilutions of Antibody			
1 : 12.5	1 : 30 36–S	1 : 60 S–S	1 : 120 S–S	1 : 240 96–S
1 : 25	1 : 60 S–S	1 : 120 S–S	1 : 240 S–S	1 : 480 84–S
1 : 50	1 : 120 S–S	1 : 240 S–S	1 : 480 S–S	1 : 960 36–48
1 : 100	1 : 240 S–S	1 : 480 S–S	1 : 960 84–S	1 : 1920 36–S
1 : 200	1 : 480 S–S	1 : 960 S–S	1 : 1920 S–S	1 : 3840 36–S
1 : 400	1 : 960 S–S	1 : 1920 S–S	1 : 3840 S–S	1 : 7680 60–S
1 : 800	1 : 1920 S–S	1 : 3840 60–S	1 : 7680 S–S	1 : 15360 60–S
1 : 1600	1 : 3840 S–S	1 : 7680 60–S	1 : 15360 36–36	1 : 30720 20–60
1 : 3200	1 : 7680 S–S	1 : 15360 S–S	1 : 30720 36–84	1 : 61440 36–42
1 : 6400	1 : 15360 S–S	1 : 30720 60–S	1 : 61440 36–48	1 : 122880 36–36

S indicates survival; numbers refer to hours of survival

antibody solution forming a geometrical series such that, with any dilution of culture used, the number of mice surviving should be the same in the different tests. As a matter of fact, there is a surprising regularity of results up to and including the culture in dilution of 1 : 800. Beyond that, that is in dilution 1 :1,600, 1 : 3,200, and 1 : 6,400 of the culture, there is a marked diminution in protective strength of the antibody in corresponding dilutions. This is found to be the same for type 1 and also type 2 as shown in tables 6 and 7. There is, however, an exception in the case of the type 2 material, that is, a culture dilution of 1 : 12.5 is quite definitely too large a dose, as is also a dilution of 1 : 25 as judged by a zone effect. It would appear from these two experiments that 0.5 cc. of any dilution between 1 : 25 and 1 : 800 of an 18-hour broth culture of maximum virulence might be used for the estimation of protective units.

EXPERIMENT 5.—COMPARISON OF ANTIBODY CONCENTRATE AS TITRATED WITH DILUTIONS OF CULTURE 1: 200, 1: 400 and 1: 800

To test further this assumption, three polyvalent lots were titrated in the same way with dilutions of culture 1:200, 1:400 and 1:800. As can be seen from the type 1 titration in table 8, quite consistent results

TABLE 7.—INFLUENCE OF SMALL DOSES OF CULTURE

POLYVALENT 24—TYPE 2

Culture Dilutions	Dilutions of Antibody			
1 : 12.5	1 : 5 20–18–20–S	1 : 10 44–60–18–S	1 : 20 20–20–60–S	1 : 40 60–36–S–S
1 : 25	1 : 10 36–36–S–S	1 : 20 S–S–S–S	1 : 40 60–S–S–S	1 : 80 60–S–S–S
1 : 50	1 : 20 20–70–S–S	1 : 40 84–S–S–S	1 : 80 S–S–S–S	1 : 160 60–36–60–S
1 : 100	1 : 40 S–S–S–S	1 : 80 S–S–S–S	1 : 160 66–S–S–S	1 : 320 60–36–S–S
1 : 200	1 : 80 60–S–S–S	1 : 160 S–S–S–S	1 : 320 S–S–S–S	1 : 640 60–S–S–S
1 : 400	1 : 160 48–84–S–S	1 : 320 36–S–S–S	1 : 640 S–S–S–S	1 : 1280 60–S–S–S
1 : 800	1 : 320 S–S–S–S	1 : 640 36–60–S–S	1 : 1280 84–60–S–S	1 : 2560 60–S–S–S
1 : 1600	1 : 640 S–S–S–S	1 : 1280 36–S–S–S	1 : 2560 18–18–60–60	1 : 5120 60–S–S–S
1 : 3200	1 : 1280 36–S–S–S	1 : 2560 44–60–S–S	1 : 5120 36–48–60–S	1 : 10240 36–36–36–S
1 : 6400	1 : 2560 60–S–S–S	1 : 5120 36–S–S–S	1 : 10240 18–48–36–36	1 : 20480 36–84–60–S

S indicates survival; numbers refer to hours of survival.

TABLE 8.—COMPARISON OF ANTIBODY CONCENTRATE AS TITRATED WITH DILUTIONS OF CULTURE 1: 200, 1: 400, 1: 800

POLYVALENT LOTS—TYPE 1

Culture Dilutions	Dilutions of Antibody				
			LOT 16		
1 : 200	1 : 1600 S–S	1 : 2000 S–S	1 : 2400 S–S	1 : 2800 S–S	1 : 3200 60–60
1 : 400	1 : 3200 S–S	1 : 4000 S–S	1 : 4800 S–S	1 : 5600 S–S	1 : 6400 42–60
1 : 800	1 : 6400 S–S	1 : 8000 60–72	1 : 9600 60–60	1 : 11200 60–S	1 : 12800 36–S
			LOT 22		
1 : 200	1 : 1600 84–S	1 : 2000 S–S	1 : 2400 S–S	1 : 2800 S–S	1 : 3200 84–S
1 : 400	1 : 3200 S–S	1 : 4000 36–S	1 : 4800 S–S	1 : 5600 S–S	1 : 6400 84–S
1 : 800	1 : 6400 S–S	1 : 8000 36–S	1 : 9600 S–S	1 : 11200 84–S	1 : 12800 36–36
			LOT 23		
1 : 200	1 : 1600 S–S	1 : 2000 60–S	1 : 2400 S–S	1 : 2800 S–S	1 : 3200 36–S
1 : 400	1 : 3200 S–S	1 : 4000 S–S	1 : 4800 S–S	1 : 5600 60–S	1 : 6400 36–36
1 : 800	1 : 6400 S–S	1 : 8000 36–S	1 : 9600 S–S	1 : 11200 20–36	1 : 12800 36–36

S indicates survival; numbers refer to hours of survival.

were obtained from dilutions 1:200 and 1:400, but definite variations from these were found from the dilution 1:800. However, in the type 2 titration, as given in table 9, the results in all three dilutions of culture were consistent.

The deduction from the foregoing titrations and others which gave similar results is that apparently there is a wide range of dilutions of culture suitable for the estimation of protective units. Consequently, the dilution chosen for the estimation of protective antibody content will be perhaps one of convenience. It is for this reason that we purpose to make a suggestion for a possible unit for the pneumococcus antibody solution and a method of estimation.

In the first place, .5 cc. has come to be a standard volume unit for test doses in work with mice, and should remain unchanged. The question of virulence should cause little trouble, but should receive constant attention. There is no doubt that strains of pneumococci can be made so virulent that a single cell will cause the death of a mouse in 36 hours. In reality even this may not be the measure of the limit of virulence, for while at least one cell is necessary, yet this cell may be so virulent that it not only kills a mouse but may kill even an animal whose resistance is a thousand times greater. Although there is some danger of using a culture of too high virulence for protective antibody titration, the common error is the use of a somewhat avirulent one. The virulence which we feel is adopted to practical work is one in which 0.5 cc. of a 1:100,000,000 dilution of an 18-hour serum broth culture, containing 3 to 5 organisms, causes the death of duplicate mice in 36 hours

TABLE 9.—COMPARISON OF ANTIBODY CONCENTRATE AS TITRATED WITH DILUTIONS OF CULTURE 1: 200, 1: 400, 1: 800

POLYVALENT LOTS—TYPE 2

Culture Dilutions	Dilutions of Antibody				
LOT 16					
1 : 200	1 : 600 S–S	1 : 800 S–S	1 : 1000 60–S	1 : 1200 S–S	1 : 1400 60–S
1 : 400	1 : 1200 S–S	1 : 1600 S–S	1 : 2000 S–S	1 : 2400 S–S	1 : 2800 60–60
1 : 800	1 : 2400 S–S	1 : 3200 S–S	1 : 4000 S–S	1 : 4800 60–S	1 : 5600 60–S
LOT 22					
1 : 200	1 : 600 S–S	1 : 800 S–S	1 : 1000 36–S	1 : 1200 S–S	1 : 1400 36–S
1 : 400	1 : 1200 36–S	1 : 1600 S–S	1 : 2000 S–S	1 : 2400 S–S	1 : 2800 60–S
1 : 800	1 : 2400 S–S	1 : 3200 S–S	1 : 4000 36–36	1 : 4800 60–S	1 : 5600 60–84
LOT 23					
1 : 200	1 : 600 S–S	1 : 800 S–S	1 : 1000 36–S	1 : 1200 S–S	1 : 1400 84–60
1 : 400	1 : 1200 S–S	1 : 1600 S–S	1 : 2000 36–S	1 : 2400 S–S	1 : 2800 36–84
1 : 800	1 : 2400 60–60	1 : 3200 S–S	1 : 4000 S–S	1 : 4800 S–S	1 : 5600 36–36

S indicates survival; numbers refer to hours of survival.

when injected intraperitoneally. This degree of virulence has been maintained in this laboratory (usual mouse passage method) almost constantly for the last two years with types 1, 2 and 3 pneumococci.

The next point is the dilution of culture in making the test. To simplify the method of calculation of the unit to a minimum, 0.5 cc. of a 1 : 200 dilution of an 18-hour broth culture of the aforesaid virulence is suggested. When a million lethal doses is used as the basis of the protective unit, the following explains the method of obtaining the number of units per cc. If 0.5 cc. of a 1 : 500 dilution of antibody solution protects against 0.5 cc. of a 1 : 200 dilution of culture, then the units per cc. equal 500 or simply the reciprocal of the dilution protecting. That is, 0.5 cc. of 1 : 200 dilution contains 500,000 lethal doses ($\frac{100,000,000}{200} = 500,000$). Since the dilution protecting was 1 : 500, it would take twice the amount or 1 : 250 to protect against 1,000,000 lethal doses; but only 0.5 cc. of a 1 : 500 dilution was used, so that in 1 cc. the amount of antibody to protect against 1,000,000 lethal doses would be one-half of 1 : 250 or 1 : 500. In other words, by using a culture of 1 : 200 and adhering to the 0.5 cc. volume throughout, the reciprocal of the fraction of the serum or antibody protecting is the number of units per cc.

This method differs only from the one used by Dr. Park and myself for the past two years, in that 0.005 cc. is the culture unit instead of 0.001, and of course 500,000 lethal doses of pneumococci for the actual test instead of 100,000. As a matter of fact, the present method is essentially what has been used by me during the 4-year study of pneumococcus antibody, that is, a dilute culture as constant against a variable serum or antibody. Although an extended comparison of the unit value in different antibody solutions as judged from estimation from culture dose of 0.001 cc. and dose 0.005 cc. has not been carried out, a sufficient study has been made to warrant the assumption that either dose will give the same unit strength. The 0.005 cc. necessitates less dilution of culture and also antibody, and the dilution protecting is the number of units per cc. of the test specimen. For these reasons we are suggesting this method as a means of standardization until a better can be developed.

In order that there can be no question as to the exact details of the method advocated, a summary is given as follows:

(1) Mice used as test animals must be healthy stock weighing about 20 grams. They should preferably be white. Colored mice may be used. However, the susceptibility of a strain must be established before use in making the estimations of unit strength of serum or antibody solution.

(2) The cultures type 1, 2 and 3, or even group 4 must be of such virulence that 3 to 5 organisms when injected into the peritoneal cavity of mice kill duplicate animals in 36 to 48 hours. An 18-hour serum or blood broth culture should contain from 3 to 5 organisms in a dilution of 1:100,000,000. In testing the number of organisms (plate method) in the 1:100,000,000 dilution it is important to make sure that the medium (blood agar) is suitable. Frequently in the case of stock blood agar, while heavy inoculation results in growth, the few organisms in the high dilutions of culture fail to grow. Virulence is maintained by frequent mouse passage. A successful procedure has been the injection of 0.5 cc. of a 1:10,000 dilution of an 18-hour serum broth culture at about 5 p. m. If the culture is of almost maximum virulence, the mouse will die by 10 a. m. A heart blood culture is taken by the usual capillary pipet technique. The different organisms must be checked for type and also for bile solubility before being used for antibody titration.

(3) The serum and antibody solution must be free from living organisms. This is an important precaution in making tests on serum. The concentrate prepared by us for several years has been preserved by the addition of tricresol to 0.2%. A higher concentration can be used, but it must be remembered that we are dealing with a water-insoluble protein which when denatured begins to become salt insoluble and precipitates—the higher the concentration of tricresol, the greater the amount denatured, and consequently the development of a troublesome precipitate. I see no reason why a concentration of tricresol of 0.2% should be exceeded as a preservative for concentrates from antipneumococcus serum.

(4) Preliminary Test: If nothing is known about the unit concentration of a given serum or antibody, a preliminary test should be made, with single mice in a geometric series of dilutions of antibody; such as 1:25, 1:50, 1:100, 1:200, 1:400 for serum; and 1:250, 1:500, 1:1,000, 1:2,000, 1:4,000 for antibody. After the approximate unit content is established, then this is checked by mice in triplicate. For example, if the 1:250, 1:500 and 1:1,000 mice survive and the 1:2,000 and 1:4000 do not, then dilutions 1:1,000, 1:1500 and 1:2000 should be run against the culture, three mice to a single dilution. The end point is judged by the last dilution in which 2 out of 3 mice survive 96 hours.

(5) Accurate pipets, of course, must be used throughout, both for culture, although this is not so important, and for the serum or antibody. In making dilutions never less than 1 cc. is used as the volume for transfer, with a clean pipet for each dilution.

(6) The actual test is carried out as follows: The dilutions of the serum or antibody to be tested are made in sterile physiological salt solution. The 1:200 dilution of culture is made in 1% sterile peptone solution which had been adjusted to P_H 7.6. (Five grams sodium chloride, 10 grams peptone, in 1,000 cc. of water, adjusted to P_H 7.6.) Sufficient culture is diluted at one time for one test fluid, and divided into as many fractions as the number of dilutions of antibody used, that is, if tests are to be made on 1:1,000, 1:1,500, 1:2,000 dilutions of the serum or the antibody, then the culture should be divided into three portions. This is done so that the residual antibody in the syringe is not mixed with the culture. Three syringes are needed for each sample of serum or antibody tested. Draw up 0.5 cc. of culture in one syringe and then 0.5 cc. of the most dilute test fluid (in the example given 1:2,000), injected immediately intraperitoneally. (Be sure there is no leak of fluid; if such does occur, discard the mouse and replace.) Do the same with the other two syringes. Then with the same syringes, take a culture from the second tube and of course antibody from the next higher dilution. This process is repeated until all the dilutions are injected in a series in triplicate.

(7) An antibody solution the unit value of which is known is always used as a control. Two dilutions, the one containing the number of units previously estimated and the other containing one-half that number, are injected in mice in triplicate. For example, if the control contains 1,000 protective units, mice are injected with .5 cc. of 1 : 1,000 dilution and also 1 : 2,000, both in triplicate. If the mice injected with the small dose of antibody survive, the culture is somewhat avirulent and the test must be repeated.

DISCUSSION

In presenting this method for standardization of antipneumococcus serum and protective antibody, its limitations are recognized. The nature of the variables, namely virulence of the organism, susceptibility of the test animals, white mice, and constituents of serum and antibody solution, preclude an accuracy comparable to the neutralization of diphtheria or tetanus toxin with the respective antitoxin. Until something more definite is known concerning the mechanism of infection of pneumococci, just what substance, substances, or activity does result in injury to the host, the development of a precise method for estimation of antibody content is blocked. For this reason and from our experience of its practicability, the present method is given as a possible aid toward further studies of the use and limitations of pneumococcus antibody.

SUMMARY

A method is outlined for the standardization of antipneumococcus serum and pneumococcus antibody concentrate. The unit is that fraction of a cc. of serum or antibody (or dilution) which will protect against one million fatal doses of an 18-hour serum broth culture of such virulence that 3 to 10 organisms injected intraperitoneally into a mouse result in death in from 36 to 48 hours. In practice 500,000 fatal doses of organisms—0.5 cc. of 1 : 200 dilution of an 18-hour serum broth culture in which 3 to 10 organisms, as estimated by the plate method, are present in a 1 : 100,000,000 dilution of culture—are used against dilutions of test serum or antibody in a geometric series. By maintaining these units the reciprocal of the dilution protecting two out of three mice represents the number of units in 1 cc. of serum or antibody.

CONCENTRATION OF PNEUMOCOCCUS ANTIBODY *

Lloyd D. Felton

From the Department of Preventive Medicine and Hygiene, Harvard Medical School, Boston

A method was given in a previous publication [1] by which the protective substance of antipneumococcus serum could be concentrated with a resulting product practically free from chill-producing characteristics. It was also stated in the same publication that the steps outlined for the purification of the water-insoluble precipitate obtained by diluting potent serum with water were applicable to the water-insoluble precipitate obtained by the common salting-out methods, using ammonium sulfate or sodium sulfate. It is the purpose of this paper to outline a method of concentration with anhydrous sodium sulfate as the precipitating agent instead of the commonly used ammonium sulfate. Sodium sulfate, rather than ammonium sulfate, is given at present because, as judged from the troublesome reaction after intravenous administration, a better product has been obtained by its use. From the standpoint of concentration of the protective antibody alone, however, ammonium sulfate has not only been used in many experiments with the same result as with sodium sulfate but also it has the advantage of greater ease in handling. The objection to its use, from our experience, is the chill-producing reaction of the final product following intravenous administration. Attempts have been made to obviate this difficulty but so far they have met with only partial success.

In the course of our investigation on the pneumococcus antibody, obtained from the serum of immunized horses, certain facts have been observed concerning the associated protein. Although details will be given in other publications a brief summary of our findings will be reported here. In the first place, in contradistinction to Avery's work,[2] the antibody has been found by us to be associated only with a water-insoluble protein; never with the water-soluble pseudoglobulin. This observation has been confirmed by Banzhaf.[3] However, the possibility should not be overlooked that the antibody when isolated may be water-soluble and also that the manipulations in Avery's work may have been such that some of the protective antibody was found with the pseu-

Received for publication, Oct. 6, 1928.

* This is one of a series of studies carried out in part under a grant by the Influenza Commission of the Metropolitan Life Insurance Company.

1. J. Infect. Dis., 1928, 42, p. 248.
2. J. Exper. Med., 1915, 21, p. 133.
3. Proc. Soc. Exper. Biol. & Med., 1925, 22, p. 329.

doglobulin. In our experience testing the serums of many horses, with a definite choice of method, all the protective substances, without exception, came down with a water-insoluble protein. It should be pointed out, nevertheless, that dilution of the serums from horses in every stage of immunization does not necessarily cause the precipitation of all the protective substance. An explanation has not been found, but seemingly it is a question of varying solubilities of the protective substance in serums of different horses. The term "varying" is used inasmuch as there seems to be in every horse a certain period during immunization at which all the protective substance is precipitated when the serum is diluted with water.

In addition, this protective water-insoluble protein is more alkaline than the well known water-insoluble euglobulin.[4] And it has also been found possible to free it from phosphorus [5] to the same degree as pseudoglobulin. These two points differentiate it from euglobin. There remain the common salting-out methods as means of differentiation. The limits of solubility with ammonium sulfate have been found to be 28 to 44% of saturation. This corresponds in the main with the findings of Avery and of Banzhaf. The results with sodium sulfate, several examples of which will be given below, have not been so definite.

If our observations are correct, the protective substance in antipneumococcus horse serum is associated with a water-insoluble protein; essentially free from phosphorus; of more alkaline characteristics than euglobulin; and at least similar to pseudoglobulin in its solubility in ammonium sulfate and perhaps sodium sulfate. It is thus seen that the protein, free or combined, or associated with the protective substance is different from any heretofore described in horse serum.

EXPERIMENT 1.—THE SOLUBILITY OF THE PROTECTIVE SUBSTANCE IN ANHYDROUS SODIUM SULFATE

This first experiment is given for the sake of orientation, an attempt to test the possibility of fractional separation of the inert from the protective protein. A sample of crude water-insoluble precipitate was obtained by diluting at the rate of one liter of immune serum to 12 liters of cold water acidulated so that the final P_H was 6.8. The mixture was allowed to stand in the ice box over night and then the supernatant diluted serum siphoned off. The precipitate was collected by centrifugation and suspended evenly in water. To 40 cc. samples heated to 40 C. was added sufficient anhydrous sodium sulfate to make percentages

4. Bull. Johns Hopkins Hosp., 1926, 38, p. 33.
5. J. Infect. Dis., 1925, 37, p. 309.

11, 12, 13, 14, 15, 17, 19, 21 respectively. After allowing the mixtures to stand for three hours at 37 C., the various precipitates with the exception of the 21% sample, were collected by rapid centrifugation, and made up to the original volume with water. A clear solution was obtained with all specimens. Due to the high salt content it was found necessary to filter the 21% sample. The supernatants of all except the 19 and 21% specimens were measured and sufficient sodium sulfate added to make the concentration in each 19%. These precipitates were collected as with the first and made up to 40 cc. with water. Each sample was then tested by standard methods for protective potency, agglutination titer, and nitrogen content. The protective potency was estimated by the survival of duplicate mice injected with 0.5 cc. of various dilutions of the protein solutions and 0.5 cc. of a 1:100 dilution of an 18-hour serum broth culture of type 2 organisms of such virulence that a dilution

TABLE 1.—SOLUBILITY OF THE PROTECTIVE SUBSTANCE IN SODIUM SULFATE

	Precipitate					Supernatant				
Sulfate %	Dilution Protecting	Nitrogen Mg. per Cc.	Nitrogen %	Nitrogen in Protective Dose	Agglutination	Dilution Protecting	Nitrogen Mg. per Cc.	Nitrogen %	Nitrogen in Protective Dose	Agglutination
11	0	.063	2.5	—	0	1:160	2.02	78.8	.0063	1:20
12	0	.161	6.4	—	0	1:160	1.79	70.7	.0056	1:20
13	1:2	.294	11.6	.0735	1:2	1:160	1.65	64.2	.0051	1:20
14	1:10	.658	26	.0329	1:2	1:160	1.32	52.2	.0041	1:20
15	1:10	1.26	49.8	.063	1:5	1:160	.798	31.5	.0025	1:10
17	1:80	1.82	71.9	.0114	1:10	1:80	.27	16.7	.0017	1:2
19	1:320	2.07	81.8	.0032	1:20					
21	1:320	2.14	84.6	.0033	1:20					
Control	1:640	2.53	100	.0020	1:20					

of 1:100,000,000 containing 3 organisms killed duplicate mice in 36 hours.

The results of this experiment, given in table 1, show in the first place that, as judged by both the agglutination and the protection, the lower limit of solubility is approximately 13% and the upper above 21%, in other words, approximately the limits given by Howe [6] and others for pseudoglobulin. There are in addition two items of interest in this experiment. The first is the difference in the yield found in the sodium sulfate precipitates as compared to the original material. Here it is seen that, although the agglutination titer of the original material is no higher than the 19 and 21% samples, the protection as judged by nitrogen content to a protective dose is higher than that of any of the various fractions except the second from 17%. The protection tests were repeated with about the same results. Our explanation of the loss with the sulfate

6. J. Biol. Chem., 1921, 49, p. 93.

fractions is the presence of some impurity in the sample of anhydrous salt; for this sample of salt was used in other experiments with a like loss. That the limiting solubility values were not altered, despite the loss in protective potency, is likely inasmuch as the same limits of solubility have been obtained with other lots of sodium sulfate. The second point of interest is the variation in the amount of protein in a protective dose. It is seen from the first precipitates that there is a gradual decrease of nitrogen or protein necessary for protection with the increase in sodium sulfate concentration, and also in the same way, the protein for a protective dose which remained in the supernatants of the lower concentration varies, the larger the concentration of sulfate the smaller the nitrogen in a protective unit. In other words, there is present an inert protein

TABLE 2.—SODIUM SULFATE FRACTIONS OF WATER-INSOLUBLE PRECIPITATE OBTAINED BY WATER DILUTION

Fractions ($NaSO_4$, %)	Volume, Cc.	Dilution Protecting (Culture 1:10)	Units Total	Units %
11.5	130	1:640	1,664,000	4.1
13	500	1:1280	12,800,000	31.9
18.5	1600	1:800	25,600,000	63.9

less soluble in the lower concentration of sodium sulfate than the protective substance. This inert protein is possibly euglobulin.

EXPERIMENT 2.—TYPE 1 PRECIPITATE FRACTIONATED WITH SODIUM SULFATE

From the standpoint of a quantitative separation of protective substance from this inert material, however, the application of the results obtained in the preceding experiment to large lots has been somewhat disappointing. For, as can be seen from table 2, in an experiment carried out with a rather concentrated type 1 precipitate, 4.1% of the total protective substance was precipitated with sodium sulfate in as low a concentration as 11.5%, and also 31.9% with the 13% fraction. Two important factors, which might have influenced this result were, however, disregarded; the first was the concentration of the precipitate, and the second was its age. It is well known that the more dilute the protein to the limit of precipitability, the better the separation of two different proteins by the common salting-out methods. It is also known that serum globulin varies greatly in its solubility in neutral salts if kept a considerable length of time, due to the process of denaturation. Because of these two facts another experiment was carried out with new precipitates diluted so that each sample contained in 1 cc. approximately 2 mg.of nitrogen. A precipitate from each type 1, 2, and 3 serums was worked up, taking out two separate fractions, one at 13% and the other at 18.5%. This latter concentration was chosen as the upper limit, as a matter of convenience for at this concentration of salt the precipitate can be collected by centrifugalization. The results (table 3) obtained in this experiment are similar to those of the first one, with the exception of the type 2 material. Here there was 17.2% of the protective substance precipitated at 13% sodium sulfate. The results of the last two experiments would indicate an impracticability of fractionating the water-insoluble precipitate directly with sodium sulfate.

As a matter of fact, the question of fractional precipitation has been taken up in numerous experiments, but inasmuch as the acid salt method [1] is used for purification of the final precipitate, the possible

TABLE 3.—SODIUM SULFATE FRACTIONS OF WATER-INSOLUBLE PRECIPITATE OBTAINED BY WATER DILUTION FROM TYPES 1, 2 AND 3 SERUMS

Type	Volume Diluted Precipitate, Cc.	Precipitate from 13% Sodium Sulfate				Precipitate from 18.5% Sodium Sulfate			
		Volume	Dilution Protecting	Units		Volume	Dilution Protecting	Units	
				Total	%			Total	%
1	10000	50	1:640	640,000	2.7	900	1:1280	23,040,000	97.3
2	8000	250	1:640	320,000	17.2	1200	1:640	1,536,000	82.8
3	8000	175	1:40	14,000	0.5	1000	1:1280	2,560,000	99.5

advantage of the use of an initial precipitation at from 11.5% to 12.5% to remove inert material is minimized. Although a slightly better product has been obtained by fractioning at 12 to 12.5% and 20%, the measure is of doubtful value. It should also be borne in mind that Banzhaf claims a loss of 8 to 10% in the 12.5% precipitate with anhydrous sodium sulfate.

THE USE OF SODIUM SULFATE FOR CONCENTRATION

While making a comparison of the yield of protective substance precipitated from serum by dilution with water, and by ammonium sulfate or sodium sulfate, it was found that practically all the protective substance was precipitated by 20% concentration of anhydrous sodium sulfate. The exact upper or lower limits for serum have not been determined, but judging from the number of protective units found in the 20% sodium sulfate protein precipitate, very little, if any, would be gained by increasing the concentration to 22.5%, the percentage which is equivalent to 50% saturation with ammonium sulfate. The possible slight increase in yield is offset by the increased difficulty in handling the precipitate due to the crystallization of the sodium sulfate. Even at 20% troublesome crystallization takes place unless filtering is carried out at a temperature between 22 and 30 C. On the other hand, less than 20% sodium sulfate may be used with only slight loss (that is, 19.5%, 19%, or 18.5%).

The method that is outlined below is one used during the last year and has proven satisfactory from the standpoint both of percentage yield and of a product essentially free from chill-producing characteristics. Although work is under way toward improving this and other methods of separation of the protective antibody from horse serum, because of numerous inquiries concerning the method outlined here, details wll be given.

Method.—To equal volumes of serum and water heated to 40 C., sufficient dry anhydrous sodium sulfate to make 20% (i. e., at the rate of 200 gm. to 1,000 cc.) is added gradually and the mixture shaken until the salt is completely dissolved. The correct temperature may be obtained by heating the water first to 70 or 80 C. and then adding it to the serum, that is, if the serum is cold. The mixture is allowed to stand preferably in an incubator room (37 C. is usual) until the precipitate breaks well, for from one to two hours.

Filtration must be carried out at sufficiently high temperature to prevent gross crystallization of sodium sulfate, 37 C. is satisfactory. The usual hardened filter paper is used, and just sufficient material poured on the filter so that it will drain dry over night. The precipitate is kept moist by the use of the customary moist cloth thrown over the funnel. The moist precipitate is then collected and pressed until quite dry. It is better to use high pressure for a short time than low pressure for a considerable length of time.

The dried cake is then dialyzed from five to seven days in running water, the time depending upon the dialyzing membrane used and the temperature of the water. Viscose membranes have been used entirely for this work and have proved very satisfactory. With this membrane five days, or even four, have been sufficient.

The sacs are emptied into graduates and the volume measured. The total volume should not be much over half the original volume of serum, preferably less, and dialysis should have been long enough so that a very heavy precipitate of insoluble protein is present. Sufficient dilute acetic acid (N/5 to N/20) is then added to make the suspension P_H 4.6 to 4.8. If the precipitate does not break readily giving a very clear supernatant, sufficient sodium nitrate should be added to make the concentration N/20 to N/40. This should stand for about one hour at room temperature, and then the precipitate collected in the centrifuge or filtered in the cold room. Too great length of time at a P_H as low as 4.6 will cause denaturation of the water-insoluble protein, and thus entail some loss of antibody. This precipitate contains very little protective substance, and is high in phosphorus and lipoids. Consequently if conditions of precipitation are optimum it can be well discarded. A practical method for adjusting the hydrogen ion concentration for optimum separation is the addition of varying amounts of N/20 acetic acid. for example 0.5, 1, 1.5, 2 cc., etc., to 10 cc. samples of precipitate. Then the most acid tube showing a clear supernatant is the one of choice. It will be found that, colorimetrically, the P_H will range from 4.4 to 4.8, i. e., colorless to chlor phenol red, about the middle range with chlor cresol green, and definitely red with methyl red.

The clear supernatant which contains the protective substance as well as all the inert pseudoglobulin (see preceding paragraph) is then neutralized to P_H 6.6 to

6.8 with N/20 sodium hydroxide, diluted four or five times with cold distilled water and held in the cold room over night. In the morning the clear supernatant is then siphoned off and the precipitate is collected in the centrifuge or filtered. The precipitate at this stage should be definitely white with an almost glossy sheen.

This final precipitate which contains the protective substance is then dissolved in 3% sodium chloride solution to which had been added tricresol to make 0.2%. The volume of salt solution used is noted (to know the amount of tricresol used), the final volume measured, and sufficient tricresol added to make the concentration 0.2%. The volume of salt solution used obviously varies with different serums, but generally a workable product can be obtained when the final volume of the concentrate is from one-twelfth to one-eighth of the original volume of serum. It has been our purpose to make the protein concentration approximately that of horse serum, that is, from 10 to 12 mg. nitrogen to one cc.

TABLE 4.—OLD TYPE 1 SERUM

Concentration with 20% sodium sulfate

Sample	Volume	Nitrogen, Mg./Cc.	Nitrogen, %	Dilution Protecting	Total Units	Nitrogen, Mg. per Unit Protection
Serum..................	10000	11.34	100	1:1000	2,000,000	.0567
Acid nitrate precipitate	440	7.67	2.9	1:4000	352,000	.0096
Final precipitate.......	1000	12.66	11.1	1:10000	2,000,000	.0063

The final product should be filtered through a coarse Berkefeld filter almost as soon as in solution, and then after being a week or more in a cold room, filtered for sterility through a normal candle. If the adjustment of the P_H has been correct and the tricresol is not unusually acid, the final product will be found to be between P_H 6.4 and 6.8, at which reaction potency remains constant, for a length of time comparable to that in whole serum. The solution should be clear, almost colorless, and have only a slight precipitate form after standing in the cold.

RESULTS OF THE APPLICATION OF THE METHOD

EXPERIMENT 3

Three examples will be given representing as nearly as possible what might be expected by the use of this method on the average lot of serum. The first experiment (table 4) is on old type 1 serum. The serum had been tricresolated (0.4%) and held in the cold room six months. From previous experience with old tricresolated serum, it would seem that the results of this experiment are exceptional. The final product was clear, the volume and protective substance were concentrated tenfold, and the nitrogen content was approximately one-tenth of the total serum protein nitrogen. It is to be understood, however, that an exact comparison of potency of two solutions is made only by many repetitions with a relatively large number of mice. In comparing the serum and the final product in this experiment, a series of dilutions was made (1:500, 1:1000, 1:2000, 1:3000, 1:4000) for the serum and the same series made for the final product from a sample diluted tenfold, the dilutions thus ranging 1:5000, 1:10,000, 1:20,000, etc. Both specimens were twice titrated with duplicate mice.

EXPERIMENT 4.—FRESH POLYVALENT SERUM

The material for this experiment was fresh unpreserved polyvalent serum. In all details the method above was carried out with the exception that the acid (P_H 4.8) precipitate was washed twice with N/20 sodium sulfate and the clear washing was neutralized and diluted fivefold with water. The insoluble precipitate was made up in the volume given in table 5. As can be seen the yield of type 1 antibody is practically ideal from the standpoint both of nitrogen in a protective unit and of the total units. It is possible that had repeated tests been carried out on the type 2 material, the percentage yield would have been found to be almost as much as with type 1. As it is, the yield of type 2 approximates 60%. It should be noted that 20% sodium sulfate precipitates protein representing 56% of the total serum protein. Of this amount it would appear that only 17.4% was water-insoluble. But it must be remembered that in the supernatant from the acid treatment of the dialyzed material, the final hydrogen ion concentration P_H 6.6 to 6.8 is sufficiently alkaline to dissolve entirely the acid euglobulin which was not precipitated in the acid treatment, providing of course the dilution in water is not too great. Thus the 17.4% of protein represents, not the euglobulin, but for the most part the water-insoluble protective protein.

EXPERIMENT 5.—A COMPARISON OF WATER-DILUTION AND SODIUM SULFATE METHODS ON SERUM FROM HORSES AFTER A LONG PERIOD OF IMMUNIZATION

A comparison of the water dilution method with subsequent purification by the acid salt method, with the sodium sulfate method was the object of this experiment. Details were in all ways like the preceding experiment. The same volume, 12,500 cc., of potent serum was used in both methods. The results given in table 6 have been a common experience with serum from horses after a long period of immunization. The yield is better with the sulfate method than with the water dilution. It is worth noting that in both methods the final product contains more type 2 protective units than were found in the original water-insoluble precipitate. The difference is of such magnitude as to be significant, and thus adds evidence to the opinion given before that there is some substance in immune horse serum which is antagonistic to protection and as a matter of fact really neutralizes the antibody.

DISCUSSION

This method is presented because of the consistently high yield of protective substance in a product which has been used for intravenous

TABLE 5.—THE SODIUM SULFATE METHOD ON SERUM FROM HORSES AFTER A LONG PERIOD OF IMMUNIZATION

Sample	Volume, Cc.	Nitrogen, Mg. per Cc.	Nitrogen, %	Type 1 Dilution Protecting	Type 1 Nitrogen per Unit	Type 1 Total Units	Type 1 % Units	Type 2 Dilution Protecting	Type 2 Nitrogen per Unit	Type 2 Total Units	Type 2 % Units
Serum	20000	10.24	100	1:1000	.0512	4,000,000	100	1:2000	.0256	8,000,000	100
Dialyzed precipitate	7775	14.8	56.2	1:2000	.037	3,110,000	77.7	1:4000	.0185	6,220,000	77.7
Acid washing	100	8.59	0.4	1:500	.0859	10,000	0.2	1:5000	.0086	100,000	1.2
Acid precipitate	700	4.6	1.5	1:250	.092	35,000	0.9	1:50	.46	7,000	0.1
Final precipitate	1520	20.9	15.5	1:15000	.0069	4,560,000	114	1:16000	.0065	4,864,000	60.8

TABLE 6.—A COMPARISON OF WATER-DILUTION AND SODIUM SULFATE METHODS ON SERUM FROM HORSES AFTER A LONG PERIOD OF IMMUNIZATION (POLYVALENT SERUM)

Sample	Volume, Cc.	Nitrogen, Mg./Cc.	% Nitrogen	Type 1 Dilution Protecting	Type 1 Nitrogen per Unit	Type 1 Total Units	Type 2 Dilution Protecting	Type 2 Nitrogen per Unit	Type 2 Total Units	Type 3 Dilution Protecting	Type 3 Nitrogen per Unit	Type 3 Total Units
Water-Dilution												
Serum	12500	11.195	100	1:2000	.0279	5,000,000	1:1000	.056	2,500,000	1:20	11.195	12,500
Water-insoluble precipitate	2500	12.045	21.5	1:10000	.006	5,000,000	1:1000	.060	500,000	1:320	.75	40,000
Acid nitrate precipitate	500	12.145	4.3	1:800	.076	80,000	1:400	.152	40,000	1:160	1.518	4,000
Acid washing	110	11.565	0.9	1:15000	.004	330,000	1:1000	.058	22,000	1:80	2.891	440
Final precipitate by water-dilution	900	16.225	14	1:15000	.005	2,700,000	1:5000	.016	900,000	1:640	.507	28,800
Sodium Sulfate												
Dialyzed precipitate	5500	15.265	59.7	1:4000	.019	4,400,000	1:1000	.076	1,100,000	1:160	.191	44,000
Acid nitrate precipitate	200	5.315	0.7	1:200	.133	8,000	1:50	.531	2,000	0	.....	0
Acid washing	14	4.285	0.4	1:8000	.005	22,400	1:1000	.021	2,800	1:320	.268	224
Final precipitate by sodium sulfate method	1500	15.935	17	1:15000	.005	4,500,000	1:7500	.011	2,250,000	1:640	.498	48,000

administration with little or no chill-producing characteristics and with apparent therapeutic activity. Many comparisons have been made of the yield of protective substance, as estimated by the mouse technique, of three methods of obtaining the initial precipitate: namely, first simply diluting ten to twelve fold with water acidulated to make a final P_H of 6.8; second, precipitating with 20% concentration of anhydrous sodium sulfate; and third, precipitating with 44% saturation of ammonium sulfate. The water-insoluble precipitate from each of the three was then purified by the method outlined above, with the result that the final products all were similar in the amount of protein to a protective unit. The concentrates from the water-dilution and sodium sulfate methods have been used for the past two years with only a small percentage of troublesome reactions following intravenous administration in pneumonia patients. On the other hand, the product from the ammonium sulfate method has produced severe reactions in a relatively high percentage of cases. It may be possible to use ammonium sulfate, but certainly not until our technique is changed so that the concentrate is practically free from chill-producing characteristics.

For those experienced in the use of anhydrous sodium sulfate, there should be no difficulty at all in following the method. There are only three points which will be emphasized. The first one is the temperature of the dilute serum before adding the sodium sulfate. It is necessary that the temperature be 37 to 40 C., otherwise the salt will crystallize and be dissolved only with great difficulty. Second, it is important that filtration be carried out at sufficiently high temperature to prevent crystallization. Dialysis is not only slower with the large amount of sodium sulfate and the volume of the contents of the sac thus greater, but also the separation by the acid treatment of the protective substance from the inert protein is not complete. The total volume of precipitate should not be over one-half the volume of the original serum. The third point is the reaction of the anhydrous salt. Some of the "chemically pure" grade of material purchased in barrels is quite alkaline. If such is the case acid may be added to the diluted serum in sufficient quantity to neutralize the amount of sodium sulfate used. That is, a preliminary test is made on a 100-gram sample of the alkaline sulfate to estimate the acid necessary to neutralize the amount of alkaline sulfate needed. The sodium sulfate must be anhydrous and free from the salts of heavy metals.

It might be well to add another precaution. The protective antibody is associated with a water-insoluble protein (i.e., relatively insoluble) not like diphtheria antitoxin which is found with the water-soluble globulin. Consequently any process which would render it less soluble interferes with the quality of the final product. That is to say, since the protein in question is readily soluble in neutral salts, only, and but slightly in water, alteration resulting in a decrease of its solubility in neutral salts renders handling from the practical standpoint impossible. For then the protein is insoluble in water and neutral salts. This change in solubilities of protein, i.e., the so-called denaturing process, has been studied rather extensively. Our interest here lies in a means of preventing the process for practical reasons. There are three common causes met with which can largely be controlled; first is bacterial contamination of the serum and also the dialyzed precipitate. Clean technique in handling the serum and precipitate, the use of fresh serum, and dialysis carried out at 8 to 10 C. minimize sufficiently gross contamination. Second is keeping the serum or precipitate at too high temperatures, especially in solutions either acid or alkaline. And third is too high a concentration of preservative in serum or antibody concentrate. These are by no means all the possible causes for denaturing of the water-insoluble protective protein, but only the more common ones encountered in the use of the method here presented for concentration.

SUMMARY

A method for the concentration of the protective substance in antipneumococcus horse serum has been given. Anhydrous sodium sulfate in 20% concentration is used as precipitating agent. The usual technique for filtering and dialyzing the "cake" is employed. The contents of the sac, euglobulin, pseudoglobulin, and protective substance, is adjusted to P_H 4.6 to 4.8, at which point a precipitate is formed containing an inert protein (euglobulin?) along with a quantity of lipoids. This precipitate is removed and the clear supernatant (pseudoglobulin, protective substance, some euglobulin and albumin) is adjusted to P_H 6.8, and diluted 4 or 5-fold with cold distilled water. A white precipitate is thrown down containing practically all the protective substance present in the original serum. This precipitate dissolves readily in sodium chloride, is high in protective power, and for intravenous injection, is practically free from severe chill-producing characteristics.

SPONTANEOUS TUBERCULOSIS OF RABBITS

Malcolm J. Harkins and Eli R. Saleeby

From Research Institute of Cutaneous Medicine, Philadelphia

As an outspoken disease of rabbits, tuberculosis occurs very rarely. Few reports appear in the literature. Aside from the value of such reports, especially to laboratory workers, we considered the two unrelated cases observed by us of especial interest because of the atypical appearance of one of the cases. Straus [1] in 1895 and Guerin [2] in 1907 each reported a case contracted under natural conditions. In both instances the lesions were found principally in the lungs. Rothe [3] later reported observing five cases in a rabbitry consisting of 80 to 90 animals. The bovine type of microorganism was isolated but he was unable to trace the source of infection, although he calls attention to the location of the rabbitry which was close to the Sanitorium Heidehaus (Hanover). Like other observers he reports the predominating lesions were located in the lungs, although foci were also present in other parts of the body.

In the wild rabbit as in other wild animals [4] there is reason to believe that tuberculosis is very rare, probably due to their environment. With the increased activity in domestic rabbit breeding for laboratory, meat and fur purposes and especially the inclusion of milk (if unpasteurized) in the diet, it is reasonable to expect the disease to become more wide-spread. It is the opinion of Wade H. Brown of the Rockefeller Institute for Medical Research [5] "that the infection is comparatively common among rabbits but it is usually localized and gives rise to no symptoms. But as an outspoken disease it is certainly rare."

The two cases observed by us occurred at an interval of 28 months and have no relationship whatever. The first case was one of a group of eleven rabbits inoculated intratesticularly with an emulsion of rabbit testicle infected with a laboratory strain of Spirochaeta pallida. The testicles of all rabbits remained normal. Twelve days after inoculation they were castrated and five and one half months later were necropsied. The eleven rabbits appeared to be in good physical condition before the

Received for publication, Aug. 1, 1928.

1. La tuberculose et son bacilli, 1895, p. 373.
2. Hygiene de la vian et lait, 1907, p. 7.
3. Veröffentl. R. Koch-Stift. Bekaemp. Tuberk., 1, 1, 1913.
4. Calmette: Tubercle bacillus infection and tuberculosis in man and animals (English translation by Soper and Smith), 1923.
5. Personal communication.

necropsy. None revealed anything unusual at necropsy except one in which small, grayish-white nodules were observed in the serous layers of the thoracic and abdominal cavities. Most of the nodules were discrete although a number coalesced and they varied in shape and size (0.1 to 15 mm.). Although most of them followed the serous layers, many of them were observed in the lung substance. The cut surface of those nodules had a smooth, yellowish-gray appearance with slight tendency towards caseation, especially in the center. Few of them showed complete necrosis.

Similar lesions were produced in other rabbits when inoculated intratesticularly and intraperitoneally. Successful transmission was made in two more sets of rabbits.

Grossly the lesions in the first rabbit did not resemble tuberculosis but by continued passage through rabbits, the lesions became more typical and more generalized, being observed in the lungs, spleen, intestines, omentum and mesenteric lymph glands.

For microscopic study, sections were fixed with a 4% formalin and stained with hematoxylin and eosin and with acidfast stain. Sections from the first rabbit were also stained by Levaditi method for demonstration of Spirochaeta pallida and were negative.

The microscopical appearance of the hematoxylin and eosin stained sections of the first animal were very atypical. The calls varied in size and stained poorly. There were no giant cells and no tendency toward tubercle formation. Several areas of necrosis were noted. However, acidfast microorganisms were easily demonstrated in the sections.

The second case observed was an eight months old pedigreed Flemish giant doe. This rabbit was one of a rabbitry of approximately 80 adult animals. According to the owner it had been in apparently good health to within a week of its death, when it was observed that the animal was not eating well and was losing weight. It had been bred 29 days previously. Necropsy revealed lesions only in the lungs which were the seat of a confluent bronchopneumonia. Acidfast bacilli were observed in smears and sections of the lung tissue. Intraperitoneal inoculation of lung tissue into other rabbits produced typical tuberculosis. Histologic sections were typical of the disease.

COMMENT

Besides the rarity of this disease in the rabbits, the most interesting feature was the atypical gross and histologic appearance of the nodules in the first animal. The distribution along the serous layers coupled with the atypical cells suggested very strongly neoplasm of the endothelioma type. A final diagnosis was made only possible by the finding of the acidfast microorganisms and by the easy transmission to the other animals with the production of characteristic lesions. The organisms were cultured and later proved to be of bovine type. We are grateful to Joseph D. Aronson of the Henry Phipps Institute for typing this culture.

The source of the infection in the first rabbit could not be traced inasmuch as it was one of a lot purchased from a local dealer.

In attempting to determine the source of infection in the second rabbit, it was learned that the present owner had purchased it eight weeks previously from a breeder, also that supposedly pasteurized skim milk was fed daily. After several months, no further cases have come to necropsy in this rabbitry and milk remains a part of the diet and it is probable the rabbit was infected before purchase by its last owner.

It is also interesting to note that in these cases the infection was apparently of quite long standing, observable effects being of short duration before death (second animal).

SUMMARY

Two cases of tuberculosis in rabbits, which is rare, are described. In one rabbit atypical nodules on the serous membranes of thoracic and abdominal cavities, together with unusual cellular response, suggested an endothelioma type of neoplasm.

IMMUNOLOGICAL INVESTIGATIONS ON TROPICAL SPRUE IN PORTO RICO

4. THE BIOLOGY OF MONILIA PSILOSIS IN RELATION TO SPRUE

CHARLES WEISS AND FRANCISCO LANDRÓN

From the School of Tropical Medicine of the University of Porto Rico Under the Auspices of Columbia University and the Presbyterian Hospital, San Juan, Porto Rico

During the past few years there has been a renewed interest in the study of monilia in relation to bronchial infections, and tropical sprue. Since the literature on these subjects has been recently summarized by one of us,[1] a repetition will not be necessary here. It will suffice to say that while Kohlbrügge,[2] Manson-Bahr,[3] and Ashford [4] consider a monilia as the cause of sprue, this opinion is not concurred in by Castellani,[5] Fairley and Mackie,[6] and others. During a two-year stay in Porto Rico we undertook an investigation of this problem and the following observations on the biology of Monilia psilosis were made in connection with other immunological and epidemiological studies to be published later.[7] It is hoped that they may throw some light on the problem.

THE P_H RANGE FOR THE CULTIVATION OF M. PSILOSIS AND THE P_H CHANGES IN MEDIUMS DURING GROWTH

Several writers have suggested that monilia obtain a foot-hold in sprue patients because of the high acidity of the intestinal contents and that the organism may again disappear when the contents become alkaline as the result of a special sprue diet. Since a search of the literature failed to reveal any work dealing with the P_H range for growth and survival of M. psilosis, nor of the P_H changes that occur in the medium during growth, it was deemed advisable to investigate these points.

Technique.—A series of plates of Sabouraud glucose agar was prepared with P_H varying from 3 to 9 at intervals of one. The surface of the solidified plates

Received for publication, July 7, 1928.

1. Porto Rico Rev. Pub. Health & Trop. Med., 1927-1928, 3, p. 367 and p. 150.
2. Arch. f. Schiffs-u. Tropen-Hyg., 1901, 5, p. 394.
3. A report on researches on sprue in Ceylon, 1915.
4. Sprue: Oxford Med., vol. 5, p. 631; Sprue, in Cecil's Text Book of Medicine, 1927, p. 350.
5. Manual of tropical medicine, 1919, pp. 1079, 1780.
6. Indian J. M. Research, 1926, 14, p. 105.
7. Immunological investigations of tropical sprue in Porto Rico, Am. J. Trop. Med., 1929, pts. 1-3, in press; An epidemiological study of sprue in Porto Rico, to be published.

were then streaked with aliquot quantities (0.5 cc.) of a standardized suspension of M. psilosis. The latter was prepared by washing off a 20 hours' growth from the surface of a Sabouraud agar slant with distilled water and diluting the resulting suspension to an opacity equal to No. 2 of the McFarland nephelometer. The suspension was now diluted 1,000 times. All Petri plates were incubated at 37 C. and the colonies were counted at daily intervals for several weeks. Similar observations were made by inoculating measured quantities of a standard emulsion of M. psilosis into several tubes of infusion broth of varying P_H to which no glucose had been added. These tubes were then examined at frequent intervals and records were kept of the number of monilia per cc. and of the actual P_H which the cultures had reached on that day.

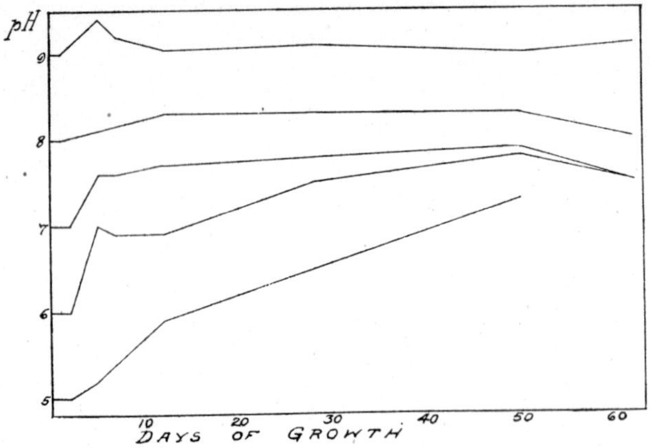

Fig. 1.—Daily changes in the P_H of infusion broth during the growth of Monilia psilosis.

TABLE 1.—GROWTH OF M. PSILOSIS IN INFUSION BROTH OF VARYING P_H

		4.0	5.0	6.0	7.0	8.0	9.0
Original P_H		4.0	5.0	6.0	7.0	8.0	9.0
The number of colonies which developed on the surface of Sabouraud agar plates after streaking 0.1 cc. of a 1:1000 dilution of the corresponding cultures	2 days	2	4	47	238	148	6
	10 days	0	0	12	450	200	2
	74 days	0	0	334	160	168	0
P_H on 74th day		5.6	6.8	8.2	8.4	8.8	8.6
P_H of unplanted broth 74th day		4.2	5.2	5.8	6.2	7.2	8.6

In another series of Sabouraud agar plates we incorporated the new colorimetric indicators of Clark (brom-cresol green, chlor-phenol red, brom-thymol blue, cresol red, and thymol blue) in order to enable us to judge approximately the changes in P_H from day to day during the growth of the organisms. The amounts of each indicator selected, after preliminary trial, was 2.0 cc. of a 0.4% solution per 100 cc. of medium, prepared with the aid of NaOH as recommended by Clark. These quantities did not interfere with the development of Monilia psilosis. Results are shown in figure 1 and table 1.

It was readily seen that when M. psilosis is planted in tubes of infusion broth and examined at intervals ranging from 2 to 74 days, the optimum for growth is found to be about P_H 7. In Sabouraud agar the optimum is at 6. Satisfactory growth is, however, observed over a wider range, 6 to 8 in liquid, and 4 to 9 in solid mediums. Each tube of broth in which the organisms have been developing at an initial P_H varying from 5 to 8 is found to grow progressively alkaline. After 74 days' growth the largest number of organisms are found in the tube whose P_H had reached 8.2. The P_H changes in solid mediums could not be as accurately studied as in liquid mediums. We observed, however, an initial production of acidity followed by a tendency to alkalinity.

THE THERMAL DEATH POINT OF M. PSILOSIS

In his article on the preparation and use of M. psilosis vaccines for the treatment of sprue, Michel [8] points out that it is difficult to kill the organism by heating at 56 C. for one-half hour, and therefore recommends a preliminary period of autolysis of several days at 37 C. It was considered therefore of interest to determine the thermal death point of the organism. Our results indicate that M. psilosis can be readily killed by heating at 56 C. for 10 minutes, if the suspension is adequately diluted, and if the volume to be heated be kept reasonably small (1.0 cc.).

THE USE OF SELECTIVE BACTERIOSTATIC CHEMICAL SUBSTANCES FOR THE RAPID ISOLATION OF M. PSILOSIS FROM THE STOOLS

Anderson [9] and Simmons [10] have suggested methods for the isolation of M. psilosis from the stools. We have not found these altogether satisfactory for routine work when several stools have to be examined daily. One has to wait several days before a pure culture is finally obtained by repeated subculturing on Sabouraud agar. Since the selective bacteriostatic action of various anilin dyes (brilliant green, gentian violet, etc.) is now being routinely applied to the rapid isolation of typhoid and tubercle bacilli from the feces, it naturally occurred to us to test these substances in connection with the present problem. After several preliminary experiments in which we made use of Churchman's technic [11] for "intrinsic" as well as "extrinsic" bacteriostasis, we found that brilliant green and gentian violet killed monilia in concentrations needed for inhibition of fecal bacteria, and hence were not suited for incorporation in culture mediums for the rapid isolation of monilia from the stool. On the other hand, whole bile as will be

8. Am. J. M. Sci., 1917, 144, p. 177; J. Infect. Dis., 1918, 22, p. 53.
9. J. Infect. Dis., 1917, 21, p 341
10. Ibid., 1926, 39, p. 209.
11. J. Exper. Med., 1921, 33, p. 569; 1923, 37, p. 543.

described, or glycerol (c.p.), incorporated in 20% concentration in Sabouraud glucose (or lactose) agar, did not interfere with the growth of M. psilosis but inhibited all, or practically all, the fecal bacteria. Hence they are satisfactory for our purpose. We therefore suggest the following:

IMPROVED TECHNIC FOR THE RAPID ISOLATION OF MONILIA PSILOSIS FROM THE FECES

Emulsify a small quantity of feces in a test tube of sterile distilled water and also in another tube containing whole ox bile in which has been incorporated glycerol in 20% concentration. By means of a glass rod bent at an angle of 30 degrees, a drop of each fecal suspension is spread over the surfaces of plates of Sabouraud agar P_H 6.3 containing 4% glucose and 20% glycerol (c.p.). After 48 hours' incubation at 35 C. a practically pure culture of M. psilosis will be found. The discrete colonies of this fungus are large (2 to 3 mm. in diameter), white or cream colored. Under the low power (1/6 objective) they resemble a mosaic of tiny glass marbles, the edges of the colony being finely serrated. For final identification a single colony may be "fished" on the various sugars in fermentation tubes and also into gelatin and slants of Sabouraud glucose agar. A full description of the organism will be found in Ashford's original article. As a general rule, M. psilosis ferments dextrose, levulose and maltose with the production of acid and gas, and often also dextrin. At times there is acid (but no gas) formed in broth containing galactose and saccharose. The organism causes litmus milk to resume a blue color a few days after the initial change to pink, and never ferments lactose. It does not liquefy gelatin but shows a growth resembling an inverted pine tree. The writer has observed that it does not ferment the various vegetable starches, (oat, bean, tapioca, wheat, rice and barley), and that it grows well under anaerobic conditions in a J. Howard Brown anaerobic jar, or under a vaseline seal.

ISOLATION OF M. PSILOSIS FROM THE STOOLS AND TONGUE OF SPRUE CASES AND OTHER PATIENTS

Confirming the work of Fairley and Mackie,[6] Ashford and others, we have been able to cultivate M. psilosis from the stools of sprue patients and also from patients suffering from various other tropical and cosmopolitan diseases. From 30 specimens from patients with sprue, 18 cultures of Monilia were isolated; from 18 of suspected sprue,

3 cultures; and from 24 specimens from various diseases (hookworm, filariasis, lues, carcinoma, diarrhea, asthma, etc.), 16 cultures of Monilia were obtained. We attempted to isolate monilia from the blood of eight patients with sprue, but were unsuccessful.

TOXIC SUBSTANCES IN MONILIA PSILOSIS

EXPERIMENTS WITH LIVING CULTURES

Several writers including Michel,[8] Ashford [4] and Smith [12] have demonstrated that cultures of M. psilosis are toxic for experimental animals. The question has been raised as to whether there is a true exo- or endotoxin in these cultures. If so, is it species-specific? And is it hemolytic, and will it help to account for the clinical picture of sprue? The following experiments were undertaken to throw light on the questions.

Comparative Immediate Toxicity of Aqueous Suspensions of Various Living Monilia.—Monilia psilosis, M. albicans and a cryptococcus from cutaneous blastomycosis * were cultivated for 5 days at 37 C. on the surface of solidified Sabouraud agar in Blake bottles. The growths were washed off with sterile distilled water and the resulting suspensions were properly diluted and then kept for 3 days in the icebox. They were now injected intravenously into rabbits weighing from 1500 to 2000 gm. in graduated doses, in order to compare their toxicity. Doses of 5 cc. of M. psilosis and of Cryptococcus were fatal, while 2.5 cc. and 1.0 cc. were innocuous.

It was readily seen that while unheated suspensions of M. psilosis are quite toxic for rabbits when injected intravenously M. albicans suspensions are also toxic, though to a less degree, while the cryptococcus is even more toxic than M. psilosis. This is confirmed by a study of the histological changes produced upon injection of the organisms into the blood stream. For the following reports we are indebted to R. A. Lambert, Professor of pathology in the School of Tropical Medicine.

M. Psilosis (2.5 cc. per Kilo): One rabbit (1) died 24 hours after injection. Lung shows marked congestion and edema with foci of acute inflammation containing eosinophiles, polynuclears and other wandering cells. The lesion seems to be embolic in origin. In the liver there is a general vacuolization of the hepatic cells, and considerable brownish pigment is scattered through the organ, some of it apparently free and some in Kupffer and hepatic cells. There is moderate conges-

12. Philippine J. Sci., 1924, 24, p. 447.
* We are indebted to Dr. B. K. Ashford for transplants of these cultures.

tion. No focal lesions are found other than slight cellular accumulations in some of the portal spaces with slight nuclear fragmentation. In the kidney marked congestion is present. Mycelial masses of large fungus are seen here and there through the kidney with little or no reaction about them, though there is some nuclear fragmentation of the cells in the vicinity.

M. Albicans (2.3 cc. per Kilo): One rabbit (2) died 24 hours after injection. In the lung a general congestion and edema are present. Focal lesions are present similar to those in rabbit 1 but less well defined, with numerous eosinophiles both in the lesions and in the blood. In the liver pigmentation and vacuolization are noted much like that in rabbit 1. In the portal spaces there is evidence of both an old and a recent inflammatory process. The acute changes are most marked just beneath the mucosa of the larger ducts. In the kidney many of the tubules contain granular debris but parenchymatous changes are slight and no focal lesions are found.

M. Albicans (5 cc. per Kilo): A third rabbit (3) died 24 hours after injection. In the lung there was marked congestion and edema. Acute focal lesions are numerous and conspicuous, much more so than in any of the preceding cases. The character of the lesions is the same, with the eosinophiles numerous along with polys and other cells. In the kidney masses of fungi like those seen in rabbit 1 are present with the same slight reaction about them.

Cryptococcus (from cutaneous blastomycosis) (5 cc. per Kilo): Rabbit 4 died 24 hours after injection. Numerous small acute focal lesions are present in the lungs with marked nuclear fragmentation. Eosinophilic reaction is not so evident as in preceding cases. Edema also is less marked. The liver shows extreme congestion. The hepatic cells in general contain a fine brownish pigment, not so coarse as in some of the preceding cases. No focal lesions are noted. In the kidney one notices with the low power lenses bluish staining masses which on higher magnification cannot be identified. They are not conglomerations of bacteria or fungi nor do they look like deposits of calcium salts. Not related to these are small focal lesions much like those seen in the lung. In some of these faintly staining fungi can be recognized.

EFFECTS OF HEATED AND AUTOLYZED SUSPENSIONS

We now proceeded to test the comparative toxicity of heated monilia suspensions or "vaccines" prepared after the technic of Michel, using the following technique: Blake bottles were streaked with suspensions of various monilia (20-hour cultures) and incubated for 5 days at 37 C. The growth was then washed off with sterile distilled water, using 75 cc. of water for each Blake bottle. These suspensions were now shaken in small bottles for two hours, incubated for 5 days at 37 C. and kept in the ice chest for another five days. They were finally killed by heating at 56 C. for one hour. As a preservative, phenol 0.5% was added. The results indicated clearly that heated and autolyzed suspensions are much less toxic than the unheated ones and that the cryptococcus and albicans vaccines are perhaps even more toxic than that of M. psilosis. When tested by intradermal injection into rabbits which had previously received intravenous doses of various types of killed monilia suspensions, none of the three showed evidence of antigenic specificity. The details are given in a separate communication.[7]

ARE THE TOXIC SUBSTANCES IN M. PSILOSIS CULTURES FILTRABLE?

Michel's experiments with filtrates of M. psilosis cultures led him to believe that there was no demonstrable extracellular filterable toxin in this organism. Our preliminary studies on guinea-pigs and rabbits gave similar results. When, however, the organism was grown for five days in infusion broth (P_H 7.6) to which freshly drawn human blood had been added in the proportion of 1 : 200, the filtrates were found to be quite toxic. This toxicity was readily shown when injections were made intracutaneously into the skin of human subjects, but not when injected into the blood stream of rabbits. M. albicans and the cryptococcus from blastomycosis yielded exotoxins similar to M. psilosis.

TABLE 2.—SUMMARY OF RESULTS OF SKIN REACTIONS IN SPRUE USING TOXINS AND VACCINES OF MONILIA

Diagnosis	Total Number Patients Tested	Percent Positive Skin Reactions: Toxin M. Psilosis	Toxin M. Albicans	Toxin Cryptococcus	Vaccine M. Psilosis	Vaccine M. Albicans	Vaccine Cryptococcus
Sprue...............	22	73	82	82	55	59	64
Control.............	26	31	35	46	23	27	27

A special investigation was made of the possible immunological relationship of the endo- and exotoxins of the various monilia to sprue. This was done by making intracutaneous injections of these vaccines and toxic filtrates into a series of 22 undoubted sprue patients and 26 miscellaneous hospital patients. These studies will be reported later, but may be summarized here as follows: While a large percentage (73) of the sprue cases gave positive skin reactions to the exotoxins of M. psilosis, a still larger percentage (82) of the same series also reacted to the toxins of M. albicans and of the cryptococcus from cutaneous blastomycosis. In the control series (26 non-sprue patients) about 35% reacted to all 3 types of toxins. The observations with the use of killed autolyzed monilia suspension (Michel vaccines), as antigens were similar. The sprue cases were 55-64% positive while the control series were 23-27% positive (table 2).

ARE THE TOXIC SUBSTANCES IN MONILIA HEMOLYTIC?

Anemia is recognized as one of the important features of sprue. At times this may be so severe as to simulate the picture of a pernicious anemia. Thus far its exact cause has not been determined. Newham, Morris and Manson-Bahr [13] think that it is secondary to a gastro-intestinal lesion which results in a lack of absorption of fats. Since the possibility of its being due to the hemolytic action of the poisons from monilia has been suggested, we proceeded to determine whether or not the toxic substances from M. psilosis were hemolytic: they were not.

Technic and Results: A dozen methods were tried in an attempt to extract a hemolytic substance from M. psilosis; and we also tried the technic employed by Abel [14] and Ford in the isolation of the hemolytic poison of the mushroom fungus (Amanita phalloides). All our efforts, however, were unsuccessful. When working with emulsions of the living organisms, it was observed that the red blood suspensions grew darker, due to consumption of oxygen by the monilia. A microscopic examination showed that the monilia had also taken up the coloring matter (hemoglobin) of the red cells. Killed suspensions seemed to show evidence of methemoglobin production. In no case was there the slightest hemolysis.

SUMMARY

The isolation of Monilia psilosis from the feces is greatly facilitated by the use of glycerol and bile to inhibit the growth of common fecal bacteria. With this technique the fungus has been obtained from a large percentage of both sprue cases and controls. M. psilosis grows in both liquid and solid mediums over a wide P_H range with an optimum of P_H 7 in infusion broth. In liquid mediums of low P_H growth brings a progressive alkalinity approaching P_H 8, the apparent optimum for survival. These observations are not in harmony with the idea that an increased acidity of the intestinal contents favors the establishment of the fungus in patients with sprue. Intravenous injection of M. psilosis kills rabbits in a few minutes to 48 hours, the time depending on the dose. In the later deaths visceral embolic lesions containing the fungus are found. M. albicans and a cryptococcus of blastomycosis act similarly. M. psilosis and the two related fungi contain endotoxins, which, however, are not hemolytic and are not specifically antigenic when tested intradermally on immunized rabbits, sprue cases, and human controls. A filtrable nonhemolytic exotoxin can also be demonstrated in each of the three fungi.

These observations do not support the theory that M. psilosis is an etiologic factor in tropical sprue.

13. Lancet, 1926, 2, p. 269.
14. J. Biol. Chem., 1906, 2, p. 273.

EXTRACELLULAR PRODUCTION OF TOXIN BY CLOSTRIDIUM BOTULINUM TYPE B

C. N. Stark, J. M. Sherman and Pauline Stark

From the Department of Dairy Industry, Cornell University, Ithaca, New York

In a previous paper [1] evidence of the extracellular production of toxin by the type A variety of the botulinum organism was reported. In the present communication we wish to record similar findings with the B type.

A culture of Clostridium botulinum Type B was grown in a 4% peptone-beef infusion broth adjusted to P_H 7.4. Incubation was at 37 C. for eight days, after which the bacterial cells were removed from the culture by passage through a Berkefeld filter. The sterility of the filtrate was verified by anaerobic and aerobic incubation tests in fresh glucose-peptone-beef infusion broth.

The bacteria-free filtrate thus prepared was immediately tested for toxin content and was found to have a MLD titer of 700. The fresh filtrate was mixed with three samples of sterile skimmed milk in the proportions of 1 part of filtrate to 9 parts of milk, 1 part of filtrate to 19 parts of milk, and 1 part of filtrate to 49 parts of milk. These filtrate-milk mixtures were incubated for four days at 37 C., after which they were tested for toxin content by guinea-pig inoculations. The sterility of the filtrate-milk mixtures was again verified after incubation. For controls, samples of the pure filtrate were incubated for four days at 37 C. and then retested for toxin content. The MLD contents are calculated in each case on the basis of the undiluted toxin filtrate.

Treatment	MLD Titer
Control: fresh toxic filtrate before incubation	700
Control: toxic filtrate incubated 4 days at 37 C.	1
Toxic filtrate + skimmed milk (1:9), incubated 4 days at 37 C.	2000
Toxic filtrate + skimmed milk (1:19), incubated 4 days at 37 C.	2000
Toxic filtrate + skimmed milk (1:49), incubated 4 days at 37 C.	5000

The tabulated results show a marked increase in toxin content when the botulinum filtrate is allowed to act on sterile skimmed milk. As was pointed out in a previous paper, this is believed to be the result of the action of the enzymes of the organism on the casein of milk.

Received for publication, Aug. 3, 1928.

1. Stark, C. N.; Sherman, J. M., and Stark, Pauline, Proc. Soc. Exper. Biol. & Med., 1928, 25, p. 742.

GLUCOSE INHIBITION OF EXTRACELLULAR TOXIN-PRODUCING ENZYMES OF CLOSTRIDIUM BOTULINUM

C. N. Stark, J. M. Sherman and Pauline Stark

From the Department of Dairy Industry, Cornell University, Ithaca, New York

Attention has been directed in previous papers [1] to certain observations which indicate the extracellular production of toxin by the enzymes of Clostridium botulinum when acting on certain protein substrates. One purpose of the present communication is to report additional observations concerning which other investigators need be cognizant should they wish to verify our findings. It is thought, in addition, that the observations here reported add further evidence of the correctness of our hypothesis concerning the extracellular production of botulinum toxin.

Cultures of Clostridium botulinum, types A and B, were grown in fresh beef infusion—4% peptone broth (P_H 7.4) with and without glucose (1%). These broths, after inoculation, were incubated for 8 days at 37 C. and then filtered through Berkefeld filters. The sterility of the filtrates was verified by aerobic and anaerobic culture tests. The toxin titers of the several fresh filtrates were determined by guinea-pig inoculations. Portions of the filtrates from the A and B types in glucose and nonglucose broths were treated as follows: the undiluted filtrates were incubated four days at 37 C.; and additional portions of the several filtrates were mixed with sterile skimmed milk in different proportions and incubated four days at 37 C. These filtrate-milk mixtures were made in the proportions of 1 part filtrate to 9 parts milk; 1 part filtrate to 19 parts milk; and 1 part filtrate to 49 parts milk. After incubation, the toxin titers of the various mixtures and of the undiluted filtrates were determined. The toxin titers of these mixtures were calculated on the basis of the undiluted toxin filtrates. The sterility of all filtrates and mixtures was verified after incubation.

The results of these experiments are reported in the table. As will be seen from preparations 1 and 2, an active extracellular production of toxin was obtained with both A and B types when the filtrates were

Received for publication, Aug. 3, 1928.

1. Proc. Soc. Exper. Biol. & Med., 1928, 25, p. 742; in press (*Author: Please state Journal)*

obtained from growth in noncarbohydrate broth. On the other hand, the data for preparations 3 and 4 indicate that this is not true (at least not to the same degree) when the filtrates were from glucose broth cultures.

These observations are not only of significance to those who wish to produce the toxin extracellularly but also because of the light thrown on our view of the mechanism of toxin formation by Clostridium botulinum. If the hypothesis is correct that the toxin may be formed extracellularly by the action of the enzymes of the organism on certain proteins, a "sparing action" of glucose would be expected. In other words, the production of extracellular proteolytic enzymes would not take place to a comparable degree when the organism is grown in a medium con-

COMPARISON OF MLD PER UNIT VOLUME OF SKIMMED MILK WITH FILTRATES OF CL. BOTULINUM TYPES A AND B GROWN IN NON-CARBOHYDRATE AND IN GLUCOSE BROTH

1. Filtrate of Cl. botulinum type A grown in non-carbohydrate broth
2. Filtrate of Cl. botulinum type B grown in non-carbohydrate broth
3. Filtrate of Cl. botulinum type A grown in glucose broth: inhibiting action
4. Filtrate of Cl. botulinum type B grown in glucose broth: inhibiting action

	MLD Titer of Different Preparations			
Treatment	1	2	3	4
Control: fresh toxic filtrate before incubation	500	700	900	700
Control: toxic filtrate incubated 4 days at 37 C.	1	1	750	500
Toxic filtrate + skimmed milk (1:9), incubated 4 days at 37 C.	2000	2000	1000	500
Toxic filtrate + skimmed milk (1:19), incubated 4 days at 37 C.	2000	2000	2000	1000
Toxic filtrate + skimmed milk (1:49), incubated 4 days at 37 C.	5000	5000	1250	500

taining a fermentable carbohydrate. This was clearly evident from the fact that the glucose filtrates did not cause such extensive proteolysis when added to sterile skimmed milk as did the filtrates of broths without glucose.

Another significant point brought out in these experiments is the fact that more stable toxin filtrates are obtained on glucose mediums than on those containing no added carbohydrate. As may be noted from the accompanying table, the titers of the fresh non-glucose filtrates decrease rapidly when incubated at 37 C., whereas the toxin contents of similar filtrates obtained from glucose broths have much greater stability. This fact is probably well known by workers in this field, as glucose broth is very generally used for toxin production. It is possible that the difference in the stability of these filtrates was influenced by their respective hydrogen ion concentrations. The P_H values of the glucose and non-glucose filtrates were 6.0 and 7.3 respectively. The P_H values of the filtrates, however, could not have influenced materially the subsequent extracellular toxin formation in milk because of the high buffer content of the milk and the small amounts of filtrate added.

From the standpoint of our own hypothesis, the relative stability of the toxin from glucose and from non-glucose broths has added significance: if the toxin results from the cleavage of certain protein molecules it would be expected that the toxin itself might be destroyed on further proteolysis. Abundant observations in support of such a view may be obtained from the literature, though such evidence is neither direct nor positive. While by no means conclusive, the data here reported add weight to that view.

SUMMARY

It is shown that when Clostridium botulinum is grown in a medium containing glucose there results an inhibition of the production of the enzymes responsible for the extracellular formation of toxin. It is also noted that the toxin produced in glucose broth is more stable than that formed in the same medium without the carbohydrate.

DESTRUCTION OF DIPHTHERIA TOXIN BY BACTERIA

C. N. Stark, J. M. Sherman and Pauline Stark

From the Department of Dairy Industry, Cornell University, Ithaca, New York

In previous papers [1] we have reported data on the destruction of botulinum toxin by certain bacteria. In the present communication we wish to report some observations of a similar nature on diphtheria toxin. This subject is not new as several observations are recorded in the literature which touch it.

Donaldson [2] in a study of septic gunshot wounds noted that, in cases where the salt bag treatment failed, no foul, pungent odor was emitted. Further investigation showed an anaerobe, which Donaldson called the "Reading Bacillus," to be the cause of the foul odor. This organism in pure culture was found capable of destroying diphtheria and tetanus toxins. Guinea-pigs were unharmed by 60 MLD of diphtheria toxin in which this organism had grown. Most workers consider the "Reading Bacillus" a strain of Clostridium sporogenes.

Dernby [3] and his coworkers conclude that diphtheria toxin is produced by the action of proteolytic enzymes on the albumoses and peptones present in the medium. They think some of the primary split products constitute the toxin. It is felt by them that further proteolysis will disintegrate the toxin. These workers found that ". . . Bacillus pyocyaneus, Bacillus proteus, and others, destroy the toxin very rapidly."

The diphtheria toxin used in these experiments was made by the method recommended by Dernby and David [4] with only minor modifications. In their procedure a veal-yeast-peptone medium with a P_H value of 7.2 to 7.3 is used. The familiar Park 8 strain of Corynebacterium diphtheriae was used by us. The sterile toxin-filtrate preparation was mixed with sterile beef infusion—2% peptone broth (P_H 7.4) in the proportion of one part of toxin solution to four parts of the peptone-beef extract broth. Tubes of this mixture were inoculated with cultures of the bacteria tested, while other tubes of the toxin-broth mixture were retained sterile as controls. All tubes were then incubated at 37 C. for

Received for publication, Aug. 3, 1928.

1. Proc. Soc. Exper. Biol. & Med., 1927, 24, p. 546; J. Bact., 1928, 15, p. 35.
2. J. Path., 1918, 22, p. 129.
3. J. Gen. Physiol., 1926, 8, p. 311.
4. J. Path., 1921, 24, p. 150.

21 days. At the end of this period the contents of all tubes were filtered and the toxin titers determined by inoculating 250 gm. guinea-pigs. The results obtained are reported in the table. In this table the MLD content reported in each case is calculated on the basis of one cc. of undiluted toxin filtrate.

These results verify and extend previous observations on the destruction of diphteria toxin by bacteria. Our results with Clostridium sporogenes are even more striking than those reported by Donaldson with the "Reading Bacillus" which he found caused a destruction equivalent to 60 MLD of the original toxin. The data here reported indicate a destruction by Clostridium sporogenes in excess of 350 MLD.

Destruction of Diphtheria Toxin by Bacteria

Material, Incubated 21 days at 37 C.	MLD Content
Sterile toxin	175
Toxin + Bacterium coli	50
Toxin + Bacillus cereus	25
Toxin + Proteus vulgaris	5
Toxin + Pseudomonas pyocyaneus	1
Toxin + Clostridium sporogenes	less than 0.5

SUMMARY

It has been shown that several bacteria have the power to destroy diphtheria toxin when grown in its presence. The data reported show this to be true of Bacterium coli, Bacillus cereus, Proteus vulgaris, Pseudomonas pyocyaneus, and Clostridium sporogenes. Especially active destruction was caused by Clostridium sporogenes.

GENERAL INDEX

A

PAGE

ABELL, ELIZABETH. See HUDDLESON, I. FOREST - 81
Abscess, lung, microorganisms of - 391
Abortus, Br., thermal death point of, in milk - 327
Abortus-melitensis organisms - 81, 232
Abortus type of undulant fever - 273
Acidophilus bacillus - 97, 218
Aerobes, action of phenol and formol on - 90
Agglutination with Salmonella pullorum, cloudy reaction in - 172
Allergy with streptococcus of rheumatic fever - 280
Anaerobes, action of phenol and formol on - 90
D'ANDREA, DOROTHY. See BENSON, HARRIET - 516
Alcaligenes, Bact. - 330
Anemia in relation to intestinal stasis - 480
Antibody, pneumococcus, protective - 531, 543
Antigens of B. typhosus - 335
Antiseptic dyes, in relation to infection - 126, 131
Antiserum, pneumococcic, from rabbits - 137
APFELBACH, CARL W. See RHODES, G. BERNICE - 215
Arteriospasm, production of, by bacterial cultures - 363
AVERY, L. W. See ROTHSTEIN, THOR - 1

B

Bacilli, lacto- - 97, 218
Bacillus, Döderlein's - 218
Bacillus, dysentery, effect of, on insulin content of pancreas - 121
Bacillus influenzae - 300, 385
Bacillus (diplo) in Mexican typhus (tabardillo) - 261
Bacillus, tubercle, "filtrable forms" of - 200
Bacillus typhous, antigenic analysis of - 335
Bacillus of white diarrhea, serologic and pullorin test for - 60
Bacteria, action of resorcinol derivatives on - 25
Bacteria, adaptation of, to acriflavine - 126
Bacteria, action of phenol and formol on - 90
Bacteria, decomposition of nitrogenous substances by - 321
Bacteria, decomposition of urea by - 67
Bacteria, destruction of diphtheria toxin by - 569
Bacteria, growth of, surface tension in relation to - 97
Bacteria, inhibition of gas formation by - 311
Bacteria from lesions from vitamin A deficiency - 407
Bacteria of dermatitis of experimental pellagra - 426
Bacteria of infected urine - 353
Bacteria of lung abscess and bronchiectasis - 391
Bacteria, psychrophilic, bacteriophage of - 403
Bacteria, thermophilic, in canned foods - 461
Bacteria, typhoid, isolation of, from feces - 345
Bacteria, production of toxic amines by - 363
Bacteriophage, action of, on psychrophilic organisms - 403
Bacteriophage, immunization with, in experimental plague - 448
Bacteriophage of infected urine - 353
Bacterium aertrycke, poison from - 507
Bacterium alcaligenes, classification of - 330
Bacterium enteritidis, poison from - 507
Bacterium fluorescens, classification of - 330
Bacterium morgani 1, infection with - 349
Bacterium, mucosus, from lesions of vitamin A deficiency - 407
Bacterium pyocyaneum, classification of - 330
B. proteus hemolysin - 458
BENSON, HARRIET, ROSE BRENNWASSER, and DOROTHY D'ANDREA. Neisseria subflava (Bergey) meningitis in an infant - 516
BIRKHAUG, KONRAD E. Rheumatic fever. 2. Allergic reactions with a toxin-producing strain of nonmethemoglobin-forming streptococcus isolated from rheumatic fever - 280
Blood broth cultures, toxic amines in - 363
Blood dextrose after injections of histamine - 117
Blood plates for identification of hemolytic streptococci - 167

PAGE

BOAK, RUTH, and C. M. CARPENTER. The thermal deathpoint of Brucella abortus - - - - - - - - - - - - - 328
BOISSEVAIN, C. H. Replacement of potassium by other elements in culture mediums - - - - - - - - - - - - - 194
Botulinus toxin, production and purification of - - 145, 152, 161, 194, 496
Botulinus toxin, extracellular enzyme in production of - - - 565, 566
BRADFORD, WILLIAM L. Mucosus organisms from suppurative lesions of rats on diets deficient in vitamin A - - - - - - - - - - - 407
Brain, histology of membranes of - - - - - - - - - - - 1
Brain, rickettsia of Rocky Mountain spotted fever in - - - - - - - 93
BRANHAM, SARA E., LUCILE ROBEY, and LOIS A. DAY. A poison from Bacterium aertrycke and Bacterium enteritidis which is active in mice when given by mouth - - - - - - - - - - - - - 507
BRENNWASSER, ROSE. See BENSON, HARRIET - - - - - - - - 516
Bronchiectasis, microorganisms of - - - - - - - - - - - 391
Bronchospasm, production of, by bacterial cultures - - - - - - 363
Brucella melitensis (and var. abortus) - - - - - 81, *232*, *273*, 327
Bulgaricus, Lactobacillus, growth of - - - - - - - - - - - 97
BURKE, VICTOR, CATHERINE ULRICH and DON HENDRIE. Bacterial adaptation to acriflavine - - - - - - - - - - - - 126
BURKE, VICTOR, M. P. JESUP and SMITH PHILIPS. Choice of antiseptic dye in mixed infections - - - - - - - - - - - - 131
BUSHNELL, L. D. Comparison of serologic and pullorin tests for bacillary white diarrhea - - - - - - - - - - - - - 60

C

CALDWELL, JANET ANDERSON. Bacteriologic and bacteriophagic studies of infected urines - - - - - - - - - - - - - 353
CANNON, PAUL R. Relationship between chronic intestinal stasis and anemia 480
CARPENTER, C. M. See BOAK, RUTH - - - - - - - - - - 327
Clostridium botulinum toxin - - - - 145, 152, 161, 496, 565, 566
Clostridium tetani, serologic types of - - - - - - - - - - 184
COFFEY, J. M. See SICKLES, G. M. - - - - - - - - - - 490
COLEMAN, GEORGE E., and JANET B. GUNNISON. Serologic types of Clostridium tetani - - - - - - - - - - - - - 184
COLEMAN, MARION B. See GILBERT, RUTH - - - - - - - - 273
COMPTON, ARTHUR. Sensitization and immunization with bacteriophage in experimental plague - - - - - - - - - - - - - 448
Conjunctivitis, Staphylococcus aureus, in newborn - - - - - - 306
CONNOR, CHARLES L. Monilia from osteomyelitis - - - - - - 108
COOPER, FRANK B., and PETROFF, S. A. "Filtrable forms" of the tubercle bacillus. A critical review and personal observations - - - - - 200
Cord, spinal, histology of membranes of - - - - - - - - - 1

D

DAY, ALEXANDER ALFRED, and WILLIAM MERRIOTT GIBBS. Surface tension in relation to bacterial growth, with special reference to Lactobacillus acidophilus and Lactobacillus bulgaricus - - - - - - - - 97
DAY, LOIS A. See BRANHAM, SARA E. - - - - - - - - - 507
DAVISON, FORREST R. Detoxifying, diffusing, germicidal and surface tension depressing properties of soap - - - - - - - - - - 292
Dermatitis of experimental pellagra, organism of - - - - - - - 426
Diabetes, noninfectivity of urine from patients with - - - - - - 399
Diarrhea, bacillary white, tests for - - - - - - - - - - 60
Diphtheria toxin, bacterial destruction of - - - - - - - - - 569
Diphtheria toxin, in vitro approximation of toxicity of - - - - - 420
Diphtheria toxin, nature of - - - - - - - - - - - - 41
Diplobacillus of Mexican typhus (tabardillo) - - - - - - - 261
Döderlein's bacillus: Lactobacillus acidophilus - - - - - - - 218
Dura mater, histology of - - - - - - - - - - - - 1
Dyes, antiseptic - - - - - - - - - - - - - 126, 131
Dysentery bacillus, effect of, on insulin in pancreas - - - - - - 121

E

ELDER, A. LAWRENCE, and FRED W. TANNER. Action of bacteriophage on psychrophilic organisms - - - - - - - - - - - - 403

PAGE
Enzyme, toxin-producing, of Cl. botulinum - - - - - - - - 565, 566
ERMATINGER, LUCILLE H. Microorganisms of lung abscess and bronchiectasis - - - - - - - - - - - - 391
ETTINGER, G. HAROLD, and GUILFORD B. REED. Absence of infectivity in filtered urine from diabetic patients - - - - - - - - 399

F

Feces, isolation of typhoid organisms from - - - - - - - - - 345
FELTON, LLOYD D. The units of protective antibody in antipneumococcus serum and antibody solution - - - - - - - - - - - 531
FELTON, LLOYD D. Concentration of pneumococcus antibody - - - 543
Fermentation, tests, use of pectin in - - - - - - - - - 475
Fever, rheumatic, allergic reactions with streptococcus from - - - 280
Fever, Rocky Mountain spotted, Rickettsia of - - - - - - - 93
Fever, typhoid, treatment of, with detoxicated vaccine - - - - - 189
Fever, undulant, in New York State - - - - - - - - - 273
Flagella, staining of - - - - - - - - - - - - - 228
Fluorescens, Bact. - - - - - - - - - - - - - - 330
Foods, canned, thermophilic bacteria from - - - - - - - - 461
FOSHAY, L. See WHERRY, W. B. - - - - - - - - - - 189
FREEDLANDER, B. L. The production of potent antipneumococcic serum in rabbits - - - - - - - - - - - - - - 137

G

GIBBS, WILLIAM MERRIOTT. See DAY, ALEXANDER ALFRED - - - 97
GILBERT, RUTH, and MARION B. COLEMAN. Recent cases of undulant fever in New York State - - - - - - - - - - - - 273
GUERRANT, N. B. See SALMON, W. D. - - - - - - - - 426
GUNNISON, JANET B. See COLEMAN, GEORGE E. - - - - - - 184

H

HAMPIL, BETTYLEE. Bactericidal properties of the acyl and alkyl derivatives of resorcinol - - - - - - - - - - - - - 25
HANKE, MILTON THEO. See KOESSLER, KARL KONRAD - - - - - 363
HARKINS, MALCOLM J., and ELI R. SALEEBY. Spontaneous tuberculosis of rabbits - - - - - - - - - - - - - - 554
HAVENS, LEON C. Antigenic analysis of strains of Bacillus typhosus - - 335
HAVENS, LEON C., and CATHERINE RIDGWAY. Comparison of glycerol and brillant green bile for treatment of feces for isolation of typhoid organisms 345
HAYS, I. M. See SALMON, W. D. - - - - - - - - - - 426
Hemolysin, pneumococcic - - - - - - - - - - - - 490
Hemolysin, proteus - - - - - - - - - - - - - 458
HENDRIE, DON. See BURKE, VICTOR - - - - - - - - 126
Histamine, effect of injection of, on blood dextrose - - - - - - 117
Histamine, production of, in bacterial cultures - - - - - - - 363
HOWELL, KATHARINE M., and MARIE WERNER. The opsonification test for the rapid identification of the streptococcus of scarlet fever - - - 525
HUDDLESON, I. FORREST, and ELIZABETH ABELL. Behavior of Brucella melitensis and abortus toward gentian violet - - - - - - 81

I

Immunization with bacteriophage in experimental plague - - - - 448
Infection, use of antiseptic dye in - - - - - - - - 126, 131
Infection, experimental focal, with streptococci - - - - - - - 215
Infection, Salmonella pullorum, cloudy agglutination reaction in - - - 172
Infection, with Bacterium morgani 1 - - - - - - - - - - 349
Infection with influenza bacillus - - - - - - - - - 300, 385
Infectivity, absence of, in diabetic urine - - - - - - - - 399
Influenza bacillus - - - - - - - - - - - - 300, 385
Insulin content of pancreas, effect of bacterial intoxication on - - - 121
ISHIKAWA, MITSUTERU. Influence of carbohydrates on bacterial decomposition of urea - - - - - - - - - - - - - 67
Chemical and bacterial inhibition of gas formation in bacterial cultures - 311
Influence of iodide on bacterial decomposition of nitrogenous substances - 321

J

PAGE
JESSUP, M. P. See BURKE, VICTOR - - - - - - - - - - 131

K

KILGARIFF, KATHLEEN J. See VAN DE CARR, F. RENE - - - - - - 442
KOESSLER, KARL KONRAD, MILTON THEO. HANKE and MARY S. SHEPPARD. Production of histamine, tyramine, bronchospastic and arteriospastic substances in blood broth by pure cultures of microorganisms - - 363
KREIDLER, WILLIAM A. Biologic and serologic studies of Streptococcus cardioarthritidis - - - - - - - - - - - - - 415
KRUGH, HELEN M. See MENTEN, MAUD L. - - - - - 117, 121

L

Lactobacillus acidophilus - - - - - - - - - - - 97, 218
Lactobacillus bulgaricus - - - - - - - - - - - - 97
LANDRÓN FRANSISCO. See WEISS, CHARLES - - - - - - - 557
LEBLANC, T. J. See WHERRY, W. B. - - - - - - - - - 189
Leishmania tropica, metabolism of - - - - - - - - - - 378
Lipoid, effect of, on botulinum toxin - - - - - - - - - 496
LOCKE, ARTHUR, and E. R. MAIN. The nature of diphtheria toxin - - 41
The approximation of the toxicity of diphtheria toxin in vitro - - 420
Lung abscess, bacteria of - - - - - - - - - - - - 391

M

MAGATH, THOMAS B. Proteus ammoniae - - - - - - - - - 181
MAIN, E. R. See LOCKE, ARTHUR - - - - - - - - - 41, 420
MCALPINE, JAMES G., and CHARLES A. SLANETZ. Studies on the metabolism of the abortus-melitensis group. 4. Effect of various concentrations of carbon dioxide - - - - - - - - - - - - - - 232
MCCOY, ELIZABETH, and W. H. PETERSON. The use of pectin in fermentation tests - - - - - - - - - - - - - - - 475
Medium, culture, potassium and other elements in - - - - - - 194
Medium for isolation of typhoid organisms - - - - - - - 345
Melitensis-abortus group - - - - - - - - - - - - 81, 232
Melitensis, Br., agglutination of, in undulant fever - - - - - - 273
Meningitis, Neisseria subflava - - - - - - - - - - - - 516
MENTEN, MAUD L. and HELEN M. KRUGH. Changes in blood dextrose after intravenous injections of histamine - - - - - - - - - 117
Insulin content of the pancreas following intoxication of rabbits with paratyphoid B filtrate and dysentery bacilli - - - - - - - - 121
Metabolism of abortus-melitensis group - - - - - - - - - 232
Metabolism of Leishmania tropica - - - - - - - - - - 378
Microorganisms of lung abscess and bronchiectasis - - - - - - 391
Microorganisms, toxic amines in cultures of - - - - - - - - 363
MONIAS, BRUNO LEO. Classification of Bacterium alcaligenes, pyocyaneum, and fluorescens - - - - - - - - - - - - - - 330
Monilia of osteomyelitis - - - - - - - - - - - - - 108
Monilia psilosis, biology of, in relation to sprue - - - - - - - 557
Morgan bacillus, septic infection with - - - - - - - - - 349
MOOSER, H. Experiments relating to the pathology and the etiology of Mexican typhus (tabardillo). 1. Clinical course and pathologic anatomy of tabardillo in guinea-pigs - - - - - - - - - - - - 241
2. Diplobacillus from the proliferated tunica vaginalis of guinea-pigs reacting to Mexican typhus - - - - - - - - - - - - 261

N

NEALON, P. J. See SOMMER, H. - - - - - - - - - - - 161
Neisseria subflava (Bergey) meningitis - - - - - - - - - 516
NORTON, JOHN F., ELIZABETH VERDER and CATHERINE RIDGWAY. The proteus hemolysin - - - - - - - - - - - - - - 458

O

Opsonification test for identification of scarlet fever streptococci - - 525
Osteomyelitis, monilia from - - - - - - - - - - - - 108

P

PAGE

Pancreas, effect of bacterial intoxication on insulin content of - - - - 121
Paratyphoid B filtrate, effect of, on insulin - - - - - - - - - 121
Pectin, use of, in fermentation tests - - - - - - - - - - 475
Pellagra, etiology of dermatitis of - - - - - - - - - - 426
PETERSON, W. H. See MCCOY, ELIZABETH - - - - - - - 475
PETROFF, S. A. See COOPER, FRANK B. - - - - - - - - 200
PHILIPS, SMITH. See BURKE, VICTOR - - - - - - - - 131
Pia-arachnoid, histology of - - - - - - - - - - - - 1
Plague, experimental, bacteriophage immunization in - - - - - - 448
Pneumococcus antibody, protective - - - - - - - - - - 531, 543
Pneumococcus antiserum - - - - - - - - - - - - 137, 531
Pneumococcus culture, hemolysin in - - - - - - - - - - 490
Proteus ammoniae - - - - - - - - - - - - - - 181
Proteus hemolysin - - - - - - - - - - - - - - 458
Psychrophiles, bacteriophage of - - - - - - - - - - - 403
Pullorin test for white diarrhea - - - - - - - - - - - 60
Pyocyaneum, Bact. - - - - - - - - - - - - - - 330

R

REED, GUILFORD B. See ETTINGER, G. HAROLD - - - - - - - 399
REIMANN, HOBART A. Rickettsia of Rocky Mountain spotted fever in the brain of the infected guinea-pig - - - - - - - - - - - 93
Resorcinol derivatives, bactericidal action of - - - - - - - 25
Rheumatic fever, allergy, from streptococcus from - - - - - - 280
RHODES, G. BERNICE, and CARL W. APFELBACH. Chronic localized streptococcus infections in dogs: experimental focal infections - - - - 215
RICHTER, R. See ROTHSTEIN, THOR - - - - - - - - - 1
Rickettsia of Rocky Mountain spotted fever in guinea-pig brain - - - - 93
RIDGWAY, CATHERINE. See HAVENS, LEON C. - - - - - - - 345
RIDGWAY, CATHERINE. See NORTON, JOHN F. - - - - - - - 458
ROBEY, LUCILE. See BRANHAM, SARA E. - - - - - - - - 507
Rocky Mountain spotted fever, rickettsia of - - - - - - - - 93
ROTHSTEIN, THOR, L. W. AVERY, and R. RICHTER. The pathology of the membranes of brain and spinal cord. 1. The histology of normal dura mater and pia-arachnoid - - - - - - - - - - - - - 1

S

SALEEBY, ELI RL. See HARKINS, MALCOLM J. - - - - - - - - 554
SALLE, A. J., and CARL L. A. SCHMIDT. The metabolism of Leishmania tropica - - - - - - - - - - - - - - - - 378
Salmonella pullorum infection, cloudy serum reactions in - - - - - 172
SALMON, W. D., I. M. HAYS, and N. B. GUERRANT. Etiology of dermatitis of experimental pellagra in rats - - - - - - - - - - 426
Scarlet fever streptococcus, opsonic identification of - - - - - - 525
SCHILLING, G. S., and S. J. SCHILLING. Incidence of cloudy reactions in agglutination tests for Salmonella pullorum infection - - - - - 172
SCHILLING, S. J. See SCHILLING, G. S. - - - - - - - - - 172
SCHMIDT, CARL L. A. See SALLE, A. J. - - - - - - - - - 378
SCOTT, JOSEPH P. The action of phenol and formol on aerobic and anaerobic organisms - - - - - - - - - - - - - - - 90
Sensitization with plague bacteriophage - - - - - - - - - 448
Serum, antipneumococcic - - - - - - - - - - - - - 137, 531
Serum in Salmonella pullorum infection, cloudy reaction with - - - - 172
Serum tests for white diarrhea - - - - - - - - - - - 60
Serum typing of Cl. tetani - - - - - - - - - - - - 184
SHAW, MYRTLE. Thermophilic bacteria in canned foods - - - - - 461
SHEPPARD, MARY S. See KOESSLER, KARL KONRAD - - - - - - 363
SHERMAN, J. M. See STARK, C. N. - - - - - - - - - 565, 566, 569
SICKLES, G. M., and J. M. COFFEY. A hemolytic substance in pneumococcus culture broth - - - - - - - - - - - - - - - 490
SLANETZ, CHARLES A. See MCALPINE, JAMES G. - - - - - - - 232
SNIPE, P. TESSMER. See SOMMER, H. - - - - - - - - - 145, 161
SNIPE, P. TESSMER, and H. SOMMER. Studies on botulinus toxin. 3. Acid precipitation of botulinus toxin - - - - - - - - - - 152
Snuffles, observations on - - - - - - - - - - - - - 442
Soaps, diffusing and detoxifying properties of - - - - - - - 292

PAGE

SOMMER, H., and P. TESSMER SNIPE. Studies on botulinus toxin. 2. Further purification by adsorption on colloids - - - - - - - - - 145
SOMMER, H., P. J. NEALON, and P. TESSMER SNIPE. Studies on botulinus toxin. 4. Dialysis experiments - - - - - - - - - - 161
SOMMER, H. See SOMMER, E. WAGNER - - - - - - - - - 496
SOMMER, H. See SNIPE, P. TESSMER - - - - - - - - - 152
SOMMER, E. WAGNER, and H. SOMMER. Studies on botulinus toxin. 5. Influence of nitrogenous and lipoid substances compounds on the potency of botulinus toxin - - - - - - - - - - - - 496
Sprue, Monilia psilosis in relation to - - - - - - - - - - 557
Stains for flagella - - - - - - - - - - - - 228
Staphylococcus aureus conjunctivitis - - - - - - - - - - 306
STARK, C. N., J. M. SHERMAN, and PAULINE STARK. Extracellular production of toxin by Clostridium botulinum type B. - - - - - - 565
Glucose inhibition of extracellular toxin-producing enzyme - - - - 566
Destruction of diphtheria toxin by bacteria - - - - - - - 569
STARK, PAULINE. See STARK, C. N. - - - - - - 565, 566, 569
Streptococcus cardioarthritidis - - - - - - - - - - - 415
Streptococci, hemolytic, identification of - - - - - - - - - 167
Streptococcus, experimental focal infection with - - - - - - - 215
Streptococcus, nonmethemoglobin-forming, of rheumatic fever - - - - 280
Streptococcus, scarlet fever, opsonic identification of - - - - - - 525

T

Tabardillo (Mexican typhus), etiology and pathology of - - - 241, 261
TANNER, FRED W. See ELDER, A. LAWRENCE - - - - - - 403
Tetani, Cl., serologic types of - - - - - - - - - - 184
Thermophiles in canned foods - - - - - - - - - - 461
THJOTTA, TH. Septic infection due to Bacterium morgani 1 - - - 349
THOMAS, ARTHUR B. Staphylococcus aureus conjunctivitis in the newborn 306
THOMAS, R. See WHERRY, W. B. - - - - - - - - - - 189
THOMAS, STANLEY. Döderlein's bacillus: Lactobacillus acidophilus - - 218
Toxin, botulinus - - - - - - - 145, 152, 161, 496, 565, 566
Toxin, diphtheria - - - - - - - - - - - - 41, 520, 569
Tubercle bacillus, "filtrable forms" of - - - - - - - - - 200
Tuberculosis, spontaneous, in rabbits - - - - - - - - - - 554
Typhoid bacillus, antigenic analysis of strains of - - - - - - - 335
Typhoid organisms, isolation of, from feces - - - - - - - - 345
Typhoid fever, treatment of, with detoxicated vaccine - - - - - - 189
Typhus, Mexican, etiology and pathology of - - - - - - 241, 261
Tyramine, production of, by bacterial cultures - - - - - - - 363

U

ULRICH, CATHERINE. See BURKE, VICTOR - - - - - - - - 126
Undulant fever in New York State - - - - - - - - - - 273
Urea, decomposition of, by bacteria - - - - - - - - - - 67
Urine, bacteria and bacteriophage of - - - - - - - - - - 353
Urine, diabetic, noninfectivity of - - - - - - - - - - 399

V

Vaccine, detoxicated, treatment of typhoid fever with - - - - - - 189
VALENTINE, EUGENIA. A method of inoculating blood plates for the identification of hemolytic streptococci - - - - - - - - - 167
VAN DE CARR, F. RENE, and KATHLEEN KILGARIFF. Observations on snuffles in rabbits - - - - - - - - - - - - - 442
VERDER, ELIZABETH. See NORTON, JOHN F. - - - - - - - - 458
Vitamin A deficiency, mucosus organism from lesions of - - - - - 407
WALKER, JOHN E. Infection of laboratory worker with Bacillus influenzae 300
Intranasal inoculation of rabbits with Bacillus influenzae - - - - 385

W

WEISS, CHARLES, and LANDRÓN, FRANSISCO. Immunologic investigation on tropical sprue in Porto Rico. The biology of Monilia psilosis in relation to sprue - - - - - - - - - - - - - 557
WEISS, EMIL. Method of staining flagella - - - - - - - - 228
WERNER, MARIE. See HOWELL, KATHARINE M. - - - - - - - 525
WHERRY, W. B., T. J. LEBLANC, L. FOSHAY, and R. THOMAS. The treatment of typhoid fever with detoxicated vaccine - - - - - - - 189